The
BODY HEALS

WILLIAM B. FERRIL, M. D.

The Bridge Medical Publishers
Whitefish, Montana

William B. Ferril, M. D.

For Billy, Hayes, Conner, and Mckenna

The Bridge Medical Publishers

Published by The Bridge Medical Publishers
P.O. Box 324
Whitefish, Montana 59937

ISBN 0-9725825-3-3
Printed in the United States of America

Cover Design by Synergy

10 9 8 7 6 5 4 3 2

Printed by Satori
200½ Wisconsin Ave.
Whitefish, MT 59937
406 862-8289

Acknowledgments

To my patients, who always point the way to better methods.

To the holistic mental giants and pioneers of the revolution, in health care freedom, that laid the clues for this book: Robert Atkins M.D; Robert Anderson, M.D.; Broda Barnes, M.D., PhD; Jeffery Bland, Ph.D.; Craig Cooney, PhD; Alan Gaby M.D.; William McKenzie Jefferies M.D.; John Lee M.D.; James Privitera, M.D.; Uzzi Reiss M.D.; Barry Sears, PhD; Norman Shealy, M.D.; Diana Shwarzbein, M.D., Andrew Weil M.D.; Julian Whitiker, M.D., Mary Stranahan, D.O.; Frank Nordt PhD; David Jones M. D.; Eugene Shippen M.D.: and Jonathan Wright M.D.

To my wife, Brenda, who loves me in a way that facilitates my passion for holistic healing.

To my layout and design expert Patty Perigo.

To Ginny Wilcox, as usual, for helping to do the final details at Sartori Publishing.

Special thanks to Rick Nagle, Esq., regarding his professional instruction for earlier versions of some of this material.

Perpetual thankfulness goes to Steven Small Salmon who patiently instructed me about the futility of being seduced into the negative emotions.

Preface to the Second Edition

It is always darkest before the dawn. The AMA recently announced its intention to restrict Naturopaths. Chiropractors endured a similar assault by the AMA in the 1960's. Yet, the health care revolution marches on because millions sense something very important missing from the mainstream paradigm.

Similarly, thousands sensed certain final touches missing in the first edition of *the Body Heals*. Over the last five years more scientific data has been woven into the original text. The first edition concentrated heavily on what was known but ignored in the medical textbooks. The second edition, in contrast, contains several hundred additional mainstream scientific literature citations that further bolster the premise for how the body heals without toxic drugs or medical procedures.

William Ferril
November 3, 2007
Whitefish, Montana

TABLE OF CONTENTS

AUTHOR'S NOTE VIII

SECTION ONE *1*

    CHAPTER ONE 4

    PRINCIPLES ONE AND TWO: PREVENT RUST AND MAINTAIN FLEXIBILITY 4

    INSULIN AND BLOOD VESSEL DISEASE...................... 24

    COUNTERING THE SECOND PRINCIPLE OF LONGEVITY: FLEXIBILITY 29

    DIABETES CAUSES RUST, HARDENING, AND USUALLY ACTIVATES AN OPPORTUNISTIC MECHANISM......... 33

CHAPTER TWO.. 40

    THE CELLS TRAVELING WITHIN THE BLOOD VESSELS40

CHAPTER THREE 53

    HIGH BLOOD PRESSURE-THE NEXT LEVEL 53

    MINERAL TABLE... 54

SECTION TWO.. *81*

    THE THIRD PRINCIPLE OF LONGEVITY: THE HORMONES GIVITH & THE HORMONES TAKETH AWAY............... 82

CHAPTER FOUR 86

    OBESITY CAN BE CURED WHEN HORMONES ARE OPTIMAL 86

CHAPTER FIVE.. 126

    ADRENAL GLANDS... 126

CHAPTER SIX 151

    OVARIES 151

CHAPTER SEVEN 172

    INFORMATIONAL SUBSTANCES 172

CHAPTER EIGHT.. 180

    STEROID TONE 180

CHAPTER NINE 209

FOUR MISUNDERSTOOD STEROIDS..209

CHAPTER TEN 215

    THYROID GLAND 215

CHAPTER ELEVEN 232

    TESTES..232

CHAPTER TWELVE...243

    HIERARCHY OF HORMONES - INFORMATIONAL SUBSTANCES243

SECTION THREE 251

    PRINCIPLE FOUR: YOU ARE WHAT YOU SUPPLY AND ABSORB...252

CHAPTER THIRTEEN..254

    DIGESTION..254

CHAPTER FOURTEEN 310

    PANCREAS 310

CHAPTER FIFTEEN 323

    AVOID THE 323

    TORTURE CHAMBER DIET...323

SECTION FOUR.. 344

    PRINCIPLE FIVE: TAKING OUT THE TRASH WATER345

CHAPTER SIXTEEN 348

    KIDNEYS 348

CHAPTER SEVENTEEN 374

    LUNGS 374

CHAPTER EIGHTEEN 399

    SKIN 399

CHAPTER NINETEEN 418

    LIVER 418

SECTION FIVE 450

PRINCILE SIX: MAINTAIN CELLULAR CHARGE 451

CHAPTER TWENTY 463

    CARTILAGE WITHIN THE JOINTS............................... 463

CHAPTERTWENTY-ONE.. 478

    IMMUNE SYSTEM 478

CHAPTER TWENTY-TWO.. 501

    IMMUNE SYSTEM AND THE JOINTS........................... 501

CHAPTER TWENTY-THREE 508

    BONES.. 508

SECTION SIX *522*

    PRINCIPLE SEVEN: ENERGIES THAT HEAL CONTRASTED TO THE ENERGIES THAT MAIM.................................... 523

CHAPTER TWENTY-FOUR 531

    BRAIN AND NERVES 531

CHAPTER TWENTY-FIVE.. 574

    HEART 574

    THE SEVENTH PRINCIPLE: THE ENERGIES THAT HEAL CONTRASTED TO THE ENERGIES THAT MAIM THE HEART.... 574

    PRINCIPLES 1 AND 2 586

    PRINCIPLE 3: THE HORMONES GIVETH AND TAKETH AWAY ONE'S HEART 587

    PRINCIPLE 4: YOU ARE WHAT YOU ABSORB 598

    THE SIXTH PRINCIPLE AND THE HEART: AVOID *LOW CELL VOLTAGE SYNDROME* 599

CHAPTER TWENTY-SIX 604

    MUSCLES AND LIGAMENTS... 604

SECTION SEVEN *617*

    100,000 MILE EXAM... 617

CHAPTER TWENTY-SEVEN 618

BIBLIOGRAPHY 627

Author's Note

Several memorable events were the inspiration for writing this book. First, many patients had documented benefit from adhering to contrary 'fringe' advice. These cases led to a growing curiosity about exploring the growing list of inconsistencies. These inconsistencies should not happen if one adheres to the official view of the medical universe. For example, back then it was beyond my education level to explain why a diet high in cholesterol and fat, but low in carbohydrate leads to a drop in harmful cholesterol parameters. Years later, I have come to understand how the different hormones that these diets promote leads to improved cholesterol profiles. The science is all there, but it largely is presented in a convoluted and fragmentary manner. The reorganization of these scientific facts is presented throughout the manual.

An additional inconsistency occurred regarding obesity. I could never figure out why no one was organizing the hormones causing obesity as they relate to one another. The science was present, but like cholesterol knowledge it was fragmented and disorganized in its presentation in the medical texts. The obesity chapter provides what science knows about gaining and losing fat.

Another learning opportunity started about sixteen years ago and occurred shortly after I married a pretty chiropractor named Brenda. Humility describes the feeling about my MD degree as my knowledge base was forced into the captive position. I watched with humility what a competent chiropractor accomplished with two hands following a multitude of musculoskeletal complaints. My world was rocked on its medical underpinnings. Thinking outside the box was the next logical step.

Later, I had the opportunity to work alongside naturopaths, other chiropractors, acupuncturists, and homeopaths. Each of their various educational perspectives provided me with additional inconsistencies for the toxic symptom control paradigm that I had been groomed into believing.

Over the last fifteen plus years I have had time to think about what is actually known about the aging process. Early on I could only come with five reasons for cellular deterioration. In the second year of this effort, it became clear that there was evidence for a total of seven mechanisms for how the body ages.

The Seven Paths to an Old Body

1. The hormones giveth and the hormones taketh away

2. Rusting processes
3. Hardening processes
4. Low cell voltage syndrome
5. Deficient and/or excessive molecular building parts
6. Failure to take out the cellular trash water
7. A preponderance of energies that maim compared to the energies that heal

This manual is about helping the reader understand ways to combat these processes. There is a lot of bad information circulating around. Without most doctors realizing it, sometimes bad information continues to circulate because the good information negates the need for help from the medical industrial complex. My definition of the complex involves the vested interest of big business that orchestrates the unseen hand of how doctors are groomed into thinking about middle-aged disease processes.

Without good information, owners will always be vulnerable to the clever advertising schemes of the medical industrial complex. These informational sound bites are dispersed through various media outlets and are usually the most profitable ways of treating an owner's disease. Unfortunately, many of these popular approaches are based in a symptom control paradigm. Symptom control has little to do with how one heals and always has side effects. Many conventionally trained physicians haven't a clue (neither did I) that their complex funded educations left out many unifying and holistic scientific principles.

Owners need to acquire a basic understanding of what is really known about the less profitable ways of treating the common diseases that begin around middle age. Accurate information about how one heals will lower gullibility. The sensationalism of what is for sale is a consequence of living in a profit driven health care system. The media and 'scientific community' collaborate and hype the latest clever symptom control measures. The common sales formula: the upside is magnified and the downside (side effects) is minimized.

I have found that most owners will make life style changes if they understand that it leads to healing. Learning is somewhat painful and depleting. This book is not for the weak minded and lazy types. This manual was written for those owners who possess enough motivation to stay focused on the goal of becoming less gullible regarding their health care choices. The reward for such commitment comes in the form of personal empowerment that allows applying the basics for how to prevent the seven processes from manifesting in our lives.

As the reader endeavors to learn each chapter, awareness will come that the profit driven approaches of mainstream medicine are about symptom control with a price. The price paid to the owner's body is evidenced by side effects and toxicities. Common examples of diseases treated today in the symptom control paradigm instead of the healing paradigm include heart disease, high blood pressure, diabetes, arthritis, asthma, obesity, and menopausal related disease.

Symptom control medicine has nothing to do with healing. True healing can only begin to occur when cause and effect are included in the decision making process. These seven processes are usually involved in this understanding. Science exists to understand and impact these seven processes that rob most owners of their vitality.

Combating these seven processes proves fundamental to achieving health that endures. This manual facilitates the reader on ways to begin accessing and applying seven correcting principles that the holism of science revealed long ago.

Do not get overly frustrated when a concept seems initially unclear. Chances are it will be explained later in a way the reader can understand. At the end of this manual a chapter for putting the entire proceeding chapters into practice begins with a more complete inquiry as to where an owner stands regarding the seven processes in the context of the physical exam. By the time the reader makes it to this section of the manual these principle will make more sense.

Disclaimer

This book is intended as an educational tool to acquaint the reader with alternative methods of understanding, preventing, and treating some common middle age diseases. The Bridge Medical Publishers hopes that this book will enable the reader to improve their well being, and to better understand, assess, and choose the appropriate course of treatment. Because some of the methods described in this book are alternative in nature, by definition some of them have not been investigated and/or approved by any government or regulatory agency.

The information contained within *The Body Heals* – Second Edition is not intended as a substitute for the advice and/or medical care of a physician. Nor is the content of this book intended to discourage or dissuade the reader from following the advice of his or her physician. The contents of this book are for informational purposes only and are not intended to diagnose or treat illness. The diagnosis and treatment of illness requires a specific exam, tests, history, and an appreciation for each individual's uniqueness of presentation. For those, the reader is advised to seek the counsel of a competent holistic physician. Individuals who desire weight loss, improved health or healing from chronic disease need close supervision and follow-up from their physician.

If the reader has any questions concerning the information contained in this text, or its application to his/her particular medical profile, or if the reader has unusual medical or nutritional needs or constraints that conflict with the advice in this book, he or she should consult his or her physician before embarking on any medical treatments advised in this text. Pregnant or nursing readers should consult their physicians before embarking on the nutrition and lifestyle programs suggested in this text. The reader should not stop taking prescription medications without the advice and guidance of their personal physician.

SECTION ONE

SECTION ONE *1*

CHAPTER ONE 4

PRINCIPLES ONE AND TWO: PREVENT RUST AND MAINTAIN FLEXIBILITY 4

INSULIN AND BLOOD VESSEL DISEASE...................... 24

COUNTERING THE SECOND PRINCIPLE OF LONGEVITY: FLEXIBILITY 29

DIABETES CAUSES RUST, HARDENING, AND USUALLY ACTIVATES AN OPPORTUNISTIC MECHANISM 33

CHAPTER TWO.. 40

THE CELLS TRAVELING WITHIN THE BLOOD VESSELS 40

CHAPTER THREE 53

HIGH BLOOD PRESSURE-THE NEXT LEVEL 53

MINERAL TABLE54

All bodies die. Some bodies accelerate on the path to premature death. This book describes a medical strategy that includes seven steps for creating longevity. The ideas in this book are scientifically sound and are supported by generally accepted medical literature. However, these ideas do not receive attention because of the nature of the medical industry. Medical industry is a profit driven business.

The medical industry exchanges health care services for money. The income from patients must exceed the cost of health care services. These business facts require medical practices and treatments that generate this income. These medical practices become the standard of practice taught in medical schools and practiced by doctors. Consequently, they become the legal standards of medical practice. Research focuses on effective treatments that will return the research cost and provide profit for the investors. Marketing campaigns create a demand for profitable medical procedures and services. In this way the media and 'science' have mutual interests.

Effective treatments that fail to provide a "reasonable" return on investment become marginalized and fail to be advertised. They are not taught. Effective, but unprofitable medical procedures and treatments remain ignored because they do not provide the appropriate inducements in a profit driven system.

This book is written for the owners who will use effective and inexpensive medical practices and procedures. These owners desire to implement medical practices that do not contain the destructive side effects of mainstream medical practices. Side effects occur because the mainstream medical standard of care largely exists within a symptom control paradigm. Symptom control always leads to side effects and has little to do with how one heals.

Some owners will do what becomes necessary for healing to occur. Healing involves understanding how certain diseases develop. Seven principles exist that explain how cells function at their optimum level. Failure to identify which ones operate inefficiently leads to disease, aging, and the need for symptom control measures. Symptom control includes prescription medications, medical procedures, and surgery. This text facilitates owners who will engage in their health and healing and renounce the convenience of mainstream medical practice.

Ground Rules

This book is organized according to seven health and healing strategies referred to as principles. Each principle is discussed, developed, and addressed in a separate section. In the first six sections the organ systems that best facilitate an understanding of a principle are grouped together. In addition, that organ system and its relationship to the other principles are discussed. The body story told in this way facilitates owner empowerment for learning about the often-omitted principles. Otherwise, the continuance of these omissions prevents healing from the common deteriorations operating in the middle age body.

The middle-aged body wants to heal. The first two principles, rust prevention and flexibility preservation within the blood vessels, have a strong relationship and are the subject of the first section. The third principle explains how one satisfies the body requirement for high quality hormones. The fourth concerns how one obtains high quality molecular replacement parts. The fifth principle involves the removal of the body's trash water by six different organ systems. The sixth principle explains the importance of maintaining adequate cell voltages. And finally, the seventh principle explains the energies that heal contrasted to the energies that maim the body cells.

More Ground Rules:

1. I call anyone in possession of a body, an owner
2. I purposely use unique and graphic medical descriptors to facilitate lay person comprehension of medical knowledge
3. Some chapters contain many single sentence facts that stand-alone. This initial format helps to build the reader's knowledge base.
4. Various types of sidebars occur throughout the text. Some of these are designed to provide the extra information that physicians need before they can believe. Anyone can try to read these but do not feel overwhelmed if they are beyond comprehension. Others arise out of my attempt to clearly denote the contained text as my personal opinion.
5. Most supporting literature to the facts in this book become obvious by persuing the bibliography. However, occasionally facts arise from well-credentialed lay-person publications. These authors are denoted in italics.

CHAPTER ONE

PRINCIPLES ONE AND TWO: PREVENT RUST AND MAINTAIN FLEXIBILITY

Health of the Blood Vessels

Each human body contains 180,000 miles of waterways that transport liquids, solids, gases, charged particles, and waste products. The waterways that flow away from the heart (arteries) carry fresh supplies of oxygen, nutrients, and recently recruited immune system cells to the tissues. The waterways that travel towards the heart (veins and lymphatics) carry waste, solids, gases, and spent immune system cells from the tissues toward their exits.

The quality and integrity of the inside inner surface of these waterways creates a powerful determinant for youth versus aging. The importance of this inner surface arises from the fact that these waterways provide the interface for exchange between the blood stream and all cell types. Healthy bodies have quality surfaces lining their 180,000 miles of waterways. Many unhealthy owners problem originates from the lost integrity of their inner waterway surface.

Nutrients, waste, solids, charged particles, and gases are selectively absorbed and eliminated through the inner-lining layer of the blood vessels. This layer distributes nutrients according to the specific nutritional needs of the tissues. An important determinant of longevity is the quality of this lining.

Blood Vessels: Rust and Hardening

The first two principles of health relate to the maintenance of the blood vessels. When these principles remain ignored the body will age. Visualize how rust corrodes when oxygen or some other molecule reacts with a surface. The inside of the blood vessels surfaces are constantly under these types of assaults. Processes that increase this assault accelerate rust formation and consequently require repair. Corroded blood vessel surfaces have either or both an accelerated corrosion rate and/or deficient repair rate. Later, cholesterol and fat debris collect where these inside surfaces have been damaged.

Loss of flexibility usually begins in the muscular layer of the vessel. Arteries have the thickest muscular layer and the highest-pressure forces. Processes that increase the muscle layer thickness increase the stiffness in the recipient blood vessel. Stiff arteries become more vulnerable to damage.

The presence of rust and diminished flexibility in the blood vessels diminishes the function of those vessels. Accumulation of rust and loss of flexibility describe processes that occur in the blood vessels, accelerate the aging process, and diminish health. Prevention or reversal of these two processes involves several steps.

Aging does not cause the processes of rust and hardening. Rust and hardening processes cause aging. When the rusting and hardening occur in the blood vessels they clog with debris and they perform inefficiently. Medicine describes these concepts as arteriosclerosis (hardening) and atherosclerosis (rust) respectively.

A common example of how rust begins will follow. After this the overall scheme between rust and hardening will be outlined. Next will be a discussion on how certain processes become opportunist and accelerate the rust and hardening damage rate. At the end of these introductory considerations, each risk factor will be discussed in regards to the development of both rust and hardening. Finally, the opportunistic mechanism will be explored in more detail.

Cells Lining the Water Ways Before Rust Damage Occurs

Visualize the cells that line the waterways appear as elaborate, shiny and flexible tiles. Each tile (cell) affixes to the others with the body's cement, the glycosaminoglycans (GAG). In health, these tiles, lining the waterways, remain intricately woven together on the inside of the tubular waterways. Each cell (tile) possesses a precise, detailed surface that interfaces with the turbulent bloodstream. On the tissue side of the cell (the side opposite of the bloodstream), the cell structure of the blood vessel depends on the body part that the blood vessel serves. Each tissue type has a specific cell structure. The purpose of a particular cell dictates structure. The structures of the blood vessel cells must be compatible with the cell structure of the tissue that the vessel it serves (explained at the end of the chapter).

Processes that harm the integrity or health of these waterway-lining cells interfere with transfer of nutrients and waste into or out of the bloodstream. Damage to blood vessels results from the initial processes of rusting and hardening. This causes the additional consequence of diminished transfer of hormones, nutritional substances, gases, and wastes and damages health.

The Basics of Rust

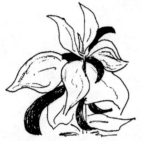

The initial presence of 'rust' in the waterway lining cells creates a 'Velcro' for debris to stick to. Picture that underlying the shinny surface, made up of GAG; each tile has an intricate surface made up of numerous types of molecular receiving stations, or receptors. These receptors detect specific molecules moving through the bloodstream. The receptors are designed to initiate the process of transferring the molecular matter from the bloodstream to the cells. The presence of rust in the vessels diminishes the exchange between the blood stream and the cells. For example, rust accumulation diminishes the quantity of nutrients transferred into the cells. When the vessels are extremely clogged, cells in the dependent tissue die.

Rust also damages the blood stream-dependent communication system by damaging the receptors. Hormones, like insulin, are informational substances that communicate specific messages to the cells. Many hormones can only be detected by a specific receptor in the blood vessel cells. Each cell has a specific types of receptors that depend on the type of tissue cell being served by a blood vessel. Rust clogs these receptors. When the clogging process occurs, the tissue cell needing insulin hormone may not be able to receive the message and consequently fails to perform.

Risk Factors for the Development of Rust

The risk factors for the production of rust are cigarette smoking, male gender, pre-diabetes and diabetes, high homocysteine level, deficiency of the anti-inflammatory essential fatty acids, obesity, excessive consumption of oxidized fats, nutritional deficiencies, and excessive exposure to oxidizing agents. In addition, the presence of abnormal hormone levels is now being considered as a factor in developing rust. Also, increased blood pressure causes hardening of the vessels and this consequence increases the rate of rust formation (explained below).

The cells lining the blood vessels are under assault from varying amounts of risk factors. Each of these risk factors contributes to the development of rust or increases the probability that rust will occur. Owners must be aware that these factors act on their blood vessels every moment and are affected by choices made during their day.

Antioxidant Retardants

Antioxidants can be better understood if one substitutes the word 'oxidation' for 'rust'. Rust is everywhere. Tissue oxidation is rust occurring in the body. When rust forms, a rough, Velcro-like cell surface remains on the waterway lining cells where debris collects. The accumulation of debris begins the clogging process.

Oxidation causes rust formation. Body cells depend on oxygen to burn fuel aerobically (from processed carbohydrates, fat and protein). Burning fuel creates the energy used for chemical reactions. Technically, the combustion of fuel involves an oxidation process. Oxygen combustion reactions share many similarities with those of a nuclear power plant. Reactor damage results when the intended reaction spills outside of the designated confinement area.

Cellular Power Plant Locations

Oxygen consumption occurs in the mitochondria of the cells, which is equivalent to the cell's nuclear power plant facility. If too much oxygen combustion byproduct intermediary's leak outside of these 'armored' powerhouses (within the cells) the equivalent of a cellular 'nuclear meltdown' occurs.

Oxygen molecules contain two oxygen atoms linked together in a high-energy bond. Paired oxygen formation proves as the only safe form of pure oxygen outside the mitochondria. Oxygen in this form makes up one component of a clean atmosphere. Air pollution leads to an increase in the unstable, chemically reactive forms of oxygen. All the other forms of oxygen oxidize (rust) body tissues. The mitochondria have the ability to withstand oxygen cleavage explosions (breaking the high-energy bond between the two oxygen atoms). These oxygen combustion reactions allow the breakdown of cellular fuels (food groups) forming energy packets (ATP), heat, water, and the chemically stable gas carbon dioxide.

However, when the unstable forms of oxygen occur outside the mitochondria in the cell, these forms need to be minimized to deter oxidation. In healthy states, these oxygen cleavage explosions take place contained within the 'armor' of the mitochondria. Very small amounts of unstable oxygen leak out of the mitochondria. This property of the mitochondria is similar to a less than perfect 'nuclear facility' containment area.

Living in clean air and practicing appropriate nutritional discretion moderates one's unstable oxygen exposure. Normally, the cell's protection team, (comprised of two enzymes, superoxide dismutase and catalase), have the ability to react with the destructive forms of oxygen and render them into harmless, stable molecules. Unfortunately, a limit exists as to their effectiveness. Consequently, environmental and dietary sources of unstable oxygen can overwhelm a cell leading to molecular oxidation (rust) damage.

Owners who become aware of the destructive effects of unstable oxygen possess a powerful tool against aging by avoiding environmental and nutritional conditions that jeopardize them. It is not difficult for an owner to decrease their exposure to unstable oxygen. For example, curtail oxygen-free radical exposure by choosing a healthy type of nutriceutical.

Some nutriceutical companies sell mineral supplements made from salts of oxygen. These salts in general are not very soluble in water so they pass like undigested gravel out of the body. However, a small portion of these salts dissolves and releases an oxygen atom with a negative charge. This describes one of the unstable forms of oxygen.

By unpaired oxygen's nature, it can't wait to react with body tissue to create rust. For this reason, owners should avoid mineral supplements that contain these reactive oxygen atoms because they defeat the purpose of taking antioxidants. Manufactures denote oxygen salt content with the term, "oxide" that occurs at the end of the product name. Common examples are calcium oxide, magnesium oxide, and ferrous oxide.

Unstable oxygen provides just one example of how rust formation begins inside the body. Some example are; excessive iron, fluoride and possibly calcium. Similarly, other risk factors interrelate in their blood vessel injuring mechanisms (see below).

Two Mechanisms That Injure Blood Vessels

Two other overall mechanisms injure blood vessels - stiffness and "sticky" cholesterol. Many factors cause stiffness, but high blood pressure proves as the most conspicuous and highly treatable mechanism. There are also many ways to develop high blood pressure, but the owner controls most of the causes (examples given throughout the first section). Stiffness caused by high blood pressure contributes to aging. Prevention of this process forms the second principle of longevity.

Sticky (cholesterol), created in the liver, describes another mechanism that damages the blood vessels. Inside immune scavenger cells called macrophages, sticky accumulates in the blood vessels as an opportunistic mechanism. It will be explained later why certain hormones direct the macrophages, lining the inside surface of arteries, to ingest blood fat slowly but surely, while other hormones promote its release. For now visualize that when rust or decreased flexibility occurs immune scavenger cells are summoned to the damaged area to form temporary patches but sometimes fail to detach and instead feed on fat and cholesterol within the blood stream. Mainstream medicine nomenclature calls sticky cholesterol, low-density cholesterol (LDL & VLDL).

Additional discussion regarding blood pressure elevation causality, rust promoting mechanisms and sticky cholesterol are noted in the parenthesis below. All three blood vessel injury mechanisms can be summarized as follows:

Rust Producing Mechanisms:
Homocysteine (chapter three)
Diabetes (liver chapter)
Nutritional deficiencies (sections three and five)
Essential fatty acid deficiencies (section three)
Cigarette smoking
Oxidant load (section three and six)
Quality of fat intake (section three)
Male gender
Obesity (section two)
Diminished hormone quality (section two)
Inflammation (heart chapter)

Blood Vessel Stiffness Mechanism

High blood pressure originates from multiple causes (chapters two and three)

Opportunist Mechanism Requires the Presence of Rust

In addition to rust and hardening, hormonal imbalance promotes the liver to manufacture sticky fats; LDL cholesterol, VLDL cholesteral, and triglycerides. These same hormonal imbalances cause a deficiency of HDL cholesterol (sections two and three).

The opportunist concept describes a mechanism that contributes to blood vessel disease when either or both of the rust forming and hardness mechanisms also operate in an owner's life. The media stresses the opportunist mechanism. However, most of the time, rust and hardening must be present before cholesterol begins the clogging process. For example, this is evidenced by the fact that only fifty percent of all heart attack victims had elevated cholesterol levels. This simple fact points to the importance of placing attention on rust and hardening processes before one can successfully lower their risk for blood vessel disease.

Blood Vessel Clogging and Cholesterol

Many physicians witness heart disease in patients with a relatively low cholesterol level. As previously stated, in at least fifty percent of heart disease cases some other factors exist that led to blockage in the coronary arteries. The mechanism of rust operates in the majority of heart disease victims. Therefore, these mechanisms need a more complete consideration. Unfortunately, these unidentified subgroups remain at increased risk for developing diseased blood vessels despite their normal cholesterol. Consequently, the true mechanisms prove important because these victims often possess a significant proportion of chemically reactive cholesterol, abnormal hormone cascades and/or nutritional deficiencies.

Science has revealed safe and effective ways to avoid these processes. However, the ways one heals provides knowledge that lacks profit potential so it remains largely ignored. This knowledge will be gradually added back into the discussion. Following this groundwork, a rationale for treatment options will be developed in section three.

Chemically Reactive Cholesterol and Rust

Cholesterol causes problems in the blood stream in three ways:

1. **There are several different types of cholesterol-fat-protein particles. The body creates each type for different purposes.**

2. **Cholesterol caused problems occur with excess gross volume of cholesterol in the blood vessels because only part of the cholesterol reduction solution lies in the composition of the different types of cholesterol.**

3. **Cholesterol caused problem is contained in the amount of chemically reactive cholesterol in an owner's blood stream.**

Cholesterol-fat Particle Chemical Reactivity

The types of fat making the cholesterol-fat particle determine the chemical reactivity. This reactivity quantifies the potential of certain types of cholesterol particles to attach to the inside of the arteries. Whenever cholesterol-fat-protein complexes attach to the inside of an artery the process to plug has begun. The previous step involves the creation of a roughened area (rust or Velcro) for the sticky cholesterol to adhere to.

Rust produced on the inner surface of the blood vessel intices cholesterol-fat particles circulating in the blood vessels to enhance a Velcro-like surface where before, the surface was shiny. Certain factors increase the clogging process.

The Body Needs a Specific Cholesterol Level

Normally, every body has about one and a half pounds of cholesterol. It is an integral component of the cell membrane and makes up some of the package that holds the cell contents together. It also serves as the building block from which all sex hormones, some salt and water regulatory hormones, and stress hormone are made.

The balance between the hormones glucagon and insulin controls the amount of cholesterol manufactured in the liver. As a consequence, processes that favor insulin will increase the liver manufacture rate of the bad cholesterol. Conversely, processes that increase glucagon lead to an improved cholesterol profile because high glucagon levels decrease the manufacture rate of cholesterol synthesis in the liver. (section three)

Types of Cholesterol-Fat-Protein Particles

The liver makes the cholesterol needed by all body cells. The blood stream transports cholesterol to the cells after the liver secretes it. It cannot circulate alone because it is not water-soluble. Therefore, it circulates in the blood steam with water-soluble proteins. If the particle created by the liver has a higher protein percentage than the associated cholesterol, then it is a high-density lipoprotein (HDL) or good cholesterol. Moderate alcohol consumption, regular aerobic exercise, female gender, low carbohydrate diet, adequate glucagon level, and taking cholesterol lowering drugs are common factors that raise HDL levels.

When cholesterol content rises on specific transport proteins in the bloodstream, it is known as LDL and VLDL, or bad cholesterol. Sedentary lifestyle, male gender, high carbohydrate diet, high fasting insulin levels, low fasting glucagon levels, Type II diabetes, low thyroid function and genetically bad luck describe factors that raise this level. In addition, sedentary lifestyles in a setting of chronic mental stress accelerate cholesterol manufacture because this combination raises insulin requirements (section two).

Three Ways Cholesterol-Fat-Protein Particle Variables Can Harm the Blood Vessel

Friendly blood vessel fats include olive oil, salmon oil, and borage oil. Eating predominantly blood vessel protective fat helps keep cholesterol-fat-protein particles from oxidizing (rusting) regardless of the type. Conversely, if the LDL and HDL particles derive from a fast food diet, the stage sets for blood vessel injury even though the cholesterol numbers look good. The worst oils are vegetable oils that have been chemically altered by hydrogenation (Tran's fats). Lastly, the worst scenario occurs when both of these harmful processes occur together: The cholesterol numbers look bad, and the wrong types of fat make up the cholesterol and fat particles.

Cholesterol Particles Made By the Liver are a Danger

The liver performs as a faithful servant to the directions it receives. Lifestyles that promote message content that direct the liver to make excessive cholesterol and fat describe a blood vessel risk factor. Conversely, some lifestyles promote message content directed at the liver that promotes blood vessel health.

When the liver receives message content directing it to make sugar (carbohydrate) into excess fat and cholesterol, a potentially dangerous situation begins. The types of cholesterol-fat-protein complexes created by the liver differ drastically in their ability to be cleared from the blood stream by metabolically hungry cells. In contrast diet derived fat enters the blood stream packaged in a way that makes it readily accessible to the metabolically hungry cells.

However, liver manufactured fat and cholesterol contains a design intended to head for the preferential absorption sites, macrophages and abdominal fat cells (a much slower process). When certain conditions arise, the liver made packages adhere to the injured areas of the blood vessels, inside the macrophages. In the genetically predisposed owner, these complexes tend to build up in the blood vessels within the macrophages at higher levels than are acceptable for lining cells health. Macrophages are immune scavenger cells that roam the blood vessels and feed on LDL cholesterol. The difference between diet derived cholesterol-fat complexes and liver synthesized cholesterol-fat complexes are explained in section three.

Now that all three mechanisms of blood vessel injury have been introduced, it is time to develop the ways that they become risk factors within their group.

The three groups of risk factors are:
1. **Rust promoting processes**
2. **Hardening processes**
3. **Opportunistic processes (including the three ways cholesterol can be harmful)**

The Individual Risk Factors of Rust Promotion

Homocysteine

Homocysteine provides a recent example where the lonely thinker lived long enough to expose a mainstream medical inconsistency. This particular medical inconsistency involves rust and is the story of Dr. McCully. While he conducted research at Harvard University, in 1969, he noticed consistent similarities between the blood vessels of patients with high homocysteine levels and in those with blood vessels that were clogged from atherosclerosis (the most common form of blood vessel disease). He postulated that elevated blood levels of homocysteine were a significant risk factor for the development of blood vessel lining cell disease. He was promptly dismissed for his preposterous theories.

Several years ago in Finland, a large double blind study confirmed, in thousands of Finish men, that elevated blood levels of homocysteine powerfully predict the development of blood vessel clogging pathology. Today, over thirty years after Dr. McCully first discovered this association, homocysteine blood levels are one of mainstream medicine's official risk factors for identifying those who are at increased risk for the development of blood vessel disease (chapter three).

Hormonal Fatty Acids as Determinants of Blood Vessel Health

Small amounts of aspirin lower the risk of heart attacks. Dr. Berry Sears, in his book, *Entering the Zone*, points out that aspirin does not lower cholesterol, blood sugar, or blood pressure. Yet it is a powerful inhibitor of the tendency for a cardiac event.

Every time an owner takes an aspirin, they alter their hormonal fats. This alteration diminishes the clotting process and increases the flow of blood over a diseased segment of coronary arteries. The increased blood flow increases the delivery of the repair molecules to the diseased section of the arteries.

Essential fatty acids determine what types of hormonal fats are possible. When owners make poor dietary choices, they make poor precursors to the hormonal fats that provide an important component of the lining of the blood vessel walls and on platelets. The anti-inflammatory hormonal fats act as lubricants for efficient blood flow. Consuming the wrong precursors to the hormonal fats produces a destructive type of hormonal fat. In this situation, the ability to keep blood from inappropriately clotting diminishes.

Clotting occurs when the hormonal fat precursors activate to full-blown hormones. These hormonal fats are only in the blood stream for a few seconds, but during their brief existence they determine the production of clotting or lubricating mechanism in a blood stream locale (like a coronary artery). Lubricating hormonal fats will become deficient when owners consistently make poor dietary choices causing the production of poor quality hormonal fat precursors.

However, the quality of the blood vessel lining hormone fat precursors can also be improved by encouraging the production of the lubricating forces. Unfortunately, most poison their good and bad hormonal fats production by taking aspirin. Aspirin poisons the clotting forces slightly more than the lubricating forces.

Regretfully, what isn't being said about an additional class of inflammatory hormonal fats (leukotrienes) that aspirin facilitates to form more readily creates another health problem. Leukotrienes are produced in the immune system and their manufacture is encouraged when substances like aspirin prevent the usual drain off of prostaglandin production. Consequently, aspirin often increases allergies and asthma conditions for these reasons. Making matters worse, the excessive presence of these inflammatory hormonal fats (leukotrienes) leads to progressive joint aches and stiffness that ensures the need for another round of aspirin when it wears off.

For this reason, aspirin, consumed regularly, increases the production of the wrong types of inflammatory leukotrienes in the blood vessels. By this mechanism, consuming aspirin also increases swelling of certain tissues including lung, sinuses, and eventually in joints. Visualize aspirin helping inflammation in certain ways but the side effect of its use creates inflammation in other ways.

The work of Barry Sears examines the natural processes that encourage the formation of good hormonal fat precursors. Dr Sears has had experience producing optimal hormonal fat precursors in a variety of body types. His work provides a broader understanding of the importance of the essential fatty acids. His years of work have shown that owners can consume the right essential fatty acids, but other dietary factors sabotage their efforts. These factors cause the wrong overseeing hormones to be secreted and prevent the desired benefit.

Some foods cause high insulin production such as high carbohydrate diets (sections 2 and 3). This first dietary factor must be addressed if the owner is going to benefit from the manufacture of the beneficial hormonal fat precursors.

Still other unfortunate owners do everything right by decreasing their insulin, but nutritional deficiencies cause them to fail in their health goals. These deficiencies are easy to remedy. If the owner fails to remedy these nutritional deficiencies, they are doomed to the frustration of becoming fatter, suffering from clogged arteries, and high blood pressure. All of these health issues are avoidable with some simple nutritional intervention and counseling.

Heart Disease Resulting from Nutritional Deficiency

Often times, blood vessel disease directly results from varying types of nutritional deficiency. Most blood vessels will heal when nutritional deficiencies correct. These deficiencies injure blood vessels through rust promotion, hardening processes and/or opportunistic mechanisms. Usually all three mechanisms are set into motion by nutritional imbalance.

William B. Ferril, M. D.

Increased Blood Fat from Nutritional Deficiency

It has been asserted in the popular media that niacin supplementation may lower blood cholesterol. A more accurate statement would be to say that niacin is one of five nutritional cofactors that need to be present before optimal blood fat to occurs. When all five of the cofactors are present, the body can absorb blood fat and burn it in the cellular power plants. When fat processes in this way, it creates the energy packets that the cells need. This combustion process ends with the release of carbon dioxide and water.

Without the presence of the other four cofactors, many owners condemn themselves to failed attempts at natural healing. These owners often return to symptom control medicine (the complex). The necessity of these factors is well documented in the medical biochemistry textbooks, but the discussion occurs in a convoluted fashion. Knowledge of these fundamental 'must have' nutrients provides another way to heal. In addition to niacin (vitamin B3), pantothenic acid (vitamin B5), carnitine, riboflavin (vitamin B2), and Co enzyme Q10 are required for fat combustion.

Without these factors, the tendency for blood fat to rise (LDL cholesterol) occurs despite efforts to optimize insulin, cortisol, epinephrine; thyroid hormones, estrogen, IGF-1, and androgens (section 2). In addition, owners who eat a low carbohydrate diet, exercise aerobically, and participate in stress reduction measures may not improve their health if one or more of these above cofactors remain absent. These motivated owners fail to achieve the desired blood fat and weight loss because no one has counseled them on these basic nutritional cornerstones.

These nutritional 'traps' can be analogous to the creation of a smaller 'drain' for fat to exit once it enters their blood stream. The drain enlarges when the cells have the nutritional mechanism to combust it (see below). Realize, optimal combustion of fat cannot occur without all of the above cofactors. When fat fails to combust, it builds within a cell and eventually spills backward back into the blood stream.

Increased blood stream fat is analogous to a drain that can no longer dispose of its contents. The contents of the blood stream contain fat. The inclusion of these factors in the diet or in some cases receiving them intravenously will allow a 'bigger drain' to form. The drain in this analogy regards the increased rate of fat removal made possible when the cells have the nutritional ability to process (combust) fat into carbon dioxide and water.

Owners who lack these five nutrients cannot properly access fat for the production of energy packets. This causes the cells to have power plant (mitochondria) problems because fat is the preferred fuel for many cell types. Sufficiency of these above factors largely depends on dietary choices.

Many owners do not receive sufficient amounts of these nutritional cofactors from their food. Multi vitamin pills may not solve this problem. In addition, when food is cooked and processed these five nutritional cofactors deteriorate. Also the absorption of nutrients proves as a critical factor in the health of an owner.

Disease processes and medications affect what the body absorbs and retains. Empowerment comes from understanding why these factors play such a crucial role in the interrelationship between cellular power plants and energy extraction. After all, insufficient energy extraction describes a disease process. For example carnitine proves necessary before any fat fuel can transport into the cell furnaces (mitochondria).

Carnitine is made from the amino acid, lysine, vitamin C, vitamin B6, and SAMe (S-adenosyl methionine). SAMe proves critical to its manufacture and becomes rapidly depleted without adequate folate, vitamin B6, vitamin B12, serine and methionine, the methyl donor system (chapter three). For each carnitine manufactured, three SAMe molecules are used. Meat contains various levels of carnitine. Severe carnitine deficiency shows up as some forms of heart failure (insufficient heart energy extraction problem).

As stated previously, carnitine is the carrier molecule that delivers fat to the cellular power plant furnace for combustion. The liver, kidney, and heart cells need tremendous amounts of energy to perform. Sometimes heart failure results solely from carnitine deficiency. When was the last time that a mainstream doctor inquired into one of his/her heart failure patients' carnitine status? Realize the cells cannot use the potential energy contained in the fat molecules without transportation by carnitine. For this reason, endurance athletes supplement carnitine to enhance in their performance.

Niacin (vitamin B3) is the second factor necessary to burn fat in the creation of energy packets. Two other cofactors, riboflavin (vitamin B2) and pantothenic acid (vitamin B5) need to be considered with niacin. These three cofactors must be present in optimal amounts just inside the outer furnace (mitochondria) compartment. When all three are present the initial oxidation of fat traps energy packets, adenosine tri-phosphate (ATP). Consequently, when any one of these three diminishes, a progressive disability to trap energy occurs. Heat production increases instead of energy packet formation.

Pantothenic acid availability limits the rate that fat combusts within the power plant. Fat can only be utilized when it breaks down two carbons at a time and attaches to a pantothenic acid containing molecular machine, Co Enzyme A. Remember, this process cannot occur until carnitine has delivered fat to the outside compartment of the cell furnace.

Pantothenic acid proves as the essential ingredient for the manufacture of coenzyme A. Coenzyme A is the carrier molecule that allows the orderly combusting of fat energy, two carbons at a time. Realize a deficiency in either carnitine or the previously mentioned cofactors disables the refining process to acetate. When fat is the raw material for fuel combustion, these cofactors are required or body fat will accumulate in the blood stream. For this reason, pantothenic acid deficiency leads to a marked slow down in burning fat calories. In turn, Co Enzyme A delivers acetate to the combustion chamber.

Unfortunately under appreciated is the fact that the type of fuel that the mitochondria accept for combustion is restricted to one processed fuel type only, acetate. Whether raw fuel starts out as protein, fat or sugar, it needs to be processed into acetate before it can be combusted in the mitochondria. Similarly, power plants of the physical world also have such limitations. They can only combust one specific fuel type for operational purposes (natural gas, coal, radio active material, gasoline, or fuel oil, etc). Realize acetate is the only fuel that the cell power plants can utilize aerobically. Only when acetate burns in the presence of oxygen, this creates carbon dioxide gas and energy packets (ATP, NADPH and FADH).

The cell power plants only accept acetate for burning within the mitochondria. Acetate is the simplest fatty acid. Cognizance, for this fact helps to elucidate the common perpetrated fallacy about sugar for fuel needs. Whatever the raw fuel, whether it is amino acids, fat or sugar, it must first convert to acetate, a fatty acid, or it cannot combust aerobically.

Co enzyme Q10 (ubiquinone) is the last nutritional Cofactor. It is similar to niacin, riboflavin, and pantothenic acid, but Co enzyme Q10 allows for additional trapping of more energy (ATP) within the cell. Co enzyme Q10 is special in that it is made from the same enzymatic machinery as cholesterol, HMG Co A reductase. Without adequate Co enzyme Q10, the cells become compromised in their ability to generate energy packets but instead make more heat energy. Energy released as heat is waste. For this reason, inadequate Co enzyme Q10 causes diminished energy packet (ATP) formation.

Extreme energetic compromise occurs within the heart when it functions without sufficient coenzyme Q10 because coenzyme Q10 constitutes a vital component, within mitochondrion. Recall it proves necessary to effectively trap energy within the power plant. This fact forms one determinant of the performance of a cell. Lowered work ability leads to lower cardiac function. The heart has the highest needs for Co enzyme Q10 in the body because each heart cell contains about 2000 mitochondria. Consequently, huge amounts of energy packets are needed here. Visualize heart cells containing thousands of power plants (mitochondria) that need all five cofactors to maintain healthy function.

Unfortunately, popular cholesterol lowering drugs, known as the statin class, inhibit Co enzyme Q10 production. Often, the presence of this factor causes further compromise because coenzyme Q10 is unstable when food is processed. Biochemistry textbooks confirm that statin drugs inhibit HMG Co A reductase. This enzyme is necessary for both cholesterol and Co enzyme Q10 production.

Suspicion exists that people on these drugs tend to die at about the same rate as the untreated groups, but for different reasons. This becomes more alarming after adding in the suspected increase in cancer rates for owners who take these drugs.

The explanation could be from the fact that initially, cancer cells possess inferior ability to generate energy compared to healthy cells. When the body remains healthy this proves as a major advantage within the immune system for destroying cancer cells at an early stage. Most immune systems continuously destroy cancer cells by generating high energy burst and targeting these packets at cancer cells. This exposes a link for why those taking statin drugs could be at increased risk for cancer: These drugs tend to deplete the body content of coenzyme Q10 and hence, cells like immune system cell types experience a diminished ability to out perform the cancer cell in energy generation.

This does not mean that statin drugs are never indicted for the prevention of heart disease. Many owners insist on taking a passive role in their disease process. For this group, their doctor has very few alternatives. However, those owners willing to take responsibility for their health can use therapies without these side effects (sections, two, three and six). These remedies can often times avoid statin drug usage and its potential side effects. The inclusion of high quality coenzyme Q10 would be a big help in those clinical situations where the statin drugs prove necessary. This need is not often in a motivated patient.

These factors need to be present nutritionally in order for fat to be utilized in the production of energy work packets (ATP,NADH, FADH). The utilization of sugar as fuel has other nutritional requirements. As with fat, unless these factors needed for cell function are sufficiently present, diminished energy delivery occurs.

Accessing Carbohydrate Energy for Cellular Needs

Carbohydrates only burn up anaerobically (without oxygen) when any of five nutritional cofactors become deficient. This leads to massive increases in lactic acid production and fatigue. Fatigued cells have difficulty defending from rusting and hardening processes. Obviously, increased acid in the blood stream causes the blood to be more acidic. Unfortunately, excessive acidity promotes rust (oxidation). In the blood vessel lining cells this leads to an increase in Velcro formation.

When any of the five nutritional factors prove deficient, the cell has no way of obtaining the necessary sugar fragment, acetate. Remember, acetate proves as the only molecule, derived from all three raw fuel types that can be combusted in the presence of oxygen.

In order to burn sugar (carbohydrate) to carbon dioxide and water, the cell needs five types of nutritional molecules in sufficient amounts plus adequate oxygen in the combustion chamber. Lipoic acid, riboflavin, niacin, pantothenic acid, and thiamine (in the presence of adequate magnesium) constitute these factors.

Inside all cells, the first part of sugar breakdown occurs without oxygen and a three-carbon fragment, pyruvate, initially forms. However, only when adequate oxygen and all five of the above factors exist can this molecule enter the power plant (mitochondria) for further energy release. Realize, with nutritional deficiency, pyruvate breaks down more readily to lactic acid. The liver usually clears this acid from the blood stream, but when its formation becomes excessive, it builds up in the muscles to prevent death. Excessive lactic acid accumulation causes pain.

The enzyme, pyruvic dehydrogenase needs these five factors to 'cut the head off' (make a two carbon molecule, acetate) of pyruvate. Only this step prevents the formation of lactic acid and stabilizes it on the carrier molecule Co enzyme A (formed from pantothenic acid). Remember, acetate is the simplest fatty acid and derives from all raw fuel sources (sugar, fat, and protein).

Unless, acetate forms and attaches to Co enzyme A, aerobic metabolism comes to a halt. Health consequences arise because the larger share of energy contained in a sugar molecule cannot be utilized unless all of these factors are present. This deficiency causes the waste product, lactic acid to build up. Lactic acid causes pain.

Many owners endure pain and experience chronic fatigue only because their cells possess a decreased ability to burn sugar energy in a healthy way. The smallest physical exertion condemns these owners to bed rest. Their tissues contain lactic acid and this creates pain. These patients need to find a competent nutritionally oriented physician or they will continue to suffer. Not all chronic fatigue and muscle aches derive from this cause, but a significant percentage originates from these types of nutritional deficiency. These deficiencies also promote the other raw fuel, protein, conversion into acetate.

Amino acids, derived from protein digestion, can be used as fuel only after the liver converts them into sugar in a process called gluconeogenesis. All amino acids contain at least one nitrogen group (the amide). This group must be removed and eventually converted into urea in the liver for excretion by the kidneys. Adequate urea helps the kidneys concentrate their waste and conserve water. Cortisol, epinephrine, and glucagon hormones encourage gluconeogenesis. Epinephrine and glucagon have little effect without adequate cortisol. Insulin and Growth Hormone oppose gluconeogenesis. Amino acids provide another source of raw fuel that needs refining to acetate before becoming combustible.

Later, it will be explained how defense of body protein content proves fundamental to lasting health. Sufficient Growth Hormone release provides for defense of body protein (positive nitrogen balance). Body protein content largely determines the metabolic rate, because protein is the only body constituent that consumes calories. Old age begins to evidence itself when metabolism slows for this reason. Paradoxically, this simple truth often remains ignored within mainstream clinical practice. For now, file away the name, Growth Hormone, and wait for its story to unfold.

Male Gender – A Risk Factor

The risk factor of male gender remains poorly understood. It was thought males lacked the protective effect that pre-menopausal females possess, secondary to their higher blood estrogen. Scientific data from postmenopausal females who took estrogen replacement therapy, fails to support this belief. Estrogen's influence increased cholesterol, triglycerides and cell division properties. For this reason, some physicians have reconsidered their prescribing estrogen therapy for supposed cardiac protection alone.

Many different types of estrogen occur in nature and each has its own unique bioactive properties. Some are strong stimulants that direct estrogen responsive tissues towards cell division. For this reason, too much message content from the various types of estrogen causes growth of uterine fibroids, breast cysts, breast cancer, increased body fat of the breast, hips and thighs, increased insulin resistance, and interference with thyroid hormone activity. Currently, all available, patented forms of estrogen replacement prescriptions are not the right ratios or type of estrogen that the healthy female will produce (section two).

Until further scientific research becomes available certain facts need to be considered. How the hormonal difference in premenopausal females confers the blood vessel protective effects needs to be clarified. Good scientific evidence exists that the patented prescription forms of estrogen increase the risk of developing heart disease. This may be due to the unnatural way that foreign estrogens or oral dosing stimulate the liver's cholesterol and fat manufacturing machinery. When this occurs, the blood triglycerides increase (section two). Second, high estrogen states also increases the risk of blood clots. This is especially true when estrogens are swallowed. Swallowed estrogen abnormally stimulates the liver into making excessive clotting proteins. Lastly, abnormally shaped progesterone substitutes are not real progesterone.

One type of progesterone exists in nature. This fact proves important because many studies have used synthetic progesterone substitutes and later falsely implicated real progesterone in the development of blood vessel disease. For this reason, some physicians feel that progesterone has been unfairly implicated in the development of blood vessel disease. When examining the designs of these studies that purport a link to progesterone and heart disease, one discovers that the authors have confused abnormally shaped progesterone substitute replacement therapies as equivalent to natural progesterone therapy.

Estrogen and progesterone types of hormones contain message content by virtue of their simple shape. However, in order to obtain a patent, substitute hormones must contain an altered shape or be contained in a mixture in an unnatural way. These alterations change the message content. Predictably, health consequences follow (explained in section two).

So if estrogen does not confer protective qualities to female's blood vessels, what explains their protection during their menstruation years? One emerging thought concerns iron. Once iron absorbs into the body it proves very difficult to leave without a blood loss event. Chronic stress promotes increased iron absorption (explained in the heart chapter). Females during their menstrual years lose iron. Excessive iron damages the blood vessel lining cells. The best screening test for excessive blood vessel iron storage levels is the serum ferritin. When found to be excessive a sequence of therapeutic phlebotomies solves the problem.

Another gender difference concerns that females have higher progesterone levels. Progesterone is a powerful fluid loss hormone. Stress promotes fluid retention and progesterone helps negate this effect. Fluid retention raises blood pressure. Females experience first hand the fluid retention effects of falling progesterone just before their periods as breast tenderness and bloating.

Smoking Facilitates Velcro Formation

Cigarette smoke injures the inner lining of the arteries. This causes damage by several different mechanisms. Cigarette smoke contains high concentrations of carbon monoxide. Carbon monoxide binds to the red blood cell's oxygen binding sites about 200 times more tightly than its competitor, oxygen. Oxygen carrying ability in the average smoker is lowered by about 15%. Lower oxygen content is sensed and the bone marrow is stimulated to release more red blood cells. This raises the solid content (red blood cell mass) of the blood to abnormal levels leading to an increased tendency for blood clots.

Second, carbon monoxide is an oxidizing agent. The presence of carbon monoxide causes rust in the inner lining cells of the waterways and lung tissue. In the lungs, oxidation of the numerous little balloons, called alveoli, leads to rupture. As the process advances this leads to emphysema. In the blood vessels, rust accumulation allows the velco necessary for adhearing deposits of cholesterol.

Finally, nicotine contained in smoke has the physiological effect of telling the artery muscle cells to contract hard in the extremities and skin. This decreases the available nutrition and oxygen delivery to those sites. For this reason, numerous patients no longer need high blood pressure medication once they successfully quit smoking. The penis qualifies as an extremity and is among the vulnerable sites. Imagine the Marlboro man's change in status if the public ever became aware of this interesting physiologic effect. It's a physiological fact that if one wants a smaller penis, he can smoke and someday the desired effect will be achieved.

INSULIN AND BLOOD VESSEL DISEASE

Hormone Opportunist Mechanism

Hormone levels and life style choices can create a vicious cycle that results in unhealthy cholesterol levels. Scientific insights reveal that hormone levels affect behavior and behavior affects hormone levels. The insulin trap is the first of several key hormone abnormalities that will be discussed in this manual.

High insulin levels turn on the fat and cholesterol enzymatic machinery (HMG Co A reductase) of the liver. Insulin promotes the type of cholesterol packages known as LDL and VLDL involved in heart disease. In contrast, high glucagon levels in the liver curtail this type of cholesterol manufacture. A tug of war occurs in the liver between the message content of these two hormones. They are both secreted from the pancreas by different stimuli. Lifestyle choices that promote a healthy balance between these two hormones will naturally improve cholesterol content. Conversely, lifestyle choices that promote more insulin and less glucagon weaken the cholesterol profile.

A simple analogy to understand insulin is this. When driving into the gas station and filling the gas tank, a nozzle is used to connect the cars tank to the fuel pump. Insulin is like the nozzle that fills the cell's fuel tank. Without a nozzle there can be no fuel delivery.

The cellular fuel tanks are just like a car fuel tank. They can only hold a finite amount of fuel before it spills on the ground or back into the blood stream. Overly nourished owners spill cellular fuel (mainly sugar) back into the blood stream. When all the cellular fuel tanks are full, the liver must clear the blood stream of the excess fuel. The liver has a finite capacity to store excess sugar fuel. When the sugar fuel level exceeds the capacity of the liver to store it (about 100 grams of carbohydrates or 440 calories worth), at the direction of insulin, the liver begins to make this sugar into fat and cholesterol.

Liver manufactured fat and cholesterol, from carbohydrate has been known for years, to be of the saturated type because it was designed with storage in mind. Saturated fats are hard at body temperature. Fact: increased insulin directs the butter-fat (saturated fat) and cholesterol to form. Other factors

cause it to prove sticky within the arteries. Fact: adequate B vitamins within the liver allow the liver to convert dietary butter fat into olive oil.

In addition, realize perfectly healthy individuals have about six grams of carbohydrate in their entire blood stream. If the blood sugar falls to around three grams of carbohydrate unconsciousness occurs. On the other extreme, if the blood sugar content rises to nine grams diabetes occurs. Cognizance here, allows one to choose foods differently.

For example, one slice of bread can be twenty-two grams of carbohydrates and one can of pop is forty-two grams! Fact: the more carbohydrates eaten, the more insulin needs to pummel the liver into butter fat type cholesterol and fat synthesis in order to return the blood sugar to normal. Unfortunately, doctors are no longer taught these facts that help one to see the real risk of carbohydrates and the advantages of healthy fats.

The newly manufactured fat particles (LDL and VLDL cholesterol) excrete into the blood stream, where they contribute to the growth of fat cells in the belly area. Some of this 'yuck' sticks in certain owner's blood vessels when other Velcro factors exist. The beer gut provides a clinical indicator about the magnitude of this process.

Picture a fuel nozzle being necessary to fill up a car's fuel tank. Similarly, the body relies on two different fuel nozzles before the body's seventy trillion cells can receive nutrition. The first, insulin, directs the cells to take up the fuel building blocks (amino acids, fatty acids, and sugar) and store them as reassembled proteins, fats and glycogen. The apparent secret is that insulin normally only provides 7% of the fuel nozzle action and, normally most of its effect occurs within the liver. Visualize the liver as an insulin trap.

For this reason, insulin requires the help of a different fuel nozzle, insulin-like growth factor (IGF-1) for fuel uptake in the other 94% of cells outside of the liver and fat. Apparently, IGF-1 is the scientific secret fuel nozzle within the body (evidence explained later). Healthy owners have over one hundred times the IGF-1 in their blood streams compared to insulin. Realize for now insulin exerts its major fuel uptake effect in the liver from the consequence of its secretion pathway. Conversely, IGF-1 exerts its major fuel uptake effect in the organs, bones and muscles.

As owners become unhealthy, IGF-1 levels fall and insulin levels need to rise (in order to keep the number of fuel nozzles constant). For example, checking the IGF-1 levels of most osteoporotics (almost always less than 100 ng/ml) shows that its deficiency is the true cause of their hungry bone cells (*hungry cell syndrome – explained in section five*).

It is important to realize that insulin preferentially facilitates the liver and fat cells in their uptake of nutrients from the blood stream. Conversely, IGF-1 facilitates the uptake of fuels by the many other body cells. It helps to think of both insulin and IGF-1 as the body's *fuel nozzle hormones*. Total fuel nozzles need to stay constant or the cells remain hungry.

Because insulin secretes from the pancreas into the portal vein, the liver always receives the highest concentration of insulin message content whatever its secretion rate. Consequently, higher insulin secretion rates lead to an exaggerated liver conversion of sugar into cholesterol and fat. Higher insulin secretion arises when IGF-1 levels fall. Many blood vessel related diseases have their origins in the fall of IGF-1 and the consequent need for excess insulin (sections two, three, four and six).

Remember, insulin directs the liver to change sugar into fat and activate HMG Co A reductase which increases cholesterol production in the liver. Insulin directed and manufactured fat and cholesterol releases into the bloodstream as the bad cholesterol-fat-protein particles (LDL and VLDL). LDL and VLDL are constructed in the liver for storage purposes. Storage of the various fuel groups describes what the insulin message content does better than any other hormone.

Consistent with this message, these particles are destined for storage sites. In certain genetically predisposed and nutrient deficient owners, the rate of their removal from the blood stream proves slow and concentrations of these particles rise. In contrast, dietary derived fat particles (chylomicrons) are easier for the body to eliminate from the circulation (section three). The more bad cholesterol (LDL and VLDL) the owner has in the bloodstream, the more tendencies exist for this sticky form of cholesterol-fat-protein complex to adhere to his/her arterial lining.

Fat cells in the abdomen area are directed by the same insulin message to take up liver manufactured fat. Macrophages that line the arteries can uptake 30% of the daily manufactured amounts of these types of liver manufactured fat-cholesterol-protein complexes. In addition, a sedentary lifestyle promotes macrophage cells, lining the blood vessels, to accumulating more of this material. Eventually these cells grow into foam cells that are affixed to the inside of the arterial wall. This development constitutes the earliest recognized lesion in the development of blood vessel disease.

Earlier it was implied that the LDL cholesterol sticks to Velcro surfaces. Actually, the macrophages accumulate LDL cholesterol over time. This fact shows that it is slightly more complicated than the introductory statement implied. Some authorities feel that the macrophages adhere to areas on the artery that are injured (Velcro has formed). Others feel that the macrophages serve a fuel storage role and the intent is to have ample fat fuel for cardiac and muscle cells the next time insulin levels drop or the owner exercises. In many owners the insulin level never drops to a level where the macrophage can release their contents. In addition, sedentary lifestyles provide little opportunity for release to sedentary muscles and heart tissues.

In America, many fine specimens of the high insulin states exist. Fast food establishments are full of these owners who have stuffed macrophages lining their coronary arteries with their accompanying expanded waistline. This excess fat creates trouble for the blood vessels because fat cells have a slow metabolic rate. The uptake of LDL and VLDL cholesterol occurs at a slower rate than the liver dumps it into their blood stream. The macrophage system was not designed to receive daily additions of fat to its cell type population.

Marked genetic variation occurs for the rate certain owners can make LDL cholesterol in their liver and how fast it can be removed from their blood stream. In general, the higher the insulin level, the higher the message content directed at the liver to increase LDL production. Certain owners have elevated cholesterol because their fat cells cannot remove the LDL cholesterol at the rate their liver dumps it into their blood stream. This chronic situation allows ample time for some LDL cholesterol to be added to the macrophages that adhere to the Velcro patches that form secondary to other risk factors.

Another useful analogy regards a high volume faucet (Morales). The faucet flow likens itself to the ability (directed by insulin) of the liver to manufacture LDL cholesterol and dump it into the blood stream. The drain is likened to the ability of the fat cells to clear this form of cholesterol from the blood vessels (the sink). Increased LDL cholesterol in the sink builds to higher levels when the drain becomes too small (fat cells in the abdomen area). The immune scavenger cells (the macrophages) ingest about 30% of these particles (grime that collects on the sides of the sink wall). They become laden and attach to places like the coronary arteries.

Sedentary people have little stimulus for their fat laden macrophages to release LDL and it continues to collect and grow into foam cells. This cycle repeats itself following each carbohydrate meal. The presence of foam cells denotes the earliest blood vessel wall change that leads to blood vessel disease. Genetics plays a role in how much carbohydrate it takes to over run the drain (fat cells). Owners can't change their genetics, but they can change the stimulus (insulin level and sedentary lifestyle) and retard the course of this type of heart disease.

Carbohydrate Overload and Increased Insulin Affect the Appetite

High insulin message content, occurring with a high carbohydrate diet, proves as a powerful appetite stimulant. The higher the insulin levels in circulation, the more behavioral stimulation exist to satisfy the increased appetite. Reducing insulin levels has a dramatic affect on the appetite cravings as well as on the amount of bad cholesterol. The effects of hormones on feeding behavior prove substantial (section two). Carbohydrates also play a role in this process. Carbohydrate, in all forms, is by far the most powerful stimulant of insulin secretion in initiating this vicious cycle.

Gonads, Thyroid and Adrenals: Firing the Engines of Life

In one way or another blood vessel disease results from the repair rate not keeping up with the injury rate. Poor gonad and/or adrenal function comprise a major risk factor that remains often overlooked in the development of blood vessel disease. These glands secretions direct rejuvenation and healthful maintenance activities of the blood vessels (repair). When optimal conditions prevail, they perform this task by secreting the appropriate types of informational substances (the steroids).

Optimal steroid mixture secretion proves as a prerequisite for good health. As the overall glandular secretion message content quality diminishes, this imbalance eventually reflects in the aging appearance of the body. When this happens in the blood vessels, rust that occurs fails to be repaired. The body tissues succeed or fail in this ongoing cellular infrastructure investment program (section two). For now realize, steroid hormones made in the adrenals and the gonads provide essential repair information for directing rejuvenation.

In addition, high normal thyroid function (thyroid hormones) benefits the blood vessels in important ways (Barnes). Broda Barnes,

M.D. PhD proved this over thirty years ago. For now, realize he showed that sufficient thyroid function proves necessary to remove nitrogen containing sugar waste (mucopolysaccharides or GAG) from the inside blood vessel lining. Failure here allows the abnormal buildup of these types of wastes, and consequently prevents cholesterol from diffusing out of the macrophages and into the hungry cells. Its buildup also eventually causes stiffening of the arteries (arteriosclerosis). If more physicians realized the simple truths contained in this man's life work, many lucrative cholesterol lowering and blood pressure lowering drugs would no longer be necessary most of the time. Imagine that.

COUNTERING THE SECOND PRINCIPLE OF LONGEVITY: FLEXIBILITY

High Blood Pressure Causes Stiffness in the Pipes

High blood pressure ages the blood vessels by promoting progressive stiffness of the artery in the muscular layer in a defensive response to the elevated pressure. As the pressure increases, the muscle layer within the artery enlarges to accommodate the resistance. Resistance increases to counter the increased pressure in the artery. This process is somewhat analogous to the fact that thicker hydraulic hoses are stiffer. The same concept applies to arteries. The thicker arteries prove less flexible and tend to have accelerated wear and tear. These changes result from the turbulent blood flow within the blood vessels that pummel the less elastic interior lining cells. This explains the injury mechanism that results from all causes of high blood pressure.

Healthy arteries remain flexible and this reduces the damage caused by the turbulent flow in the blood vessel. As the wear and tear occurs, weakened areas appear. Small breaks occur in vulnerable small arteries leading to leakage of trace amounts of blood into the surrounding tissues. These small bleeds continue until there is an irreversible loss in function in the affected organ. The most vulnerable sites to these silent small bleeds are the hearing apparatus, retina, brain, heart, and kidney areas. Injured blood vessels are another way of describing Velcro. The more Velcro that exists, the more repair necessary to keep macrophages from adhering as temporary patch jobs against the injured blood vessel lining. Adding in the high insulin states, the macrophages uptake some of the extra LDL cholesterol, manufactured in the liver, and this process accelerates blood vessel disease even more.

High blood pressure proves as a silent and symptom free enemy until late in the disease process. Patients in the early stage of this disease process insist that they feel fine and are less compliant with their high blood pressure medication. Most high blood pressure prescription medications work by poisoning an enzymatic process that results in a lowered blood pressure. Until recently, physicians justified medicines' inevitable side effects because there was no better way.

Recently, an old scientific truth was reasserted. Magnesium proves as a powerful smooth muscle relaxant. Arteries generate pressure by contracting their smooth muscle layer. Some evidence suggests that intracellular depletion of magnesium content tends to make these smooth muscle cells sometime 'contractile prone' which leads to an elevated blood pressure. Adequate supplementation with magnesium can restore the natural balance and the blood pressure will come down without poisoning an enzymatic process.

Taking 500-700mg elemental weight of magnesium per day will significantly drop blood pressure readings in seven to fourteen days for some owners. Magnesium absorption depends on the manufacture of adequate stomach acid. Magnesium tends to open the airways and make the bowels more regular. The effect of magnesium on bowel movements varies with the ingestion of different types of salt. The most powerful form is magnesium citrate, a laxative. Many different causes exists that lead to high blood pressure. Magnesium has a beneficial effect on some hypertensive owners. Several other abnormalities can lead to high blood pressure (chapters two and three).

Magnesium supplements come in the form of a salt. The magnesium salt weight contained in the pill, capsule or powder is usually stated on the front of the bottle and is always more than the actual content of the weight of elemental magnesium (active ingredient). Usually in the small print on the back of the bottle is the weight of the elemental magnesium content per dose. This amount ranges from 15-150 mg depending on the brand.

All magnesium supplements are not equally effective. Some have a small amount of elemental magnesium per dose and this requires ingesting a handful to receive what other brands contain in a single pill. There are some brands that poorly absorb, which diminishes their therapeutic value. Finally, some companies manufacture magnesium with salts of oxygen (oxide), which is unacceptable. 'Source Naturals' and some other manufacturers make an excellent line of magnesium products. Magnesium deficiency provides only one example of how mineral imbalance can affect blood pressure.

Mineral Imbalance Can Cause High Blood Pressure

The larger problem of mineral imbalance results from a processed food diet. Processed foods contain drastically altered mineral composition when compared to real food (see mineral table in chapter three). In contrast, real food (unprocessed food) tends to be high in magnesium and potassium and intermediate in its calcium content. Real food is usually low in sodium. Bottom line: Processed food (food from a box, bag or can) contains reversed mineral content compared to real food with the exception of calcium.

The body energizes by an electrical system that maintains itself by potential differences across trillions of cell membranes in the body. The body requires specific mineral proportions. A real food diet supplies these and a processed food diet does not. Around middle age cells begin to lose their electrical pizzazz. It is a miracle that the body can tolerate reversed minerals (electrolytes) ratio intake for as long as it does before it begins to fail.

The car battery electrolyte (minerals) composition provides an analogy that demonstrates the effect of mineral imbalance. Like the body cells that charge themselves by concentration differences around cell membranes, so it is with car batteries. Car batteries contain a maximum charge only when the different minerals exist at a maximal difference across the membrane. For this to occur, the battery manufacturer adds the proper minerals into the battery fluid.

The chronic consumption of processed food is analogous to dumping battery fluid on the ground and reversing the proportion of electrolytes in battery fluid. Most owners would see this behavior as foolish. Yet, this is what they are doing every time they eat processed food. Around middle age the 'battery fluid' in the body begins to alter despite the best effort of the kidneys to compensate for the reversed ratio of mineral intake. This process describes the origin of many diseases. One common disease that results from this imbalance is high blood pressure.

Most owners need about 4000 mg of potassium, 1000 mg of sodium, 1000 mg of calcium and 500 mg of magnesium every day. Profuse sweating increases sodium needs. Altered kidney and adrenal function will also alter these amounts. Most Americans obtain about 6000 mg of sodium a day and much less potassium and magnesium than they need (mineral table).

By this simple mechanism, around middle age the cells have usually sacrificed much of their potassium to maintaining the blood potassium level. The cost to health occurs when potassium leaks from cells and this decreases the electrical charge. This means that the afflicted cells perform less work because of fatigue. Early fatigue is a sign of aging.

98% of body potassium sequesters inside the cells. Realize, the inside the cell potassium sacrifices itself to maintain the potassium level in the 2% tank (floating in the blood stream). For this reason, many owners are misled when they have their blood drawn and their potassium result comes back normal. The blood test says nothing about the sufficiency of potassium content inside their 70 trillion cells.

Potassium Deficiency and Sodium Excess and High Blood Pressure

Many owners have had the experience of receiving instructions from their physician about the benefits of a low salt diet. However, very few are counseled about the importance of a healthy potassium to sodium ratio. The optimal ratio between potassium and sodium proves as a minimum of three-to-one.

Unfortunatley, most Americans ingest the opposite proportions between these two vital minerals. Food manufactures add many types of sodium to processed foods to preserve its shelf life. Most of this added sodium does not taste salty. Sodium only tastes salty when it occurs as the salt of chloride (table salt). Monosodium glutamate, sodium aspartate, sodium benzoate, sodium nitrite, sodium alginate, and sodium sulfate are examples of added sodium. In addition, sodium oxide is added to soften water.

Ways a chronic potassium deficiency will harm the body and raise blood pressure:
  1. **Kidney damage (sections two, three, four, and five)**
  2. **Insulin resistance (sections two, three, and six)**
  3. **Increased cholesterol (sections two, three, and six)**
  4. **The choice of normal testosterone and high blood pressure or a lower testosterone and normal blood pressure (chapter three, sections two, three, four, five, six)**
  5. **Irritable nervous system (sections five and six)**
  6. **Weakened cell force field (sections three, four, and five)**

7. **Slower metabolism (sections two, three, and six)**
8. **Loss of protein (sections two, three, and four)**
9. **Chronic stress accelerates potassium deficiency (sections   two, three, four, and five)**

The majority of high blood pressure problems partially relate to mineral imbalance. Potassium is the major mineral deficiency that is responsible for the high blood pressure of middle age. Several other significant nutritional causes exist for high blood pressure.

These factors are proven mechanisms for the development of blood pressure elevation: Methyl donor depletion syndromes, nitric oxide deficiency, stiff red blood cells, a processed food diet, the wrong balance of essential dietary fats (hormonal fats), and inappropriate attention to the 'tug of war' occurring between the biogenic amines. All of these contribute significantly to blood pressure elevation. Yet, they are rarely discussed (chapters 2 and 3).

Weaning off blood pressure prescription medication involves a tricky process. A competent physician needs to oversee the transitional period. In this period, less hypertension medication will be needed after the implementation of magnesium and/or other methods and supplements (see chapters two and three). A sudden or premature cessation of prescription anti-hypertensive medications can produce dangerous rebound effects that place the owner at increased risk for complications.

So far introductory statements have been made about rust, hardening and opportunistic mechanisms that cause blood vessel damage. These blood vessel damaging mechanisms all interrelate. There are disease processes that employ all three mechanisms on how it injures the blood vessel. Diabetes is such a process.

DIABETES CAUSES RUST, HARDENING, AND USUALLY ACTIVATES AN OPPORTUNISTIC MECHANISM

Diabetes

Diabetes diminishes health by injuring the blood vessels. Diabetes exemplifies a disease process that includes all three blood vessel injury mechanisms. High blood sugar injures the blood vessel lining cells by promoting Velcro formation. In turn, most diabetic's high blood insulin levels promote high blood pressure and thus the stiffening mechanisms (chapter three). High blood insulin also creates the abnormal amounts of LDL cholesterol, which provides the opportunistic mechanism (sections two and three). All three combined together creates an accelerated path to blood vessel disease.

Until recently, medical approaches aimed at the prevention of blood vessel injury, from diabetes, were a disappointment. The treatment success of a diabetic depends on three variables. If these three variables are addressed squarely and honestly, the complications of diabetes slow down. In some cases, the complications can be avoided almost entirely. The first variable concerns "who" the diabetic patient consults for advice. The examples of Dr Richard Bernstein, MD and Steven Gordon, ND demonstrate the significant results that can be achieved by the application of effective treatments.

A fresh scientific perspective is heard from Dr. Richard Bernstein, MD, who developed diabetes at age twelve (*Diabetes Solution*, Little and Brown Co.). When he was in his late twenties, he had many complications from the disease process including moderately severe kidney disease. His engineering background allowed him to approach his disease methodically and rigorously. He carefully noted his dietary intake and daily intake weight of the different food groups. He also carefully followed any changes in his diet and the effects this had on blood sugar.

Finally, he confirmed a simple concept and through rigorous dedication he reversed his kidney disease entirely. At the age of sixty-nine he is in better health than many of his peers. In this informative and well-written book he outlines a plan of healing from the potential complications of diabetes and the genetic tendencies to change carbohydrate into LDL cholesterol.

He discovered that since diabetes involves a disease primarily of abnormal sugar metabolism then if one strictly curtails sugar (carbohydrate) the complications of diabetes diminish. Dr. Bernstein concluded that strict adherence to a low carbohydrate diet brings about a lowered insulin level (need) and this favorably affects cholesterol parameters.

While Dr. Bernstein has insulin dependent diabetes (10% of diabetics) this program is equally beneficial for the adult onset diabetes patients (90% of diabetes patients). Realize, most adult onset diabetics suffer from excessive insulin in their bodies (the exceptions to this are discussed in the liver chapter). Diabetes occurs when their body mass reaches their pancreas' upper limit of insulin production.

The more body fat, the more insulin needed to maintain it. Excess insulin exposure also causes the majority of heart disease (liver chapter). This program identifies a huge percentage of people on the road to developing heart disease (prediabetes stage) because they suffer from chronically elevated insulin levels (liver chapter). Chronic elevated insulin secretion rates, secondary to increased insulin need (explained later), cause excessive cholesterol and triglyceride to form. For this simple reason, by following, Dr. Bernstein's program, these at risk owners can dramatically lower their heart disease risk.

This author was initially skeptical about Dr. Bernstein's findings. It was difficult to accept that eating high levels of fat and cholesterol could result in a dramatic reduction of those substances in the blood stream. Approximately ten years ago this author observed different patients who had followed various versions of low carbohydrate diets. Some of them had heart disease, some had cerebral vascular disease, and some had diabetes. In most cases there was an agreement achieved about their obtaining a cholesterol profile at the start of the diet and then again in thirty days after trying their seemingly ridiculous diet. This author was shocked when the results began coming back thirty days later. With few exceptions, the cholesterol profiles for these disease types were dramatically improved. ***According to the mainstream medical dogma this should not have happened***.

Years ago, this author began working with a naturopathic doctor, Steven Gordon. Dr. Gordon persuaded the author to buy Dr. Bernstein's book and study it for a likely explanation why these contrary diets work. Dr. Gordon began to treat his own insulin dependent diabetes with a low carbohydrate diet and has used the recommendations of Dr. Bernstein in his treatment program over the last ten years. Dr. Gordon has reported immense benefits to himself and his patients. For example, his hemoglobin A1C runs consistently between 5-5.5! Normal is considered less than 6 (but optimum is less than 5).

The second variable that will predict the outcome of the diabetes treatment concerns the motivation of the patient to comply with taking an active and consistent role in changing his/her diet and lifestyle. Only those patients willing to commit to positive changes have a high probability of treatment success. In contrast, patients who remain unwilling to take responsibility for their lifestyle and insist on a passive approach to their disease process condemn themselves to symptom control medicine. These treatment modalities litter the owners' body with side effects and result in unreasonably limited outcomes.

The third variable that will predict treatment success involves correctly classifying the type of diabetes, its root. This discernment is important because a minority of diabetics exist whose true origins of their disease process fails to be comprehended correctly. Here, their elevated blood sugars are measured, but the cause fails elucidation. Appropriate treatment modalities cannot be suggested when the cause of the elevated blood sugar remains unknown. Consequently, this group of diabetics (explained in the liver chapter) suffers rampant disease complications. Fortunately, accurate diagnosis allows the exploration for ways to heal.

Remember, an important common fact exist between most diabetes and heart disease patients: In the majority of these illnesses a high insulin level occurs. The difference between these two diseases is that the adult onset diabetic's have reached a body mass that exceeds their genetic ability to make even more insulin. The more body fat, the more insulin needed to maintain it. When the upper limit of a pancreas' insulin output occurs blood sugar increases.

However, in both heart disease and adult onset diabetics, high blood insulin feeds fat accumulation in their arteries. For this reason, by the time an owner develops obesity to the point of a rising blood sugar; their blood vessels already evidence atherosclerotic disease. In fact, by definition, mainstream medicine now states that at the time of diagnosis for adult onset diabetes heart disease is already presumed to exist. The mechanism: Unfortunately, chronic elevated blood insulin encourages their macrophages that line their arteries to ingest fat for many years before their blood sugar finally rises (the silent killer years).

Realize, the greater the body fat, the more insulin required to sustaining it. For those that doubt this fact, consider how the opposite situation of childhood diabetes presents. Childhood diabetes presents with a rapid loss of body fat because insulin proves deficient. Contrast this situation with the majority of adult onset diabetics who are obese. Obese diabetics suffer from an excess body exposure to insulin. However, their obesity has exceeded their genetic ability to increase insulin further (later the IGF-1 component to this problem will be discussed).

Different bodies have their upper limit of maximal insulin production. When body mass exceeds the pancreas ability to manufacture ever more insulin, the blood sugar will rise beyond normal and diabetes manifests. This variability between different owners explains why some owner's obesity is not extreme when they develop diabetes. In others, obesity is marked before their blood sugar rises.

Visualize, years before this, their high insulin state encourages their blood vessel lining cells to silently fill with fat long before their pancreases' failed to continue increasing its insulin production. In fact, some owners never reach their upper limit of insulin production despite becoming obese. However, their high insulin levels will usually cause blood vessel disease at an early age. As a general rule, the greater the obesity, the higher the insulin level required to sustain the fat mass.

The association between increased insulin levels and blood vessel disease illuminates another important point: Mainstream medicine sometimes treats adult onset diabetes by raising insulin levels. While this approach will lower blood sugar, it is paid for with the price of further feeding the blood vessel macrophages more fat. Consequently, this approach arguably corrects the rusting processes, but raises the stiffening and opportunistic processes rate.

The reader is cautioned to recall the group of diabetics that are neither type one nor type two, but victims of some other abnormal hormone process (liver chapter). As was mentioned, this small group of diabetics does poorly because they fail to receive the correct diagnosis for why their blood sugar elevates. A more complete hormonal assessment will identify these patients. The trouble arises in that many physicians receive scant training for how to interpret the test results needed to identify this subgroup of diabetics. The above provides, yet, another prelude for the later explained evidence that many owners needlessly suffer at the hands of the complex.

This concludes the introductory level discussion of rust prevention and hardening processes. In the next chapter, how these same processes injure the red blood cells will be explored. Rusted and stiff red blood cells cause many complications in diabetes. If the blood vessels also have opportunistic processes in operation (high LDL cholesterol), the added insult of stiff and rusted red blood cells exaggerates the severity of the disease process (chapter two). Before chapter two begins a mental picture of the different body cells proves useful.

The Basic Unit of the Human Form is the Cell.

The numerous body cell types are analogous in some ways to the many different varieties of fruits and vegetables. Different fruits and vegetable types are composed of different textures of skin, color, shapes, sizes and consistency.

Extending this analogy one can envision the different skin types of these foods as analogous to the different types of environments that surround the cell types. For example, cartilage and bone cells that are widely spaced between the hard outside the cell matrixes that they create are like coconuts. In contrast, red blood cells are like sponges in consistency (technically not an edible food, but the consistency and resiliency are accurate.).

Some owners have health problems because their cell types are like overly ripe fruit or vegetables. Fruits and vegetables deteriorate for the same reasons as human cells, diminished GAG (glycosaminoglycan) content. The amount of GAG whether it's in a fruit or human cell largely determines its water content. Old cells and shriveling fruit occur as their water content diminishes. When cell types shrivel they are observed in humans as old age. Old age since antiquity is known to involve a drying out process.

The goal is to keep all the body 'fruits and vegetables' in their most appealing state. The supporting architecture for the cell's interior is called the cytoskeleton. The supporting architecture for the cell's exterior is called the extra-cellular matrix. When the supporting architecture diminishes the body assumes the shrunken and flattened look of old age. The science exists to perform a much better job at explaining why GAG diminishes and how it can return (section five).

Almost all cells have a complete 'computer program' (DNA), but only certain programs (genes) activate within a cell type. In turn, gene activation leads to a specific protein's manufacture. Consequently, which genes activate determine what a cell looks like and the products that its different cell factories produce.

The specific gene activated directs the manufacture of a certain protein. Realize, protein is the metabolically active component of the body. Therefore, the quality and amounts of the different proteins constitute an additional determinant of youthfulness. Specific hormones defend body protein levels. Section 2 is about these hormones and how one determines whether they have them or not.

For now simply summarize that the activity of the DNA program (genes) determines; the types and amounts of the different cellular machines (enzymes) that perform different assembly line activities; the sufficiency of mineral pumps that line one's 70 trillion cells to create a cell voltage and the active segments of muscle (actin and myosin proteins). Note that all the above examples of gene products are proteins.

In general the multiple enzymes that create a metabolism by burning energy segregate into specific cellular factories. Examples of cellular factories are: Golgi apparatus, endoplasmic reticulum, and peroxisomes. Each cell factory needs a power supply to draw from for their activities.

This energy is supplied by the cellular power plant (mitochondria). When a cell remains healthy the energy packets (ATP) created by the combustion of fuel and oxygen exist sufficiently in the cell. Many cells have additional waste incinerator facilities (peroxisomes). All living cells create a cellular force field (cell membrane voltage).

The cell membrane voltage supplies energy for work. The strength of its charge is determined by the amount of membrane pumps, the ratio of minerals available and the amount of ATP available. The membrane energy also acts like a force field because it shields the cell from harmful, foreign molecules. Harmful molecules always lurk outside the cell and only the electrical charge contained in the membrane prevents their penetration. For these reasons, processes that harm the strength of the electrical charge (voltage) contained in the membrane accelerate the aging process (section five).

A cognizance for these basic dynamic mental pictures helps in one's healing quest. The cells in the blood vessels, in the next chapter, help to begin this journey. The red cells also provide the simplest example of what cells need to function.

CHAPTER TWO

THE CELLS TRAVELING WITHIN THE BLOOD VESSELS

The previous chapter's discussion concerned the amount of stiffness and rust formation within the blood vessels. Whether or not healthy cells travel within these vessels (the pipes) form another very important determinant of the body's condition. The cells which travel within the blood vessels can efficiently perform their purpose only when they are both flexible and without rust.

Many chronic degenerative diseases are made worse or arise completely from these two destructive processes that damage the blood cells. Examples include: high blood pressure, fibromyalgia, complications from diabetes, peripheral vascular disease, brain deterioration syndromes, cardiac ischemia, kidney injury, and splenomegaly. When the blood cells sustain damage restoring their flexibility and integrity restores the body's health.

The cells that flow through the blood vessels perform some of the body's most vital functions. First, no matter where in the body that oxygen is delivered (organs, muscle, bone, etc.); it is delivered by the red blood cells. The red cells deliver oxygen to the cells at the capillary level.

Capillaries are the smallest vessels and are only one cell thick. One cell between the blood and the organ it penetrates. The capillary is the level where oxygen disengages from the red cell. The red blood cells arrive at the capillaries and literally compress by their squeezing through the narrow capillaries.

This squeezing action releases the oxygen gas from the red blood cells. Once freed it passes into the body cells serviced by the capillary. This squeezing action occurs because the average capillary is slightly smaller than the diameter of a single red blood cell. When a red cell remains healthy, the ability to deform and squeeze through the capillary happens smoothly. After the red blood cell traverses the capillary the healthy red cell quickly recovers its shape.

Visualize trillions of red blood cells within the body's blood stream having the consistency of a sponge. Consequently, at the level of the capillary where oxygen unloads, a stiff sponge causes problems. A Stiffened red blood cell will tend to clog the capillary and will not compress sufficiently to deliver the oxygen, nutrients, or remove wastes as well.

The re-inflation of the 'sponge' creates a vacuum effect. This vacuum causes the red blood cell to absorb waste molecules created by the body's tissue cells. A pressure wave propels the red blood cells forward.

The heart's beating creates the pressure wave. The pressure wave created by the heart propels these sponges forward through these tight spaces within the body tissues. Stiffened or rusted red blood cells possess less elasticity to accomplish this important task of oxygen delivery in an optimal manner. For these reasons, owner's become more vulnerable to degenerative disease as the volume of sickly red blood cells increases within their body.

The analogy of the stiffened sponge describes a mechanism of high blood pressure. The heart pushes harder to move stiff red blood cells through the tight capillaries. To accomplish this blood pressure must go up. This explains why one of the most popular classes of blood pressure medicines is the calcium channel blocker. Calcium channel blockers make stiff red blood cells more flexible by increasing the red cell's magnesium level. Rather than physicians' educations providing the fact about increased magnesium intake naturally acting as calcium channel blocker they are only taught about prescription type calcium channel blockers. However, prescriptions always have side effects and toxicities.

The red blood cells have unique energy requirements. The red blood cells are analogous to a man buried to his neck in the sand with flasks of water all around him. The water is analogous to oxygen within the red blood cell. The water content within flasks by the man's head cannot do the man any good because he lacks the appendages to get the water to his lips. The situation for oxygen usage within the red cells proves similar. Even though they transport huge amounts of oxygen, they lack the machinery to combust oxygen for their own energy needs.

This is true because red cells lack mitochondria. Without mitochondria, red cells remain unable to burn fuel aerobically. Consequently, the red cell is forced to burn fuel anaerobically, which enfeebles their ability to perform normal cellular work. Cellular work within the red blood cell dramatically decreases because without oxygen less energy creation occurs per gram of sugar consumed. In addition, anaerobically consumed sugar creates a constant source of lactic acid as a waste product.

The fact that dead blood cells can still transport oxygen is important. This unfortunately happens in transfused blood because keeping blood alive for longer than about seven days proves a difficult process. The practice of transfusing dead blood into post surgical patients may be responsible for the massive organ destruction that is commonly called DIC (diffuse intra-vascular coagulation). Problems arise with dead red blood cells because without life they are unable to generate the energy necessary to remain as flexible. Not all dead red blood cells plug the capillary, but with other dietary and lifestyle bad habits that are practiced by the donor of the blood the risk increases (see below for details).

During the red blood cell's one hundred and twenty day lifespan it must remain flexible. Mainstream medicine sometimes offers prescriptions, like pentoxyphyline, that have a beneficial effect on red blood cell flexibility. However, these medicines are expensive and often have side effects. In contrast, known nutritional and life style choices exist that will positively affect the flexibility of red blood cells.

Factors that Determine Red Blood Cell Flexibility

1. **Electrical cell membrane potential (the strength of the force field)**
2. **High cellular magnesium content**
3. **Low cellular calcium content**
4. **High cellular potassium content**
5. **Low cellular sodium content**
6. **Adequate cellular zinc levels**
7. **Optimal ferrous hemoglobin with minimal ferric hemoglobin**
8. **Optimal blood sugar**
9. **Healthy dietary fat choices**
10. **Quality of steroids transported within the red blood cell**
11. **Quality of enzymatic machinery within the cell**
12. **Copper levels**
13. **The level of the completeness of the methyl donor system**
14. **Adequacy of vitamin C**
15. **Waste level within the blood stream**
16. **Thyroid status**

17. **Cholesterol status**
18. **Availability of glucosamine and galactosamine**
19. **Glutathione levels and other anti-oxidants**
20. **Level of exposure to oxidants, rust promoters, in the environment (ozone, volatile acids, and inappropriate blood metals, smoking)**

1) The electrical potential contained in the red blood cell membrane (the strength of the force field)

Red blood cells protect themselves and perform useful cellular work by maintaining an electrically charged membrane. However, unlike other body cells, the red blood cell is more vulnerable because its electrical charging ability is greatly reduced. Red blood cells are energetically weak. They cannot use oxygen because they lack mitochondria and are therefore forced into anaerobic metabolism.

One of the determinants of the cell's flexibility is contained in the strength of their cell membrane voltage. Consequently, processes that weaken the voltage will make the red cell contents vulnerable to hostile invasion forces and this causes a loss in flexibility (read on).

2) High inside-the-cell magnesium content

Adequate magnesium within the red blood cells causes the red blood cells to become more flexible. The blood pressure will be reduced as a result. Adequate magnesium within the red blood cell, past middle age in America, is unlikely if an owner eats a diet of processed food instead of real food (section three).

Magnesium is also required by the red blood cells to create energy by the combustion of glucose in an anaerobic fashion. The red blood cell cannot create the energy packets (ATP and NADH, NADPH, etc.) to perform their work without adequate levels of magnesium.

The correct proportion of magnesium and potassium within the red blood cell creates the best possible energy content within the cell membrane. In contrast, there is the additional benefit of also having a low concentration of both calcium and sodium inside the red blood cell. The red blood cells require a constant level of energy supply in order to; maintain the optimal ratios of these minerals. These four minerals relative concentrations form a powerful determinant for the health of any body cell. When one mineral within the red blood cell becomes deficient or excessive, their proportional relationship with one another becomes altered. When the mineral relationships are altered within a cell, health consequences follow (section five).

3) Low inside the red blood cell calcium concentration

Red blood cells contain less calcium than most of the other cell types in the body. This probably protects the hemoglobin content within the red blood cell or the enzymatic machinery that burns sugar for energy creation. As the magnesium content decreases inside the red blood cell more calcium can get inside. If the amount of calcium within the body cells is too high the calcium tends to injure the other cellular contents. This fact underscores the need for adequate magnesium relative to calcium content within the body (sections three and five).

4) High inside the cell potassium concentration

Potassium, like magnesium, is needed within the red cell in high concentrations for many reasons. Adequate potassium within the body is necessary for proteins to remain stable. Red blood cells will often sacrifice their potassium content for the blood streams needs. The price paid for this donation is a weakened electrical charge of the red blood cell membrane. A weakened electrical charge means the red blood cell has less energy for both work (flexibility) and protecting itself from the invasion of hostile ions.

However, the body prioritizes the potassium in the serum over the potassium in the red blood cell. Eventually, the deficient potassium situation recruits other body cells to sacrifice their potassium content, as well. The trouble here arises from, in part, that all body cells need adequate potassium in order to stabilize their protein content. For example, in muscle cells potassium is needed to make larger muscle tissue. Muscle tissue derives largely from protein. Therefore, owners that desire youthful vitality need adequate potassium within their red blood cells and other body cells.

Adequate potassium is also necessary for insulin to effectively deliver fuel to the cells. For this reason, high carbohydrate diets tax the potassium within the blood stream because as sugar goes inside the cellular fuel tanks it also must pull potassium with it (one for one ratio). The blood steam plasma must keep plasma concentrations of potassium relatively stable. In this situation, the red blood cell becomes forced to give up too much of its potassium. The red blood cell is first in line for donating some of its potassium when potassium levels decrease within the blood stream. Refined sugars come largely devoid of potassium content and therefore these types of meals can create this situation. As the problem becomes more chronic other body cells will donate potassium to prevent further drops in the serum potassium level (chapter 3).

5) Low inside the cell sodium content

Stress greatly increases the tendency for sodium content to rise inside the red blood cell. This occurs until the body is near death and then sodium content begins to fall off. The human body was not designed for chronic stress. Modern life can be stressful.

Part of the stress response causes the increase of inside the red blood cell sodium because stress causes sodium retention and potassium loss via the kidney. The problem exaggerates for those under stress when they chronically consume a processed food diet. In these situations, the red blood cell is forced to compromise its own well being in order to improve the way the blood plasma appears.

The appearance of the blood plasma improves as the red cells donate potassium lost in the stress response and take in sodium. This explains why the blood test, which measure serum potassium, can be misleading as to the true inside the cell status for potassium content (explained better in the next few sections). For these reasons, chronic stress and high sodium diets provide another mechanism for the compromise of red blood cell integrity.

6) Adequate zinc levels

Adequate zinc is needed within the body cells types that make acid (hydrogen proton) or base (bicarbonate) from carbon dioxide gas. To do this they need the enzyme carbonic anhydrase. Carbonic anhydrase needs zinc for activity. Red blood cells, stomach, pancreas, brain, prostate, kidneys and the testes all need to do this. In some tissues like the stomach, this enzyme splits carbon dioxide to secrete acid. In others, like the pancreas, the opposite reaction occurs in that it secretes bicarbonate instead. In other cases, carbonic anhydrase is crucial to prevent excessive body acid from accumulating and consequently damaging intracellular structures. Preservation of the red blood cell's architectural integrity is only possible when there is just the right amount of pH. This enzyme is fundamental within the body for pH balance. In the case of red blood cells it allows a continued oxygen carrying capacity. These facts explain why owners' cells that lack adequate zinc levels are vulnerable to many harmful processes.

7) Adequate ferrous hemoglobin

The iron contained on the hemoglobin is necessary for the red blood cell to carry oxygen to the body's cells. When the ferrous (+2 charge) iron contained on hemoglobin oxidizes to ferric (+3 charge) hemoglobin then it becomes unable to transport oxygen. Less oxygen transport means less of it is available to the tissues. Fortunately, the healthy body contains an elaborate and multi layered system to prevent this oxidation from occurring in more than nominal amounts. When this oxidation occurs in less than excessive amounts the body has multiple systems to remedy the problem. This fact is better explained below [See the methyl donor system (13) below, vitamin C (14), and glutathione levels (19) also below].

Unfortunately, certain medications irrevocably damage the red blood cell's ability to bind oxygen. Medications like sulfa drugs, acetaminophen, nitroglycerin and phenacetin all have the potential to irreversibly form sulf-hemoglobin. Also mal-digestive states can allow hydrogen sulfide gas (rotten egg smell of farts) to become absorbed into the blood stream and combine with the red blood cell. The occurrence of this process ensures that hemoglobin will never carry oxygen again. If one is suspicious they can order a sulf-hemoglobin level and see what percentage of their blood is unable to carry oxygen.

8) Both a high and low blood sugar can injure the red blood cells flexibility

Uncontrolled diabetes (high blood sugar) has long been known to cause the red blood cells to become stiffened. This process describes a powerful mechanism for the etiology of the micro-vascular complications found in diabetes. Conspicuous examples of the cell hardening are demonstrated when stiffened red blood cells become wedged in the capillaries of a diabetic's foot or retina.

Hypoglycemia has an adverse effect on red blood cell function. Because the red cell can only burn sugar anaerobically for its energy needs a fall off of its delivery rate profoundly influences its energetics in a negative fashion. Low blood sugar renders the red blood cell vulnerable to penetration from ions like calcium. These ions will irreversibly bind with cellular contents such as proteins, causing deformation. Deformation of cell proteins causes diminished function. When the low blood sugar becomes severe enough the possibility exists for killing some of one's red blood cells off and therefore decreasing their flexibility permanently. Realize that dead red blood cells still carry oxygen. However, numerous hostile forces within the blood stream rapidly damage dead red blood cells.

9) The adequacy of healthy fat choices in one's diet

The fats contained on and within the red blood cell are unique when compared to most other body cells. They are more similar to the brain's fat make up. These types of fats require huge amounts of the vitamins and nutrients contained within the methyl donor system (see 13) below). When these vitamins and nutrients prove sufficient the fat content of the red blood cells is optimized. Optimized fat makeup forms a additional powerful determinant of red blood cell flexibility.

Unfortunately, owners that eat processed foods cause, around middle age, varying levels of nutritional deficiency. In many ways the red blood cell is more vulnerable than other body cells because it has a more limited ability to repair itself once damage has occurred. The red blood cell's limited ability to repair itself arises from three main sources. First, because it lacks a cell nucleus (DNA) it cannot manufacture new proteins once protein damage occurs. Second, because it lacks mitochondria, energy generation becomes greatly reduced even in the best of circumstances. Reduced energy generation leads to less ability for the work of repairing damaged fat. Third, the blood stream is a hostile environment in many life situations and the red blood cell fat is therefore possibly exposed to these forces at a high rate of occurrence. Damaged fats on the surface of the red blood cell accumulate and compromise the flexibility of the blood cell. Certain dietary habits and nutritional deficiencies provide another mechanism to injure the flexibility of the red blood cells (explained in sections two, three, four, and five).

10) The quality of the body steroids forms a determinant of flexibility

Many of the body steroids are transported within the blood stream by intermingling with the fats contained within the red blood cell membrane. High levels of cortisol tend to decrease flexibility while high levels of estrogen increase it. Many steroids rely on an interaction with the red blood cells as part of their delivery strategies to their target cells. In fact, enzymatic machines exist within the red blood cells that convert the original steroid hormone to more powerful and different steroids. An example of this process is the enzyme 17hydroxy steroid dehydrogenase that converts estriol into 16hydroxy estrone.

11) The quality of the enzymatic machinery within the red blood cell

While the red blood cell was being constructed within the bone marrow, its enzymes levels (cellular machines) were determined. The construction phase is the only time that a red blood cell contains DNA. DNA (genes) is necessary to instruct the manufacture of proteins which makeup the red blood cell. The type and amount of the different enzymes that were made during this process are largely determined by the quality of the message content (types of hormones). The type of hormone message content determines the instructions that the DNA program receives. Message content directs the DNA program. Only a few specific hormones deliver message content to the DNA. In turn, the DNA program activity determines which proteins express within a cell. All enzymes are made from protein. Therefore enzyme content within a cell is determined by what hormones instructed the various DNA programs (section two).

This is the last chance a red blood cell will ever get in regards to what it is equipped with, to perform metabolically, because its own genetic program (DNA content) gets destroyed shortly after it releases into the circulation. In contrast, all other body cells have their DNA program still present. DNA content allows these cells to create new proteins, when older proteins become damaged. As a consequence, owners who experience poor informational directions at the level of their bone marrow crank out inferiorly equipped red blood cells. Remember, the lack of genetic material (DNA) within the red blood cell, after it releases into the blood stream causes it to have unique needs and vulnerabilities.

12) Adequate copper proves necessary for an important enzymes manufacture within the bone marrow during a red blood cell's construction phase.

One of the enzymes that are created while the red blood cell is being constructed within the bone marrow is called catalase. This enzyme protects the red blood cell from oxygen radicals by neutralizing them. Some owners are copper deficient and this is a critical trace mineral that is needed to make the enzyme catalase. When this enzyme is deficient, a red blood cell ages quickly and its flexibility becomes compromised.

13) The level of completeness of all the molecular components of the methyl donor system constitutes a big determinant of red blood cell flexibility

One billion times a second the body relies on the methyl donor system to prevent breakdown in molecular structure or improve biological messengers throughout the body (Cooney). Specialized fats found in the brain and red blood cells require extremely high amounts of the nutrients that make up the methyl donor system. This fact explains why people who fail to eat enough fat in their diet tend to become deficient within this system. The low fat diet adherents use up tremendous amounts of their methyl donor system nutrients in order to manufacture these specialized fats. The continued need for these types of fats is routinely included in a more healthful diet. However, the eventual depletion of the methyl donor system caused by the low fat diet increases the likelihood for a deficiency of these specialized fats as well.

Choline (lecithin building block) provides an example of the debilitating effect of the low fat diet. Choline is a specialized fat building block. Specialized fats are needed in high concentrations within both the red blood cell and nervous system. Choline synthesis requires three methyl groups for manufacturing it one time. Realize, these specialized fats, like choline, are needed by the gazillions within both the brain and red blood cell. Eggs are nature's best source of choline. The methyl donor system depends on numerous vitamins and amino acids. Depletion of this system is sometimes the root cause of many degenerative diseases, like: high blood pressure, neuro-degenerative disease, and blood vessel disease (chapter 3).

14) The adequacy of vitamin C in the body

When other anti-oxidants become deficient (glutathione, trimethyl glycine, and ergothioneine), vitamin C levels can become rapidly depleted. Vitamin C is required for the maintenance of ferrous hemoglobin (see above) within the red blood cell. Recall, this is the only form of iron that can transport oxygen to the body tissues. When vitamin C is used up in this fashion the total daily requirement increases tremendously. Some clinicians claim that the signs of scurvy (vitamin C deficiency) can develop when other anti-oxidants become deficient. The signs of scurvy occur because the rate of usage of vitamin C is many times greater than normal when other anti-oxidants become scarce. Glutathione serves as the major anti-oxidant within the red blood cell. Its sufficient presence prevents the rapid depletion of vitamin C. This simple peptide is made from three amino acids. Certain prescription medications tend to deplete this important substance from both the red blood cell and the liver. Certain prescriptions and nutritional bad habits tend to deplete vitamin C more quickly (see liver chapter). When these situations occur it is important to increase one's vitamin C intake. Ample vitamin C within the red blood cell will allow continued ferrous hemoglobin content. Remember, ferrous hemoglobin is the only form of iron that transports oxygen.

15) Waste level within the blood stream (this discussion will be deferred until section four)

16) Thyroid status and red blood cell flexibility

The amount of thyroid message content (hormone level) affects the amount of cholesterol inside the red blood cell. Cholesterol within the red blood cell competes with the specialized fats. Specialized fats, like phospholipid, give the red blood cell the maximum of flexibility. Just like increased thyroid states tend to lower the serum cholesterol the same trend appears to be true with the red blood cell fat composition. High thyroid function increases the proportion of phospholipid relative to cholesterol in the red blood cell membrane. Conversely, low thyroid function retards flexibility. Thyroid hormone plays an important role within the body in facilitating waste removal activities from the cells, including red blood cells. The colon, immune system, kidney's, lung, skin and liver depend on adequate thyroid message content for their waste removal activities.

17) Cholesterol status (see above and digestion section)

18) Availability of glucosamine and galactosamine to the red blood cell

The availability of glucosamine and galactosamine is one of the significant determinants of flexibility of red blood cells. These substances promote the process of "gelation". This process is what allows the red blood cells to temporarily compress within the capillary. Jell-O is composed of both galactosamine and glucosamine. These are obtained from grinding up and partially digesting animal cartilage. The same molecules that give jell-O its consistency also creates the flexibility of the red blood cells. These are the building blocks of the all important glycosaminoglycans (GAG) that hydrates the body tissues.

19) Glutathione levels

This important antioxidant keeps the preformed enzymes and oxygen carrying capacities intact for the life of the red blood cell. Prescription drugs could possibly deplete this important anti-oxidant. One common medication ingredient, which requires glutathione for metabolism is acetaminophen (Tylenol). There are many other medications that deplete glutathione. Glutathione is found mainly in the liver and the red blood cells. Quality protein intake proves necessary to increase production of this important anti-oxidant.

20) The level of exposure to oxidants (rust promoters) such as environmental ozone, volatile acids in smog, inappropriate blood serum levels of metals and minerals (aluminum, fluoride).

The more the blood cells are exposed to rust promoters, the greater the need for the anti-oxidants within the blood stream. (Ideally, one should also be thinking about ways to reduce chronic exposure to rust promoters.)

For example, increased blood fluoride and/or iodide levels will poison the energy metabolism of red blood cells. Consequently, excessive exposure to these minerals jeopardizes red cells' energy production abilities. Red blood cells whose energy production has been compromised are more vulnerable to the rust and hardening mechanisms (#'s 1-19). Fluoride being a powerful rust (oxidizing agent) promoter ion within the body gives the average owner something to think about the next time while shopping for toothpaste.

The medical media's focus has largely been on the blood vessel but the cells within it are of equal importance in one's pursuit of healthful longevity. The sensationalism of what is for sale by the complex has largely excluded the important consideration of how flexible one's red blood cells are within the pipes. The ongoing exclusion for the abilities and needs of the trillions of microscopic 'sponges' coursing within the blood stream has cost owners in America plenty. This is evidenced by both the quality of life lost and in the need for symptom control medicine with all it's side effects and diminished out comes.

When these microscopic sponges remain pliable their ability to carry oxygen, nutrients, and deliver important body hormones enhances. This process can be thought of as similar to when a sponge is efficiently wrung from its water content. Likewise, when red blood cells encounter the capillary and experience squeezing out of their contents of hormones, nutrients and oxygen, their flexibility forms a crucial determinant of how efficiently one receives the molecules that prove necessary for life to continue. For these reasons, processes that stiffen the red blood cell predictably will lessen this life giving process and the owner will get a little bit older.

There is no need to worry about the details mentioned above because throughout the remainder of this manual these will be thoroughly explained and ways to heal will also be discussed. In addition, the immune cells are also within the blood vessel and will be discussed in section five. Earlier in this section an introductory discussion of how blood pressure elevation hardens the vessels was mentioned.

The goal of the next chapter is to offer pause when the diagnosis of high blood pressure arises. During the pause one needs to consider their level of motivation. Without motivation, symptom control medicine is all that is possible. However, when one truly feels motivated to explore possible ways to heal their blood pressure elevation little risk exists with placing some attention on what caused the pressure problem. Healing paths have no health side effects. However, many times when healing paths are explored the need for the complex's symptom control approach evaporates.

CHAPTER THREE

HIGH BLOOD PRESSURE-THE NEXT LEVEL

Mainstream medicine claims that more than ninety percent of all high blood pressure arises from unknown causes (essential hypertension). The implication usually leads doctors and patients to believe it is largely genetically determined. It is as if whenever the genetics receives blame the next step involves how clever science provides symptom control approaches.

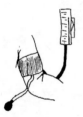

At the same time, very little discussion occurs for how the survival of the fittest led to the aberrant genes being selected down through the ages. Healing paths open up when one begins to look at these outdated survival advantages as the root cause of their blood pressure problem. The examples of insulin production and sodium conservation are both obsolete survival advantages carried over from the ancestors of primitive times. The case of insulin will be discussed at an introductory level here and more completely throughout the text. The case of sodium retention was introduced in chapter one and will be further developed in this chapter.

The ancestor who could make insulin during times of plenty was at a big advantage during times of scarcity. A survival advantage occurred because insulin caused both a behavioral effect and a metabolic effect. Insulin stimulated within the owner a behavioral pre-occupation with food. This behavioral preoccupation focused the owner on feeding. Insulin message content creates a preoccupation with the next feeding event. However, today in the developed world of the haves, food scarcity never comes and owners with this survival trait tend to become fat and have high blood pressure, as well (see below).

Eventually, continued exposure to high insulin message content directs their liver to turn carbohydrate into excessive fat and cholesterol. The old survival advantage has become a curse in today's world of high carbohydrate foods. This curse occurs in today's world because the owner who can make more insulin than the next owner will make extra fat, as well. One can heal their insulin caused high blood pressure problem when they are motivated and understand a way to heal.

The second outdated genetic trait concerns the ability to retain sodium better than the next owner. In prehistoric times sodium was rare. Natural food has many more times potassium than sodium. The owner during times of low sodium availability that could conserve body sodium obtained a survival advantage. However, today it often causes the curse of high blood pressure because processed food has a reversed mineral content from that of natural food. Natural food has high potassium and low sodium. However, processed food has very high sodium and much lower potassium content (sections two, three, four and five).

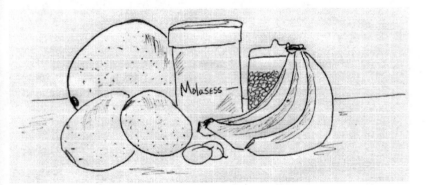

MINERAL TABLE

All mineral amounts are in milligrams below

Breads, Rolls, Etc	Amount	sodium	potass.	calories	mag.	calcium
White Bread	1 slice	142	29	76	0	32
Rye Bread	1 slice	139	36	61	0	20
Whole Wheat Bread	1 slice	132	68	61	0	20
Biscuit	1 (2"dia.)	185	18	104	0	0
Cornbread	2 1/2 sq.	263	61	178	0	133
Pancake	1 (6" dia.)	412	112	164	16	60
Waffle	1 (7" dia.)	515	146	206	13	143
Graham Cracker	2(2 1/2" sq.)	95	55	55	14	12
Brown Rice	1 c + salt	550	137	236	86	20
White Rice	1 c + salt	767	57	223	26	24
Bran Flakes	1 cup	207	137	106	108	26
Corn Flakes	1 cup	251	30	92	16	6
Oatmeal	1 c (cooked)	523	146	132	57	22.5
Pufffed Rice	1 cup	148	33	140	0	10
Wheat Flakes	1 cup	310	81	106	108	100
Wheat Flour	1 cup	130	0	499	0	0
*Egg Noodles	1 cup	3	70	200	31	19
*Macaroni	1 cup	1	103	192	20	8
*Spaghetti	1 cup	1	103	192	0	0
Beverages	**Amount**	**sodium**	**potass.**	**calories**	**mag.**	**calcium**
Coffee, Instant	1 Tblspn	3	87	3	*80	*50
Coffee, Regular	1 cup	2	65	2	10	3
Beer	12 oz	25	90	150	46	36
Gin, Rum, Vodka	1 oz (80 proof)	0	1	65	0	0
Sweets	**Amount**	**sodium**	**potass.**	**calories**	**mag.**	**calcium**

Angel Food Cake	1/6 cake	340	106	322	0	88
Brownie	small	50	38	97	0	0
Chocolate Bittersweet	1 oz	1	174	135	30	6
Chocolate, cupcake	1 piece	74	35	92	0	0
Chocolate chip cookies	10 (2.5" dia.)	421	141	495	0	32
Chocolate Syrup	1 oz	20	106	92	24	3
Gelatin, sweet	3 oz	270	0	315	0	1
Honey	1 Tblspn	1	11	64	0	1
Jelly	1 Tblspn	3	14	49	trace	4
Sherbert, Orange	1 cup	19	42	259	16	104
Sponge Cake	1/6 cake	220	114	196	0	42
Sugar, Brown	1 cup	44	499	541	0	187
Sugar, White	1 cup	2	6	770	trace	trace
Sugar, powdered	1 cup	1	4	462	trace	0

Fruits	Amount	sodium	potass.	calories	mag.	calcium
Apple	1 (2 1/2" dia.)	1	116	61	6	10
Apricots, Fresh	3 medium	1	301	55	8	15
Apricots, Dried	5 lg halves	6	235	62	11	10
Banana	1 medium	1	440	101	33	7
Blackberries	1cup	1	245	84	28	46
Cantalope	1/2 (5" dia.)	33	682	82	28	28
Cherries, Sweet	10 count	1	129	47	8	10
Dates	10 count	1	518	219	29	27
Figs	1 piece	1	126	52	8	18
Grapefruit	half	1	132	40	10	13
Grapes	1 cup	3	160	70	3	9
Honeydew Melon	half (6 1/2" dia.)	90	1881	247	9	8
Orange	1 medium	1	290	66	15	56
Peach	1 (2 3/4" dia.)	2	308	58	6	5
Pear	1 (2 1/2" dia.)	3	213	100	5	10
Pineapple	1 cup	2	226	81	22	12
Plum	1 (1"dia.)	0	30	7	<1	1

Prune, Dried	10 medium	5	448	164	51	58
Raisins	1 tablespoon	2	69	26	3	5
Raspberries	1 cup	1	267	98	22	28
Strawberries	1 cup	1	244	55	16	22
Tangerine	1 (2 3/8" dia.)	2	108	39	10	12
Watermelon	1 cup	2	160	42	18	14
Avocado	1 medium	21	1097	324	70	19

Fresh Vegetables	Amount	sodium	potass.	calories	mag.	calcium
Asparagus	1 cup	3	375	35	22	30
Beans, Lima	1 cup	3	1008	191	126	54
Beets	1 cup	81	452	58	28	22
Broccoli	1 cup	34	868	72	38	72
Carrot	1 medium	34	246	30	11	19
Celery	1 stalk	50	136	7	4	16
Corn, Sweet (no butter, no salt)	1 ear	0	131	70	34	2
Cucumber	1 large	18	481	45	33	42
Eggplant	1 cup	2	300	38	10	30
Lettuce, iceberg	1 head (6" dia.)	48	943	70	48	102
Onion	1 cup	17	267	65	16	32
Peas	1 cup	3	458	122	34	62
Potato, Baked	1 medium	6	782	145	55	20
Potato, Boiled	1 medium	4	556	104	30	7
Radishes	10 large	15	261	14	4	9
Spinach	1 cup	39	259	14	158	244
Sweet Potato	1 medium	15	367	272	32	70
Tomato	1 medium	4	300	27	13	6
Watercress	1 cup	18	99	7	8	40

Canned Vegetables	Amount	sodium	potass.	calories	mag.	calcium
Asparagus	14 1/2 oz can	970	682	74	22	34

Beans, Green	8 oz can	536	216	41	18	36
Beans, Lima	8 oz can	1070	1007	322	94	50
Beets	8 oz can	535	379	77	40	34
Carrots	8 oz can	535	272	64	22	62
Corn, Creamed	8 oz can	585	241	203	44	8
Peas	8 oz can	569	231	159	22	44
Spinach	8 oz can	519	550	42	132	144
*Tomatoes	8 oz can					
Dairy Products	**Amount**	**sodium**	**potas.**	**calories**	**mag**	**calcium**
American Cheese	1 oz.	322	23	105	6	124
Blue Cheese Dressing	1 Tblspn	164	6	76	0	0
Cheddar Cheese	1 oz.	147	17	84	8	204
Cream Cheese	1 oz.	80	25	110	2	23
Cottage Cheese	1 cup	580	144	172	14	154
Parmesan Cheese	1 oz.	208	42	111	14	390
Swiss Cheese	1 oz.	70	29	105	10	272
Butter (salted)	1 stick	1119	26	812	2	27
Butter (unsalted)	1 stick	<1	<1	812	2	27
Buttermilk (cultured)	1 cup	319	343	*88	27	285
Skim Milk	1 cup	127	355	*88	28	302
Whole Milk	1 cup	122	351	159	33	291
Evaporated Milk	1 cup	297	764	345	60	658
Heavy Cream	1 Tblspn	5	13	53	1	10
Ice Cream (no salt)	1 cup	84	241	257	9	88
Hot Chocolate	1 cup	120	370	238	24	93
Hot Cocoa	1 cup	128	363	243	0	0
Egg Yolk	1 medium	8	15	52	1	23
Egg white	1 medium	42	40	15	4	2
Egg Broiled	1 medium	54	57	72	5	25
Yogurt, Plain	1 cup	115	323	152	26	274

Meat and Poultry	Amount	sodium	potas.	calories	mag.	calcium
(Beef)						
Corned Beef Hash	1 cup	1188	440	398	14	9
Frankfurter	1 med.	627	125	176	6	7
Heart	1 oz	29	66	53	0	0
Hamburger	2.9 oz	49	221	235	5	2
Liver	3 oz	156	323	195	0	0
Rib Roast	6-9 ribs	149	680	1342	22	11
Flank Steak	3 oz	45	207	167	26	7
Porterhouse Steak	11 oz	155	680	1400	28	9
Sirloin Steak	11 oz	173	793	1192	32	12
T-Bone Steak	11 oz	152	660	1431	28	9
(Lamb)						
Chop	1 med.	51	234	341	27	28
Roast	3 oz	60	273	158	36	16
(Pork)						
Bacon	1 slice	123	29	72	<2	<1
Chops	3 oz	47	214	300	15	6
Ham, baked	3 oz	770	241	159	18	5
Roast	3 oz	698	218	281	0	0
Spareribs	2 pieces	65	299	792	0	0
(Veal)						
Loin cut	3 oz	60	570	220	9	10
Roast	3 oz	57	259	229	21	23
(Chicken)						
Broiled	4 oz	75	310	154	28	19
*Light Meat	4 oz	60	240	120	25	18
*Dark Meat	4 oz	45	100	180	27	19
(Turkey)						

White Meat	4 oz	70	349	150	29	29
Dark Meat	4 oz	42	169	87	26	26
Fresh, Fish & Seafood		**sodium**	**Potass.**	**calories**	**Mag.**	**calcium**
Bass, striped	3 oz	0	0	168	69	27
Clams	4 clams	144	218	56	52	12
Cod	3 oz	93	345	144	16	36
Crab	1 cup	0	0	144	78	0
Flounder	3 oz	201	498	171	15	27
Haddock	3 oz	150	297	141	27	33
Halibut	3 oz	114	447	144	37	72
Lobster	1 cup	305	261	138	138	80
Mackerel	3 oz	0	0	201	9	63
Oysters	3 small	21	34	19	39	45
Salmon	3 oz	99	378	156	180	29
Shrimp	3 oz	159	195	192	45	30

Mineral Imbalance Caused High Blood Pressure

The larger problem of mineral imbalance is caused by a processed food diet. Processed foods deliver drastically altered mineral composition when compared to real food. Real food tends to be high in magnesium and potassium and intermediate in calcium content. Real food is usually low in sodium. Processed food has reversed mineral content compared to real food.

The body is energized by an electrical system that maintains itself by potential differences across trillions of cell membranes in the body. Logically, it follows that the body requires specific mineral proportions in order to accomplish an optimal cell charge (voltage). Guess what: A real food diet supplies these and a processed food diet does not. This fact explains why around middle age, body cells begin to lose their electrical pizzazz. It is a miracle that a body can tolerate reversed mineral ratios intake for as long as it does before it begins to fail.

Recall, the car batteries' mineral composition analogy, this demonstrates the effect of mineral imbalance. Like the body cells that charge themselves by concentration differences around cell membranes, so to it is with car batteries. Car batteries maximally charge only when the different minerals are at extreme differences across the membrane. For this to occur, the battery manufacturer adds the proper minerals into the battery fluid.

For this simple reason, the chronic consumption of processed food is analogous to dumping battery fluid on the ground and replacing it with a reversed proportion of minerals. Most owners would see this behavior as foolish. Yet, this is what they are doing every time they eat processed food. Around middle age the 'battery fluid' in the body begins to alter despite the best effort of the kidneys to compensate for the reversed ratio of mineral intake. This process describes the origin of many disease processes. One common disease that results from this imbalance is high blood pressure.

As stated previously, most owners need about 4000 mg of potassium, 1000 mg of sodium, 500 mg of calcium and 300 mg of magnesium every day. Profuse sweating increases sodium needs. Altered kidney and adrenal function will also alter these amounts. Most Americans obtain about 6000 mg of sodium a day and much less potassium and magnesium than they need.

Around middle age, the cells have usually sacrificed much of their potassium to maintain the blood potassium level. One consequence to health when potassium escapes from cells concerns a decreased energy charge (voltage) within the cells. This means that the afflicted cells perform less work because of early fatigue. Early fatigue often serves as a sign of aging.

Recall, 98% of body potassium sequesters inside the cells. However, this larger tank sacrifices its potassium content to the 2% tank, the blood stream. Without this knowledge, many owners are misled when they have their blood drawn and their potassium result comes back normal. Their normal blood test result says nothing about the state of potassium content inside their cells. Only when the 98% percent tank contained within the body cells outside of the blood stream severely depletes, will the blood stream amount begin to fall off. At this point, the heart rhythm irregularities that follow create a real medical emergency.

Visualize that because potassium is highest inside cells its sufficient presence pulls water into the cells. However, sodium is highest inside the blood stream and consequently pulls water here. It helps to appreciate this ongoing tug of war of where water ends up because excessive sodium allows extra water in the pipes, which increases the pressure! An appreciation for this simple fact allows one to see the foolishness of continually eating the wrong mineral balance in a setting of blood pressure elevation.

The overall point is that owners who desire optimum health past middle age must consume the proper mineral ratios consistent with body design. The only diet that provides the proper ratios is the real food diet. Real foods are fairly obvious in the above mineral table. The fairly consistent trend concerns the fact that these foods are in their natural state. In other words, they are not generally processed into a box, can and bag or found in a fast food restaurant. Section 2 will begin the journey of how specific hormone abnormalities encourage mineral imbalances in certain owners that cause the heightened hypertension vulnerability. In turn these facts are further developed in the kidney chapter. For now, it is only important to realize that mineral imbalance logically extends to blood pressure problems.

High Blood Pressure and Nutritional Remedies

The subject of this chapter is high blood pressure. The discussion will continue to explore the causes of high blood pressure, and some simple supplements and methods that can be used to reduce high blood pressure. The owner who uses these methods suggested may avoid the need for prescription medications and their unavoidable side effects. The earlier in the disease process that nutritional intervention is implemented then the higher the success rate for blood pressure reduction. When the owner addresses the nutritional cause of their elevated blood pressure, the need for prescription medication will decrease and further damage to their organs will diminish.

Recall, chapter 1 and this chapter, describing three common imbalances that cause elevated blood pressure (magnesium, sodium and potassium). Chapter two described how stiff red blood cells contribute significantly to blood pressure elevation. The remainder of this chapter will describe other nutritional events that affect elevated blood pressure. It is important to emphasize that the discussion in this chapter will rely on information already provided in chapters one and two. The information in chapters one and two will be discussed in light of the new factors that are introduced in this chapter. The goal of this chapter is to provide some additional insight into ways to heal from high blood pressure. The ways one can heal is the goal instead of the acceptance of symptom control medicine's paradigms.

When the adrenals become deficient in certain molecular parts, blood pressure will rise.

Specific deficiencies in the adrenal gland can initiate the hypertension disease process. The owner using nutritional strategies can successfully treat these deficiencies. These nutritional strategies can reduce the owner's blood pressure and lower the owner's heart disease risk profiles, as well.

This first adrenal deficiency is called the methyl donor deficiency syndromes. Deficiencies of the various components of the important methyl donor system induce both high blood pressure and heart disease states.

Differences exist in the message content between epinephrine (adrenaline) and nor-epinephrine (nor-adrenaline). Both are known as catecholamines or biogenic amines. Unfortunately, when certain nutritional deficiencies develop epinephrine becomes the first to decrease and concurrently more nor-epinephrine occurs. This situation leads to significant physiological consequences within the blood vessel. The altered blood vessel performance then increases the risk for heart disease from the resulting high blood pressure.

The adrenal gland is divided into two components, the cortex and medulla. Biological, emotional, and environmental stresses are hard on both compartments of one's adrenal gland. Stress constantly triggers the steroid producing outer section of the adrenal gland. This causes cortisol to be secreted (among other steroids). Important point: sufficient cortisol is needed in the blood stream before the cell receptors recognize epinephrine and nor-epinephrine message content.

Epinephrine and nor-epinephrine are released by the adrenal medulla under stressful stimuli. This fact is important because without the cortisol message directing the manufacture of the receptors for these adrenal medulla hormones (epinephrine and nor-epinephrine) their message content will go unrecognized (see the hierarchy of hormones of section two). This subsection will only address the nutritionally induced imbalance between epinephrine and nor-epinephrine.

Normally the adrenal medulla secretes 90% epinephrine and only 10% nor-epinephrine. Epinephrine is preferred because it opens up the blood supply to the heart, skeletal muscles, and the liver. In contrast, nor-epinephrine does not do this. All other blood vessels (except the brain where blood flow is kept constant in the healthful state) are directed to clamp down when nor-epinephrine is the message (hormones contain message content inherent in their precise shape). The net effect of epinephrine message content (because the muscle and liver blood vessel beds are so large) is a lowered peripheral vascular resistance. This effect is commonly referred to as a lower diastolic blood pressure. Epinephrine has this effect within the body even when the epinephrine level within the blood stream is relatively high. Epinephrine also increases cardiac performance, which may result in a slight rise in systolic blood pressure.

However, the effects of epinephrine within the heart, liver and skeletal muscle vessels are in direct contrast to the message that nor-epinephrine delivers to these same blood vessels. Nor-epinephrine's message content directs the vessels to clamp down on everything except the blood supply to the brain. Consequently, nor-epinephrine's message causes the blood supply within all the vessels in the body (except the brain where the blood flow is kept constant in health) to constrict. When blood vessels constrict without a corresponding dilation somewhere else blood pressure elevates.

Realize when owners are healthy the adrenal medulla (inner adrenal layer) manufactures 90% epinephrine and only 10% nor-epinephrine. However, when the adrenal medulla becomes deficient in certain vitamins and cofactors this ratio changes for the worse. For this simple reason, a nutritionally caused inability to make epinephrine will tend to raise blood pressure when nor-epinephrine secretes instead of epinephrine!

Both of these hormones act rapidly and effectively for the redistribution of blood flow. This effect causes the blood stream to maintain an adequate flow of blood within the brain during normal movement of the body. Without the outpouring of epinephrine or nor-epinephrine unconsciousness would result. For example, when an owner gets out of bed the forces of gravity cause the blood pressure to suddenly drop. Within healthy owner's adrenal medullas epinephrine secretes in sufficient quantities to deliver a smooth machine that goes from lying flat to standing upright with grace and ease. Normally these hormones have a lifespan of about 2 minutes within the blood stream. Because of this very short lifespan of these two hormones a constant need arises for these hormones when one is either upright or under stress.

An additional process occurs during body movement that affects the blood pressure level. When an owner stands up or experiences stress, the sympathetic nerves discharge nor-epinephrine out of their endings. The endings of these nerves exist on the blood vessels' muscle layer. Here, these nerves release nor-epinephrine only, onto the motor end plate of the smooth muscles of the blood vessels. The release of nor-epinephrine causes these muscles to contract and thereby constrict the affected blood vessels.

Hence, nor-epinephrine released from the sympathetic nerves exerts an additional and direct effect on the blood vessel muscles. Concurrently, as discussed above, nor-epinephrine released from the adrenal medulla into the blood stream diffuses towards the same muscular layer but from the other direction.

Important point: The additive effect between the sympathetic nerve activation that releases nor-epinephrine into the smooth muscle and the adrenal secreted nor-epinephrine and deficient epinephrine in the blood stream describes a powerful mechanism for elevating blood pressure. Here, the only moderator of high blood pressure in healthy people is epinephrine. Recall, epinephrine increases blood flow to the heart, muscles, and liver. For this reason, adequate epinephrine release proves cornerstone in the prevention of high blood pressure.

Normally, this results in a tug-of-war between the full contraction and full relaxation of the blood vessel. Where a blood vessel ends up on the continuum is determined by the sum of the informational substances within the blood stream and the nervous tone instructions that reach that blood vessel. For this simple reason, when a sub-optimal or unbalanced release of adrenal medulla derived epinephrine occurs, increased blood pressure becomes likely. However, owner awareness for this process allows a nutritional strategy to be implemented to reduce blood pressure and the exacerbations of the symptoms of heart disease.

In order to obtain epinephrine, adequate molecular building parts and all of the nutritional cofactors must be present within the adrenal gland (discussed specifically below). These factors form a necessary pre-condition for the biosynthesis of epinephrine within the adrenal gland. Epinephrine and nor-epinephrine are derived from adequate supplies of the amino acid tyrosine. Tyrosine can also be obtained from the amino acid phenylalanine.

The adrenal gland cannot convert tyrosine to epinephrine unless all of the nutritional cofactors are present within the adrenal medulla (see below). Each step of the assembly line that eventually leads to the end product of epinephrine requires a scientifically validated cofactor before the next step in the assembly process proceeds. If any one of these nutritional cofactors depletes, assembly stops and epinephrine synthesis becomes impossible.

The most common deficiency, which occurs in the adrenal medulla, involves the methyl donor system. The conversion of nor-epinephrine to epinephrine requires the molecular components in the methyl donor system (explained shortly). The last step in the assembly process is the conversion of nor-epinephrine to epinephrine. This last step cannot occur without a particular cofactor that degrades with each epinephrine molecule made.

Scientists call this cofactor, S-Adenosyl methionine (SAMe for short). SAMe functions as part of the methyl donor system. The SAMe cofactor donates its one methyl group to make one new epinephrine molecule from nor-epinephrine. This spent cofactor has to be recharged. If it is not recharged it is called S-adenosyl homocysteine. This deactivated molecule will further degrade into adenosine and homocysteine within the blood stream. As was previously stated a methyl group is needed within the body one billion times a second.

Unless adequate SAMe remains available in the body, epinephrine biosynthesis curtails. For this reason, insufficient epinephrine biosynthesis leads to an increased biosynthesis of nor-epinephrine. Increased release of nor-epinephrine will raise the blood pressure. Additional exacerbating factors for blood pressure elevation arise when SAMe becomes deficient.

When SAMe depletes a marked decrease in the body's ability to clear both epinephrine and nor-epinephrine from the blood stream also occurs. In other words, making matters worse, not only does the body have the wrong hormone secreting (nor-epinephrine) because of the SAMe deficiency, but because of this same deficiency a decreased ability to remove nor-epinephrine from the blood stream occurs! These hormones clear from the body when other SAMe in the circulation methylates them.

When nor-epinephrine has these types of methyl additions it becomes inactive and readily exits from the kidney into the urine. These relationships describe the nasty process that traps certain owners in a vicious cycle of high blood pressure. High blood pressure occurs because their body becomes deficient in its ability to manufacture epinephrine and in the clearance of the sub-optimal nor-epinephrine. Remember, without inactivation from other SAMe in the circulation, abnormal amounts of this hormone remains free to continue spreading its message.

Nutritional attention for the ways to recharge one's methyl donor system (SAMe is one of the members in this group) often has the ability to heal the epinephrine deficiency and the nor-epinephrine excess. The correction of epinephrine deficiency is important because only epinephrine can oppose the clamping down of the sympathetic nerves during stressful times (see above discussion). For this reason, a deficient epinephrine output during adrenal medulla activation causes dramatic increases in the blood pressure.

The blood pressure rises dramatically because all information is contraction information at the blood vessel level. Remember, only epinephrine moderates the contractile response. Epinephrine can do this because its message content directs the liver, heart and skeletal muscles blood vessels to dilate. Conversely, nor-epinephrine cannot do this because it contains all contractile message content. Here, all blood vessels in the body, except the brain, are being directed to contract, therefore, the blood pressure rises dramatically. Recall, the same deficiency that diminishes synthesis of epinephrine also causes the diminished breakdown of elevated nor-epinephrine (see above). This is because additional SAMe is necessary for the inactivation of epinephrine and nor-epinephrine.

Only epinephrine has the special message property of opening up the blood vessels within the heart, skeletal muscle, and liver. Consequently, when sufficient epinephrine occurs the body directs blood into important areas and this prevents dramatic blood pressure elevation. Blood pressure does not rise dramatically because the increased blood flow within these areas offsets the decreased blood flow elsewhere within the body. Within the rest of the body (excluding the brain) epinephrine directs the clamping down of blood vessels (constriction raises the pressure).

Usually the net effect is a slight rise in the upper blood pressure value (systolic) and a slight lowering of the lower blood pressure reading (diastolic). This is called a widened pulse pressure. A widened pulse pressure indicates an increased cardiac output.

In contrast, the stress response directed from the sympathetic nerves directs the constriction of all blood vessels except the brain. For this reason, adequate epinephrine release is crucial in times of stress to prevent the sky rocketing of the blood pressure. Sky rocketing blood pressure means that blood flow delivery to heart, muscle and liver decreases. Here, the concurrent sympathetic nerve activation coupled with the constriction effects of nor-epinephrine from the adrenal medulla will increase blood pressure.

The below listed cofactors are well documented in basic biochemistry textbooks as all being necessary for epinephrine to be manufactured. Basic medical physiology textbooks point out the marked difference between the effects on blood flow patterns and blood pressure between epinephrine and nor-epinephrine.

The biosynthetic sequence of catecholamines is tyrosine-dopamine-nor epinephrine-epinephrine. The necessary cofactors that are needed in the synthesis sequence of tyrosine to the end product epinephrine are: tetrahydrobiopterin (made from folate), pyridoxal phosphate (vitamin B6), vitamin C, and SAMe.

Additional cofactors and vitamins exist that SAMe needs in order to reform after it donates a methyl. These cofactors and vitamins which reform SAMe are called the methyl donor system. The molecules that make up the methyl donor system are; methionine, serine, vitamin B6, vitamin B12 and folate. These factors are involved in the remanufacture of SAMe once it degrades into S-adenosyl homocysteine.

The methyl group addition converts nor-epinephrine to epinephrine. All of these cofactors, which are involved in recreating SAMe, are known collectively as the methyl donor system. Depletion of this system has predictable consequences but paradoxically has been largely ignored by mainstream medicine in the clinical setting. It should be emphasized that the consumption of extra methionine without proper attention to the adequacy of the other methyl donors will lead to elevated blood homocysteine levels because of the inability to recharge SAMe after the manufacture of each epinephrine.

Summary of vitamins and cofactors for the conversion of tyrosine to epinephrine

> **Tetrahydrobiopterin (made from folate)**
> **Vitamin C**
> **Vitamin B6**
> **SAMe**

A real food diet will provide most of these cofactors and the methyl donor group, especially if one eats eggs. Eggs contain substantial amounts of methionine. However, a processed food diet will likely lack one or more of these vitamins and cofactors. In addition, many B-vitamin formulations are often deficient in folate content. Without adequate folate the methyl donor system will not function. All members of the methyl donor system need to be present or SAMe levels fall and homocysteine levels will rise.

The rise of blood homocysteine levels has been documented to signal a powerful risk factor for blood vessel disease (chapter one). However, if one applies basic biochemical principles to the analysis of homocysteine for it to play a role in

the development of heart disease, it reveals it to be an unlikely agent in the direct injury of blood vessels. Rather it is more probable that it serves as a biochemical red flag that something is wrong within the owner's nutrition status. When blood homocysteine rises epinephrine synthesis will decrease proportionately.

Elevated homocysteine levels denote a malfunction within the methyl donor system that leads to decreased epinephrine production and increased nor-epinephrine production. For this reason, elevated blood homocysteine levels may reflect a convenient biochemical marker to identify a depleted methyl donor system.

One of the consequent pathologies of a depleted methyl donor system is that it causes high blood pressure to develop (among other things). Elevated blood pressure and diminished blood flow to the heart muscle will result whenever nor-epinephrine occurs in the blood stream in higher than normal amounts compared to epinephrine. Dr. Steven Gordon of Whitefish, Montana, points out that finding an elevated blood homocysteine level may provide high blood pressure's etiology and its solution as well.

When one appreciates the fundamental role that both a highly functional and interrelated methyl donor system plays a way to treat blood pressure becomes possible. When this approach is considered in disease prevention strategies it begins to make sense why the adrenal medulla nutritional state is important.

This brings up the beauty of healing paths versus symptom control medicine. Prescriptions are all about symptom control and contain all the inevitable side effects as well. Healing does not have negative side effects. This is because once a problem is fixed it is over with.

None of these cofactors is more risky than if one takes of a multiple vitamin, in the general population (not very risky). Each of the above listed cofactors has proven biochemical necessity in the synthesis of the epinephrine hormone. Healing involves working with the body to correct unbalanced states. Healthy owners' adrenals predictably contain optimal amounts of each of these cofactors and produce adequate epinephrine to maximize bodily function.

The caution concerns the avoidance of allergic reactions, which some owners have to the fillers and trace contaminants in certain brands of nutritional supplements. In general, one should choose the best brand and quality (pharmaceutical grade). Once in a while there will be an owner who proves allergic to vitamin C. Obtain the advice of a competent physician who will work on natural healing of the adrenal function and reduce the blood pressure naturally.

It turns out that the sympathetic tone is often increased in hypertensives and this central nervous system effect contributes greatly to the observed increase in blood pressure. The neurotransmitter involved in this case is nor-epinephrine. However, what is often under appreciated with regard to blood pressure is the tug of war between the sum of the hormones' message content within the blood stream and the message content delivered by the central nervous system. Visualize this dynamic equilibrium because it provides insight into the consequences of epinephrine deficiency.

Nor-epinephrine is a more powerful messenger (has more effect) when delivered within the nerves to the blood vessel (these nerves end in the muscular layer and when firing direct contraction here) than when it is acting within the blood stream. In other words, nor-epinephrine has more ability to raise blood pressure at a given concentration of secretion within the nerves than it does when it is secreted into the blood stream. This is a subtle but important point. For this reason, epinephrine deficiency can cause blood pressure elevation merely because there is an insufficient counter balance to the powerful nerve secreted message contained in nor-epinephrine.

In contrast, within the blood stream epinephrine has powerful vascular effects starting at 50pg/ml, but nor-epinephrine doesn't exert its vasoconstrictor effects (within the blood stream) until 1500pg/ml! Realize, nor-epinephrine's ability to raise blood pressure is mainly through its affect as a neurotransmitter within the sympathetic nervous system. Take home point: In the healthy body, epinephrine is needed as a counter response to the sympathetic nervous system's tendency to raise blood pressure.

The second deficiency syndrome that leads to high blood pressure.

The second deficiency syndrome, often overlooked in many owners that suffer from high blood pressure, is nitric oxide deficiency. The lack of nitric oxide gas in certain situations can raise blood pressure. The blood vessels manufacture nitric oxide. This gas serves as a powerful artery and vein relaxant. Healthy owners produce nitric oxide in the right amounts and locations. This process needs to happen to keep the blood flow optimal.

A deficiency in the production of this powerful and locally acting messenger gives the green light to many nasty blood pressure raising substances. These blood pressure raising substances in the presence of adequate nitric oxide otherwise would not be manufactured within the blood vessel lining cell. Nitric oxide is a powerful blood vessel wall relaxant. Nitric oxide is also a powerful suppressor of the insulin-induced manufacture of the blood pressure raising hormone, endothelin. Both nitric oxide and endothelin are informational substances that act exclusively locally (they are type 4 informational substances in the hierarchy of hormones, see section 2).

The enzyme, nitric oxide synthase, makes nitric oxide gas from the amino acid arginine. It needs four cofactors or it cannot perform this task. The absence of any one of these cofactors causes a nitric oxide deficiency and the blood pressure rises.

Nitric oxide synthase needs the presence of the cofactors arginine, Thiol, tetrahydrobiopterin (made from folate), flavin mononucleotide (FMN), and flavin dinucleotide(FAD) in order to produce nitric oxide. FMN and FAD are made from riboflavin (vitamin B2). A deficiency of any one of these cofactors, within the numerous cells that line the body's waterways, causes diminished nitric oxide production. For these reasons, diminished production tips the 'antique weight scale' in the direction of unopposed blood pressure elevation.

The above menu of cofactors required for the production of nitric oxide explains one of the reasons that garlic lowers blood pressure. Garlic contains thiol, which is one of the cofactors necessary for the production of nitric oxide. One also obtains the other cofactors from nutritional sources. Tetrahydrobiopterin is obtained by consuming royal bee jelly or is manufactured within the body from folate. FAD and FMN are obtained by having adequate riboflavin (vitamin B2) in the diet. Lastly, arginine is an amino acid that needs to be adequately consumed in the diet or made from Krebs cycle intermediates. Krebs cycle intermediates are mostly found within the mitochondria of cells.

In some instances, oral replacement proves inadequate for these types of deficiencies. Some cases occur, where owners for one reason or another, lack the ability to absorb optimal vitamin nutrition orally. These cases warrant the extra precaution of intravenous or intra-muscular vitamin replacement therapy.

Most of the above vitamins and cofactors are contained in conventional chelation protocols. Perhaps this fact provides a partial explanation for their continued devotees despite the ongoing vicious mainstream medicine criticism. The addition of thiol by consuming garlic would complete the supplementation of the above necessary cofactors needed by nitric oxide synthase. In the case of methyl donor deficiency, mentioned in the previous subsection, the addition of folate, methionine and serine would possibly prove of further benefit in the chelation setting.

Prescription medications which raise nitric oxide levels, but it is a secret.

An additional insight now arises about nitric oxide production and its relationship to a popular blood pressure lowering medication called, the angiotensin converting enzyme inhibitors (ACE inhibitors). These types of medications affect the histamine like content of the body, which also happens to powerfully lower blood pressure. The mainstream textbooks say very little about this powerful association. Instead, they discuss in great detail the blood pressure lowering effects as being the result of lowered angiotensin two levels.

It is really quite a shock to most physicians when they encounter evidence that the touted mechanism for a drugs action is not always the only way that they have an effect on the body. The ACE inhibitors provide such an example. The drug literature focuses almost exclusively on the supposed powerful role that angiotensin two plays in tightening up the blood vessels directly. However, very little of this literature discusses the well-documented fact that inhibition of this very same enzyme raises the total body content of a histamine like substance, bradykinin. This explains why a dry nagging cough remains these recipient patients' number one side effect. In addition, bradykinin itself lowers blood pressure but the price paid involves increased leakiness of the capillaries in areas like the lungs and kidneys.

Maybe there was a marketing problem if this mechanism was related to increased histamine like substance content within the body. No one will probably ever know for sure. Nonetheless, these facts prove instructive for one seeing a bigger problem with other drugs in how the physician gets 'groomed' into thinking about how drugs work.

Because these drugs increase bradykinin within the body they also increase nitric oxide production as well. Increased bradykinin powerfully stimulates the turning on of its enzymatic synthesis machinery within the endothelial cells lining the arteries. Bradykinin and histamine share the same receptors in the body. They also act in a similar manner. They contain similar message content. In addition, once bradykinin elevates it tends to stimulate the mast cells to release histamine, as well.

The other touted benefit of these angiotensin converting enzyme inhibitors (ACE inhibitors), is their documented benefit in the preservation of kidney function. To understand that this benefit is both a circuitous and expensive solution in many cases one needs to recall four things. First, ACE inhibitors conserve body potassium and this has a known kidney protective effect on the tendency to become potassium deficient. This medication then lowers blood pressure despite the elevated sodium in the body by the less realized mechanism of increased bradykinin within the body. Second, a bradykinin-increased presence also lowers blood pressure by powerfully stimulating nitric oxide production.

Third, if a given patient was correctly counseled about a real food diet instead of a processed food diet, before kidney damage occurs from chronically low potassium intake (hypokalemic nephropathy), blood pressure medication in these cases would no longer be needed.

The fourth fact to understand about the consequences of decreased angiotensin two production concerns its affect on the adrenal glands. Rather than get all lost in the inconsistent evidence that these ACE inhibitors have on aldosterone levels it becomes more instructive to look at the consistent evidence: Decreased angiotensin two will directly correlate with a decreased ACTH output.

A decreased ACTH output will decrease stimulation to the adrenal glands release of aldosterone, cortisol and DHEA. This little detail has powerful implications for another mechanism for how these medications lower the blood pressure. It also has powerful implications for why diseases like autoimmune disease intensify when owners take these types of medications.

Owners are made worse with autoimmune disease because they already have a wounded adrenal system (adrenal chapter). The addition of an ACE inhibitor will only exaggerate the diminished adrenal function, which operates in these diseases by decreasing ACTH (the major stimulant for adrenal steroid secretion). This also provides a clue as to why these same types of owners will be at increased risk for neutropenia and lymphocytosis (explained in the adrenal chapter).

Now it is time to turn the analysis on its head. The biggest mental road block is in the realization that people who consume high potassium and magnesium diets relative to total sodium intake are also going to have a high aldosterone (a increased potassium intake will powerfully stimulate aldosterone release). However, in these cases a diuresis ensues because total body sodium is not excessive.

Conversely, stress (ACTH) alone will tend to raise both aldosterone and cortisol secretion and in the situation, of a high sodium diet, this proves inappropriate. Cortisol occurs at levels many times that of aldosterone and powerfully promotes sodium and hence water retention. When this happens blood pressure rises. The point to consider is that perhaps a little effort spent counseling an early hypertensive on how to change their mineral intake ratios by eating 'real foods' (section three) would have some merit before condemning them to medication with all its side effects.

The additional intellectual roadblock to these facts occurs because physicians are not taught about the simple but drastic proportion differences between sodium and potassium, between the blood stream and cells. Recall, potassium occurs many more times prevalently than the sodium concentration amount within cells. Conversely, sodium is many times more plentiful within the extracellular space including the blood stream. Thinking these ratios through allows one to more clearly see why potassium promotes a normal blood pressure beyond its direct hypotensive effects.

Like any dominant mineral, potassium pulls water into cells because it remains low outside of cells (in the blood stream). Therefore its amount in the blood stream has very little extra cellular space expansion effect here. In contrast, because sodium is the dominant mineral of the blood stream anything that promotes its elevation will powerfully affect blood pressure. Realize sodium retention requires that the body compensate this with fluid retention so as to dilute down sodium to a normal value. The increased fluid in the vessels elevates the blood pressure.

Understanding this important relationship between the differences of where these two minerals pull water allows for seeing the difference when aldosterone elevates with a high potassium/low sodium diets rather than the reverse. Follow where water moves to understand the most common cause of high blood pressure. Remember, aldosterone and cortisol both promotes potassium loss and sodium retention. Consequently, owners that experience chronic stress (with capable adrenals) and eat reversed mineral content year after year usually suffer from high blood pressure for these reasons.

ACE inhibitors have been shown to improve a patient's clinical situation while in heart failure. What is not said concerns the fact that histamine like substances delivers a powerful strengthening action on the heart muscle's performance abilities. This effect is obviously one benefit of these medications beyond the increased histamine like content within the blood stream reducing the effort of the heart pumping the blood with each beat. Trouble is there is a lot of money in anti-histamines and this creates a marketing problem.

Steroids have a role in blood pressure

Certain steroids increase the calcium concentrations within the cells and therefore alter cell functions. The trigger to synthesize nitric oxide within the cells lining the blood vessels involves the increase of calcium concentrations within those blood vessel lining cells, the endothelium. Additionally, low insulin levels, high bradykinin levels, and high levels of certain steroids all lead to increased calcium influx into the cells that line the arteries, the endothelial cell.

The ability of certain steroids like progesterone to increase cell calcium content is well documented. For example, when sperm encounters the progesterone molecule, within the cervical mucus, this promptly triggers the rise in its intracellular calcium content. High intracellular calcium will disable a sperm. This process describes one of the reasons that high progesterone levels prevent pregnancy.

Calcium modulation routinely occurs within the central nervous system, as well. Progesterone affects the nerve cell's intracellular calcium concentration and also changes its operational properties. In fact, progesterone, at very high levels produces anesthesia. At more physiologic levels it produces a calming effect. Nerves become calm when they can charge up their membrane (increase the voltage about the membrane). Generally, nerves are less irritable when the membrane voltage increases.

DHEA occurs at the highest concentration of any steroid within the blood vessels in the healthy body. Because certain steroids increase cellular calcium it is not too far fetched to speculate that they are also one of the triggers that increase calcium influx pulsations within the endothelial cell. No one has specifically studied which steroid does this within the blood stream. However, it is probably progesterone or DHEA.

The message of DHEA, bradykinin, and insulin direct an increase in these cells' calcium content. This effect of certain steroids is believed to be non-genomic. Non-genomic mechanisms mean that these steroids act outside of generally accepted steroid message delivery methods. They occur without interacting with cellular DNA programs. The non-genomic method describes an additional ability besides the other methods that steroids control cell function (turning off and on different DNA programs within a given cell).

The emerging data suggests that steroids play an important role in blood vessel health. The effect that certain steroids have on cellular calcium concentrations will probably turn out to be another way that the body controls blood pressure. The ability of steroids like progesterone or DHEA to encourage nitric oxide formation could be a powerful determinant in blood vessel longevity. If the data proves to be accurate it would be another method of encouraging blood pressure back to optimal levels.

Syndrome X

Increased insulin need describes a subset of people that have embarked on an accelerated path to premature death. These people are often thought of as the typical Syndrome X types (metabolic syndrome or insulin resistance syndrome). One of the consequences of a low potassium diet concerns the fact that low potassium intake leads directly to more insulin need. More insulin need occurs because sufficient potassium needs to be available for sugar to leave the blood stream under insulin's direction (one cause of insulin resistance). The increased insulin exposure and the consequent destructive hormonal cycle that follows worsen when chronic mental stress occurs, as well. High insulin also powerfully stimulates fat cell growth.

Gerald Reaven MD, of Stanford University, coined the term, Syndrome X. This term describes those owners who are on an accelerated path for blood vessel rust production and fatty arterial growths. Dr. Reaven believes that Syndrome X derives secondary to having high blood insulin. He explains the clinical signs of this syndrome as the result of the high insulin state. His opinion of the clinical signs of the high insulin state are: increased abdominal fat, high blood pressure, increased blood triglyceride level, elevated LDL cholesterol, increased skin tag growths on the neck and under the arms, increased blood clotting tendency and an accelerated rusting (oxidation) rate within the blood vessels.

In addition to Dr. Reaven's findings, this author feels that the signs of high blood pressure and increased rusting rate are better explained by two additional factors. One is the chronically elevated production of cortisol caused by a hectic lifestyle in those that possess heightened adrenal secretion ability. The second is that these owners often consume a processed food diet.

Syndrome X owners exist on an accelerated tract to an old body. Their fundamental defect often concerns both elevated insulin levels and increased mental stress (section two). For now realize, increased stress will accelerate potassium and magnesium loss. For this reason, low potassium, low magnesium diets and elevated sodium intake accelerate the disease process (chapter one). In many ways a high stress hormone output could help explain how Syndrome X patients age so quickly and have high blood pressure as well.

This is better illustrated by the fact that chronically elevated cortisol delivers the message to the body that an emergency situation exists. When the body perceives an emergency (real or imagined) the body's energy redirects into survival pathways. In syndrome X owners the survival pathway becomes the norm instead of rejuvenation activities. This clue ties in the connection between premature heart disease and the Type A personality individual. Type A personalities excessively worry about their next deal, are driven and tend to be intense. These traits chronically activate the stress response.

When body energy chronically directs energy into survival pathways, the wear and tear changes become more likely. Wear and tear changes become more likely secondary to the chronic stress response deferring cellular repair activities. This helps to explain why Syndrome X owners tend to age so quickly. Not only do they tend to have high insulin exposure derived disease but also high cortisol derived disease. Recall, cortisol directs body energy into catabolic pathways. Too much catabolism within the blood vessels leads to wear and tear changes

The severity of the Syndrome X exacerbates from the consumption of processed foods.   Excessive sodium relative to potassium intake greatly exacerbates blood pressure elevation for the reasons listed at the end of the previous subsection. Remember, the interplay between chronic stress and reversed minerals intake.

Dr. Reaven is right about insulin having some role in the blood pressure elevation of these owner types. One of the reasons that elevated insulin raises blood pressure results from its ability to powerfully stimulate the blood vessel lining cells production of endothelin. When endothelin production increases blood pressure then rises. High insulin levels also diminish the ability of the blood vessel lining to produce nitric oxide. The diminished production of nitric oxide further reduces the body's ability to maintain an appropriate blood pressure level.

Large amounts of insulin within the blood stream require huge amounts of cortisol to effectively counter insulin's behavior of moving every last sugar molecule out of the blood stream. Cortisol counters the effect of insulin by increasing the blood sugar levels. Cortisol, however, directs body energy and molecular building parts into survival (catabolic) pathways and out of repair and rejuvenation (anabolic) pathways. Consequently, anti-oxidant synthesis and blood vessel repair defer with chronically high cortisol levels. The stressor effects exacerbate the effect which insulin has on cortisol levels.

Chronically high levels of cortisol release rates cause the body energy to move away from cellular rejuvenation activities. Syndrome X causes the inefficient use of molecular building parts for repair activity by the body. The correction of this dysfunctional process begins when the healthy and appropriate ratio of cortisol and insulin realigns within the blood stream. This can be substantially accomplished by nutritional rather than symptom control treatment plans. Before a description of those strategies occurs a syndrome closely related to Syndrome X will be emphasized: Type A personality can be treated by very similar nutritional strategies used for the treatment of Syndrome X.

Recall, the description of syndrome X provides an insight into the tendency for people with Type A personalities (hard driving and aggressive types) to develop heart disease. One, or both, of two different processes, could cause this tendency. The first process involves the predictable increase of cortisol that occurs when the owner experiences the stress to perform and achieve during their daily activities. In turn, the increase in cortisol directs the blood sugar to rise as part of the survival response.

The big difference between mental and physical stressors concerns the fact that in the former the released sugar has nowhere to go. These inappropriate increases in blood sugar demand a corresponding rise in insulin levels that facilitate the uptake of blood sugar into the liver. Realize also that the catabolic effect of cortisol generates extra sugar by sacrificing protein and converting it into sugar (gluconeogenesis).

Recall; defense of body protein forms a powerful determinant for subduing the aging process (further explained in section two). The liver cleans up the mess because insulin secretes from the pancreas and always arrives within the liver in the highest concentration via the portal vein. This anatomical fact means that mental stress promotes fat and cholesterol synthesis because increased insulin in the liver turns on the fat and cholesterol machinery. For these reasons, elevated blood

insulin, caused by sedentary type A behavior, has the identical effect on the body as the elevated insulin need caused by the previously mentioned excessive carbohydrate intake.

The second process, found in both Type A personalities and Syndrome X is the development of blood vessel disease. Evidence exist that additional blood vessel disease results from the continued demand for more epinephrine secretion. Epinephrine secretion normally increases as part of the stress response. The excessive demand for epinephrine can increase both the blood pressure and blood sugar raising tendencies. Blood pressure will tend to rise when the adrenal stimulation becomes chronic. When the adrenal stimulation becomes chronic, in the setting of nutritional cofactor deficiencies, the blood pressure raising nor-epinephrine begins to secrete instead (see above discussion for why this situation has blood pressure elevating consequences).

With the above two considerations in mind, add in the understanding of how exercise may benefit hard driving and over achieving types (type A personality) undo some of the metabolic aberrations mentioned above. This is accomplished in part by utilizing the blood sugar released by the direction of increased stress hormones, both cortisol and epinephrine (section 2). In addition, attention to rebuilding nutritional vitamin and mineral status will help alleviate the nutritionally derived causes of high blood pressure.

Finally, in order to complete the introductory discussion of syndrome X, the importance of IGF-1 levels needs mention. Healthy owners predictably have high normal IGF-1 levels. IGF-1 is synthesized within the liver in response to DHEA. Sufficient, Growth Hormone release causes the IGF-1 stored within the liver to secrete it into the blood stream. Normal owners have at least one hundred times the IGF-1 in their circulation as they do insulin. IGF-1 acts like insulin for the cells outside the liver and fat. Consequently, high IGF-1 levels lower the amount of insulin needed within the body. IGF-1 levels provide a mechanism for fuel uptake by cells outside the liver and fat cells between meals. In contrast, insulin is designed to facilitate the liver and fat cells to remove fuel out of the blood stream following meals.

Troubles start around middle age in sedentary and stressed owners. These two lifestyle traits combine to diminish IGF-1 levels (section two, the muscle chapter and the liver chapter). A lower IGF-1 level means that insulin secretion must rise abnormally during the fasting state in order to attempt to offset the decrease in IGF-1 levels. This detail explains why Syndrome X types present with elevated fasting insulin levels. Healthy owners have greatly diminished insulin levels in the fasting state. Insulin has a half-life of ten to twenty minutes. Fasting insulin therefore provides a pretty good marker for diminished IGF-1 levels (excluding type-one diabetes). One primary health effect arising from falling IGF-1 levels and rising insulin levels concerns the activation of the fat and cholesterol making machinery within the liver. The additional consequences of these facts are explained in the next chapter.

For now, hopefully the reader is asking: If IFG-1 level is as important as a predictor for heart disease, Syndrome X, diabetes, obesity and old age, why do the textbooks and journal articles mostly ignore its fuel nozzle role? Why not even a cursory discussion about these facts? Why do they increasingly mention it as the villain in diminished survival and cancers' development? All of these are very good questions and deserve honest answers. Read on in section two and begin to hear the other side of the scientific story of what is known about the hormones that control lean body mass versus fat mass.

SECTION TWO

SECTION TWO.. *81*

    THE THIRD PRINCIPLE OF LONGEVITY: THE HORMONES
    GIVITH & THE HORMONES TAKETH AWAY 82

CHAPTER FOUR 86

    OBESITY CAN BE CURED WHEN HORMONES ARE
    OPTIMAL 86

CHAPTER FIVE 126

    ADRENAL GLANDS.. 126

CHAPTER SIX 151

    OVARIES 151

CHAPTER SEVEN 172

    INFORMATIONAL SUBSTANCES 172

CHAPTER EIGHT.. 180

    STEROID TONE 180

CHAPTER NINE 209

    FOUR MISUNDERSTOOD STEROIDS........................ 209

CHAPTER TEN 215

    THYROID GLAND 215

CHAPTER ELEVEN 232

    TESTES 232

CHAPTER TWELVE 243
    Hierarchy of Hormones - Informational Substances243

William B. Ferril, M. D.

THE THIRD PRINCIPLE OF LONGEVITY: THE HORMONES GIVITH & THE HORMONES TAKETH AWAY

Balanced hormones equal a youthful state of being. Imbalanced hormones arise from either their excess or deficiency. Body cells' optimal function depends on the adequacy of specific hormones. In addition, the body's most powerful hormones deliver fundamental messages to the genes. These most powerful hormones are secreted out of hormone producing glands; the thyroid, adrenals and gonads.

Unfortunately, accumulated toxins, nutritional deficiencies and chronic stress are hard on one's glands. Consequently, eventually these important glandular secreted hormones (messages) become sub-optimal. Imbalanced hormones mean that the message that the genes receive is off kilter. Gene activity adequacy determines much about one's ability to repair the wear and tear of life. However, if the optimal message (hormones) fails to arrive, the traumas that life delivers fail to be repaired. Eventually this manifests as an older appearing and feeling body.

Unfortunately, Western medicine largely overlooks this fundamental truth causing dietary failure, brittle bones, blood vessel disease, changes in body stature, diminished organ function, decreased mental ability, muscle loss, joint dysfunction, immune dysfunction, refractory depression, and shriveled or flabby skin. The alert reader needs to be aware of the discrepancies often missed by the conventional approach to hormonal imbalance.

Mainstream medicine panders numerous treatment strategies. Regretfully, these treatment strategies often only address the consequences of hormonal deteriorations in peripheral ways. However, the above middle-aged afflictions largely arise because the wrong hormones secrete out of these few important glands. Important point: Only a few body hormones control gene activity.

Fundamental truth: Which genes turn off or on determines the quality of protein content within a cell. Defense of body protein, the metabolically active constituents of the body, must occur or aging effects begin. In one-way or another, the above afflictions have in common, protein deficiency. Consequently, the above diseases cannot begin to retreat until an adequate consideration occurs as to what hormones prove excessive or deficient.

Contrast this deeper consideration to the fact that physicians are taught to focus on the 'symptom control' paradigm. Symptom control has little to do with how one heals and also causes side effects. This leads to the need for more medicines and procedures. It also suggests the mechanism for why one who blindly follows the symptom control methodologies of the complex often suffers from copious amounts of medicine and many procedural scars.

Medications and a history of medical procedures often reflect failed attempts for regaining healthy physical function. Healing insights begin with the realization that the quality of one's hormones most substantially impacts the owner's health and ability to age gracefully. Regretfully, the primacy of this truism often fails full comprehension.

Thankfully, the holistic approach to degenerative processes includes the medical data necessary to restore hormonal health. Through a more complete investigation into the owner's hormonal status and by applying the latest scientific insights to hormone replacement, healing many chronic-degenerative diseases becomes possible.

It is important to emphasize that mainstream medicine also possesses the medical data necessary to restore hormonal health. Most readers' will now ask: If this is so then how come their doctor doesn't know about it? Unfortunately, traditional medical texts present this medical data in both a convoluted and disintegrated format. Compounding the problem concerns the removal of old scientific truths from newer textbook editions (see evidence in *Healing has One Side Effect* book).

These facts create substantial consequences. First, textbooks offer incomplete scientific holisms. This maneuver isolates knowledge for the root causes of many chronic-degenerative diseases (read on for evidence). Consequently, many physicians receive little training for how to apply on Monday morning, the more complete and congruous scientific data. Secondly, even if hormones are prescribed, the insufficient hormone testing methodologies, so prevalent today, often causes patients to receive an abnormal or altered hormone mixture. The wrong proportionate hormonal mixture leads to side effects and toxicities. In both common methods of practice; ignoring hormonal imbalances or prescribing inferior replacement hormonal strategies derived from suspect testing methods, the owner ages more rapidly.

Imbalanced hormones eventually manifests by an ongoing deteriorating body appearance. **Visualize that the genes provide nothing until the right hormone arrives.** Thankfully, science provides data to re-establish an effective and appropriate hormone balance. The natural process of healing begins when the hormones within again achieve an improved quality and proportionate relationship.

This is all good news but before hormone quality can be understood, one needs a workable and concise definition of what qualifies as a hormone: Each hormone, by virtue of its unique shape, carries a message through the blood stream to specific cells.

Each hormone type's precise shape activates change within a range of receptors when it arrives at the recipient cell. For this reason, a very slight alteration in the shape of the hormone changes its message content. Simple science discussed here, yet not commonly taught in a way that doctors can understand the desirability of real hormones.

Hormone messages direct the cell on how to spend its cellular or behavioral energy. It helps to consider that a musical note arises only after an accurate vibration within a piano string occurs. Visualize the true note as the accurate message and the flat note produced by an altered tug on the string as the inaccurate message. Again it is the precise tension-induced vibration that creates a certain piano string's musical note. The note arises from a specific vibration frequency within the string. In contrast, the flat altered piano string tension changes the musical quality because it changes its vibration frequency.

Similarly, the body operates within a vibrational system of molecular communication: Certain molecular shapes create specific hormones that after binding specific genes vibrate in their optimal way. Realize these accurate vibrations create specific messages. For this reason, change the molecular shape, even a little bit, and the message content that a gene receives changes.

In the search for more profit, a problem arises because unless a hormone's shape is changed no patent is possible. However, realizing that changing the shape alters its message helps one to see the often overlooked vulnerability: For this reason, changed message content arriving at the genes carries the high probability of eventually evidencing itself clinically as side effects and toxicities.

Remember, the quality of the hormones secreted determines the efficiency of the information carried within the blood stream (message content). The message content received determines how a cell will spend its available energy. With this in mind, confusion can be avoided while studying medical literature.

Medical literature is uniformly disorganized in making it easy for doctors and patients to grasp the hierarchy between the different hormone classes. It is the goal of this section to help one become more knowledgeable about the hormone hierarchy. Competency here diminishes gullibility for the next time one reads a sensationalized version about the latest patented hormone.

CHAPTER FOUR

OBESITY CAN BE CURED WHEN HORMONES ARE OPTIMAL

With sensationalism in mind, obesity serves as a constant example of medical strategies that fail. In contrast, through addressing hormonal factors like restoring their appropriate proportions and quality, obesity can be healed.

Inadequate attention is given to the influence hormones have on regulating body weight. Each diet addresses some of these issues, but ignores others. Nutrition experts counsel those with large weight to frame ratios on the need to reduce their caloric intake. Most of the time, they omit facts about certain hormones facilitating or inhibiting fat's combustion. These approaches also tend to ignore the role hormones play in feeding behaviors. The seven main hormone imbalances, which perpetuate obesity, can be thought of as a **Torture Chamber effect.**

An effective weight loss strategy must include a method of obtaining and maintaining the proper relationship between the body's hormones. Other considerations exist for long lasting weight loss. These will be discussed in other sections of this manual. Below is the overview of an effective weight loss plan and the part of this manual that discusses it.

Obesity: Deactivating the Fat making Machinery

Six factors activate the fat making machinery:
1. **The glandular component (section two)**
2. **Reversed mineral ratios diet component (sections three and five)**
3. **Lack of exercise (section six)**
4. **Unmanaged stress (section two)**
5. **High carbohydrate diets (the torture chamber diet in section three)**
6. **Vitamin and trace mineral deficiencies (nutritional deficiencies which propagate fat's accumulation and impede its usage, sections one and three)**

Overview of the problems associated with other popular diets

The Glandular component

> **Six glands control the amount of body fat:**
> **Pituitary**
> **Thyroid**
> **Liver**
> **Pancreas**
> **Adrenals (adrenaline and steroid compartments)**
> **Gonads (the ovaries or testicles)**

Notice that most overweight owners have not had these glands' function checked in a scientifically sufficient manner. Obesity always has a glandular component to its causality. Until the glandular component is identified and corrected the owner stays stuck within the torture chamber of worsening obesity.

Popular diets available today are incomplete for various reasons. The first problem concerns their incomplete attention to the fat making hormones. Successful weight loss requires considering seven basic fat maker related hormones - insulin, cortisol, androgens, estrogen, insulin-like growth factor type one (IGF-1), thyroid and epinephrine. In addition, indirect but important influences occur from the amount of Growth Hormone and prolactin secreted by the pituitary. One needs to consider these hormones first before starting any weight loss plan. Imbalances in the pituitary secretions cause disproportioned amounts in the basic seven hormones listed above. Obesity propagates as the result of inappropriately proportioned relationships between these basic seven hormones. Weight loss becomes prevented and fat production becomes promoted when these seven hormones imbalance.

Theoretically, there are even more fat-maker related hormones. The jury is still out on how they really relate to the overall fat making machinery in the body. Rather than add in these mysterious and so far without-weight-loss-benefit hormones to the discussion, the tried and true hormones listed above will be the focus of this book. Meanwhile, the academicians can fight about these theoretical and peripheral hormones for gaining and losing fat.

Popular low fat / high carbohydrate diets fail to manipulate all seven basic hormones that are a determiner of obesity. A successful diet must affect the hormone-based urge to consume food.

In addition, it must inhibit the fat making hormones and encourage the fat burning hormones. The power of these hormone messages constitutes an important concept for weight loss and other health successes.

High protein/good fat and low carbohydrate diets improve the probability for weight loss by partially addressing hormone imbalance. Eating protein and good fats instead of carbohydrates reduces insulin exposure, the fat maker. Using this principle also turns down the appetite center in the brain. The seven basic hormones for fats creation and the glands that secrete them are explained in this section.

The Mineral Component

High protein diets often fail by creating a mineral imbalance between sodium and potassium. When mineral imbalances occur, weight loss curtails because the body then requires increased insulin secretion for even a small amount of carbohydrate intake (explained in section 3). In this case, the failure rate becomes secondary to overlooking the importance of mineral balance. Mineral balance and its effect on weight loss are explained in sections one, three and five.

The weakness in the high protein diet turns out to be the strength of some of the other diets. The high fruit, vegetable and unprocessed grain diets often have superior mineral balance content. However, these diets fail because of the other hormonal imbalances they perpetrate in the already obese owner.

Correcting these diet defects will be explored throughout this manual. The ideal diet combines the best of each diet and eliminates the part that sucks the owner back into the *torture chamber*. Understanding how the seven different body hormones either help or hinder weight loss proves essential. The mineral needs of the body are explained as noted above. Implementing these interrelating factors allows overweight owners to start on a healing path.

The Stress filled lifestyle component

Chronic mental stress provides another fat maker messenger. Unlike physical stress, mental stress causes an increased insulin need within the body. Recall, certain owners inherit strong adrenal secretion ability for a given stressor (section 1). Couple this to type A personality behavior and the weight gain propensity increases many fold. Until the obese owner receives counseling on the ways to side step this hormonal havoc, weight loss efforts will fail. How stress affects fats accumulation will be explained throughout this manual.

The Movement Component

Weight loss success cannot occur without an increase in body movement. Move or die. The body was designed to move around and resist the forces of gravity. Sedentary owners succumb to the shrinking forces that lead to old age: little muscles, little organs, weakened bones and loosened skin. The same lifestyle habits that lead to shrinkage in the above organ systems also contribute to an increase in body fat. However, less commonly appreciated is the fact that obesity is a wasting disease hiding amongst the fat. In other words, the functional tissue, which is protein, wastes away but it hides its dimunition amongst the fat.

Recall, only proteins create metabolism because this is the only part of the body structure that consumes calories. This fact explains why sedentary owners doom themselves to defeat until they assimilate an active lifestyle into the equation. The muscle versus fat chapter explains this important relationship (section six).

The Nutritional Deficiency Component

The final component of the successful dietary approach concerns the necessity of certain vitamins for the removal of body fat. The science is all there but it paradoxically collects dust. One of the reasons it remains largely ignored arises from the disjointed and circuitous manner in which it is organized within the medical textbooks. However, until these nutritional facts are organized in a way that both doctors and patients can understand, fat will continue to accumulate from nutritional deficiencies.

Ironically, the industrial societies often are the land of the nutritional deficiency diseases: obesity, heart disease, high blood pressure and diabetes.

Each of the above component's contribution to making body fat is reviewed in the chapters noted above. Owners that understand the interconnectedness of these components are empowered to heal. Diets fail but insight heals. Healing often involves nothing more than a heightened awareness of how one became fat and how one loses fat. Awareness allows focus. Getting fat did not occur overnight. Likewise, shedding fat takes

awhile. **Most owners that follow the program outlined below will shed between fifty and one hundred pounds in the first year. In addition, they will gain back muscle, organ size, bone mass and skin health. In each success case it all started with a brave first step into a new life of healing. Many other steps of awareness follow the first step. This section begins the healing process by creating awareness for an individual's hormonal solution to heal their weight problem. Fact: until the hormones improve the liver will be the nutritional hog of the body, turning nutrition into fat, while other body cells starve (explained below).**

The Glandular Component

Glandular secretions play a powerful role in the creation of body fat and constitute the starting point for a successful weight loss plan.

Glands secrete information (hormones) into the blood stream. The types and amounts of these various secretions determine how the body's 70 trillion cells spend their energy.

Optimal secretions facilitate the right amount of 'raw blood fuel' (amino acids, fat, and sugar), cell nutrition and cell function.

Poor secretions facilitate manufacturing excess fat, decreased organ function and accelerate the aging process.

The glands, listed on the next page, secrete various hormones that affect the gaining and losing of fat. Hormones carry information to the body cells via the blood stream. Visualize the blood stream as containing a 'sea' of information that changes, as the body needs change.

All hormone message content (information) concerns how the cells channel their energy.

Obese owners have the problem in one way or another of too much body energy being directed into the storage of energy. In addition, because obese owners have too much food energy directed into storage as fat, their cells are always hungry. These owner's cells will remain hungry until their hormones change into a message of fuel availability. Available body fat becomes fuel that combusts in the cell power plants.

The body stores energy mostly as fat.

The ideally weighted person stores about 80,000 calories as body fat. However, the obese person stores many times this amount.

No matter what the body weighs, only 2000 total calories can be stored as sugar within the liver and muscle cells, as glycogen. A cognizance of these relative amounts of storage abilities between these two fuel groups helps to elucidate the fundamental fat making problem. Many pinheads pontificate the platitude about losing weight being a simple matter of restricting calories. Oh if it were only that simple. Hormones direct whether fuel stores or fuel burns up in the cell power plants. By definition pinheads, are those that do not remember their basic science.

Losing weight requires redirecting fuel energy away from storage as fat.

The hormones giveth and the hormones taketh away. Hormones direct how the body treats raw fuels (sugars, proteins, and fat). The right hormones within, minute to minute, create a balance between storage and combustion of these fuels. Also important, the right hormones minute to minute defend body protein from excessive breakdown. Remember, proteins are the metabolically active component of the body. Therefore, healthy owners always enjoy hormone balance. Conversely, unhealthy owners always suffer from hormone imbalance. Regretfully, American health care often overlooks this basic fact for how one becomes fat.

Until the quality of the hormones within improves, weight loss efforts end in defeat.

Fortunately, out of the over 100 body hormones only 7 types centrally affect the making and losing of body fat. Two other hormones influence the central seven.

The glandular composite hormone report card is essential at the beginning of any weight loss effort.

The initial hormone report card includes:
1. **Fasting insulin and C-peptide levels**
2. **Fasting insulin like growth factor type 1 (IGF-1) levels**
3. **Adrenal steroids (including aldosterone) and their metabolites**
4. **Androgen type gonad steroids (from the ovaries or testes) and their metabolites**
5. **Thyroid hormones' levels (including reversed T3)**
6. **Estrogen steroids status for both men and women**

7. **Epinephrine urinary output (metanephrine and normetanephrine) alternatively obtain a homocysteine level**
8. **Prolactin level in certain cases**
9. **Growth Hormone levels (surmised by looking at the amount of androgens and IGF-1 levels)**

Each of the first seven hormone types has a specific role in the overall message that directs the manufacturing of fat (energy storage). Prolactin has special fat making properties through its effect on some of the first seven hormone types listed above. Lastly, Growth Hormone directly influences the amount of IGF-1 released. For this reason, in practice it makes more clinical sense to measure IGF-1 levels instead of Growth Hormone levels.

Another fact about some of the obesity causing hormones becomes important: Steroids and thyroid hormones are among the most powerful class of body hormones. These are the most powerful body hormones, with the addition of vitamin A, because they are the only body hormones that possess the ability to directly instruct the DNA (genes) within the 70 trillion body cells. All other body hormones cannot directly instruct the genes inside cells. Remember, gene activity determines which proteins are made. Recall, protein constitutes the metabolically active component of the body. Metabolism burns calories.

A few specific hormones control gene activity. In turn, gene activity determines whether or not body cells spend energy wisely or unwisely. Obesity results from the unwise use of available body energy. The hormone message content that the cells receive determines body energy usage.

Message content (information) to all body cells conveys by the body hormones via the blood stream. The blood stream can be thought of as a sea of information that changes, as the body's needs change. Bad information within the blood stream results when the wrong hormones secrete. Hormones direct how the body spends or saves energy. For this reason, too much energy storing-hormone secretion (energy storage message content) causes excessive fat.

It will be explained in this section how many of the obesity causing hormones are amongst the most powerful type because they uniquely direct the DNA (genes) into activity or silence. Remember, the activity or silence of the DNA within one's 70 trillion cells powerfully determines calorie expenditure. It is very important to realize that gene activity also determines repair versus disrepair within a cell. Part of the reason certain owners' gain fat derives from imbalances in their most powerful hormones instructing their genes.

Here lies the central explanation for why obesity associates with an accelerated aging rate. The hormone mismatch, which either allows or creates obesity are among the most powerful body hormones.

Out of kilter powerful body hormones, not only encourage obesity but also other health problems arise because body energy moves in misdirected ways.

For example, instead of rejuvenation hormone message content arriving at the body cells excessive body energy channels into to fuel storage activities (fat manufacture). Realize there is a big difference to ongoing overall health between energy storage versus cellular rejuvenation activities.

This fact partly explains why obesity increases the risk of heart disease, diabetes, high blood pressure, and arthritis (middle age related disease). Each of these diseases often has a large component of causality in the abnormal hormones associated with obesity. This is good news because it means that by correcting the obesity-causing hormones it will also impact middle age related diseases as well.

The basic seven hormone types that when imbalanced cause obesity (note: these are all glandular secretions)

> **Thyroid hormones (T3 and T4)**
> **Insulin**
> **Insulin like growth factor type one (IGF-1)**
> **Cortisol**
> **Androgens**
> **Estrogen**
> **Epinephrine**

The additional two pituitary secreted hormones, prolactin and Growth Hormone, which influence the amounts of the basic seven.

2. **Thyroid hormones** (T3 and T4) direct the DNA to increase the manufacture rate of cellular mineral pumps and furnace combustion chamber components. Its sufficiency arriving at the pituitary also determines how

much Growth Hormone this gland manufactures (a key longevity pearl so read on to see why).

The lack of thyroid message content within an owner's body diminishes the furnace flames within his/her 70 trillion cells. Hence, the most reliable indication of low thyroid gland function is a low body temperature upon awakening (basal temperature). Low thyroid also accelerates the aging rate because Growth Hormone secretion rates decline and this sets off a cascade of abnormal hormone levels.

Only Growth Hormone defends body protein content during fasting and exercising. For this simple reason, insufficient amounts of it logically extend to shrinking muscles (sarcopenia), organs, sagging skin that hides amongst the fat. Thought of in this way, obesity is really a wasting disease. Wasting disease is the accurate descriptor because functional tissue, protein, diminishes, while fat increases (explained below).

A poorly functioning thyroid gland leads to a decrease in its message content to the numerous body cells. One component of the thyroid hormone message concerns its directions to invest in furnace component upgrades. Scientists call the furnace or power plant of the cell the mitochondria. Poorly functioning mitochondria are analogous to heating one's home with a furnace that contains worn out components and plugged air filters. For the same reasons that these homes remain cold, an owner with worn out mitochondrion components in his cells stays cold.

Most body cells prefer fat as their fuel source

Recall, all body cells need certain key vitamins to process raw body fuels (protein, carbohydrate, and fat) into a processed fuel called acetate. Acetate is the simplest fatty acid. No matter what the raw fuel (protein, sugar or fat) consists of before it can burn up in the cell power plant it needs refining into acetate. The different raw fuels need specific and numerous vitamins to process into the refined fuel, acetate. Many owners have weight gain simply because they lack the necessary vitamins to turn raw fuel into refined fuel.

The cell furnaces can only burn acetate within their combustion chambers. This last fact is analogous to the requirement for refined fuels within power generators of the physical world. For example automobile engine designs usually require the refinement of raw oil into gasoline. In general the combustion chamber of each power generator is designed to work with one fuel type.

Similarly, the numerous body cell furnaces can only combust one fuel type. Therefore many thyroid problems worsen from specific vitamin deficiencies that impede the processing of raw body fuels into acetate. A diminished delivery of the refined fuel, acetate, will exaggerate weight gain because it tends to also contribute to hungry cells (section one).

Membrane pumps require thyroid

There is an additional message that thyroid hormones deliver to the body cells beyond the thyroid hormones' heat creating effect within the numerous cell furnaces. The additional message involves its ability to direct the genes into creating membrane pumps that trap some of this heat energy for useful work. Each of the body's 70 trillion cells needs to create a cell voltage to remain alive. The strongest cell voltage occurs in the nerve cells and the weakest in the red blood cells. The more mineral pumps embedded in the cell membrane, the higher the voltage possibilities. Membrane pumps burn calories through the act of creating a cell's voltage.

Again this is similar to a car engine creating heat but some of the energy is used to move the car down the road by engaging the drive train. Power plants also lose energy to heat but again some of this energy is trapped in the form of electricity.

The body cells also operate on an electrical system. A cell's ability to charge its membrane proves critical to life. The energy needed to charge the cell membrane derives from the energy trapped within the mitochondrion combustion chamber in the form of ATP. The more ATP available determines one aspect of how high a cell can charge up its membrane.

Another determinant of how high a cell voltage can rise is the number of membrane imbedded mineral pumps on its surface. Membrane pumps charge the cell membranes' voltage. Membrane pumps need the energy contained in ATP to pump up the electrical charge (increase the voltage) contained in the cell membrane. For this reason, the constant supply of ATP needs to occur or the electrical charge contained in the membrane diminishes and if severe the cell dies.

The thyroid hormone's message content provides the informational direction that instructs specific DNA programs (genes) to activate. In turn, these activated and specific DNA programs direct the manufacture of more membrane contained mineral pumps (specific proteins). Realize the gazillions of membrane pumps within the membranes of all cells of a body consists of proteins. General scheme: A specific DNA program (gene) codes for each body protein.

More mineral pumps within the cell membrane allows one more determinant for higher membrane electrical charge to become satisfied. **The greater the 70 trillion body cell's cumulative electrical charge is, the more calories burned to maintain it.** In fact, the cell membrane mineral pumps amount comprise the reason that most calories burn up within the body in the sedentary state. Fewer mineral pumps lead to fewer calories burned. Fewer calories burned leads to a lower metabolic rate. This fact provides an example of protein being the metabolically active constituent of the body. Mantra: Its defense proves paramount to continued metabolism.

Body cells utilize the electrical charge within the membrane to perform the cellular work of living. The more work performed then the more calories combusted. This is analogous to the charge within the membranes of a car battery, which can be drawn upon to power the electrical gadgetry within the automobile. Similarly, the cell power plants recharge the cell membrane like the cars engine recharges the car battery.

All body cells protect themselves and perform work by utilizing the energy contained in their membranes. Fully charged cells are maximally alive. Fully charged cells burn more energy (fat). The more energy consumed, the more calories consumed. Later, in section five, it will be explained how the body cells cannot fully charge without the proper proportions of mineral intake within the diet (the third determinant of cell membrane charge).

For now, it is important to summarize the three main messages that the thyroid hormone conveys to many different body cells. 1) Carries to the DNA the message to invest in furnace component upgrades. 2) Carries to the DNA the additional message to create more mineral pumps within the membrane, which charges the cell electrically. 3) The amount of it arriving within the pituitary determines how much Growth Hormone is created. Other lifestyle habits determine how much Growth Hormone releases (explained later in this chapter) but thyroid hormones levels retain primacy for the above reasons. Only when all three of these processes occur smoothly can a normal amount of calories burn.

Certain DNA programs need the additional presence of sufficient vitamin A message content to activate what the thyroid hormone message started. In this way, vitamin A and thyroid hormones work synergistically (see the misunderstood steroids).

2. **Insulin** Carries the Fat Maker Message and IGF-Competes with the Fat Maker Message

Insulin is made and secreted by the pancreas
IGF-1 within the blood stream is made and secreted by the liver

There are only two hormones that allow the cell fuel tanks to fill up. Recall, it helps to think of these two hormones as fuel nozzle hormones. Just as in filling a car with fuel, requires a fuel nozzle, so it is with most body cells, a molecular 'nozzle' is necessary to fill the 'tanks' of the cells with the fuel circulating in the blood stream.

Remember, the two 'fuel nozzle' hormones are insulin and insulin like growth factor type 1 (IGF-1). As stated previously, healthy people have at least 100 times more IGF-1 compared to insulin in their blood streams. Each of these two fuel nozzle hormones has a preference for the cell types it prefers to fill up. Because there are roughly 100 times more cells that prefer IGF-1 it makes sense that healthy people have at least 100 times this hormone as compared to insulin. Only when the body becomes unhealthy and IGF-1 levels consequently fall off, will the body attempt to raise insulin hormone production rates so as to keep the total amount of fuel nozzle hormones constant. Hungry cells result when fuel nozzle hormones become scarce.

However, the insulin hormone, because of its secretion pathway, delivers message content that the IGF-1 hormone does not share. Insulin delivers the fat maker message. Overweight people have a problem with too much fat maker message. Until the fat maker message decreases they will continue to gain weight year after year.

Body fat is not possible without enough insulin message content to maintain it.

The other six hormone types of obesity, when unbalanced, facilitate the amplification of the insulin message.

Healthy people have almost no insulin in the fasting state but have high amounts of IGF-1.

Unhealthy and obese people have higher fasting insulin and/or C-peptide and lower IGF-1. C-peptide blood levels derive from insulin formation and because it is more stable it serves as a better marker of true body insulin exposure.

Therefore at the start of any dietary program obtain these values for a baseline.

Insulin's major message concerns fuel storage.

Key point: Ideally insulin levels only increase following meals. Unhealthy people, however, need insulin to stay alive between meals, while fasting and attempting to exercise. Cognizance here allows for healing paths to open up (read on to see why).

The majority of the insulin message directs the liver to store energy. The liver can store up to 100 grams of glycogen. When the liver already has enough glycogen stored, the insulin message then directs the liver to convert the additional sugar into fat and cholesterol.

The opposite situation occurs between meals because blood fuel tends to drop off. In these situations blood fuel needs to be released from the liver and not stored. New supplies of fuel need to be present in the blood stream to constantly provide nourishment to the body cells. Blood fuel content delivery, into the body cells, is not possible without adequate *fuel nozzle hormones* available to facilitate this process. In healthy people, when the blood fuel levels begin to fall off, the re-supply of fuel occurs via the other *fuel nozzle hormone* called insulin like growth factor type 1 (IGF-1). Important point: **IGF-1 occurs at levels many times greater than that of insulin in healthy people.**

This hormone's design helps the body cells outside the liver and fat cells procure the fuel they need. The high IGF-1 levels, within the blood stream of healthy owners remain so compared to insulin levels even following meals because its half-life is 15 hours up to four days. In contrast insulin's half-life is about ten minutes. IGF-1 levels increase slightly between meals, while exercising and in the fasting state. Two other hormone types and two lifestyle habits need to occur for adequate IGF-1 levels to be maintained beyond middle age.

The two hormones are: Growth Hormone and androgen. Ideally, Growth Hormone releases from the pituitary gland, when blood fuel levels fall off. Growth Hormone release instructs the liver to release more IGF-1 and fuel (sugar and fat but not protein). Notice that ideally no insulin is needed as the blood fuel falls off in the between meal, fasting or exercising state. This allows health to continue (read on as to why).

Androgens, like testosterone and DHEA, instruct specific liver cell genes to activate and hence manufacture more IGF-1. Summarize, androgen causes IGF-1 creation and Growth Hormone causes IGF-1 release. Remember that the pituitary manufacture rate of Growth Hormone depends on sufficient thyroid hormones. Therefore, normal blood stream IGF-1 levels require: optimal thyroid hormone, which allows normal Growth Hormone manufacture rates. Finally, there needs to be adequate androgen levels (testosterone or DHEA) arriving at the liver to instruct IGF-1 synthesis. The above discussion elucidates the interdependence of several hormones or health deteriorates. When was the last time a conventionally trained physician inquired into their patients' level of these important hormones?

Summary:

Sufficient androgens, like DHEA and testosterone, direct the liver to make adequate IGF-1.

Sufficient Growth Hormone secretion causes the liver to release the manufactured IGF-1 into the blood stream.

Sufficient thyroid hormones need to instruct the pituitary to manufacture adequate amounts of Growth Hormone.

The lifestyle habit concerns the fact that a fall in blood fuel that occurs between meals (fasting) and when one exercises triggers Growth Hormone release. Consequently, these two habits encourage adequate levels of Growth Hormone. This knowledge explains why chronically underfeeding (fasting) both in animals and humans results in a lengthened life span. The underfed human will tend to secrete more Growth Hormone (protein sparing). In addition, increased Growth Hormone arriving at the healthy liver chronically will help promote elevated IGF-1 levels (no insulin is needed to deliver fuel during the falling blood sugar state).

It is important to emphasize that sufficient Growth Hormone defends body protein because it encourages the liver to release stored sugar and fat but inhibits protein processing for fuel generation (inhibits gluconeogenesis) In addition, elevated

IGF-1 levels provide the nutritional advantage to the organs, bones and muscles of the body. Whereas, elevated insulin provides the nutritional advantage to the liver where more fat and cholesterol manufacture occurs (read on to find out why).

Remember, adequate IGF-1 in the blood stream facilitates the body cells outside of the liver in their procuring nutrition. Adequate insulin, but not too much, facilitates the liver and fat cells in storing fuel following a meal. Healthy owners, in the between meal state and while exercising, draw down the stored fuel within their liver and fat cells. Because they also simultaneously deliver this fuel with released IGF-1, no insulin is needed and this prevents obesity.

In contrast, some unhealthy owners suffer from decreased Growth Hormone secretion rates and hence a diminished IGF-1 level follows. Death is prevented between meals, when their blood fuel falls off, because two other hormonal aberrations save them (health consequences follow however). First, excessive stress response hormones releases and this activates catabolic pathways. Catabolic means that body structure dismantles to free up more fuel. Catabolically vulnerable body structure is composed of sugar, fat and proteins. Unfortunately, proteins become fair game. Second, concerns the exaggerated amounts of insulin needed to help the body cells procure nutrition because IGF-1 levels have fallen.

Remember, the unhealthy body attempts to provide a constant amount of total "fuel nozzles" in its desperate effort, to fill hungry cell fuel tanks. Only when the pancreas secretes insulin in large amounts (commonly described by the smoke and mirrors term of insulin resistance) can some of it spill past the liver and into the general circulation where it acts much like IGF-1 (explained below).

Important anatomical point: Unfortunately, when insulin secretes in large amounts, the highest concentration still arrives at the liver. Ideally, insulin is only needed when the blood sugar rises following a meal. Here, its sufficient presence diverts a certain proportion of the meals nutritional content into liver storage in preparation for the next time the blood fuel falls off. Remember, the insulin message within the liver also instructs the fat and cholesterol making machinery to activate.

Realize the abnormality of needing insulin while the blood fuel falls off and it only results after IGF-1 fuel nozzles have become scarce. Visualize a falling blood fuel level and the competing process of excessive insulin hitting the liver first. The unhealthy body has no other choice than to promote this aberration because fuel nozzles are scarce beyond the liver and hence these important body cells are hungry.

This anatomical fact means that falling blood fuel in unhealthy people is compounded because the anatomy of insulin secretion instructs the liver to make the low blood fuel worse by pulling fuel out of the blood stream and then turning it into more cholesterol and fat. This fact is true because insulin within the liver always instructs it to store fuel. (see diagram on page 125)

Realize, unless there is an excessive counter regulatory stress response to the falling blood fuel these owners' lives are over with. It is the excessive insulin need that makes them fat. It is the excessive need for the counter regulatory stress hormones that viciously dismantles precious protein to save their butt by making sugar quickly. Visualize the violence at the level of the liver.

High insulin and/or C-peptide in the fasting state provide a good laboratory marker for these types of obesity prone owners. Realize that as Americans become more obese what the laboratory calls normal fasting insulin and C-peptide must be distilled upward. This fact occurs because healthy people have almost none of these markers in the fasting state.

Unfavorable cholesterol profiles also provide an initial clue but in some the best one seems to be the expanding waste line. Modern literature calls these people Syndrome X, Metabolic Syndrome or Insulin Resistance Syndrome (heart chapter).

Interestingly the fact that these individuals have at the root of their problem a falling IGF-1 level remains almost universally ignored. In its place, peripheral approaches like cholesterol lowering drugs, drugs that whip the pancreas into even more insulin production and high blood pressure medication are prescribed. All these accepted approaches do little to heal the underlying problem and inflict side effects to these owners' health. Until steps are taken to raise these owners IGF-1 levels both obesity and accelerated aging will continue to propagate (read on as to why).

Pivotal longevity point: Healthy owners have the ideal balance between insulin and IGF-1. In these situations insulin increases following meals and the IGF-1 stays unchanged. Balance between these two hormones allows the liver to uptake a proper proportion of fuel compared to the amount that other body cells are allowed to procure with the assistance of IGF-1 following a meal. In addition, the fuel stored by the liver in a healthy person becomes readily available between meals, when exercise or a fast occurs. In all three of these situations blood fuel begins to fall, Growth

Hormone releases, which directs the liver to release the stored fuel (sugar and fat) and more IGF-1. Recall, as well, that sufficient Growth Hormone inhibits the liver from processing precious protein into sugar (encourages positive nitrogen balance).

Ideally, sufficient IGF-1 release serves as the fasting and exercising fuel nozzle for the hungry body cells uptake of nutrition. Notice, here insulin is not needed. Realize the Growth Hormone mediated release of IGF-1 along with the sugar released negates its initial diabetogenic action (it initially raises the blood fuel level by instructing the liver to release stored fuels). Only when excessive Growth Hormone releases or the liver is unhealthy will it cause an uncompensated increase in blood sugar (fuel release but the simultaneous compensating IGF-1 release fails). Unfortunately, the connection between these facts is routinely ignored in most literature and textbooks.

Remember that only Growth Hormone prevents the catabolism of body protein for fuel between meals. Here lies the chronic weakening mechanism when unhealthy people are between meals, fasting or exercising. As their blood fuel falls in these situations the wrong hormones make body protein available for their fuel needs because Growth Hormone release proves inadequate. This leads to the wasting process mentioned earlier that hides its assault amongst the increasing fat.

Summarize: Unhealthy owners have diminished IGF-1, as a consequence of diminished Growth Hormone release, following meals and between meals. Alternatively, something happens to the livers ability to manufacture IGF-1. In both situations this sets up the need for abnormal secretion rates of insulin (commonly referred to as insulin resistance). Remember insulin delivers the fat maker message simply because of the anatomy of its secretion pathway heading straight into the liver. Consequently, the higher the insulin secretion rate, the higher the fat maker message within.

Syndrome X owners are doomed until their need for insulin decreases. One of the ways insulin-needs fall off involves IGF-1 levels increasing to normal. IGF-1 contains none of the fat and cholesterol stimulating message content that insulin contains. Rather, IGF-1 message content concerns itself with the procurement of nutrition (fuel) by other body cell types, outside of the liver and fat cells.

This all being said, it remains rather curious to this author that even a cursory discussion about the importance of IGF-1 in sugar metabolism and insulin needs remains ignored. Instead, the modern literature contains numerous articles disparaging high IGF-1 levels on many fronts. These half-truths will be ferreted out through out this manual in attempt to include the other side of the story that science has revealed.

(Nerd corner) The Myth of Insulin Logic

Mainstream medicine's propaganda dogma grooms physicians and patients to focus on insulin as the nutrition uptake hormone. Meanwhile they ignore the scientific fact that IGF-1 occurs at levels many times greater than those of insulin in the healthy individual. The disconnection between optimal ratios maintains itself by arbitrarily measuring insulin in micro units or micromoles and IGF-1 in nanograms throughout the medical texts. More disconnection results from the fact that numerous different names describe IGF-1. For example, the older medical literature describes IGF-1 in the following additional three ways: Nonsuppressible insulin like activity of the blood, sulfation factor, and somatomedin C. In order for a physician to appreciate the important role that IGF-1 plays in the cells for obtaining nutrition he/she would need to be aware of and have time to look up all four of these alternative descriptors for the same hormone. Reconnecting all four different names with the facts associated with them and a common measurement method allows the important role of IGF-1 to emerge.

Simple logic shows that there is not enough insulin to go around to all body cells. One liver or fat cell contains 200,000 pure insulin-type receptors. The over 100 times more IGF-1 compared to insulin makes up the volume discrepancy needed to deliver fuel uptake message content to the other body cells. Furthermore, IGF-1 binds liver and fat cells at 1/1000th the affinity of insulin. The highest IGF-1 receptor concentration is found in the muscles. Also important concerns the textbook fact that during exercise (in well trained athletes) insulin levels fall to zero. Why isn't anyone asking what serves as a fuel nozzle during exercise?

The 200,000 pure insulin-type receptors per liver cell illuminate another important point: Whatever the insulin secretion rate, the liver always receives the highest amount of insulin message content because the pancreas secretes into the portal vein. The portal vein heads straight into the liver. Consequently, before any pancreas secreted insulin spills out of the liver it traps huge amounts for these

---

anatomical reasons alone. Visualize the liver as an insulin trap.

Add in the biochemical fact that the amount of insulin arriving within the liver determines the cholesterol and triglyceride manufacture rate and the almost ubiquitous need for the statin drugs starts becoming suspicious. This follows because a cognizance of this anatomy helps one to visualize why high insulin exposure within the liver leads to deranged metabolism such as increased cholesterol and fat synthesis, and increased hogging of blood stream nutrition within the liver relative to other body cells. It is important to visualize that the root of the problem in these individuals concerns the need for insulin while the blood fuel is falling in order to stay alive between meals or while exercising (explained more deeply later on).

It was briefly mentioned above that unhealthy owners have other hormone increases, which facilitate resupplies of blood fuel between meals. **However, there is a price paid from this aberration to the body structure in the form of lost muscle and organ mass. This largely ignored medical fact explains another consequence of the unhealthy body's lack of sufficient stimulus for Growth Hormone release and/or sufficient IGF-1 release**. Only when adequate Growth Hormone release occurs will a sufficient counter message to prevent protein destruction for fuel needs follow. The functional constituents of muscles and organs are made from protein. Growth Hormone's presence prevents the excessive combusting of protein when blood fuel levels fall. Instead, Growth Hormone preferentially directs the liver and fat cells to dump sugar, fat and IGF-1 into the blood stream. Important longevity point: its message spares protein. This fact partially explains why healthy owners have nice muscles while unhealthy owners do not.

Summarize mentally the basic sequence of protein destruction, when unhealthy owners find themselves between meals and their blood fuel begins to fall. Now concentrate on the fact that their very survival depends on the excessive release of blood fuel elevating hormones. The entire group consists of glucagon, cortisol and epinephrine. Like Growth Hormone they all facilitate the release of sugar and fat into the blood stream. Unlike Growth Hormone, excessive body protein dismantling (gluconeogenesis) becomes fair game when Growth Hormone levels prove insufficient.

Here again, another vicious process destroys the physiques of countless middle-aged owners. **The importance of protecting**

their body protein content needs to be explained to them. One of the central determiners of body protein content relies on adequate Growth Hormone levels for the above stated reason.

The other consequence of a falling Growth Hormone secretion concerns the fact that less IGF-1 releases into the blood stream from the liver. Less IGF-1 release means that the optimal 100:1 ratio between IGF-1 and insulin diminishes. When IGF-1 falls then insulin levels must rise to facilitate a way for the other body cells to procure nutrition. Remember that the body desperately attempts to keep total *fuel nozzle hormone* levels, between insulin and IGF-1, adequate or the body cells become hungry. Therefore a fall in IGF-1 necessitates a corresponding rise in insulin to attempt total *fuel nozzle hormones* constancy within the blood stream.

Recall the anatomy of this imbalance: portal vein connection between the pancreas and the liver. Secondary to this relationship the liver will always receive the highest insulin message content for a given secretion rate from the pancreas secreting into the portal vein, which leads directly into the liver. Recall, as well, the liver contains 200, 000 pure insulin receptors per liver cell. Visualize the liver as an insulin trap. Huge amounts of it therefore need to secrete out of the pancreas before a tiny amount can escape beyond the liver and serve as a *fuel nozzle* to the hungry body cells. Hungry body cells occur whenever IGF-1, the main *fuel nozzle*, levels fall off because of the liver insulin trap.

Remember, the insulin message concerns itself with storing food energy in times of plenty (following a meal). However, realize that insulin arriving within the liver while the blood fuel falls is abnormal. This fact occurs because the higher the insulin, the more that body fuel tilts towards the liver as the nutritional hog of the body from simple anatomy of its release pathway. Visualize 200,000 insulin receptors within each liver cell. Recall the insulin message within the liver concerns energy storage.

For this simple reason, insulin release while the blood sugar falls compounds the blood fuel scarcity and an excessive presence of the other counter regulatory hormones (glucagon, epinephrine and cortisol) becomes necessary to stay alive. Picture the conflict at the level of the liver. Visualize the violence because although these hormones compete with the excessive insulin within the liver they also make protein dismantling fair game. Here lies the dirty little secret ruining many middle aged body's health.

In contrast, healthy owners release sufficient insulin that directs the important process of allowing enough fuel storage within the liver following meals in order to provide fuel for the next between meal state (fasting and exercising). However, the 100 fold greater amounts of IGF-1 present in healthy owners' blood streams tips a proper proportion of the blood fuel towards the body cells outside the liver and fat following meals as well. For this reason, only an optimal *fuel nozzle* ratio facilitates the sufficient nutrition of the cells throughout the body.

Picture the tug of war between these two *fuel nozzle* hormones. Hungry cells occur when insufficient amounts of either insulin or IGF-1 occur. In addition, when insulin must increase to compensate for a falling IGF-1 then the fat making machinery abnormally activates. This fact arises because of the anatomy of its secretion pathway arriving within the liver trap (200,000 pure insulin receptors per liver cell) first before even a tiny bit of it can make it beyond the liver.

The additional troubles within obese owners, such as other hormone abnormalities, nutritional deficiencies, dietary indiscretions and/or mineral deficiencies all diminish IGF-1 levels as well (discussed later). The fall in IGF-1 levels means that the peripheral cells suffer from a decreased ability to uptake nutrition following meals because of the anatomical secretion pathway of insulin.

This anatomical fact means that the liver always receives the highest concentration of insulin message content. Bottom line point: Abnormally high insulin levels, with low IGF-1 levels, cause cells outside the liver to possess a diminished ability to obtain nutrition and fuel. Instead the liver, secondary to excessive insulin exposure in these cases, becomes the nutritional hog of body energy and directs it into the storage pathways (fat).

This means that because insulin levels increase, their livers are making more fat and cholesterol for the same amount of caloric intake. Healing obesity involves facilitating a rise in IGF-1 levels. Weight can then be lost as insulin needs fall off.

Recall, Insulin has a half-life of 10 to 20 minutes. IGF-1 has a half-life from 15 hours up to four days. Healthy people contain adequate IGF-1 levels, while fasting or between meals, they therefore have no need for insulin during these times. **Here lies another valuable clue: why would a body elevate insulin levels in the fasting state?**

By definition an elevation of fasting insulin levels is called Syndrome X, Insulin Resistance Syndrome or Metabolic Syndrome. Unfortunately, the fact that IGF-1 levels diminish in this syndrome is almost completely ignored. Unfortunately, the common approach causes the prescribing of blood pressure

medication, cholesterol lowering medication, and insulin increasing medication. All of these prescriptions only treat the symptoms of this disease process. Symptom control has nothing to do with how the body heals.

Insulin increases brought on by certain diabetic drugs only worsen the obesity problem. The pancreas design was not intended to produce massive amounts of insulin to shore up falling IGF-1 levels. The pancreas is little and the liver is large. IGF-1 at amounts one hundred times insulin levels is easily produced and secreted by the large liver when the right hormones instruct it to do so. In contrast, the pancreas however has to work itself to death when IGF-1 levels fall even a little bit. Unfortunately, these owners can eventually exhaust their pancreas (beta cell burn out) and this leads to one form of diabetes (see liver chapter).

Simplistically, two hormones determine the amount of IGF-1 available and released (there are others but for now the all important first two are discussed). First, the amounts of androgen steroids like testosterone and DHEA secreted. Second, concerns Growth Hormone secretion rates.

Basically, the pituitary secretes Growth Hormone when the brain senses a falling blood fuel.

Blood fuel levels tend to fall with 2 situations
1) Fasting (between meals)
2) Exercise

The trouble with a sedentary lifestyle and obesity concerns two things:
1. Other associated hormone abnormalities prevent the fall in blood fuel
2. Exercise does not happen

Because of these two processes Growth Hormone secretion rates drop off. This leads to a decreased secretion rate of IGF-1. The fall in IGF-1 increases the need for more insulin. More insulin message content arriving within the liver increases the production rate of changing sugar into fat and cholesterol (the butter fat variety).
Scientific fact: high insulin levels turn on the cholesterol and fat making machinery.

Normal insulin secretion rates leads to a normal cholesterol and fat manufacture rate.

This simple relationship is largely forgotten within the hysteria to sell more cholesterol lowering prescription medication. Cholesterol lowering medication has side effects. Some authorities liken these side effects to the acceleration of the aging process.

3. Androgen steroids: made in the adrenals and gonads (ovaries and testicles). Their message content always concerns rejuvenation and repair of body cells.

Two major androgen types, one secretes from the gonads and the other from the adrenals.
DHEA secretes from the adrenals
Testosterone secretes from the gonads

Remember that steroid hormones are among the most powerful hormone class. Only the most powerful body hormones directly instruct the 70 trillion cells' DNA programs. Depending on the steroid type, certain DNA programs (genes) activate or shut down. What the message involves for a given steroid type results from its precise shape. Gene silence means that protein synthesis ceases for which that gene codes. Gene activation results in protein synthesis specific to the gene activated.

Recall, proteins constitute the metabolically active component of body tissue. In other words, proteins, when active, burn up calories. Examples of metabolically active protein types are: enzymes, mineral pumps, muscle components and cell receptors.

This subsection begins the discussion of the first two types of steroid message content: Anabolic versus catabolic.

The androgen message (anabolic) concerns itself with rejuvenation (cell repair and build up) activities. Scientists denote this anabolic property of certain steroids as causing a positive nitrogen balance. Nitrogen balance can be thought of as a shorthand way for denoting protein adequacy because the summation of all proteins contains the lion's share of body nitrogen.

The catabolic steroids deliver the opposite message. Catabolic message concerns itself with consuming body structure for the creation of energy. Catabolically vulnerable body structure is made up of fat, carbohydrate and protein. Realize, high levels of catabolism make all three raw fuel sources fair game.

One facet of high levels of catabolic steroid's message concerns energy channeling for a perceived survival threat whether it proves real or imagined. The stress response activates this system. **Body structure dismantles when the stress response activates in order to maximize available energy.** Stress steroids (the catabolic type) are only made in the adrenal glands. Both the adrenal and gonads manufacture the androgen steroids.

Healthy owners have a balance between survival message content and rejuvenation message content.

Unhealthy owners are out of balance between these two opposing messages.

This subsection concerns the androgen message and how it curtails obesity. In the next subsection, the survival message (catabolism) elicited by stress will be reviewed in regards to its perpetrating obesity.

A few words on why only real hormone shapes carry accurate information

Hormones carry information via their precise shape. Steroid hormones are relatively small and simple in the world of other much larger hormones. The smaller the hormone then the more the message will change with even a slight change in shape.

In order to obtain a patent advantage, drug companies must change the shape of the natural body hormone. Natural body hormones deliver precise messages. Unnatural hormones, such as being patented by drug companies, create profit but because their shape has been altered their message content changes as well.

One prominent example concerns horse estrogen collected from pregnant horse mares' urine. There is some human type estrogen within this mixture of horse estrogens given to millions of women. Remember, the pharmaceutical

companies cannot obtain a patent advantage without selling the whole mixture.

However, the mixture contains unnatural shaped estrogens that one does not find in the human body. Consequently, the altered shaped estrogens contain different message content. The message content differs because the shape differs. Unfortunately, the unnaturally shaped horse estrogens deliver an altered message to the ingesting owners trillions of cellular DNA programs (genes).

Uzzi Reis, M.D. Ob/Gyn author of the book, *Natural Hormone Balance for Women* says it very well. "Are you a horse? Do you eat hay? Then why take horse estrogen?"

Estrogen's role in creating body fat will be discussed more completely in a following subsection. For now realize that estrogen promotes anabolism for fat cells in the body by a circuitous route. As a consequence, the higher estrogen becomes relative to androgen hormones the larger a women's breast and hips.

For now, it is only important to begin to appreciate that the different types of steroids need to occur in the proper amounts and timing or the message content reaching the DNA alters.

Unnatural hormones carry inaccurate message content to the trillions of body cells. Unnatural hormones carry faulty information because their shapes deviate from the natural hormone's shapes.

It is importanat to emphasize that steroid hormone's shape needs to change in order to get a patent. However, the different shape causes the message content to change. Cells that receive altered directions on how to spend their energy eventually manifest as side effects and disease.

One of the side effects when the androgen message becomes diminished concerns the fact that the afflicted owner's body becomes older. Bodies become older when their cells receive diminished instructions to repair and rejuvenate. Androgen type steroids carry the rejuvenation message content to the body cells. Remember, the androgen message concerns rejuvenation instructions within the trillions of cell contained DNA programs. The lack of rejuvenation message content accelerates the aging process. Some components of the aging process are the loss of muscle and bone but also the gaining of body fat.

The androgen message contained in testosterone and DHEA shed fat in one important way. Androgens direct the liver DNA programs (genes) to synthesize IGF-1. High IGF-1 blood levels mean that one requires less insulin for their cells, outside the liver and fat, to procure its nutritional needs.

Less insulin means that the fat maker message diminishes.

Many women notice weight gain after removal of their ovaries. Some of this tendency can be explained by the loss of androgen message content. Healthy ovaries and adrenals make androgens.

Weak adrenals incompletely compensate for the removed ovaries. Menopause also brings on diminished ovarian function. Health after menopause depends on healthy adrenals, which produce significant androgens.

Many postmenopausal diseases have a component of causality in poorly functioning adrenals. Examples are: osteoporosis, osteoarthritis, obesity, fibromyalgia and chronic fatigue.

A well run 24-hour urine test can check the status of the thyroid hormones, adrenal steroids and gonad steroids. Over a twenty-four hour period in a typical day the peaks and valleys of hormone release will average out. In contrast, the standard mainstream approach entails a blood drawn sample for measuring one or two of these important hormones. However, the instant of the blood draw only measures that instant in time of where the body directs its energy. Whether the values obtained prove the high or low for the day is not discernible with this approach.

For example, if drawing blood for the test causes stress then the rise in stress hormones, like cortisol causes the displacement of the bound thyroid hormone fraction and thus artificially increases the true average of this hormone in one's blood stream. Forgetting this fact doctors often falsely reassure low thyroid functioning patients that their thyroid tested normal when it is not. However, taking the time to measure thyroid hormone production over a twenty-four hour period averages out these peaks and valleys.

The volatility of the blood stream levels makes sense when one realizes that all hormones direct how the body spends its energy. The many different activities and situations of life demand different message content to direct body energy appropriately. For example, the resting state predominantly provides a time when body energy directs into rejuvenation activities. The right hormones need to occur to oversee this process. Conversely, exercise demands different body hormones to direct the freeing up of energy that allows this activity to continue. As a consequence, a blood sample taken in either of these situations would show entirely different results.

Remember that thyroid hormones, all steroid hormones and vitamin A comprise the most powerful body hormones because only they directly instruct the trillions of cells' DNA programs (genes). Only these most powerful hormones directly determine a cell's genetic program activity. In turn, the genetic program activity determines which proteins are made. Bottom line: The amounts and types of proteins made by a cell determine its productive capacity, overall integrity, and repair rate. Finally, these are the most powerful hormones because all the many other body hormones cannot directly instruct the DNA programs.
Keeping these facts in mind it becomes more logical for why the overall mixture of hormones within constitutes an important determinant of health. The overall mixture of hormones within determines the informational direction of how the body spends its energy. Some bodies spend energy wisely and there occurs a continuum all the way down to those bodies that spend energy foolishly.

Healthy body cells receive the proper proportions of the important hormones directing them in the wise use of available energy. The opposite situation exists, in that unhealthy bodies spend their energy unwisely because their hormones are wrong. The wrong hormones result from nutritional habits, lifestyle habits, patented forms of unnaturally shaped hormones and glandular failure.

All hormone message content concerns how the body directs energy expenditure. Healing an unhealthy body cannot occur until better informational direction occurs, via the hormones, on how their body spends its energy. Remember, obesity has a component of too much message content directing body energy into storage. Hungry body cells result when too much energy channels into storage (fat).Similarly, unhealthy owners always suffer from poor hormone message content. Their health will continue to deteriorate until improvement to the quality of the message that directs their cells occurs.

"Steroid tone" provides a basis that helps quantify the quality of the mixture of information carried in the blood stream. Recall, the steroids are among the most powerful body hormones because they each carry specific message content, inherent in their unique shapes, directly to the DNA. Important point: Each specific type's message uniquely directs the trillions of cell DNA programs (genes). Consequently, too much or too little of a particular steroid causes the cell to experience either excess or deficiency for that message respectively.

Realize healthy people always enjoy the proper amounts of these most important hormones because the genes provide nothing until the right hormone arrives. Conversely, middle age begins to occur when the quality of the information delivered to the cells by these most powerful hormones begins to deteriorate. Again, good genetics provides nothing if one's glands begin to fail. One of the consequences of middle age with a large component of causality in the deteriorating message content concerns obesity.

Almost all the body cells have a complete genetic program. Gene activation sufficiency determines the adequacy of that cell's protein makeup. Recall, proteins comprise the metabolically active constituent of the body. Logically it then follows that the genetic program (genes) activity determines much about the cell repair rates, rejuvenation rates, functional ability and the overall integrity of the cell. Paradoxically, mainstream medicine often overlooks the central importance, for continued youthfulness, of bodies possessing correct message content directing their cells.

"Steroid tone" is measured by a well-run, 24-hour urine test. It provides a "hormone report card" for these most important body hormones. The more optimal amounts, of the different steroids proportional to one another, the higher the "steroid tone" becomes. Adequate rejuvenation and repair activity occurring requires a sufficient amount of "steroid tone". A high "steroid tone" signifies that there are optimal proportions of message content among the various steroids.

In other words, the catabolic message content balances with the anabolic message content. Unhealthy owners suffer from poor quality hormone message content. Their health will continue to deteriorate until improved message content delivery occurs.

"Steroid pressure" provides another useful basis that helps to visualize the behavior of steroids once released from their glands of origin. Only the most powerful hormones (steroids, Vitamin A, and thyroid) can access all body tissues and chambers. There are essentially no barriers to their penetration. Consequently, the amount of their presence within the body periphery (the joints, bones and skin) is determined mostly by their initial amount of release from their gland of origin.

Like smoke in a room, which moves from a high concentration to a lower concentration peripherally, steroids similarly, diffuse towards the periphery of the body kingdom.

A poor steroid generation rate at the source (the adrenals and gonads), diminishes the pressure head. It is the peripheral tissues that suffer first. Therefore, falling "steroid pressure" manifests as wrinkled skin, painful joints and osteoporosis.

The periphery of the body kingdom is the most vulnerable because the presence of rejuvenation message content falls off here most severely because these tissues are furthest from the source of this information.

"Steroid tone" quantifies the quality of the steroid message content reaching the body cells. Different types of steroids have unique and precise shapes. It is the unique shape that conveys the message. Change the shape and the message content changes.

"Steroid pressure" quantifies the amount of a specific steroid reaching the body cells. For example an adequate androgen message directs sufficient rejuvenation activities. In contrast, inadequate androgen message content leads the body's cells to fall into disrepair.

The signs of disrepair show up first in the periphery:

The skin
The joints
The bones

4. Stress Hormones and Weight Gain

The stress hormones cortisol and epinephrine are both made and secreted by the adrenal glands. This subsection

concerns the cortisol component of the stress response. High levels of cortisol, as seen in the stress response, consume body structure to maximize energy, a catabolic effect.

The first facet of the stress response and weight gain

Sadly, the association between the chronic activation of the stress response and its tendency to promote obesity is often not mentioned within the mainstream medical approach. Even though the fact is that when owners remain sedentary and they continually experience mental stress, whether real or imagined, more insulin needs to be released. The more insulin released the greater the message content to create fat. How does increased mental stress create increased insulin need?

Well the first part of the answer arises because the body cannot discern the difference between mental and physical stress. Therefore the physiological changes in both instances are the same. The physiology of the stress response largely involves outdated energy channeling when mental stress occurs. Even though mental stress does not need increased blood fuel (sugar, fat and amino acids) to survive, the body responds by dumping fuel into the blood stream as if a physical challenge was forthcoming. In prehistoric times the extra fuel was advantageous because the fuel allowed increased strength within the muscles for running from the jaws of some large animal.

In contrast, modern stress is largely mental in nature. The extra fuel released consequently has nowhere to go. The body eventually figures out that it has been fooled into dumping massive amounts of sugar (some of it derived from protein breakdown) into the blood stream. Prolonged elevated blood sugar eventually mandates that insulin secrete out of the pancreas. Remember insulin always arrives in the liver first and directs it to suck up the sugar out of the blood stream to rectify the situation. In addition, the more insulin within a liver the more fat making machinery activated.

Magnifying the chronic damage concerns the fact that increased cortisol secreted out of the adrenals, during mental stress, makes protein breakdown fair game. Remember the body thinks an emergent situation exists so that it sacrifices functional tissue, protein, to increase blood fuel (gluconeogenesis describes this process of converting protein into sugar). However, mental stress day in and day out provides a chronic wasting mechanism directed against precious body proteins.

The process described above elucidates how chronic mental stress slowly depletes body protein and increases body fat. Visualize the overall hormone directed shift of body energy away from functional tissue, protein, and into storage as fat: A wasting disease hiding amongst the fat describes this process.

These mental stress induced hormonal consequences elucidate why the old adage about walking it off has merit: Exercise causes the extra fuel within the blood stream to be sucked into the muscles and combusted for the creation of energy. Exercise also increases androgen production, Growth Hormone output and IGF-1 secretion rates. All these hormones combat the need for insulin (see previous discussion).

The stress response and the second facet of weight gain

The major hormone of the stress response is cortisol. Remember that cortisol is from the steroid class called catabolic. Catabolic hormone's message content concerns the consuming of body structure for fuel release into the blood stream. Making matters worse, unhealthy owners suffer from other hormone increases as well which facilitate fuel delivery but are paid for with the consequence of consuming body structure between meals and when stressed. The detrimental consequences occur towards body structure in the form of lost muscle, bone and functional organ mass.

This largely ignored medical fact explains itself again by the fact that unhealthy bodies lack a sufficient stimulus or ability for Growth Hormone's release. Only when adequate Growth Hormone secretes, from the pituitary, will there be a sufficient counter message to prevent protein destruction for fuel needs. Muscles and organs are made from protein. Growth Hormone's presence impedes the combustion of protein when blood fuel levels fall. Instead, Growth Hormone preferentially directs the liver and fat cells to dump sugar and fat into the blood stream while sparing protein. Realize, this fact partially explains why healthy owners have nice muscles while unhealthy owners do not.

The basic sequence of unhealthy owner's body protein's destruction when they experience stress, are between meals or when they attempt to exercise depends on other hormones. The entire group consists of glucagon, cortisol and epinephrine. Like Growth Hormone they all facilitate the release of sugar and fat into the blood stream. However, unlike Growth Hormone body protein dismantling becomes fair game when Growth Hormone levels prove insufficient.

Here again another vicious process destroys the physiques of countless middle-aged owners until they understand the importance of protecting their body's protein content.

A deeper insight into the abnormal stress response occurring in the unhealthy owner

As if the body structure consumption facilitated by cortisol when Growth Hormone levels diminish wasn't bad enough, there is an additional obesity perpetuator and muscle loss facilitator to consider: Middle-aged and obese owners have an increasing tendency for their adrenal glands to make more cortisol and less DHEA.

Healthy owners secrete approximately two times the DHEA compared to cortisol during the stress response. This fact prevents the catabolic message contained in cortisol from becoming too aggressive. In this way some of the body cells give up structure during the stress response while others continue repairing and rejuvenating.

Around middle age a steep fall off in this optimal ratio between the adrenally released opposing steroids occurs: Cortisol tends to greatly increase relative to DHEA. In other words survival ability (the stress response involving cortisol) maintains itself at the expense of the repair and rejuvenation rate (DHEA). Hence, most middle-aged owners' adrenal secretion lacks sufficient rejuvenation ability and this is why the 'wear and tear' look begins to accelerate after age 40.

Remember, DHEA is the major androgen steroid that instructs the liver to make IGF-1. Although testosterone levels also contribute to the IGF-1 manufacture rate within the liver it proves less important, in females because it usually is one hundredth the DHEA blood levels. Conversely, men's testicles secrete about 33% of the androgen as testosterone and thus enjoy a backup system not available to women.

Remember, IGF-1 facilitates muscle nutrition and impedes fat accumulation. A fall off of IGF-1 will necessitate an increased release of insulin. Insulin contains the fat maker message.

This last fact, taken together with the need for increased insulin whenever mental stress occurs (without a compensatory walk off the stress experience) explains how the fat maker message amplifies. A falling DHEA secretion rate from the adrenal gland accompanies middle age. A chronic stress response amplifies this problem because more cortisol secretes relative to the DHEA released.

Until these owners improve their DHEA levels, manage their stress and increase their Growth Hormone promoting activities these owners' muscles and organs will shrink while their metabolic loss (proteins) hides amongst the ever-increasing fat mass.

5. High Estrogen Levels Can Promote Obesity

Estrogen: a steroid hormone made in the adrenals, ovaries and very small amounts are also made in the testes. Fat cells can also make significant estrogen from the testosterone floating its way. The estrogen message contains a component for instructing cells to divide. High estrogen levels also initiate a circuitous message to increase body fat when its levels become too high compared to androgens (testosterone and DHEA).

When estrogen levels increase above normal, the potential arises to promote two of the hormonal factors creating obesity: The ability of estrogen to raise insulin and lower androgens, in certain females, describes these two factors.

Three main clinical situations promote estrogen induced weight gain. Not all female owners will express these tendencies equally. This variability may have a genetic basis. Not all women with increased estrogen states tend to gain weight equally. However, high estrogen states tend to promote weight gain in many female owners. This fact will be the focus of this subsection. Compounding the problem concerns the fact that excessive fat increases the rate of testosterone turning into estrogen!

The first clinical example for estrogen induced weight gain results from birth control pills. They predictably increase insulin in the body. The first mechanism for this situation arises from an abnormal hormone tandem that high estrogen levels cause.

The first part of the hormone tandem involves the high estrogen induced increased release rates of Growth Hormone from the pituitary gland. This occurs in the increased estrogen states that result from birth control pill usage. Recall, Growth Hormone release initially raises the blood sugar level. However, it is the second hormone in the normal tandem that estrogen simultaneously inhibits, which alters the normal pattern of events.

So when estrogen levels remain optimal, the release of Growth Hormone directs the simultaneous release of insulin-like growth factor (IGF-1, the second hormone in the tandem) along with the liver stored sugar and fat. As was previously discussed, IGF-1 has powerful insulin-like blood sugar lowering message content. Consequently, IGF-1 released lowers the blood sugar that the secreted Growth Hormone initially caused to elevate. Notice, here extra insulin is not needed.

Normally, this tandem hormone effect provides an effective way between meals for the cells to receive fuel from the blood stream, without raising insulin levels. Conversely, high estrogen states, although they initially stimulate Growth Hormone release, counteracts the normal tandem by inhibiting insulin-like growth factor release (IGF-1). **Realize the normal hormone tandem interrupts because excessive estrogen causes the simultaneous inhibition of IGF-1 release.**

It was previously mentioned that IGF-1 is an insulin-like hormone that acts almost exclusively in the cells outside the liver and fat. Consequently, its presence lowers the amount of insulin needed by the body. The IGF-1 released assists insulin by taking sugar out of the blood stream and into the cells outside the liver and fat. However, when IGF-1 levels diminish, the Growth Hormone released is uncompensated and this elevates the blood sugar. As a consequence, more insulin needs to be secreted from the liver to make up the deficit of total *fuel nozzle* hormones. The more insulin secreted, the more message content arriving within the liver to make body fat.

The second clinical situation of estrogen-caused obesity involves increased prolactin levels caused by the increased estrogen state of birth control use and/or stress filled lifestyles. Prolactin inhibits ovarian hormone formation and release. Mentally summarize that when prolactin increases the ovary thinks the body is pregnant or survival is at risk.

Fortunately, this hormone-induced mechanism, favoring obesity, generally does not operate in pregnancy because this physiologic state possesses a growing placenta. The growing placenta, in the pregnant state, more than offsets the prolactin induced inhibition of the ovaries by its serving as a hormonal factory for steroid production.

However, birth control pill usage fools the body into thinking it is pregnant. Prolactin levels rise in response to either increased estrogen or cortisol. However, in either of the above cases, there is no placental hormone factory to make up the prolactin caused androgen deficiency.

In a real pregnancy, the placenta manufactures androgens even though the ovaries become relatively dormant by the fifth month of gestation. When a female owner takes birth control pills, their body thinks it is pregnant. During birth control pill usage, prolactin levels rise because estrogen levels approach pregnancy levels. However, with birth control pill usage there is no placenta to manufacture the androgen lost when the ovaries become inhibited by excessive prolactin.

Potential obesity problems occur because, like pregnancy, the birth control pills increase prolactin levels. Unlike pregnancy, there is no placenta (hormone factory) to correct the inhibition of steroid production within the ovaries. The potential for problems compound due to the fact that the birth control pill does not contain androgens, only estrogen and progestins (abnormally shaped progesterone substitutes). Androgen production can fall within these owners because their adrenals are left all alone for this task. Some female's adrenals fail at the challenge of increased androgen production and obesity ensues.

The third clinical situation of high estrogen-induced obesity is beyond the level of this discussion. For those who are curious, it involves the dramatic increase of sex hormone-binding globulin that high estrogen levels direct. Androgen that may be produced by the ovary or adrenals, in high estrogen states, binds to a carrier protein in the blood stream at 98% of the efficiency level. Until some other metabolic change occurs, 98% of the measurable androgens, like testosterone cannot exit into the cells. Instead, this fraction circulates around and around bound to its carrier protein.

6. Adrenaline deficiency as a cause for obesity

Adrenaline message delivery depends upon its completed receptor being present on the recipient cell. The adrenaline receptor is a protein that requires both sufficient cortisol and thyroid message content instructing the appropriate genes coding for its manufacture. Realize, adrenaline activates the receptors that these two more powerful hormones directed to be manufactured. Consequently, only when there are sufficient receptors can adrenaline's message be heard by the target cells.

Adrenaline that releases under these normal circumstances causes metabolism to increase. When metabolism increases, fuel consumption increases. In addition, sufficient adrenaline proves as a powerful inhibitor for insulin release. Because the popular weight loss nutriceutical, ephedra, is molecularly similar to adrenaline, this explains its continued demand.

Some owners suffer from various forms of adrenal insufficiency. It is of little use to manufacture sufficient thyroid hormone and cortisol when the body experiences inadequate adrenal function from the lack of adrenaline. The manufacture of thyroid hormone takes place in the thyroid gland. The manufacture of cortisol takes place in the adrenal cortex. When the cortex fails, the diminished ability to make one or more adrenal steroids becomes the problem. Adrenaline manufacture needs to follow up on what both the thyroid and cortisol message started in the creation of adrenaline receptors.

Overtaxed adrenal glands can often masquerade as a thyroid problem. These owners walk like a thyroid problem and talk like a thyroid problem, but they are not a thyroid problem. Patients feel lousy and intuitively sense something is wrong. These owners' standard fatigue work-ups come back normal at their doctor's office.

A superficial inquiry leads to superficial platitudes and the statement that nothing is wrong. Some of these owners end up on antidepressants. How can this be? Further intrigue occurs when one includes the many depressed and overweight owners who note a marked lifting of their depressive like symptoms while taking ephedra (probably the real reason it gets bashed as dangerous while the more dangerous drugs, like aspirin, still sells over the counter).

A common example is revealed when one understands where adrenaline (epinephrine) derives from. Twenty different amino acids occur that, when arranged uniquely in sequence, type, and amount become the various proteins. The body manufactures most of these de novo (from scratch). Eight essential amino acids must be obtained in the diet. The egg provides the only food source that contains all eight. All other protein sources are deficient in one or more amino acids. Adrenaline derives from the essential amino acid phenylalanine.

The above discussion explains the importance of attaining adequate phenylalanine in the diet but there is a subtle and often overlooked reason for adrenaline deficiency.

Protein disassembly requires adequate stomach acid and digestive juices if essential amino acid supply lines are to be maintained. Owners who lack sufficient stomach acid and/or digestive juices tend to become deficient in essential amino acids necessary for the reactions of life. Deficient adrenaline manufacture describes one of the problems that can ensue due to ineffective digestive ability to dismantle protein into its individual amino acids.

A quick recap (chapter 3) of another cause of adrenaline (epinephrine) deficiency concerns the failure to obtain the necessary molecular building blocks for its manufacture. Most adrenaline is made from phenylalanine or the closely related amino acid, tyrosine. Physicians understand this much. Unfortunately, vitamins and cofactors, which are necessary to make either one of these amino acids into adrenaline, often go unnoticed. Deficiency of any one of these halts this critical hormone's biosynthesis. The nutrients necessary for the manufacture of adrenaline are: tetrahydrobiopterin (folate derived), vitamin C, vitamin B6, vitamin B12, folate, methionine, and SAMe (S-adenosyl methionine). The most common deficiency arises from a deficiency of SAMe which clinically evidences by an increase of blood homocysteine levels. SAMe is part of the important methyl donor system and was explained in the high blood pressure chapter.

A deficiency in one or more vitamins and cofactors results in health problems. These additional health problems develop because the adrenal secretes partially manufactured adrenaline (dopamine or nor-adrenaline) into the blood stream. When this occurs, deficiencies of one or more vitamins exist. Dopamine and nor-adrenaline have different shapes, therefore, a different message. A different message results when altered molecules bind to the adrenaline-like receptors.

When elevated amounts of nor-adrenaline enter the blood stream instead of adrenaline, a drastic increased tendency toward high blood pressure occurs. A single, simple vitamin deficiency can physiologically be the cause of elevated blood pressure. Some of these hypertensive owners may prefer taking vitamins. In this case, vitamins instead of blood pressure medicine lead to healing without the predictable side effects (see chapter three).

When was the last time a mainstream medical doctor inquired about these possibilities before prescribing medication? Please note, it is not the intent of this discussion to cast disparaging remarks on the many caring and kind physicians in practice today. It has been quite a shock to this author, while researching this work, the numerous holes in physicians (and this author's) educational exposure addressing healing versus symptom control. Usually the physician is not the one to blame, but rather, the way that simple concepts continually and knowingly continue to be withheld. The motive is money.

7. Insulin-like Growth Factor Type 1 (IGF-1)

The Seventh Hormone to Consider for Healing Obesity

Insulin like growth factor type-1 has been discussed earlier in relationship to how it lowers total body insulin requirements. Also discussed was how normal levels of it keep the fat making machinery, within the liver, quiescent. Before leaving the glandular component of obesities' propagation a few summary statements need to be made about the important role IGF-1 has towards the body cell's nutrition status.

As long as, a sufficient amount of liver manufactured IGF-1 releases into an owner's blood stream daily, there will be less need for insulin. Insulin release in healthy owners falls to very near zero between meals. However, unhealthy owners often need massive increases in their insulin levels between meals because IGF-1 levels have fallen.

When IGF-1 levels fall, increased amounts of insulin are needed outside of the liver and fat so that other body cells can receive nutrition. The trouble with increased insulin exposure, needed to make up for the nutritional message deficit within the other body cells, regards its additional fat maker role. Whatever the insulin release rate, the liver always receives the highest message content via the portal vein. Unlike IGF-1, insulin delivers a powerful message within the liver and fat cells to uptake excessive sugar and changes it into fat and cholesterol.

Healthy owners gain weight less readily because their cells, like muscle and heart, receive their nutrition with the help of adequate IGF-1. Conversely, unhealthy owners suffer from diminished IGF-1 levels so they will need excess insulin in order for their cells to uptake nutrition. By this mechanism, high insulin release rates make an owner fat.

Healthy insulin levels cause the liver to store just the right amount of fat and sugar within the liver and fat cells following meals (a blood sugar rising event). In addition, healthy owners between meals or while exercising (a blood sugar falling

event), release this stored fuel and IGF-1 under the direction of increased Growth Hormone. In this way the healthy owner has sufficient blood fuel and *fuel nozzle* hormones to feed his/her cells from one meal to the next.

The liver chapter explains more of the particulars on how important a high IGF-1 level is in regards to body health. Here it is only important to understand how, when IGF-1 falls, the insulin level needs to rise. Insulin needs to rise because when the other *fuel nozzle* hormone becomes scarce hungry cells scream out for fuel. Insulin on the rise means fat making will also be on the rise. Conversely, IGF-1 levels (at healthy levels) facilitate muscle and organ development from sufficient nutrition. Well-fed cells greatly diminish the amount of insulin needed.

IGF-1 is the villain or youthful marker?

Finally, it is important to again acknowledge the numerous unfavorable articles currently in print about IGF-1 and its supposed role in cancer development. The holistic picture about IGF-1 would acknowledge that ample cell nutrition plays the role of a double-edged sword. Once cancer forms, a normal IGF-1 level helps with the tumor's nutrition needs. This explains why emaciated types of individuals, despite their weakened and deteriorating body habitués, would tend to have a lower tumor growth rate. Left out of the discussion concerns their quality of life within their aged body. The body that has both low insulin and IGF-1 describes a body that has starving cells. Here tumor cells starve as well.

On the other side of this double edged sword concerns the facts that adolescents, athletes, pregnancy, regular fasting, nice muscles and a lean body mass, a good nights sleep and youthful vigor all associate with the highest IGF-1 levels. Yet, these conditions are certainly regarded as desirable by mainstream medicine. In addition, epidemiologically collected data regarding the desirability of the above states powerfully contradicts the popular scientific campaign to vilify adequate IGF-1. They cannot have it both ways. High insulin levels are the true culprit in determining poor outcomes once cancer occurs. How can this blatant statement be defended?

Well, by comparing the similarities of an infant's body and hormones to those of a typical Syndrome X type, insight follows. Both the healthy infant and the middle aged Syndrome X body have abundant abdominal fat. They both have excessive insulin exposure and low IGF-1 levels. But in the infant it is advantageous and in the Syndrome X it is deleterious. How can this be?

The difference is explained by the fact that the infant contains cells that are supposed to be dividing (growing). In contrast, the middle aged Syndrome X owner doesn't need to increase his/her cell division propensity. Cell division propensity forms a primary determinant of tumor growth. Obesity requires high insulin exposure. Tumors of the breast, pancreas, lung, colon, and prostate metastasize more readily in the obese owner. Rather than simply acknowledging this fact about obesity and its relationship to insulin, IGF-1 receives the blame by circuitous methodologies. As more physicians become aware of these facts they will begin to ferret out these shenanigans.

Lastly, physicians need to keep in mind the lack of even a cursory discussion for IGF-1's role in glucose metabolism in the syndrome X body. Along with this cognizance they need to also realize that the healthiest of owners contain the highest IGF-1 levels. In addition, realize that IGF-1 levels increase through childhood and finally peak around adulthood as the muscles, organs and bones reach their prime. The rise in DHEA levels parallel these changes. The onset of middle age witnesses a fall in IGF-1 and hence increased insulin need. Those middle aged owners that possess a pancreas capable of secreting excessive insulin, at this time in their lives, notice an expanding waistline much like infancy. Think about these facts before succumbing to the complex's confusing tactics.

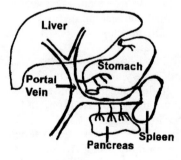

CHAPTER FIVE

ADRENAL GLANDS

The adrenal glands sit on top of each kidney. They are about the size and shape of an acorn. The 'seed' makes the adrenaline and is directly wired into the sympathetic nervous system. This sympathetic nerve connection facilitates the release of adrenaline. Adrenaline conveys an overall body message of both alertness and increased metabolism. The 'cap' makes the adrenal steroid hormones (aldosterone, DHEA, progesterone, androstenedione, and cortisol) from cholesterol. Aldosterone proves as a key hormone in the regulation of salt and water balance and its amount also controls the rate of all other steroid's manufacture rates. DHEA and cortisol can be thought of as counter regulatory opposites.

As cortisol levels rise, the message that directs cellular energy into survival pathways increases. Recall, the primitive survival response is the same whether a stress proves real or imagined. It is also the same whether it proves physical or mental in nature. The fallout of this truism means that whatever the stress, massive fuel dumps into the blood stream. Physical stresses need extra fuel to survive them but mental stress does not. Cortisol provides blood fuel by dismantling body structure. The fuel generating vulnerable body components consists of sugar, fat and protein. By definition hormones that dismantle body structure for fuel needs are called catabolic.

This redirection of cellular energy occurs whenever cortisol levels rise beyond a very low threshold. In the healthy state low levels of cortisol (below the threshold) provide anti-inflammatory, cellular rest, sodium and fluid retention, and maintain blood vessel responsiveness to adrenaline's message.

Conversely, DHEA and androstenedione are from the androgen class of hormones that direct body energy into cellular infrastructure investment activities that lead to cellular rejuvenation. Note that the androgen steroids provide the opposite message compared to the catabolic hormones. As an aside, insulin proves anabolic for fat and cholesterol accumulation (explained later).

True anabolic steroids build up the protein component of the body tissue (muscles, joints and organs functional components).

Proteins comprise the metabolically active component of body tissue. In other words, their presence burns up calories. Examples of proteins that consume energy while they function are: enzymes, some hormone types, cell receptors, muscle proteins (actin and myosin) and membrane pumps. The more of these one has, the more calories burned. The more calories burned, the faster the metabolic rate.

The role of progesterone within the adrenal also seems to counter the salt and water retaining effects of cortisol and aldosterone. Progesterone in women is manufactured in both their adrenals and ovaries. Some women have weakened adrenals and when ovarian progesterone production slows just before their menstruation their progesterone levels fall too far. These women, just before their menstruation, experience first hand the fluid retaining effects that occur when progesterone levels suddenly plummet. They can also experience anxiety and mental irritability (PMS).

These symptoms shed light on the calming effect of progesterone within the central nervous system. In fact it has been known for many years that high doses of progesterone produce anesthesia from the increased GABA that results within the neurons of the brain and spinal cord. Progesterone rises considerably during pregnancy. Pregnant women also possess a calming beauty and note frequent urination as well. Both of these facts further elucidate progesterone's powerful message content within the body.

An ongoing 'tug of war' exists between adrenal androgen and cortisol message content. Modern life complexities often cause chronic stress that increases cortisol output relative to other adrenal androgens. Typical modern stress comes in the form of deadlines, job insecurities, complex multiple task responsibilities, and incessant noise, to name a few. If one adds in the increased consumption of carbohydrate, which increases the need for more cortisol in many middle-aged owners, gland exhaustion becomes possible.

Increased cortisol becomes necessary to balance the effects of increased insulin within the blood stream of unhealthy owners (explained below). One gains insight, about this modern day problem, by considering the excessive counter-regulatory response necessary to keep extra insulin behaving within the blood stream.

Low blood sugar often provides the first clinical sign that the adrenal glands are beginning to fail in the output of cortisol (stress hormone). Increased cortisol becomes necessary in order to deal with the stress of modern life and the stress of having extra insulin. When the cortisol level becomes inadequate the first symptom is often 'brain fog'. 'Brain fog' provides a warning sign that something is wrong with the hormonal balance. The loss of balance incrementally leads to an amplification of the mental problem.

Balanced hormonal responses create a cellular communication harmony that underlies the healthful state. As the adrenals lose their ability to respond to the demands for balance, 'brain fog' ensues.

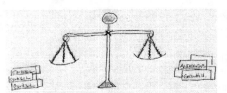

As stated above, the androgen class of steroid hormones within the adrenal glands is DHEA and androstenedione. While DHEA is mostly secreted by the adrenal gland, androstenedione is made by the ovary, testicle and adrenal gland. DHEA only will be discussed here, but the reader can also extend this as applicable to androstenedione.

Cutting edge scientific thought: Different body tissues prefer to interact with different androgens. DHEA proves particularly important in females as it displays the utility of peripheral conversion into the more powerful androgens like testosterone once inside the recipient cell (muscle, ligament, bone). Peripheral conversion spares females the masculine effects of dumping straight testosterone into their blood streams. DHEA and androstenedione (steroid precursors) are much weaker androgens than testosterone. Peripheral conversion denotes the process of where steroid precursors initially secreted into the blood stream later convert into more powerful steroids within the target cell. This process is particularly important for women.

Over the last several years it has come to be realized that women, pound for pound of functional tissue, need just as much testosterone as men. However, women derive 99% of their testosterone in a sex neutral fashion (the process of peripheral conversion). Conversely, mens' testicles release testosterone (33%of total androgen) straight into the blood stream and this masculinizes them. The other 66% in men comes from the peripheral conversion process (sex neutral). Bottom line: peripheral conversion describes a process where powerful androgens arise from weak androgens within the recipient cell. Androgens determine much about the ability to repair the wear and tear of life.

DHEA, once it converts into powerful androgens, directs cellular energy into cellular infrastructure investment activities (an anabolic effect). Regular infrastructure investment proves necessary for continued health. Testosterone and DHEA differ in the strength of their message content to direct masculine traits. Brilliantly, the female body initially secrets the much weaker androgen, DHEA and later peripherally converts it to testosterone within the recipient cell. This approach leads to sufficient repair but allows diminished masculine message carried within the blood stream. It also allows the body's wisdom to activate or ignore it. For example, the endometrial cells cannot activate DHEA and hence this steroid precursor cannot stimulate uterine bleeding.

Unfortunately, as the adrenal loses its ability to keep up with the demands for its hormonal products, DHEA manufacture can be the first to drop off. This imbalance is often missed clinically. At this level of dysfunction there are only subtle clues. Realize, females are more vulnerable to the ravages of diminished DHEA production because there is less androgen output from the ovaries (1%), relative to the male testes (33%). These patients tend to present with increased fatigue, some with increased fat and the earliest signs of deteriorating musculoskeletal structures.

As stress continues, the adrenal glands of some owners cease to make adequate cortisol to counter balance insulin's blood sugar lowering message and this causes "brain fog". "Brain fog" often indicates adrenal imbalance has continued long enough for moderate body cellular damage to occur. Cellular damage arises secondary to the prolonged survival message that directs the body's energy away from rejuvenation activities.

At a cellular level, the lack of rejuvenation activities leads to old cellular components - old cell factories (organelles), old cellular machines (enzymes), and diminished cellular charge (the battery) – plainly, old age.

The body possesses a backup system within the gonads for specific steroid type hormones (not cortisol or DHEA). The amount of DHEA produced within the healthy adrenal gland can be 100 times more than the amount of testosterone produced within the ovary. The amount of androstenedione production within female ovaries, under the best of circumstances, approaches one-fifth the adrenal amount of DHEA normally produced. The ovary functions poorly for secreting DHEA. For these reasons, internal havoc is probable when the adrenal becomes wounded. The wounded adrenal gland led to the description of diminished adrenal reserve over fifty years ago.

Diminished Adrenal Reserve Syndrome

In the 1950's John W. Tintera, MD, pioneered the concept of early adrenal exhaustion. He noted that early adrenal exhaustion often results from prolonged stress and added this to the previously accepted causes. Some of the other causes were various infections, hemorrhage, and genetic defects for certain adrenal steroids manufacture and medication side effects. The focus here regards how stress leads the way to diminished adrenal function and how this will always manifest with a tendency for low blood sugar episodes.

In 1955, he published a paper in the New York State Journal of Medicine that included over 200 cases of patients with sub-optimal adrenal function. He discovered that 100 percent of these patients had low blood sugar episodes along with their other complaints that occur with the diagnosis of adrenal insufficiency. He called this state of sub-optimal adrenal function, hypo-adrenal-corticism.

Years later it was established that cortisol, secreted from the adrenal gland, proved as a powerful counter regulatory hormone to the blood sugar lowering effects of insulin. As the adrenals in these patients began to fail in their ability to counter the message of insulin, these patients would present with low blood sugars. The low blood sugars result from too much insulin and not enough cortisol to balance out the message content.

The body design includes a system of counter balanced hormones. When secreted, a given hormone always needs a counter balancing response from an opposing hormone or group of hormones. The balancing hormones direct energy expenditure so energy never moves too far in any direction.

Recall, diminished IGF-1 requires the abnormal increase of insulin in the fasting state (a blood sugar falling event) in order to stay alive. Insulin always arrives in the liver first. However, this anatomical fact compounds the falling blood sugar. The abnormal need for insulin, in the fasting state, causes the excessive need for counter regulatory hormones to offset the anatomical fact that insulin arrives within the liver first before any of it makes it beyond the liver to help deliver fuel to the hungry cells. Within the liver, insulin powerfully instructs the liver to remove sugar from the blood stream but realize that this exacerbates the falling blood sugar occurring in the fasting state.

Out of the counter regulatory hormones, cortisol most effectively moderates the effect of insulin. The balance between these two hormones avoids going too far in any one direction for energy expenditure. Disease results when this balancing system impairs. Dr. Tintera correctly deduced that when prolonged stress depleted the ability of the adrenal to respond as a counter balance to insulin, blood sugar regulation diminished. Patients with impaired adrenals are unable to secrete sufficient cortisol so their blood sugars become unstable. For these reasons, these patients remain more vulnerable to the threat of hypoglycemia.

In general, an important point to remember about these patients: Many years before their adrenals' lost the ability to produce sufficient cortisol, these glands sacrificed their ability to make sufficient anabolic steroids. This explains the emaciated appearance of most of these patients. Visualize the severe loss of functional tissue preceding the loss of blood sugar balance. Begin to consider the many faces of glandular failure.

Over fifty years later, new hormonal understandings about the ideal blood sugar regulator between meals being Growth Hormone come into play for the youthful body to continue (explained in the liver chapter). For now it is only important to realize that first Growth Hormone levels fall in these patients. This fact exaggerates the need for insulin within the body (insulin resistance).

In the between meals state, instead of Growth Hormone causing the continued secretion of blood fuel, cortisol needs to pick up the slack. **Dr. Herb Joiner-Bey** points out (private discussion) that increased cortisol secretion proves violent to body structure because it accelerates protein dismantling where Growth Hormone does not. In fact, Growth Hormone proves as the only hormone to protect body protein content between meals and while exercising. Healthy bodies have ample protein content within their muscles and organs. Unhealthy bodies do not.

Again, hormones always need opposition from counter hormones to maintain balance. It helps to understand balance if one envisions an antique weight scale. In general, whenever there is a hormone secreted (weight), an adequate counter hormone response (counter weight) needs to occur or health cannot continue. Healthy owners have balanced 'weight scales'. Their bodies secrete the very best hormones in their optimal amounts. Their counter response hormones also secrete in the optimal amount and with appropriate timing.

Thankfully, improved laboratory testing developed over the last 40 years has led to more accurate testing of patient's hormone profiles. Unfortunately, owners in America live in a profit driven health care system. The profit motive results in the inferior $25,000

131

solution receiving press coverage while the more effective $1,000 solution collects dust or remains ignored. The basic knowledge of what science has revealed empowers an owner who suffers from diminished adrenal function.

For example, the technology of gas chromatography mass spectometry (GC mass spec) accurately measures hormones and their important metabolites spilling into the urine. Unfortunately, the increasingly suspicious and doubtful salivary and serum assays remain the standard of care. This inferior practice continues despite the scientist of the world increasingly laughing at any doctor that makes hormonal treatment decisions based on these suspect methods. In contrast, the more accurate method of using GC mass spec technology approach opens up options that can lead to healing instead of symptom control. In addition, this knowledge allows awareness of some inconsistencies perpetrated by the profit motive of the medical industrial complex.

Diminished adrenal reserve steps off of the path of health. The body wants to heal from adrenal insufficiency. The adrenals of some owners will never fully recover. After understanding some basics, the owner arrives at a place to begin on a journey towards renewed wellness. A competent, loving physician or health practitioner can coach the owner in this next step. This problem lends itself to a change in one's lifestyle and nutritional habits and often a need for real steroid hormonal support. Real hormones are the only treatment that leads to healing, not the fake hormones that always have side effects and toxicities.

Alternatively, all is not hopeless if one includes the consideration of certain plants that possess the ability to stimulate adrenal steroid production. Further research is warranted, but encouraging results have been achieved with high quality ginseng. Panax ginseng root, that is at least 7 years old, possesses a class of substances called the glycosides. By definition all glycosides possess the ability to form suds (foam). In order to avoid confusion, ginseng is best thought of as a steroid contained in a package. While this steroid is still in its 'package', it possesses properties of the surfactant class (helpful for asthmatics). The intelligence of the body decides whether it needs ginseng as the glycoside or as the broken down (package removed) steroid building block for the production of other steroids.

An interesting degree of inconsistency in the medical literature occurs, when inquiring into the utility of the plant glycosides as surfactants. Medical dictionaries and textbooks go on about how all plant glycosides are not orally absorbable. They further go on to caution the reader that if given intravenously they lead to rupture of cell membranes. The inconsistency of this statement is revealed when one understands that a very important oral heart medication being used for over 200 years comes from this class of plant substances. When looking up the class of drugs coming from the foxglove plant that make the various digitalis derivatives, it is stated that they are from the class of substances called the glycosides. It is further stated that absorption of most glycosides is almost 100% orally. There is nothing about the need to worry about these drugs causing cell membrane rupture. This information saves the inquiring reader from the common pitfalls that are holding back the usage of this valuable group of plant substances in the treatment of asthma and adrenal insufficiency.

The additional confusion over what ginseng will do for aging adrenals provides further insight into the deceptive scientific duplicity of using different vocabulary to hide common concepts. For years, as this author studied the peculiar biochemistry of ginseng, he came upon the names of the active ingredients in ginseng - saponins and sapogenins. Finally, he read Dr. John Lee's progesterone biochemistry text only to discover that some of the saponins and sapogenins were only a few molecules away from testosterone contained within a 'package'. The conceptual roadblock lifted and the explanation for all those fertile and gracefully aging Asians regularly taking ginseng began to make sense.

The duplicity of scientific vocabulary surfaces when one realizes that for prescription related drugs, these same plant substances are referred to as 'plant glycosides'. In contrast, when they are considered herbal substances they are referred to as containing saponins. When a curious physician inquires into the molecular makeup of the saponins, he finds a scientific roadblock. However, once he becomes aware of the duplicity, he can access a whole wealth of data. For example, the plant glycoside, digitalis, is related to testosterone in a package. If a curious physician ever got this far in the analysis, he would see how ginseng and digitalis share similar powers in their ability to provide the body with steroid precursors within a 'package'.

Ginseng stimulates gonads and adrenals in the aging body by virtue of providing ample steroid-like precursors as the critically needed steroid building block. If there is any life within the gonad, libido rises considerably as does male prowess. This is probably due to increased testosterone production. However, without certain nutritional factors being present in adequate supply an owner will see little effect from ginseng.

Some authorities feel that ginseng has an effect on stimulating the master hormone gland, the pituitary, in a beneficial way. This makes sense as Chinese medical theory purports that ginseng is an 'adaptogen' in the face of life stress. It may be that when the pituitary gland, located at the base of the brain, activates, there will be multiple benefits to the endocrine glands throughout the body. Examples would probably include thyroid, adrenal, gonads, and possibly the thymus. Ginseng is worth considering when ones' adrenals begin to fail. Ginseng may act on the body at other body locations beyond the adrenal.

Hormone Mimics

Hormone 'mimics' diminishes the health of adrenals and gonads. Pervasive and insidious effects of hormonal mimics surface as the worldwide phenomenon of falling sperm counts in men. Androgen levels are the primary determinant of a man's sperm count. Hormone mimics surface from environmental and nutritional sources. Around the world chemicals like DDT and Agent Orange have been implicated in the estrogen mimic effect. These mimics compete with men's androgen tone causing sperm counts to drop increasingly each decade.

The numerous common chemicals that exert a biochemical message effect along various degrees of estrogen mimicry initially sounds fantastical. However, when one considers that all estrogen mimics share a similar molecular shape with their estrogen counter part, it becomes conceptually consistent. The common shape in the 'key' of estrogen is technically called the aromatic ring. Trouble starts because these diverse chemicals also all contain this estrogen 'key' shape and once inside the body they lead to unnaturally high estrogen message content.

In many ways, estrogen and estrogen mimics are counter regulatory to the effect of androgens like testosterone. The most frightening aspect of turning up the estrogen message, in both men and women, is the powerful cell division message that certain estrogen and estrogen mimics deliver. For example, this property causes abnormal growths in the prostate tissues of some men - a prime cause of benign prostatic hypertrophy (BPH). In women, estrogen dominance (relative to progesterone) leads to an increased tendency towards developing fibrocystic breast disease, uterine fibroids, breast cancer, PMS, and others.

Plastic wrap, plastic food containers, and the liners inside canned foods all contain estrogen mimics. As a general guide, the higher the fat content, the greater the tendency for hormone mimics to migrate into the food. Prime environmental hormone disrupters are DDT, PCB's, and dioxin that are widely dispersed throughout the environment. DDT (a suspected carcinogenic in mammals), is an environmentally persistent insecticide that causes fragile and broken eggshells in wild birds. Estrogen-like substances stimulate cell growth in estrogen sensitive tissue.

Though banned in the late 1970's, PCB's used in transformers and other electrical components still persist throughout the environment.

The list of detrimental effects includes severe birth defects in people and animals, cancer in animals, as well as a link to intellectual deficits in children. These mimics clearly tend to stimulate cell division inappropriately.

Dioxins have been shown to cause cancer in both animals and humans and have acted like estrogen in animal studies. In 1979, the environmental protection agency banned some herbicides because they were contaminated with dioxins, but there are still numerous additional sources including paper bleaching facilities, polyvinyl chloride factories and trash incinerators. The EPA and industry modified industrial practices with some success, but it has proved difficult to eliminate them all.

Plasticizer compounds may leech from landfills into the environment, but do not seem to linger in human bodies. Two types of plasticizers suspect in causing problems are phthalates and adipates. In lab animals phthalates cause liver cancer and testicular damage. Adipates in animal studies link to shortened life spans and decreased fertility. Bisphenol A, a building block of plastic manufacture used in dental sealants and in food can liners causes enlarged prostates in animals.

There are several low cost strategies to avoid ingesting estrogen mimics. Reduce consumption of suspect compounds by avoiding plastic containers and wrappers. Consider using alternatives to pesticides and insecticides on both lawn and pets. Wash fruits and vegetables thoroughly or buy organic foods. Limit consumption of suspect fatty foods where these compounds accumulate in the food chain. Watch for local fish pollution possibilities. When reheating food, don't use plastic. Heat accelerates transfer of the hormone mimics into the food.

The adrenals and gonads share many similarities in their abilities to rejuvenate the body's cells. However, the adrenals perform unique roles in the maintenance of certain organ systems. The immune system provides an example of how the adrenals maintain health.

Adrenal Health Determines Immune Systems Appropriateness and Readiness

Many owners in America wake up tired, catch colds and cough frequently, and deal with stress poorly. Many have diffuse aches in their muscles and joints. The majority of these afflicted individuals suffer from depression and this often expresses as a lost zest for life. Most have allergies or asthma that worsens with prolonged stress and fatigue. In the more severe cases of diminished adrenal function, chronic degenerative diseases like rheumatoid arthritis, systemic lupus erythematosus, ulcerative colitis, Crohn disease, and fibromyalgia syndrome surface. Many of these ailments appear to be from divergent sources. However, often, each of these afflictions traces back to a poorly functioning adrenal system.

The science behind the dysfunctional adrenal-gland-system conflicts with the symptom control medicine approach. The complex panders the symptom control, medicinal philosophy. As a consequence, many physicians have no idea that a deeper understanding of adrenal function can often lead to considerable improvement in the above disease processes. Patients continue to suffer needlessly because their physicians have been groomed to think of the adrenals in a very superficial and piecemeal way.

Medical textbooks are curiously deficient in their discussion of interrelated consequences of a diminished adrenal reserve. Their discussion instead focuses only on the most extreme examples of adrenal dysfunction. Examples of these extremes are Addison's disease (cortisol deficiency) and Cushing's disease (cortisol excess).

A peripheral discussion might surface regarding the role of the adrenal hormone, cortisol, and its role in the prevention of hypoglycemia. Cortisol is the major player in the prevention of hypoglycemia for many middle-aged owners. Most textbook discussions concern hormones within the adrenal gland, but fail to unite the fact that adrenal steroid hormones secrete together in a preformed ratio. Making matters worse, a reoccurring tendency within the medical textbooks exists that completely ignores the concept that some owners may have diminished adrenal function under stressful conditions. However, these owners' level of dysfunction is not as severe as those of an Addisonian patient.

Doctors are taught to think about disease of the adrenal gland in a piecemeal fashion. Cushing's disease exemplifies this. A hallmark of this disease involves losing muscle and gaining body fat. Unfortunately, a consistent failure exists for emphasizing the reason body fat goes up and that it is not directly related to the markedly elevated cortisol levels that are present with this disease.

Cortisol initially promotes fat and sugar dumping into the blood stream. However, this property of cortisol fails to explain how increased body fat proves secondary to elevated blood sugar spikes (explained below). The elevated blood sugar results from the high cortisol message content, which then directs the liver to dismantle protein (gluconeogenesis) and glycogen. These processes allow the release of sugar into the blood stream. The body eventually realizes that the blood sugar has elevated inappropriately.

Unfortunately, elevated blood sugars suppress Growth Hormone secretion while it promotes the excessive release of insulin into the blood stream to counter this situation. The increase in insulin required to make the blood sugar normal leads to the increased making of body fat. Remember the pancreas secretes insulin into the portal vein and it heads straight into the liver connection (200,000 pure insulin receptors per liver cell).

Lost protein results from two other abnormal hormonal processes that occur with chronic stress and elevated insulin levels. The first part occurs secondary to the fact that elevated cortisol levels leads to increased prolactin release. Increases in prolactin levels inhibit the gonads release of androgens that constitute a counter weight to the high level of insulin's ability to make patients fat. Remember that the androgens promote muscle and organ growth and repair. The inhibition of the gonads is often left out of the textbook discussion.

Also left out of the discussion, concerns the additional fact that a slight elevation in the blood sugar, which cortisol causes, will inhibit Growth Hormone release. In turn, diminished Growth Hormone release will lead to a diminished ability to hold onto body proteins (liver chapter) and diminish IGF-1 release. Recall that IGF-1 is insulin's helper and occurs at levels one hundred times those of insulin in healthy owners. As Growth Hormone secretion falls off less IGF-1 secretes and this leads to excessive insulin need (insulin resistance). **This last little detail ties in Syndrome X (also known as metabolic syndrome or insulin resistance Syndrome) patients to a variant of Cushing's disease pathology (explained in inflammation and heart disease, heart chapter).** This specific disease example points to the incongruous discussion between the various hormone abnormalities occurring in these patients. Consequently, physicians are incompletely educated on how to think about adrenal disease.

Cushing's and Addison's disease exemplify extreme examples of adrenal dysfunction. Cushing' disease sufferers produce extremely high cortisol production rates. Conversely, Addison's disease describes an extreme deficiency of cortisol. In these cases, the deficiencies are so significant that viability can only be maintained by taking cortisol supplements.

What about those owners whose adrenal abnormality lie somewhere between these two extremes of adrenal dysfunction in stressful situations? Both of these situations have health consequences. Unfortunately, mainstream medicine most often recognizes only the extremes of adrenal dysfunction. *The consequence of this is that there are owners suffering, but not in immediate danger of death. This common medical practice is analogous to only considering thyroid dysfunction if it is on either extreme that puts the patient at risk for death.*

Science could help those owners with the above disease's improve their adrenal systems function. Curiously, this is not the case. Medical educations do a better job at alerting physicians to the subtleties of altered thyroid function and the diseases that follow. Before ways to heal from these diseases are discussed, there needs to be a discussion about two important facts. First, steroids have a powerful nature when compared to other body hormones. Second, different disease presentations result from the same common deficiency of cortisol and/or DHEA. Much is known about the first fact and an introductory discussion follows. Very little is understood about the second fact and this awaits further scientific investigation before a plausible explanation can be given. Be aware of this current mystery.

The common property of steroids, vitamin A and thyroid hormone deserve emphasis: These hormones are the most powerful of all hormones in the body. The steroids include testosterone, estrogen, DHEA, androstenedione, cortisol, progesterone, and aldosterone. Other steroids of less importance occur. The power of this group lies in the fact that only these hormone types carry their message directly to all the DNA

***programs throughout every cell in the body. No other hormones
directly influence the DNA program (genes).***
    These hormones interact with the genetic program. They
directly determine which genes turn off or on. Gene activity
determines which body proteins manifest. Healthy bodies have the
exact amount of protein types needed. Consequently, the only way
to possess the right amount of protein types involves one's cells
receiving the right amounts of these powerful hormones.
    Remember, the genes provide nothing until the right
hormone arrives. Therefore, the quality, type, and amount of these
powerful hormones determine how wisely the cells will spend their
available energy. These hormones carry their message by virtue of
their unique and precise shape. The steroids, vitamin A and thyroid
hormones differ from other hormones by binding directly with many
DNA receptors. They also access every body chamber.
    The unique properties of each of these hormones allow them
to be the determinants for which DNA programs activate or repress.
For this reason, owners that have the proper quality, amounts, and
timing of these hormones receive a tremendous health advantage.
The effectiveness of these hormones relates on into the quality and
amounts of the lesser hormones manufactured (see hierarchy of
hormones at the end of this section). Therefore, these hormones
prove as the most critical to consider out of all the hormones in the
body. Ways to heal begin with sufficiently considering their quality
within an owner.
    Remember, the power of these hormones lies in their control
of the genetic program. An excess or deficiency provides abnormal
message content to the DNA of the cells. When the wrong DNA
programs activate or repress, the cell spends energy unwisely.
Energy used foolishly on the wrong proteins, wrong repair to rest
ratios, wrong immune activation level, wrong amount of cell
product, etc. describes a disease process.
    Though the above diseases have somewhat predictable
abnormal hormone results, identical excesses or deficiencies will
initiate different diseases in different owners. This is only partially
understood and the understood portion is complex. Any of the six
links in the adrenal system chain will cause disease when it becomes
defective.

    In today's world of harried physicians and managed care, the
owner needs to be aware of the six levels where the adrenal system
can fail. Erroneously, most attention toward adrenal health inquiry
limits the focus to one or two levels only. Consequently, many

owners diagnosis are incorrect and/or they receive symptom control treatments. Thus owners miss out on ways to heal themselves. The next subsection explores the six levels of the adrenal system and how any one of these being defective leads to the above-mentioned adrenal system related diseases.

Uniting high stress and a defect within the adrenal system make any of the adrenal system diseases worse.

1. **Allergies**
2. **Asthma.**
3. **Colitis**
4. **Systemic lupus**
5. **Rheumatoid arthritis**
6. **Crohn's disease**

In this subsection the reasoning will be explored. Attention will be given as to why many well-meaning physicians looking for a diminished adrenal system function fail to find it. Often, they have not been trained to evaluate all six links in the adrenal system. **The chain in the adrenal system includes:**

1. **Hypothalamus in the brain**
2. **Master control panel gland for hormone glands, the pituitary, which hangs on the underside of the brain**
3. **Healthy adrenal gland function**
4. **Blood stream transport system**
5. **Complete, intact characteristics of the DNA receptor waiting for something to do within the target cell**
6. **Other DNA programs activation also results in the manufacture of certain protein-composed receptors for the 'lesser' hormones.**

A defect at any of the six levels behaves clinically as if the adrenal system functions improperly. Most physicians receive little instruction for evaluating the integrity of the entire system. The profit in treating symptoms of the above diseases overrides the incentive to educate physicians about the other side of the story. Unfortuantely, some lonely thinkers clunk along with some really good healing insights while the complex supports effective ways of marginalizing their scientific discoveries.

One of the heroes in the 'lonely thinker/scientist' category is William McKenzie Jefferies MD. Dr. Jefferies, the author of *Safe Uses of Cortisol,* 1996, brings over 45 years of clinical insight to the discussion of illness secondary to a malfunctioning adrenal system. His career in Endocrinology included professorships at both Case

Western Medical School and more recently at Virginia Medical School. All of the above diseases are discussed and reviewed in his book. This book is a must read for an owner with any of the listed diseases secondary to a poorly functioning adrenal system. Education is necessary to step beyond symptom control and into healing.

Many physicians have been effectively taught to fear cortisone like treatments over the long haul. This training has been so well performed that many physicians automatically respond negatively to hearing the word cortisone or steroid. This effect results from successfully confusing physicians and the public between the effects of cortisol within physiologic doses versus higher doses.

Further confusion results from failing to educate physicians on the basics of how the precise shape of the steroid delivers accurate message content. Once again, to repeat, only altered steroid shapes receive patent advantages. However, altered steroid shapes deliver inaccurate message content to one's DNA programs. Inaccurate message content leads to side effects and toxicities.

Additionally, the omitted fact that the optimal adrenal secretions contain pre-formed ratios between the different steroids listed earlier is perhaps even more damaging to overall middle-aged health. To only replace one when several prove deficient recreates even more message content disharmony. The above diseases arise from an adrenal deficiency. Each unique deficiency means the optimal proportions of the various adrenal steroids fail to arrive at the afflicted owners DNA programs.

The six links in the adrenal health chain follow and this discussion will elaborate on why this occurs. Without a complete inquiry into all six links, these diseases continue to smolder until they erupt. Diseases that erupt require symptom control and symptom control has side effects.

Successful media campaigns have persuaded physicians and owners into fearing even small doses of the natural body manufactured cortisol. This occurs despite the fact (evidence to be discussed shortly) that the diseases mentioned before have in common a deficiency of one or more adrenal steroids. In other words, these diseases often directly result from the failure to receive adequate adrenal steroids directions to their cells DNA programs.

An extension of Dr. Jefferies' work addresses the emerging realization that healthy, activated adrenals secrete a mixture of steroids in pre-formed ratios. This optimizes the message content of a healthy owner whenever the stress response activates. For this reason, only giving cortisol in all instances of the above diseases results in the potential for a lessened healing response. A lessened healing response follows from the exclusion of the other adrenal steroids, which the healthy adrenal normally produces.

To understand how the adrenal system becomes compromised, a brief review of the break down mechanisms amongst the different links is explained below. All links need to be performing at a basic level or the clinical manifestation of adrenal dysfunction caused disease manifests. Keep in mind that other, less recognized, adrenal steroid imbalances may contribute significantly to a disease process. Consequently, the twenty-four hour urine test for adrenal steroids often proves as the best method for detecting these defects in steroid production. Unfortunately, many physicians remain unable to interpret these tests results correctly. Until physicians receive education here, they will remain unable to prescribe the optimal replacement of the missing message content (steroid hormones).

First Link-Hypothalamus - the top of the Adrenal System

Almost fifty years ago, multiple autopsies were performed on victims of various flu epidemics. Analysis during autopsy of the adrenal glands proved that these victims's adrenal tissue was unstressed and even looked inactive. This pathological discovery contradicts all other known diseases or causes of shock.

A normal adrenal will damage itself trying to combat a disease process if that is required. In all other stress producing infections or traumas that lead to death, signs exist, at autopsy, within the adrenals of extreme adrenal depletion and hemorrhage (except flu and mononucleosis).

Strong evidence (Jefferies) suggests that some viral illnesses diminish the ability to activate the hypothalamus, the first 'link' in the adrenal health 'chain'. Failed hypothalamus activation causes the entire adrenal system to remain quiescent. The hypothalamus is the first link in the adrenal chain of health. Nothing starts in the survival message release (cortisol and other steroids) until the hypothalamus activates. Viral illness, like the flu, damages this ability.

The symptoms of flu are commonly: fever, chills, malaise, body and joint aches, weakness, anorexia, and a general grouchiness. Is it just a coincidence that these happen to be the same symptoms of cortisol deficiency in the acute state? For this reason, some physicians administer low dose cortisol when the flu first appears

142

(Jefferies). The flu symptoms quickly abate and the illness often retreats. It is important not to misdiagnose a bacterial infection as the flu because this treatment can make certain infections worse.

One current thought - there are some owners with autoimmune disease that originates from a prior viral illness. The viral illness somehow damages their hypothalamus from turning on the adrenal system properly (the first link in the adrenal chain of health). In some, the decreased direction from the hypothalamus evidences itself only during times of extra stress. Extra stress increases the body requirement for cortisol. When the hypothalamus fails to deliver the message to the second link, the pituitary, the increased production of cortisol becomes impossible. The impossibility arises because the first link underperforms and therefore all successive links suffer a sequential lack of stimulus.

This example demonstrates how a virus can decrease the ability of the hypothalamus to perform its function and activate the successive links in response to an illness or stress. When the hypothalamus function diminishes, stress can cause one to exceed the level of their adrenal gland's functional ability. For this reason, it may be prudent to supplement these owners with adrenal products during times of increased stress or disease activation.

Second Link - Pituitary -Hangs Off of the Underside of the Brain

This pea-sized gland secretes hormones that stimulate the growth of many endocrine glands and the release of their hormone contents. One of the secretions it releases, in a healthy state is called adrenocorticotropic hormone (ACTH). ACTH is derived from a larger precursor hormone called proopiomelanocortin. This hormone cleaves into numerous fragments producing ACTH, the body's natural opium (endorphin), and pigment producing hormone (MSH). The natural pigment-producing hormone in people with poor health of their adrenal glands, tend to cause pigmentation changes on their skin (see below). The pituitary secretes the message content that directs the adrenals to secrete its preformed steroid mixture. In these situations, the pituitary releases all three of the above hormones. This leads to increased skin pigmentation when pituitary secretions rise to abnormal levels secondary to the need to 'whip' a failing adrenal.

Third Link -Adrenal Health Determines the Mixture and Amounts of Adrenal Steroids

The adrenal gland secretes a concoction containing six basic types of steroid hormones:

Cortisol	**Aldosterone**
DHEA	**Androstenedione**
Estradiol	**Progesterone**

Steroid production within the adrenal glands depends on many different vitamins. Consequently, steroid production compromises unless all the needed vitamins are present. For example, the adrenal gland contains the highest concentration of vitamin C in the body. Steroid biosynthesis critically requires vitamin C. The need for large amounts of vitamin C might explain why this vitamin seems to be so effective in activating the immune system. B vitamins are also needed. In addition, vitamin A is necessary to activate the adrenal glands DNA program properly (see misunderstood steroids later in this section).

Several factors influence the ability of the adrenal gland to produce its steroids. For example, the level of aldosterone proves as a powerful determinant of the body's steroid synthesis rate. In addition, several genetic defects lead to a diminished ability to produce one or more steroids.

Aldosterone levels determine the rate of all the other adrenal steroids production. Steroid production rates within the adrenal are controlled by aldosterone because it controls the rate-limiting step of steroid biosynthesis. This step concerns the conversion of cholesterol to pregnenolone. Aldosterone activates the enzyme that performs this conversion, side chain cleavage enzyme (also known as cholesterol desmolase).

High potassium intake (live food diet instead of dead food) relative to sodium intake will increase aldosterone levels. However, here, blood pressure tends to remain normal when the sodium content in the diet stays low. Aldosterone, a steroid hormone, activates the DNA programs within the adrenals and gonads for increasing steroid manufacture within these glands. When specific DNA programs activate in this way it directs the manufacture of side chain cleavage enzyme. Consequently, certain blood pressure lowering medications that decrease aldosterone levels will therefore tend to cripple steroid production (the ACE inhibitors in chapter three).

Still other owners suffer from genetic weaknesses causing an excess or deficiency of specific adrenal steroids. Fortunately, physicians who can piece together clues allowing a specific diagnosis can supplement with the deficient steroid and the excessive ones will return to normal. Enzymatic deficiencies cause diseases such as: some cases of polycystic ovary syndrome, adrenogenital syndrome, salt wasting hypotension, cystic acne, hirsutism, and menorrhagia.

Fourth Link–Adrenal Steroids within the Blood Stream

Once, the adrenal receives the message from the pituitary, link two, its pre-formed steroids concoction dumps into the blood stream. Adrenal steroids transport within the blood stream in three different ways. The first mode involves transportation as the free hormone within the liquid component of the blood stream. The second is within the red blood cells and the third is attached to carrier proteins. The proportions of each of these three ways to transport steroids powerfully determine the availability of the released adrenal steroids to the 70 trillion cell's DNA programs (genes).

Unfortunately, American laboratories completely ignore the amount of steroid transported within the red blood cells. In addition, the amount of steroids bound to the carrier protein is sometimes poorly evaluated. Sadly, these two common errors lead doctors to falsely reassure their patients that their adrenal gland is functioning normally.

The adrenal system level most commonly evaluated is the blood stream. This incomplete mainstream approach overlooks what is actually known about the steroids in transit within the blood stream because the majority of certain steroids transport within red blood cells. Realize this method allows a powerful mechanism for these dominant hormones to squeeze into tissue at the capillary level. For this simple reason, over relying on serum (the liquid component of the blood that is devoid of cells) for determining one's level of active hormone is wrought with difficulty. It is now known that steroids within the red cell are actually more representative of the 'steroid pressure' driving their message into cells.

For example, when the body needs cortisol, the blood stream supply depletes rapidly. Ingle, in the 1940's, demonstrated that cortisol levels in the blood stream did not rise when extra amounts were given during times of stress. During times of stress, rapid movement of cortisol into the tissues (cells) occurs, where it is needed to survive the stress. For this reason, the increased need for cortisol is not measurable within the blood stream.

In addition, the clinician must consider, while measuring the cortisol level of those with the potential for diminished adrenal reserve that borderline patients tend to have deceptively normal blood cortisol levels while low stress prevails. However, during stress their adrenals' production of cortisol diminishes relative to need in order to remain symptom free. In these cases of diminished adrenal reserve, blood testing or a twenty-four hour urine test for cortisol production can be deceptively normal.

Usually, the 24-hour urine results offer powerful clues because the all important cortisol metabolites appear below the mean of the reference range (a trend towards lower than normal). In this culture of deadlines, job insecurities, troubled economy and world strife, a below the mean result should at least merit monitoring the clinical situation. Some of these patients will require an ACTH challenge test before their diminished reserve shows up on laboratory tests.

The ACTH challenge test measures the ability of the adrenals to increase cortisol production when stimulated. Since ACTH is the actual hormone that stimulates the adrenal to release cortisol, a challenge with this hormone should increase cortisol, in the blood stream, within thirty minutes. A normal response is two times greater than the blood level before the adrenals were challenged with ACTH.

Many owners, with diseases related to adrenal deficiency, fail to achieve this increase in cortisol production. For this reason, many of these diseases intensify when an owner experiences stress. Realize stress increases the need for cortisol within the cells. The cell DNA needs cortisol to survive various stresses of life. The above diseases come about when certain cell DNA programs receive defective amounts of the adrenal steroid message. If any of the six links of the adrenal system break, a deficiency can result. A broken link causes a defect for all levels below it. All six links need to be intact or the above types of diseases begin to manifest.

Physiologically, the ability to handle stress depends on adequate increases in cortisol penetrating into the tissues (cells). Adequate increases in cortisol direct energy into survival pathways. Surgeons witness first hand the importance of cortisol production as a determinate ability to survive the stress of surgery. Following the stress of surgery, a patient will die if their adrenals prove incapable of increased cortisol production. However, when cortisol release skyrockets into the body,

potassium loss increases. **Consequently, these two facts are routinely provided for post operatively. Potassium and cortisol are administered in the post-operative period. This precaution prevents severe complications in case a post-surgical owner's adrenal glands are not up to the task or their total body potassium falls below critical levels.**

One of the best ways to screen for defects in the first four links of the adrenal health chain involves obtaining a twenty-four hour urine test. Unfortunately, the urine test misses the last two links in the adrenal health chain (see below). Regretfully, very few physicians can interpret the complex issues that arise from the results of this test. Also, the standard method on which the twenty-four hour urine test is calibrated is to give the patient instructions regarding a normal stress day. This raises the question about missing those patients that only become adrenal compromised during times of stress (when there is an increased need for cortisol that they cannot provide).

Fortunately, there are valuable clues that suggest a deficiency in the adrenal system (all six links in the 'chain'). These clues can occur whenever a white blood cell differential is performed. If the eosinophils, (a type of white blood cell), are elevated, the adrenal system may be deficient. In addition, when neutrophils decrease and lymphocytes increase (a right shift), this raises another red flag suggesting adrenal insufficiency. When either clue occurs, the physician should thoroughly consider the six levels of the patient's adrenal system. A cortisol deficiency will allow abnormalities of these white blood cell types. Realize, all of the diseases (listed at the beginning of this section), have a high likelihood of increased eosinophils within their clinical picture.

Another valuable clinical discovery indicates that patients with an adrenal system deficiency consistently wake up tired. This is especially true when their disease process activates. This contrasts to the low thyroid patient who usually tires in the afternoon.

Occult infections and hidden malignancies can present with some of the same clinical findings as adrenal deficiencies. As a precaution, rule these out before initiating a treatment plan for an adrenal problem.

Fifth Link – DNA Associating Nuclear Receptor Must Be Complete and Undamaged or No Message Can Be Delivered

For a steroid to deliver its message content to cells, a nuclear receptor must be present to receive it. The nucleus of a cell is the part that contains the genes (DNA programs). The resulting shape of the receptor plus the exact shape of the steroid creates a message within the DNA to activate or repress the bound gene. Logically, unless a receptor is present, the cell cannot receive its message.

Owners who suffer from this problem will have a deceptively normal lab test. At times they can have normal eosinophils and neutrophils in certain clinical situations. Sometimes a disease behaves like an adrenal problem, but the lab values come back normal. Unfortunately, commonly available lab values only check steroids to the fourth link. Although level five and six are often suspected when one looks at the white blood cell abnormalities, they are not always abnormal despite adrenal dysfunction driven disease.

No one knows how many patients suffer from this type of defect. When a level five defect happens, the right hypothalamus input, the right pituitary input, the appropriate adrenal response, and the proper transport within the blood stream all occur. However, for example, cortisol, without a pre-formed nuclear receptor, does not activate the DNA properly, which causes the problem.

Nuclear receptors differ for different steroids. Thyroid, vitamin A, and optimal steroids are all necessary to make each other's DNA receptors. Unless a physician is aware, even the twenty-four hour urine tests will look deceptively good in some cases. Realize what the physician tests for fails to identify the level of the problem, when link five is the culprit for adrenal system disease.

There is much to be learned about the fifth link of adrenal system malfunction. Recent scientific insights have the potential to help solve the 'why' for receptor defects within the DNA. These results point to the increased understanding that many of these 'big daddy' hormones depend, in an interconnected way, for activation and manufacture of their various DNA receptors. There is agreement that vitamin A, thyroid, and cortisol all contribute to the manufacture of certain receptors. Since many Americans are vitamin A deficient, could this be the cause of some of these diseases?

It is worth some investigative work to try and assess the status of these powerful hormones by means of a well-run twenty-four hour urine test. If the clinical situation proves suspicious, a careful trial of some of these hormones is warranted as long as frequent follow up occurs and the patient stays properly motivated.

Sixth Link–Result of DNA Program Activation is the Manufacture of Specific Receptors for the Lesser Hormones

Steroid activation of a DNA program (gene) results in protein synthesis. The DNA sequence activated determines which protein eventually occurs. Some of the steroid message directs certain DNA programs to produce receptors for the lesser hormones. Lesser hormones are all hormones not included with thyroid, vitamin A, or steroids (secondary receptors). How the hierarchy works between hormones will be explained at the end of this section. The primary hormones (big daddies) are the focus at this point and include the adrenal cortex hormones.

The bodies of some owners make antibodies to the 'secondary' receptors that are made by the message of certain steroids delivered to the DNA program. Antibodies bind these receptors and essentially deactivate the lesser hormones ability to bind their receptor. These receptors for the lesser hormones comprise the sixth link of the adrenal chain of health.

Caution should be taken not to confuse the previous nuclear receptor (link five) with these secondary receptors (link six). The nuclear receptors can only bind thyroid, vitamin A and steroids. Only when the steroids bind to the DNA programs (level five), can the manufacture of the next level of receptor occur. In contrast, a level six receptor results from the message content of the steroid hormones, vitamin A and thyroid hormones that activate a specific DNA program (gene).

In turn, the steroid message results in synthesis of specific receptors for specific 'lesser' hormones that follow within the blood stream (see hierarchy of hormones). The integrity of these 'lesser' hormone receptors needs to be considered at the sixth link for adrenal health. Problems at this level of the adrenal chain can cause or contribute to disease. Like level five problems, the lab tests can look deceptively normal.

This has probable merit in the production of adrenal system related disease (see above list) due to finding antibodies to various 'lesser' hormone receptors. In these cases even though these 'big daddy' hormones designate that the receptors be built, they are inactivated by the immune system.

All hormones need their specific receptors intact before recipient cells can receive their message. Said in another way, a cell understands the message content, only when these receptors that exist on the cell surface function properly. 'Lesser' hormones receptors tend to be on the cell surface. This contrasts to the 'big daddies' hormones. Their receptors are near the DNA program.

When antibodies disable the 'lesser receptor' before the 'lesser hormone' (i.e. adrenaline) arrives, that cell can't receive the 'lesser' hormone's message content. This creates adrenal deficiency in the clinical situation, even though the first five 'links' in the adrenal system are intact. These unfortunate patients will almost always have normal blood values for adrenal steroids and normal twenty-four hour urine values for those steroids involved. Their disease results from the message not being able to activate when the lesser hormones arrive because the lesser hormone cannot activate its receptor when the immune system has disabled it. In these cases the steroid directed and manufactured receptor has been disabled by the immune system.

The antibodies to the cortisol directed manufacture of the adrenergic B2 receptor (adrenaline) demonstrates this. Antibodies to these receptors have been found in patients with asthma and allergic rhinitis (hay fever). The development of an antibody test for B2 receptors would help to identify some of these patients who suffer these two diseases. The inclusion of testing for antibodies to the nuclear steroid receptors is also appropriate as it would evaluate antibody production against either a level five or a level six problem as well.

The accuracy of this last suggestion needs to be confirmed by further research. Until then, it will be up to their physician to follow both the owner's steroid hormone profiles and also clinically for signs of excess or continued deficiency.

The six links in the adrenal health chain provide a way to conduct an initial inquiry as to the status of an owner's endocrine function within these glands. Many additional diseases result from an imbalanced interrelationship between adrenals and ovaries. The next chapter introduces this interrelationship. Like the adrenals, the ovaries can be best understood by considering the multiple levels (links in the chain) of ovary health. The testicle chapter is also similar and is found near the end of this section.

> Cutting edge scientific thought: Autoimmune disease not only involves defective repair hormones (steroids and thyroid hormones) but also an increased injury rate secondary to IgG mediated food allergies. Identify and eliminate these food allergies and replacing the deficient adrenal and /or thyroid hormones leads to a high probability of healing from asthma, colitis, Crohn's disease, lupus, rheumatoid arthritis and MS.

CHAPTER SIX

OVARIES

Modern Female's Dilemma

A defective ovary system can lead to the same clinical picture as the adrenal system. However, the origins of these diseases differ because of different defects in the 'chain links'in the ovary system of health. When the physician fails to consider all six links in the 'chain' then these types of disease will be treated within the symptom control paradigm. However, physicians and female owners interested in healing require an organization of what science knows about how these glands work in the context of the ovarian system.

Healthy females have highly functional ovaries and/or highly functional adrenal glands. Unfortunately, around age thirty-five, many female owners begin to experience various levels of hormonal decline. The clinical clues are there, but the physician needs to know how to look for them. Sadly, the standard of care involves prescribing abnormally shaped hormones or abnormal mixtures and these replacement strategies cause problems. Problems occur because these types of hormones do not contain the intended body message content that female owners require.

Recall, it helps to consider that a musical note arises only after an accurate vibration within a piano string occurs. Visualize the true note as the accurate message and the flat note produced by an altered tug on the string as the inaccurate message. Again it is the precise tension induced vibration that creates a certain piano string's musical note. The note arises from a specific vibration frequency within the string. In contrast, the flat altered piano string tension changes the musical quality because it changes its vibration frequency.

Similarly, the body operates within a vibrational system of molecular communication: Specific molecular shapes create specific hormones that after binding specific genes vibrate in their characteristic way. These vibrations create messages. For

this reason, change the molecular shape, even a little bit, and the message content that a gene receives alters.

A problem arises because in the search for more profit because unless a hormone's shape is changed no patent is possible. However, realizing that changing the shape alters the message helps one to see the often overlooked vulnerability: Changed message content arriving at the genes carries the high probability of eventually evidencing itself clinically as side effects and toxicities.

Remember, the quality of the circulating hormones determines the efficiency of the information carried within the blood stream (message content). In turn, the message content received determines how a cell will spend its available energy. With this in mind, confusion can be avoided in medical literature.

Medical literature is uniformly disorganized in making it easy for doctors and patients to grasp the hierarchy between the different hormone classes. Recall, it is the goal of this section to help one become more knowledgeable about the hormone hierarchy. Competency here diminishes gullibility for the next time one reads a sensationalized version about the latest patented hormone.

This chapter contains scientific revelations on this subject. Other pertinent information relates how natural female hormones keep middle age at bay. Both the decline in natural hormones within and ingesting the patented unnatural ones with their altered shapes, cause diminished outcomes. Alternatively, the common practice of prescribing excessive replacement doses, even with bio-identical varieties, proves damaging as well. Diminished outcomes predictably occurs whenever the message content disrupts or imbalances at the level of the genes.

How one heals revolves around replacing the lost message content by nutritional, lifestyle, and correctly dosed real hormone replacement. This chapter discusses the problem of symptom control, why real hormones are better, how nutrition affects the ovaries health, and the six links in the ovary chain of health.

Introduction to the Imbalanced Hormonal States of Female Owners

The general imbalance, in pre-menopausal female owners today, results from too much and the wrong types of estrogen message content. Too much estrogen occurs relative to the availability of the counter regulatory hormone, progesterone. For post-menopausal females the imbalanced hormone situation can be more variable but progesterone deficiency is almost always present (see below).

The important difference between natural progesterone and the fake progesterone substitutes (commonly called progestogens and progestins) remains not widely understood. Lack of this knowledge has led countless female owners to suffer from unnecessary chronic disease. Natural progesterone plays an important role in maintaining female health.

Because Estrogen and progesterone belong to the steroid class of hormones, they are some of the most powerful body hormones. Logically it follows because both their quality and amount directly instruct trillions of genes it is in the owners best interest that their doctor be careful. Sloppy or careful practice decisions still determine which genes turn off and on. Gene activity, in turn, determines which proteins are present or absent. Metabolism depends on specific proteins. Mess with these and it leads to a sure fire path to an old body. Simple science being discussed here, yet, not taught in ways that the average physician comprehends.

Different types of unnatural estrogen substitutes compound the problems created by fake progesterone by creating additional poor message content. Realize, health consequences occur when DNA programs (genes) receive poor directional information. The abnormal monthly cycle of a female describes the effects that occur when DNA receives poor message content.

Steroids, like estrogen and progesterone, are relatively simple molecules compared to the larger hormone molecules like insulin. The smaller the hormone (message carrier), the more exact shape the hormone needs to be in order to preserve its message content.

Consequently, in the size class of the steroids, changing a single angle in one chemical bond between carbon and oxygen changes the message content and/or strength. For example, it has been known for almost fifty years that changing the angle between one carbon and oxygen in estradiol changes the potency of the message content by a factor of thirty. Chemists denote this change as beta to alpha angle rotation (beta-estradiol versus alpha-estradiol).

Importantly, the most powerful estrogen type in humans is Beta-estradiol. However, common estrogen replacement prescriptions contain Alpha-estradiol that is thirty times more powerful than the naturally occurring human form, Beta-estradiol. In addition to the alpha type estrogen that horses make, these animals also make other horse specific estrogen message content. Unfortunately, many estrogen prescriptions contain these additional horse specific estrogens (described as equilin and equlinin in the package insert). The general class of these prescriptions is called conjugated estrogens.

Sadly, many women still ingest these powerful and altered message type estrogens in the prescriptions given to them as their hormone replacement. These altered hormones are collected from the urine of pregnant horses or made synthetically from soy or yams. They are marketed to women under the vernacular of conjugated estrogens.

The Monthly Cycle and Imbalance

Normally, estrogen stimulates cell division in estrogen sensitive tissues (breast, uterus, fat, and liver) for the first half of the female menstrual cycle. However, if left unopposed, the stimulant effects of estrogen lead to common ailments such as fibrocystic breast disease, uterine fibroids, breast cancer, uterine cancer, and unnatural growths in other estrogen responsive tissues.

Ideally, in the second half of the menstrual cycle, with optimal health, progesterone counter regulates much of the estrogen message content. Progesterone directs influence over DNA programs in the same cells that estrogen influences. Unfortunately, progesterone deficiency is a common problem.

The first of four reasons for this deficiency concerns the multitude of pervasive 'estrogen' mimics within the environment (discussed in previous chapter). This increases the total estrogen message for many women when compared to their ability to manufacture progesterone.

Second, the progesterone part of hormone replacement therapy intensifies the problem by using unnatural progesterone substitutes (fake hormones). Unnatural progesterone substitutes can inhibit natural progesterone production that women's bodies need in the counter-regulation of estrogen and other youth preserving processes.

Third, progesterone deficiency relates to a nutritionally poor diet. Certain nutritional elements are necessary for adequate progesterone production. Each of these factors that contribute to estrogen dominance will be explained shortly.

The fourth factor relates how female hormones become imbalanced and eventually suffer from disease. This common situation results when female owners are prescribed the wrong types of estrogen (in contrast to factor two above, which is caused by the prescribing of abnormal shaped progesterone substitutes).

Many different natural and unnatural estrogens are prescribed to women by mainstream medicine adherants. When the estrogen message content tips out of balance, the wrong cellular message chronically occurs.

Four Factors Leading to Estrogen Dominance Relative to Progesterone

1. **Estrogen mimics in the environment (see hormone mimics in the previous chapter)**
2. **Unnatural progesterone in hormone replacement therapies decreases real progesterone levels.**
3. **Nutritional deficiencies exacerbate the progesterone and estrogen imbalance (discussed within the six links in the ovarian chain of health, link three).**
4. **Hormone prescriptions commonly contain abnormal estrogen message content**

In order to understand how prescriptions commonly disrupt the natural message in a woman's body, the natural state needs to be defined. When treatment strategies facilitate a recreation of the natural state, healing becomes possible. There is wisdom in the power of the female body to heal.

Three natural estrogens produced within the human body allow balanced health (beta-estradiol, estrone and estriol). Each natural human estrogen type has an optimal percentage of the total estrogen message content within the body. When balanced, a coherent cellular message occurs. Conversely, a deviation from the optimal relative percentages leads to an imbalanced hormone message with cellular consequences. For example, estriol has weak cell division stimulation tendencies, but it is the major natural form of human estrogen initially released from the ovary.

Good reasons exist for the weakest estrogen to initially release within the pelvic cavity in the highest concentration (see below). Estriol proves very powerful in the maintenance and health of the vulva and vaginal tissues. For this purpose, it does not need to be converted into the more powerful estrogen types.

This contrasts to Beta-estradiol and estrone, which contain powerful cell division message content directed at estrogen responsive tissues. This fact helps one begin to see the advantage of their minority position. Many physicians miss the fact that some of their postmenopausal females contain high levels of estrone and its metabolites. Usually they miss this risk factor because they fail to obtain a 24-hour urine test for steroids where it shows up best.

Unfortunately, the patented pharmaceutical estrogens prescribed to women contain the powerful cell division message type. Fortunately this situation is completely avoidable if the patient obtains a prescription intended for a **compounding pharmacist**. Natural estrogens prescriptions are commonly designed for delivery via a patch, cream, capsule, sublingual drops, or vaginal gel. Ideally, the dosage is determined by a well-run 24-hour urine test result. This cautionary step facilitates the goal of achieving a natural cellular message in the estrogen responsive tissues.

Symptom control medicine largely ignores the natural estrogen message content found in the human owner. This practice evidences itself over and over again when women receive their 'conjugated estrogens' without the benefit of a scientifically valid inquiry. Realize that over the last few years the standard practice of utilizing serum or saliva sampling to guide hormone treatment strategies has been called into question by several scientific authorities. Yet, it still drums on as the standard of care.

It is important to emphasize that conjugated estrogen prescriptions contain abnormally shaped versions (nonhuman estrogens) derived from either horse urine concentrate or wild yams. Also remember that relatively speaking, steroids, like estrogen and progesterone, are simple molecules compared to larger hormone molecules like insulin. The smaller the hormone (message carrier) the more exact the hormone needs to be in shape to preserve the message content. As was previously mentioned, the changing of a single angle in one chemical bond between carbon and oxygen can alter the message content and/or strength significantly.

The earlier example concerned the futility of attempting to make even a slight change to human estrogen by changing the angle between one carbon and oxygen in estradiol. This very small alteration in one bond changes the potency of the message content by a factor of thirty. Chemists denote this change as beta to alpha angle rotation. In addition to the most powerful estrogen type in the human, Beta-estradiol, these prescriptions contain, Alpha-estradiol, which is thirty times more powerful than the natural human form, Beta-estradiol.

Remember that horses make the more powerful alpha type along with some beta types and in addition, they also make horse estrogen message content, equilin and equlinin. Many women consume these powerful, altered message type estrogens in the prescriptions given to them for their hormone replacement. These altered hormones are collected from pregnant horses' urine or are made synthetically from soy or yams.

In contrast, in the natural condition, humans make small amounts of the much weaker Beta-estradiol. This alone is a very powerful estrogen in the scheme of things. Imagine the potential consequences when the message content is multiplied by a factor of thirty. Yet, this is happening to millions of women who are taking unnatural mixtures of estrogen or abnormally shaped versions. This fact leads to estrogen imbalances (number four factor). The fourth factor is the topic of this subsection. Physicians may be unaware of this chemical fact because they receive their medical information through sources that are 'friendly' to the interests of drug companies (medical schools and journals).

If women are healthier with natural estrogen, why aren't more pharmaceutical companies manufacturing it? Natural prescriptions cannot be patented and hence, are less profitable. In order to obtain a patent, the natural estrogen or progesterone shape needs to be changed in some way. Small changes in molecules of this size prove impossible without changing the message content inherent in the precise shape.

Recently, slick delivery systems have been patented for delivering at least one human estrogen, estradiol via a cream or gel. This is a start in the right direction but the common failure to first properly test all steroid output and the consequent metabolites, prescribe the steroid precursor foundation first and then add in estrogen later lead to excessive estrogen need.

Realize both alternative and conventional doctors still prescribe oral estrogen dosing regimens. However, recent scientific papers call into question the wisdom of this route of delivering estrogen. The concern arises because oral estrogens pummel the liver first and stimulates it to manufacture abnormal amounts of important proteins. For starters, some of these abnormal protein secretion changes increase the blood vessel inflammation and blood stream clotting tendencies (increased fibrinogen and CRP respectively).

Making matters worse concerns the fact that within the various birth control pill formulations, the shapes change alters even more radically compared to the natural shape of estrogen and progesterone. Also alarming is that most of these birth control pill formulations are designed for oral ingestion, which increases the recipients risk for increased blood vessel inflammation and blood stream clotting tendencies (see above discussion). These first few examples site the estrogen molecule alterations from the natural human shapes, but what about the consequences of altering progesterone, the counter hormone to estrogen?

Abnormal Shaped Progesterone Substitutes as a Factor in Real Progesterone Deficiency for Its Message Content.

Synthetic alteration of progesterone's natural shape profoundly affects a woman's health for two reasons (factor two above). First, only one type of progesterone exists in nature. The natural form proves necessary to serve as the building block molecule for the creation of many other steroids.

Second, like other natural hormones, the exact inherent shape of progesterone carries an exact message that women need in the second half of their monthly cycle. It counters many of the effects started by estrogen in the first part of the menstrual cycle. The progesterone content, which rises in the second half of the female cycle, counters the cell division and fluid retaining effects of estrogen.

Without adequate progesterone, females will tend towards estrogen dominance based disease such as fibrocystic breast disease, breast cancer, uterine cancer, premenstrual bloating, uterine fibroids, and migraine headaches. Unfortunately, shape alterations, found in patented progesterone substitutes (called progestins and progestogens), changes the message content. Hormonal balance occurs when the balance-counter-balance mechanisms function properly. This includes proper timing and an adequate amount of real progesterone and estrogen.

In addition, progesterone serves as a building block molecule for other important steroids manufactured within the adrenals and ovaries. For example, progesterone, provides the building block for cortisol. For this reason, owners with synthetic progesterone prescriptions in their body increase the likelihood for creating an imbalance in the synthesis of other steroids.

Remember that the message content of molecules the size of steroids, like estrogen and progesterone, depends on their precise shape. The precise shape binds the gene and causes a specific vibrational event. Similarly, musical notes arise from precise vibrations and this describes how these precise shaped steroids deliver messages to genes by the accurate vibration that results.

Consequently, when the shape changes minutely so does the message delivered to the DNA.

Healthy people have real hormones that deliver accurate message content to their DNA programs (genes). Conversely, unhealthy people are often the consequence of unnatural message content being delivered to their DNA. Recall, the genes provide nothing until the right hormone arrives. Realizing this truism allows one to be more mindful of whether or not the message content arriving at their 70 trillion cells' DNA programs proves adequate, deficient or excessive.

Oral Hormones and the Liver

The "first pass" effect, in the liver of orally ingested steroids complicates steroid hormone replacement. Oral supplements are required to pass through the liver once they have been absorbed by the digestive tract. On average, about 70-80% of an ingested steroid is removed from circulation following oral administration. The ingested steroid remains inside the liver.

There are two important concepts regarding the liver first pass effect. First, the liver itself is rich in steroid hormone receptor sites. Failing to comprehend this can lead to a powerful message to liver cells altering their function (including liver cancer in some cases). Second, sometimes synthetic steroids are not well metabolized. Poor metabolism of certain steroids within the liver leads to sequestering of these hormones. When steroids sequester within the liver, they promote liver congestion phenomena.

Some physicians have substantiated this congestion phenomenon clinically. The observation that a large percentage of blue eyed females who chronically take birth control pills witness a gradual change of their original eye color to green. The Chinese medical theory associating liver health with eye color makes this clinical observation acutely disturbing.

In summary, taking steroid hormones orally, without thinking about liver health, is potentially dangerous. Safer alternatives are available in the forms of patches, creams, and injections in some cases. These routes bypass the liver first pass effect allowing the liver to use its energy for more constructive tasks, like disarming environmental toxins.

Estrogen Dominance

Conspicuous clinical signs of estrogen dominance:
1. **Pre-menstrual breast pain**
2. **Poor sleep quality**
3. **Fluid retention more than twenty four hours before the onset of the menses**

4. Increased tendency toward premenstrual tension (increased irritability and combativeness) up to fourteen days prior to the onset of menses.

As was previously mentioned, estrogen dominant imbalance that persists, leads to an increased likelihood for the development of diseases like: fibrocystic breast disease, uterine fibroids, breast cancer, shortened menstrual cycle, endometrial cancer, menstrual cycle migraines, osteoporosis, and weight gain. Being mindful of what the female body is saying will create awareness about estrogen dominance.

These clinical signs deserve attention into the 'why' and the 'how' of estrogen dominance. A brief review of the six links in the 'chain' of the estrogen and progesterone system will follow in the ovary system. Within this discussion there is an explanation for how estrogen dominance accelerates the deleterious changes of middle age. Attention to these six links will increase the odds of a female owner having the best hormones that align with good health.

Six Links in the 'Chain' - Good Health of the Ovarian System

Six links in the health of the ovarian system include:
1. **Hypothalamus**
2. **Pituitary**
3. **Ovary**
4. **Blood stream transport system**
5. **Nuclear receptor at the DNA level within the ovarian hormone responsive tissues**
6. **Receptors manufactured as a result of ovarian hormones activation of certain DNA programs causing direction for the manufacture of new receptors (other steroids and the 'lesser' hormones)**

Different female owners suffer from different points of break down in the six links of the 'chain' within their ovarian system. For example, menopause results from a broken link at level three, the ovary. Also, some systemic illnesses affect level one, the hypothalamus. In Addition, some hormone abnormalities at the pituitary (level two) inhibit the ovary. The broken link must be correctly identified to restore hormonal balance.

Link One - Hypothalamus

The hypothalamus controls all the other links within the ovary system. Under activity of the first link creates under activity of all successive links of the chain. The amount of ovary stimulant information that the hypothalamus sends out is largely determined by the amount of estrogen it senses. Too much estrogen reaching this level weakens the link at this first level. When the hypothalamus turns down its informational direction of the ovarian system, other important hormones are affected. As long as the female ovarian system maintains balance, turning down the volume is appropriate. However, when women take certain estrogen prescriptions, this fools the hypothalamus and consequently it fails to direct the manufacture of other important hormones.

For example, sometimes doctors prescribe various estrogens without considering how this practice will decrease testosterone like steroids. The ovary, while releasing progesterone and estrogen, also releases testosterone and androstenedione (important androgens) steroids as well.

Realize rejuvenation requires the androgen message. In this way, female owners who take too much estrogen can short circuit powerful androgen messages needed to combat the wear and tear of life. The androgen message decreases because artificially high estrogens within certain female owners' bodies have fooled link one, the hypothalamus.

In the example of estrogen replacement, the androgen deficiency results because hormonal replacements usually do not contain androgens. However, the hypothalamus assumes when estrogen elevates that testosterone has elevated as well. In the subsection 'steroid tone' the central role that androgens play in rejuvenation will be explained (next chapter).

Remember that larger amounts of estrogen inhibit the amount of stimulatory information, which the hypothalamus sends into the ovary chain of health. Only when the ovary remains healthy, will it produce optimal progesterone, estrogen, androstenedione and testosterone. Realize, estrogen replacement strategies usually do not contain the androgen that is lost when estrogen levels elevate artificially. As a consequence, both androstenedione and testosterone constitute ovarian androgens that fall off when the hypothalamus is fooled by the above mechanism.

Link Two - Pituitary

The master gland, the pituitary, regulates the other hormone glands. It manufactures many competing hormonal messages and releases each one under specific body circumstances. Unfortunately, hormone replacement all too often fools this important gland that all is well.

Hormones contain message content. A glands importance lies in which hormone messages it releases. The quality of the mixture that the master gland, the pituitary, secretes instructs the ovary how to expend energy. This becomes the dominant message. Adequate and rhythmic release of leuteinizing hormone (LH) and follicle stimulating hormone (FSH) released from the pituitary, nourish the ovary by giving specific direction to continue its natural cycle.

In addition, adequate release of adrenal corticotropic hormone (ACTH) also stimulates the ovary to increase its steroid biosynthesis rate. Also, the release of aldosterone provides an additional circuitous but important pathway, as well (see informational substances chapter). The main point to consider now, regarding these last two hormonal alternate pathways concerns the concept of glandular interdependency. The goal of this entire section is about organizing these interdependent processes into a grand design that facilitates healing strategies.

Conversely, within the master gland (the pituitary) exists another powerful hormone, prolactin. The ovary becomes inhibited when prolactin releases beyond low levels. Even though many physicians have been groomed into the 'knee jerk' summary that prolactin stimulates milk production, the evidence clearly implicates prolactin as a powerful inhibitor of ovarian function.

Confusion arises because they know that during the pregnant state, steroid production becomes very high and the prolactin level also elevates. One solves this false discrepancy about pregnancy and prolactin inhibition of the ovaries when the additional placenta hormone factory receives recognition. Even though prolactin eventually inhibits the ovaries, after the fourth month in the pregnant state, the placenta cranks out huge amounts of steroids, which explains the increase.

Unfortunately, there are four common clinical states, without the benefit of a placenta, where prolactin, produced within the pituitary, induces ovary inhibition. Unfortunately, in these cases, no placenta exists to make up the difference in the lost steroids produced by the ovary.

The four states that stimulate the pituitary to release high levels of prolactin include: low thyroid function, birth control pill usage, chronic stress, and high serotonin. In these cases, the production of the ovarian component of body steroids greatly diminishes because these situations lead to increased prolactin. Steroids are so powerful if any one of them diminishes, the DNA content of the body will go either dormant or hyper. Most people have a pretty good feeling that when the DNA misbehaves a danger to over all health exists. Fortunately, with an appropriate prolactin level, healing transpires.

Mechanisms for the increased pituitary release of prolactin:

> **Birth control pill usage**
> **High serotonin levels**
> **Chronic stress**
> **Low thyroid gland function**

Increased prolactin levels result from the increased estrogen contained in birth control pills. Prolactin inhibits ovarian hormone formations and release. This fact provides another hormone-induced mechanism associated with obesity that does not operate with pregnancy. The pregnant state contains the growing placenta that generates needed steroids. The placenta manufactures androgens even though the ovary becomes relatively dormant by the fifth month of pregnancy. When female owners take birth control pills the body thinks it is pregnant and prolactin levels rise. Prolactin levels rise when estrogen levels approach pregnancy levels.

Potential obesity occurs because like pregnancy, the birth control pills increase prolactin levels. Unlike pregnancy there is no placental hormone factory to correct the inhibition of the ovaries steroid production. Additional potential problems exist. Birth control pills do not contain androgens, only estrogen and progestins (abnormally shaped progesterone substitutes). Consequently, androgen production can fall and some females' adrenals fail in the challenge to increase androgen production, thus obesity ensues.

Also, high pituitary serotonin levels can occur when SSRI type anti-depressants are taken (section six). Serotonin, in the pituitary, encourages prolactin release but inhibits Growth Hormone release. For now, realize that these prescriptions are very popular.

However, their number one side effect, sexual dysfunction is explained by this mechanism.

In addition, chronic stress tends to raise prolactin levels. Prolactin levels elevate when increased cortisol release stimulates prolactin as part of the stress response. By this mechanism, chronic stress causes even more havoc towards one's ability to repair the wear and tear that life inflicts.

Finally, low thyroid gland function will stimulate the hypothalamus to chronically release thyroid-releasing globulin (TRH). TRH proves as a very powerful secretogogue for prolactin release from the pituitary. The deep husky voice occurring in women with long standing low thyroid function occurs because their estrogen levels fall for the reasons mentioned above. This situation allows a relative increase in unopposed androgen message content coming from their adrenals. The vocal cords respond to the increased androgen message content and the voice becomes huskier.

Link Three - Ovary

Healthy females possess ovaries that make appropriate amounts of androgens. In addition, the healthful state involves proper levels of estrogens, which are cycled with proper levels of progesterone. Each month a new cycle begins and her cells receive the right amount of message content directing them to invest in rejuvenation activities. Rejuvenation activities keep the body young.

Around menopause her ovaries begin to fail and give up their steroid production role to their middle aged adrenal glands. Many years prior to this, steroid production begins to diminish within their ovaries. When clinicians miss this or treat with fake hormones, their female patients jump on an accelerated path to an old body.

Nutritional deficiencies play a major role in ovarian disease. Common factors include a chronic tendency for the consumption of a 'processed food' diet versus a 'real food' diet. Ovarian steroid production provides an example of how nutrition affects ovarian health. One central facet of ovarian function is determined by the rate at which cholesterol is converted to pregnenolone. Aldosterone levels determine the rate of this important step in all the body steroids' creation. This fact about the steroid manufacture rate is true for the adrenals, testicles and ovaries. Specifically, in the ovary, testicle and adrenal DNA programs, adequate aldosterone is needed to start production of cholesterol desmolase. This initial enzyme involved in steroid manufacture is also known as a side chain cleavage enzyme.

A high potassium diet ('real food') stimulates aldosterone release. Fresh meat, vegetables, and fruits provide high potassium. Unfortunately, processed food diets are deficient in potassium and pave the road for dysfunctional ovaries. Processed food constitutes any food that comes in a box, can, and bag or from a fast food restaurant. This fact provides an example of steroid interdependence for ovary health to be possible. Along with aldosterone, the healthy ovary needs vitamin C, vitamin A and vitamin B complex for adequate steroid production capabilities. The mineral zinc allows steroid synthesis to occur at high levels. Adequate zinc also prevents the excessive conversion of testosterone to estrogen.

The mineral content contrast between these two types of diets shows drastic differences. Real food contains minerals in the proportions required for health. In contrast, processed foods contain drastically altered mineral content. Minerals like, magnesium and potassium, become depleted by processing natural foods. Unhealthy amounts of sodium, calcium, hydrogenated fats, and sugar are added to extend shelf life. This equals profits for the food industry.

Processed food doesn't contain the proper ratio of the four minerals - magnesium, calcium, potassium, and sodium. Ovaries need the correct mineral ratio more than other body tissues to maintain the aldosterone message content (informational substances chapter). Aldosterone message content determines the rate of all steroids synthesis within the adrenals and ovaries. For this reason, natural food diets facilitate an increased aldosterone level.

As a consequence, owners who eat 'dead food' diets become potassium and magnesium depleted around the onset of middle age. Making matters worse, a deficiency of potassium creates the need for an increase in insulin exposure in order to process the same amount of sugar (sections three and five). In addition, potassium and magnesium deficiencies lead to high blood pressure, irregular heart rate, diminished adrenal and ovary steroid production, diminished red blood cell flexibility and decreased cell voltages (a weakened cell force field). The 'why' and the 'how' of these facts is discussed in the appropriate sections throughout this manual (see especially section five). For these reasons, proper mineral intake equates to a better ovary and adrenal gland function.

Link Four - Bondage Fraction versus the Free Level of Ovarian Hormones within the Blood Stream

Transport of ovarian steroids is the fourth link in the ovarian system chain of health. Three different ways exist that transport ovarian steroids within the blood stream.

1. Binding the red blood cell membrane (major fraction).
2. Trapped on bondage proteins (binding proteins). Western owners are often misled because of an incomplete inquiry into the level of ovarian hormones released and trapped within this compartment (see below).
3. Small amounts travel by themselves free within the blood stream.

The majority of ovarian steroids (estrogen, progesterone, testosterone, and androstenedione) are usually transported within the red blood cells. Estrogen, while in transport within the red blood cell, can be acted upon by enzymatic machines and transformed into more powerful types of estrogens. By this mechanism, the initially released estrogen types changes in the periphery. For this reason, the initial types of estrogen secreted from the ovaries, can be altered while in route to the distant target cell.

The liquid coponent of blood, the plasma, also transports some ovarian hormones (testosterone, androstenedione, estrogens, and progesterone). However, the majority of plasma transport of steroids requires binding proteins (bondage proteins) because they are very insoluble in water. Also, the higher the thyroid hormone and estrogen level within the body, the higher the transporter ('bondage') protein levels. This consequence results from these hormone classes stimulating the liver to manufacture excessive binding proteins when their levels rise beyond healthful parameters.

Both thyroid and estrogen hormones, when they occur at high levels, instruct the liver to make binding proteins for all steroids within the blood stream. Some physicians are misled into thinking a blood drawn laboratory test looks good, where in actuality the proteins, being abnormally high, captivate the steroids within the blood stream. Remember steroids need to bind to the DNA before they deliver message content. For this reason, trapped messages circulating around and around within the blood stream prove worthless.

A higher bondage protein level means that a hormone measured within an owner's blood may be misleading if the transport (bondage) protein level is either higher or lower than normal. The name of the binding protein for testosterone and estrogen is referred to as sex hormone binding globulin (SHBG).

The blood stream must contain this important protein for ovarian function. However, deviations from normal levels do two things to steroid message content. First, they alter the rate at which the liver can inactivate steroid levels. The higher the levels, the less readily the liver inactivates them. Conversely, the higher the level, the less readily the body cells access their informational content. When levels are high, they slow the ability of steroids to get into target cells (DNA programs).

Only the blood cells content and free fraction of the various steroids have the ability to flow into the 'target' cells. Only when the steroids make it into the target cells can they activate the various DNA programs. When the DNA programs receive message content (the gene activated or repressed) modifies the direction of cell energy expenditure. Energy expenditure modifies because gene activity or silence changes which proteins are manufactured. The type of proteins present determines where energy flows within a cell. Healthy bodies contain appropriate protein that reflects optimal cell function. Unhealthy bodies suffer from a diminution of this important process.

Conversely, 'bondage' binding protein (SHBG) levels determine the amount of steroids that can't escape from the blood stream. Steroids, trapped onto bondage proteins, remain unable to deliver message content into cells until another hormone event changes their equilibrium. This last detail is beyond the scope of this book. These are basic variables to consider concerning steroids when interpreting blood test results.

Remember, to look at only steroid levels in the blood can be misleading. A modest improvement in accuracy can be achieved with obtaining a SHBG level. When this protein level is high, large amounts of steroids could be circulating without a destination. For these reasons, a twenty-four hour urine test for steroid hormone excretion and a SHBG level adds predictive value.

Remember, only the GC mass spec derived 24-hour urine test offers quantitation of the important metabolites. Metabolites occur after the native steroid binds specific genes. To ignore the proportion of steroids secreted that actually delivered message content to the DNA is folly for this reason. In addition, the level of effectiveness of a steroid to bind and activate its DNA associated receptor (link five) is a concern. Failure to consider the links that make up the ovary system chain has led many clinicians to falsely conclude that all is well.

Link Five - Integrity and Amount of Functional DNA Associated Nuclear Receptors within the Target Cell

Once an ovarian steroid successfully travels within the blood stream and enters the target cell, it needs to activate its DNA binding receptor. Without binding its receptor it cannot activate or repress a cell's DNA program. Something wrong with the receptor link means that the message content of a steroid cannot be heard. A simple example of level five-associated receptor formation regards the interdependence between progesterone and estrogen to manufacture each other's DNA associated receptors.

A dysfunction in the fifth link can mislead clinicians because patients often have normal blood and urine tests for different ovarian steroids. The prematurely aged female body will warn an astute physician that a level five problem most likely operates.

Whenever hormonal dysfunction happens at this level, the preceding four levels operate effectively. However, diagnosis proves difficult. Even the best, most thorough tests available remain not sophisticated enough to measure dysfunction in the message content the DNA receives (level five). Specific accuracy requires better scientific methods that so far await development.

Sidebar - It takes a brave physician to prescribe the powerful natural steroid hormones without a lab test to back up their need. Yet, this practice is exactly what happens when post-menopausal females ingest unnatural and abnormally shaped hormones without checking to see what this will do to other hormone systems. Inferior scientific thinking is acceptable. However, where 'contrary' thinkers, dare to think about the different links in the chain of ovarian dysfunction, is not. A legal medical 'witch hunt' occurs when any physician thinks differently from the 'herd'. The herd determines the standard of care. The herd learns its viewpoint from the pharmaceutical darlings. How convenient; withhold basic science from the educations of doctors but make them think they are in the scientific 'know'.

Physicians resist sticking their neck out medically or legally even though scientific revelations tend to back up the practice. This describes one more way that the complex effectively controls its best interest. Ideally, consumers will begin to demand more honesty about how doctors are taught to think about hormones. Politicians are scared to death of angry voters. Voters need to be scared to death of fake hormones before change even begins to come about.

Natural hormones are safer than their fake counterparts (see above discussion). However, when dealing with level five problems, safe dosages for patients are currently unknown. One in nine female owners will suffer from breast cancer. If her physician uses a natural approach and breast cancer develops, it sometimes constitutes an excuse for the licensing board to prosecute or even results in a malpractice claim. However, if the physician uses fake hormones, even in excessive doses, and performs only a superficial hormone inquiry, the medical legal standard has been upheld even if a patient develops cancer. This reoccurring theme demonstrates how sound science remains suppressed. The concern of the complex involves exposing that a contrary physician's patient has breast cancer.

The physician that suspects he/she has a level five problem operating within a patient is caught between medical legal concerns and a patient who shows clinical signs of accelerated aging.

Adequate zinc plays an important role in preventing improper steroid receptor interaction, once the steroids arrive at the DNA associated receptor. The DNA associated receptor contains Zinc. Zinc is to steroid receptor activation as oxygen is to burning fuel within the mitochondria. Just as oxygen deficiency diminishes the power plant flame, zinc deficiencies prevent steroids from activating the different DNA associated receptors. Many owners have zinc deficiencies. DNA associated receptors refers to the types of receptors for all steroids, vitamin A, and thyroid hormone. If the owner experiences a level five problem they should ask their physician about their zinc status.

A properly functioning fifth link forms a prerequisite for the sixth link to function. The sixth link concerns protein receptors that are manufactured or repressed, on additional DNA segments, when the DNA activates or represses by a specific ovarian steroid. These activated or repressed DNA segments result in the increase or decreased amounts of receptors for the 'lesser hormones'. In contrast, the fifth level (this subsection) concerns hormone receptors manufacture levels determined for the most powerful hormones only (the steroids, vitamin A, and thyroid hormones).

Link Six - Receptor Manufacture, for the Lesser Hormones, Depends on the Success of Ovarian Steroids Activation of certain DNA Programs

The sixth link concerns the receptor formation amounts for the lesser hormones. These lesser hormone receptors only occur as a result of successful activation of the DNA associated nuclear receptor. As the result of DNA activation by a specific steroid, this directs recipient cells to manufacture specific proteins. The instructions for the manufacture of specific proteins are contained within the genetic code - the DNA segment activated. Some of the specific proteins directed to be synthesized lead to new receptors being made from these proteins. These specific receptors are manufactured for other steroids and other 'lesser' hormones. Hormones can't deliver message content without specific receptors.

Most of the discussion at this level is beyond the scope of this book but a basic appreciation is warranted. At the sixth level interdependence of the different steroids, vitamin A, and thyroid hormone takes place. However, the final hormone receptors created at level six are constructed to receive the messages contained within the lesser hormones. An example of the lesser hormones receptor being decreased by estrogen's influence on the DNA program occurs within the liver.

High estrogen states influence the liver DNA to suppress Growth Hormone receptors' manufacture associated with IGF-1 release. Realize when these receptors diminish because they trigger the release of IGF-1, then Growth Hormone will tend to raise the blood sugar without compensation by increasing IGF-1 levels. This increased estrogen caused defect leads to an increased insulin release in order for the Growth Hormone caused blood sugar to return to normal (one cause of insulin resistance). The increased insulin then turns on the fat making machinery within the body. This cascade provides an example of a level six problem, which leads to a fatter female owner until someone helps her to normalize her IGF-1 again.

To eliminate confusion of the ovarian system, visualize six links in a chain. If one of the links breaks, the ovarian system failure profile appears. Common examples of this dysfunction include: hot flashes, irritability for up to two weeks prior to the onset of menses, insomnia, forgetfulness, breast tenderness, cyclical migraine headaches, fibrocystic breast disease, uterine fibroids, some breast cancers, some uterine cancers and some cases of obesity. Also the consequences of diminished androgen eventually present as joint aches, osteoporosis, premature wrinkles and fatigue. These occur clinically regardless of which link fails. Even a well-run battery of ovarian steroid tests including urine and blood can be deceptively normal. In these cases, listen to the body and find a doctor who will look carefully for clinical clues.

The content of this section should alert the owner to the complexity of inquiry necessary to establish the level of ovarian function. Superficial inquiries have side effects; involve little about how the body heals, and lead to symptom control medicine. With opportunities for healing in mind, the time has come to discuss how various hormones interact as informational substances.

CHAPTER SEVEN

Informational Substances

The amount of communication that occurs between different cells via the informational substances (hormones) proves critical to health. These substances secrete at numerous sites within the body and exert distant cellular communication. Glands secrete specific informational substances into the blood stream. The blood stream carries the 'information' towards the target cell. Upon binding its specific receptor, the shape that results from this combination causes a specific vibration that generates a message within the target cell. In this way, the blood functions as a stream of information molecules.

Informational substances are of two types, rapid response and delayed response. The term delayed denotes the ability to affect the activity level of a cell's DNA program. Activated DNA programs make new cell proteins possible. One of the proteins made possible by DNA activation is the manufacture of certain receptors for the rapid response hormones. Consequently, all of the rapid types depend on proper amounts of the delayed type of informational substances activating enough DNA programs. Unless this happens there will be defective receptors when these 'lesser' hormones release (the rapid response type).

The term 'rapid' denotes informational substance types that only affect existing receptors and cellular machinery's activity levels. By far these are the majority of total body hormones. These types of informational substances prove rapid in their message delivery since they have no ability to directly instruct the DNA programs. When DNA programs activate or silence, the protein levels are affected only after a delay within the target cell. Rapid response informational substance side steps this and stops short by having message effect on what already exists within a cell. **Mainstream medicine adherents often fail their patients because they have forgotten this sequence of primacy: Only a select few body hormones determine the activity of the genes. In turn, all other hormones ability to deliver message content depends on the adequacy of these select few hormones performance.**

Adrenaline and insulin provide common examples of the rapid response type of informational substance. In general, rapid acting informational substances affect existing cellular machinery. In other words, adrenaline and insulin only affect the activity level of preexisting cellular machines (enzymes).

In contrast, delayed informational substances determine the types of cellular machinery and receptors created. Cellular machinery types and amounts are only created when the delayed informational substances instruct the DNA programs (genes). Consequently, only when DNA programs receive instruction will cellular machines and new cellular structural components be manufactured. These delayed types of informational substances act by binding specific genes directly and turning them off or on. Examples of delayed informational substances are thyroid hormones, vitamin A, and all steroid hormones.

The rapid response informational substances are generally made from amino acid metabolites, amino acid combinations, or hormonal fat precursors. The final shape carries information. The precise shape is created from these variously arranged molecular building blocks. Molecular building blocks, when processed into the manufactured hormone, carry information by virtue of the final shape. There are numerous sites of manufacture for each of the different types of rapid response hormones. Once released, the closest target cell receives the highest message content and the farthest the least. In this way the site of release sometimes controls the response.

Remember, without proper activation by enough types and amounts of delayed response type of informational substance, to the DNA programs, the rapid response hormones confer diminished ability to deliver message content. For this reason, rapid response informational substances depend on the delayed informational substances for their receptor formation. Without a receptor they remain unable to deliver their message content. The rapid response informational substances can only affect the activity level of existing cellular machinery and structural cell components. One of the structural cell components involves the receptor types it contains.

In general, only the delayed informational substances determine the manufacture rate of cell repair, cell structures, and new cellular machinery. All healthy people contain the proper amounts and timing of release of these gene-controlling hormones. In contrast, all unhealthy people lack or suffer excesses of these important hormones. Recall, the genes provide nothing until the right hormone arrives. Yet, paradoxically, mainstream medical educations spend insufficient time in instructing doctors on how to best assess and augment these important factors.

Basic medical physiology texts are full of molecular and metabolic pathways that describe the individual rapid response type of informational substances. These descriptions detail the rapid response informational substances. However, it is more practical to simplify things down to the overall big picture. In this case, the big picture of the rapid response type of hormones means that they only affect existing cellular 'infrastructure and machinery'.

All rapid and delayed response hormones transport within the blood stream. The blood stream is the mode of transport for the messages contained via hormonal type of informational substances (within the nerves these same substances are called neurotransmitters and the blood stream is not involved).

Communication occurs amongst the cells via numerous informational substances that flow within the blood stream. Factors that improve the quality of the 'tone' in this informational highway reflect themselves in improved owner health. Conversely, factors that decrease the quality of the informational 'tone' within the bloodstream predictably decrease health.

Traditional scientific dogma states that the central nervous system is the center of communication. This dogma erodes by the introduction of new data. Contemporary biochemical studies have revealed that information from numerous cells can direct the central nervous system. The classical notion of the central nervous system still has some truth in the control of its command of conscious thought processes, body movement, and tissue tone (as far as the nerve part of the central nervous system goes). Examples of nervous system movement include voluntary and involuntary types. Voluntary movements include ambulating (walking), the mechanics of talking, and conscious urination. Involuntary movements directed by the classical nervous system are the heart's beating, most unconscious breathing, and digestion. Blood vessel tension, airway tension (bronchial tone) and intestinal tone evidence tissue tone that is orchestrated by the central nervous system.

Not all cells have a nervous system connection. All cells have an informational substance connection (see below). All body cells depend on the quality of informational substances. Informational substances direct the cells in their energy expenditure. Consequently, whether or not one's cells receive quality information proves central to his/her longevity.

Quality informational substance content forms a prerequisite to health. Healthy owners have optimal types and amounts of informational content flowing through their bloodstreams. This occurs at appropriate times and intervals and allows maximal cellular efficiency and harmony. Conversely, unhealthy owners have reflective poor qualities of types and amounts of informational content within their blood streams.

Their informational tone is out of sync with the needs of their cells that need proper informational direction on how to expend available energy. The quality of the informational substances within the blood stream determines energy usage patterns.

Good health cannot occur if the informational substances circulating in the blood stream are not the types and amounts that promote maximum cellular efficiency and vigor. Stressed owners carry and secrete informational substances that communicate stress messages to every cell. Common negative emotional energies such as fear, anger, guilt, and sadness communicate to cells. Unhappy owners communicate 'unhappiness' messages to their cells via their informational substances. Chronically sad owners secrete informational substances that decrease the readiness of their immune system cells. This decreases the ability to defend against rogue cancer cells, foreign invasion from yeast, bacteria, or virus' and from toxins.

Conversely, happiness, love, thankfulness, forgiveness, and hope stimulate the immune system to increase its effectiveness and this communicates through informational substances.

Scientists call informational substances hormones. Some of these same substances are also called neurotransmitters when secreted by nerves. Numerous cell types secrete hormones. Each hormone conveys a specific message. The message content depends on the shape of the hormone plus the cell receptor type that it interacts with. Informational substance can convey varied message content by binding different receptors it is designed to interact with. The combinations of shapes between the hormone and receptor creates message content. There are many different receptors a hormone type can interact with. The resulting message depends on the hormone / receptor combination.

For example, cortisol (a steroid) molecule conveys different types of message content depending on which type of receptor it interacts with. When cortisol binds to the DNA program of the gonads, the message to direct energy away from androgen production and reproduction conveys. However, when cortisol binds to the DNA of a blood vessel smooth muscle cell, its message directs the manufacture of adrenaline hormone receptors. In other cells, it instructs DNA programs in their conservation of energy. Directing these cells to stop their cellular infrastructure investment and rejuvenation activities conserves energy. This maximizes energy for survival. As a final introductory example, cortisol in the liver importantly instructs the liver to manufacture the enzyme, glycogen synthase. The amount of this enzyme here, determines the ability to store glycogen while the blood sugar is rising. In turn, only with adequate glycogen breakdown during falling blood sugar will hypoglycemia be avoided. This explains why owners who suffer from insufficient cortisol fail to maintain their blood sugars (hypoglycemia) between meals, while fasting or attempting to exercise.

All hormones message content centers around how the body directs the expenditure of available energy. Energy usage determines which enzymes activate and which ones remain quiet. Plus which hormones release within the body.

The numerous, different enzymes contained within the body are analogous to molecular machinery. The different types of enzyme machines are contained within specific work areas. These different work areas can be thought of as cell factories.

The different cell factories are called organelles. Organelles are best thought of as different types of cell factories. Mitochondria, endoplasmic reticulum, Golgi apparatus, and nucleolus provide examples of specific organelles.

Different types of cells contain different types of enzymes (cellular machines). Many different additional enzyme machines exist within the blood stream, in the area around cells, and on cell membranes. The enzyme types within a cell depend on the products and functions of each cell type. Each cell type generates specific products.

The integrity of the following three components prove as crucial determinants for preventing the aging process: 1) Cell support structures (cell membrane, GAG integrity and organelles), 2) the sufficiency and integrity of enzymes (cellular machines) positioned within cells and 3) the adequacy of the membrane imbedded mineral pumps that create the cell voltage. It is the overall hormone mixture that determines whether energy directs toward repair and rejuvenation of these vital components or instead into chronic survival mode.

Hormones direct energy expenditure. As a consequence, the hormones present reflect how wise a body directs its energy expenditures. The quality of the hormone message forms one of seven main determinants of aging quickly versus aging gracefully. If the informational content contained in the blood stream remains optimal, youthfulness continues. Youth can only be maintained when the cells receive proper direction on their wise use of energy

Wise use of energy involves adequate energy appropriation towards cellular maintenance, repair, toxin removal, and adequate cellular product formation. All of these processes depend on cells receiving appropriate informational direction. Cells direct energy toward rejuvenation and cellular infrastructure investment when they are given the appropriate informational substance message. Only the correct informational message will direct them to do so. The types and amounts of informational substances determine how the body spends energy. For these reasons, hormone quality significantly effects healing and the slowing down of the aging process. Thankfully, the science exists to assess and improve the body's hormone profile.

How Delayed Informational Substances Affect Energy Management

Testosterone is of the steroid hormone class. Its excess or deficiency serves as an example of appropriate versus inappropriate hormone directions delivered by informational substances. The steroid hormone class is part of the delayed onset type of informational message content. Testosterone, because it is a delayed type of informational substance, alters the types and amounts of cellular energy available by its influence over a cell's DNA program (genes). The sufficiency of DNA program activities or silencing determines the maintenance and rejuvenation adequacy within the cell. Testosterone's presence directs anabolic activities.

Scientists denote the cellular buildup and repair message content as informational substances that are called anabolic. Anabolic means to build up. Alternatively, scientist denote anabolic adequacy by discussing positive nitrogen balance. Because proteins constitute the majority of nitrogen containing molecules in the body, this is a short hand way of saying the protein content is adequate.

In contrast, catabolic processes mean to use up. Alternatively, scientists discuss catabolic hormones as causing a negative nitrogen balance. They cause a negative nitrogen balance because they promote the combusting of body protein as fuel.

Logically, balance between these two forces, anabolic versus catabolic, proves paramount in the struggle to maintain body function.

Realize, catabolic steroid hormones (delayed informational substances) cause some of their catabolic effect by suppressing gene activity because gene activation is a prerequisite for protein synthesis. In contrast, 'lower level' catabolic hormones cause loss of protein only by encouraging combusting it as fuel. But before one can understand where the message of testosterone fits, an overall picture of steroid message content is helpful.

Within the steroid class there are three basic types of metabolic activities controlled at the level of the DNA.

1. **Water and salt content of the body**
2. **Cell survival (deferred cellular maintenance)**
3. **Cellular infrastructure investment and rejuvenation activities**

The steroid, testosterone, activates rejuvenation and infrastructure investment (anabolic or positive nitrogen balance). However, cortisol provides an example of the steroid class that directs body energy into maximizing the survival response (catabolic or negative nitrogen balance). Part of the survival response makes fuel available by its release into the blood stream for survival needs.

Recall, stress, whether real or imagined, involves a catabolic process because fuel is made available by dismantling body cell structures for perceived fuel needs. Catabolically vulnerable body structure is built from sugar, fat and amino acids. In turn, all of these raw fuels need to convert into acetate before the mitochondria power plants incinerate them in the presence of oxygen.

Cortisol frees up these three raw fuel sources by directing body structure to dismantle. Also recall, protein is the metabolically active constituent of body structure. Consequently, run away catabolic message content powerfully ages the body by this mechanism.

In addition, with the help of cortisol, aldosterone controls salt and water balance (kidney chapter). Furthermore, aldosterone controls the rate at which steroid producing glands manufacture other steroids like testosterone. Steroids are some of the central 'players' in how the DNA programs of cells direct the expenditure of energy. Thyroid hormones and vitamin A complex also work in this capacity (at the DNA level).

It is important to emphasize that the testosterone cellular message is one of cellular buildup and restorative integrity activities in both male and female owners. To avoid confusion testosterone will be discussed as representative of anabolic steroids. The anabolic class of steroids is known as the androgen class collectively and includes testosterone, dihydrotestosterone, DHEA, androstenedione, and progesterone. Many of these can be peripherally converted to the others to varying degrees (ovary chapter). This allows for an increase in initially secreted potency without the masculine message in women (intracrinology).

Testosterone-like steroids direct buildup of the integrity of cellular components, in male and female owners by directly switching off or on DNA programs (genes). Testosterone gives the cell the message that cellular infrastructure investment and rejuvenation are important. This message results in increased repair rates, strong bones, increased organ size and function, increased red blood cell production, increased immune cell production and function, increased bulk to muscles, and increased mental functioning abilities.

Certain energetic and lifestyle qualities promote testosterone production and secretion. Certain other energetic and lifestyle qualities decrease its secretion and production. Good information coursing through the blood stream is important. Testosterone is one of many necessary informational substances that help revitalize cells.

The intent of this subsection was to introduce the reader to the importance of containing sufficient anabolic message content. Without anabolic message content the cells lack direction to invest cellular energy in rejuvenation activities. Rejuvenation activities lead to healing. Healing requires an understanding of the three roles that the steroids message serves within the body. The quality of representation of these three roles of steroids determines the steroid tone.

CHAPTER EIGHT

Steroid Tone

As was previously introduced, *steroid tone* serves as a useful construct to help predict the youthfulness of an owner's cells. Optimal steroid combinations and relationships promote cellular health. Unhealthy steroid mixtures diminish cellular function. Cellular dysfunction accelerates the aging process. Cellular health improves as steroid tone improves. The appropriate amounts of steroids in the proper proportions create *steroid tone*. Optimal steroid mixtures direct cells to perform at maximum energy efficiency. Precise combinations of testosterone, DHEA, progesterone, cortisol, and aldosterone direct energy efficiently.

Maximum function and efficiency at the cellular level equals healthy owners through correct steroid mixtures. These appropriate steroid mixtures direct cells towards the efficient use of resources. Wise use of body energy equates cellular efficiency. Only when cellular efficiency occurs is youthfulness possible.

Highest Quality of Steroid Types and Proportions Instructing DNA Programs = Optimal Steroid Tone

Optimal steroid tone only remains possible when the catabolic message content balances with the anabolic message content.

Remember, steroids constitute as powerful hormones because they turn the DNA program on and off. The cells health depends on the quality of informational directions (hormone types and amounts) they receive. The other hormone types (immediate response type), if they act at all, influence the cellular DNA activity by indirect means. In general, immediate response hormones can only direct what already exists within a cell.

In contrast, delayed hormone types determine what exist within a cell because they turn on and off the DNA programs (genes). When DNA programs turn on, certain proteins that are coded for within the activated DNA program are manufactured.

Different body barriers in where they deliver message content generally limit the immediate response hormones. However, the delayed type hormones penetrate everywhere within the body. It is only the steroid class, vitamin A and thyroid hormones that penetrate everywhere (simplified in the case of thyroid hormone because the testes, spleen and lymphatics fail to let it inside parts of their cells).

A youthful, physically fit owner operates in optimal hormone balance. Some owners are youthful physically at age 80 while others are prematurely aged at age 30. The choice is made by the sum of daily decisions and lifestyle behaviors that either promote wellness or accelerates the rate of the aging process.

If one desires youthful vigor the enhancement of steroid tone constitutes a major principle. Healthy owners possess optimal steroid tone without exception. Optimal steroid tone requires balance between the steroid forces that oppose one another (catabolic versus anabolic forces). High quality steroid mixtures direct cells to spend energy wisely between cellular maintenance, rejuvenation, product formation (unique to each cell type) and appropriate rest.

Stress unbalances steroid tone. Stress increases the release of certain survival steroids inherent in the stress response that are catabolic. Under stress the body perceives a threat and directs energy into survival activities. These same steroids direct body energy away from cellular maintenance and repair activities (decreased anabolism). Chronically stressed owners exist in a chronic survival pathway. These pathways predictably decrease steroid tone.

As a consequence, the steroid-tone-fall-off leads to diminished health. Health decreases because stress hormones direct energy away from cellular maintenance, build up, waste removal, and repair activities needed to maintain the youthful state. The youthful state gradually diminishes as the stress steroids proportion increases above normal because the quality of steroid message content has deteriorated

One of the stress response steroid hormones is cortisol. Cortisol is necessary in small amounts for proper cell function. In normal amounts, cortisol directly influences many cellular processes such as: immune regulation, maintenance of blood pressure (especially in moving from sitting to standing), limiting the inflammatory response from the mechanical strains occurring in muscles, ligaments, and joints, and in the counter-regulation of insulin's message. In these situations the cortisol proportion of steroid tone is normal.

However, the chronic survival messages (stress) causes cortisol levels to increase. Chronically increased cortisol secretion creates an imbalance of steroid content within the blood stream. This leads to more survival message content (cortisol) and less rejuvenation message content (testosterone like). In other words, higher cortisol content lowers the proportional contribution of other steroids in their direction of body energy.

For these reasons, the body that stays in survival mode channels energy away from rejuvenation activities and into catabolic pathways. These pathways increase the blood fuel by dismantling body structure components. Simply put, the consequence of mounting a stress response results in lowering the *steroid tone*. By definition, *steroid tone* is high when rejuvenation activity stays high. *Steroid tone* becomes low when rejuvenation activity stays low. *Steroid tone* is a construct to help conceptualize the adequacy of the body steroid mixture, carrying information within the blood stream, for maintaining youthfulness.

Remember, steroid mixtures that deviate from optimum, leads to consequences to the message content and this effects steroid tone. Without optimum types and amounts of steroid mixtures cellular injury and breakdown occurs. For this reason, developing one's knowledge for how breakdown occurs and ways to promote healing proves imperative.

Cells need the correct informational message to heal. The function of cells depends on the hormone instructions they receive. Steroids turn on and off DNA programs within the cells and therefore comprise a primary consideration to maintain youthfulness. Steroid tone attempts to quantify the importance of the quality of instructions that cells receive from steroids.

Six Determinants of Steroid Tone

1. **Health of the adrenal glands and gonads**
2. **Genetic inheritance**
3. **Environmental adrenal and gonad toxin exposure history**
4. **Nutritional adequacy for manufacturing the right steroids**
5. **Emotional lifestyle quality**
6. **Secretogogue influence on the adrenals and gonads. (amount of anabolic enhancement from the secretogogues)**

Five of the six determinants of steroid tone remain under the influence of the owner and respond to healing strategies. The remainder of this chapter describes how to improve steroid tone. Section four develops further the concept of *steroid pressure*. Section five explains how to improve both steroid tone and pressures.

Five of these six determinants can be manipulated to create healing. Female owners need more information about how the modern medical complex depresses their steroid tone. After this, the discussion will apply to the steroid tone of both sexes.

Health of Adrenals and Ovaries Influence the Steroid Tone of Female's

As females age their steroid tone depends more on properly functioning adrenals. Females make less androgen in their ovaries than males make in their testes. For this reason, their ovarian derived androgens fall off more quickly than a man of the same age.

Healthy ovaries manufacture estrogens cycled with progesterone in a balanced and cyclical fashion. However, significant amounts of androgen (androstenedione and testosterone) are also manufactured here. Different female owners have different rates of decline in their ovary-produced steroids.

The adrenals are the backup system for androgen steroid production in females. The female, like the male, needs adequate androgen production to maintain her steroid tone. Only by maintaining steroid tone can the youthful human body be realized.

While the adrenals remain healthy, they are capable producers of androgen-like steroids. DHEA (an androgen steroid) is only produced in adrenal glands. Significant androstenedione production also occurs within the adrenal gland. Cortisol, the stress steroid, production takes place in the adrenal glands. Adrenals also produce the steroid aldosterone that proves vital for mineral and water balance (adrenal chapter). In addition, the aldosterone secretion adequacy determines the rate of production for all other steroids produced within the adrenals and the gonads (ovaries and testes). Consequently, a low aldosterone level will diminish all other steroids production rates for this reason.

With these facts in mind the next level of steroid tone understanding is:
Steroid tone = adrenal (androgen steroids + stress steroids - excess stress steroids + aldosterone steroids) + ovary or

testicle (androgens + progesterone + estrogens (-excessive estrogen).

Very few physicians receive training in assessing steroid output (**24 hour urine and sex hormone binding globulin levels**). Fewer still practicing physicians attempt to replace lost androgen production that results from the post-operative state of a hysterectomy. After uterus removal, even if the ovaries remain left in place, they tend to die off in their steroid production role within two years. This fact results from the dependency of the ovaries for over 80 percent of their blood supply being derived from the uterus. How many female owners receive false reassurance about their ovaries following their hysterectomy? It should be acknowledged that some females possess remarkably strong adrenal glands that adeptly pick up the slack in steroid production following hysterectomy. However, the majority does not evidence this ability within their adrenals.

A progressive decline in muscle mass, increased tendency for weight gain, decreased libido, decreased mental acuity, and premature osteoporosis all result from this omission in the treatment plan. These consequences result from a decline in steroid tone.

Abnormal types of estrogens and progesterone substitutes make the androgen deficiency worse (ovary chapter). These substitutes describe the standard of care for hormone replacement therapy amongst mainstream physicians. Most of these estrogen prescriptions are made from the urine of pregnant horses. Alternatively, some prescriptions are made synthetically from yams or soy by a chemical process and the same chemical mixture results. These abnormal mixtures of estrogens are not healthy. They are also inadequate substitutes for replacing the lost human estrogen message content.

The optimal estrogen message is created by healthy ratios of three different estrogens (estriol, estradiol, and estrone). Optimal estrogen ratios occur within healthy females. In contrast, recall common prescriptions of estrogen substitutes contain an overabundance of alpha estradiol that amplifies the message of cell division by a factor of thirty within estrogen responsive tissues. The estrogen responsive tissues include the breast, uterus, cervix, vulva, vagina, ovaries, and fat cells (located within the breast, hips and thighs).

These prescriptions also contain horse estrogens (equilin and equilinin). Horse estrogen sends out horse estrogen messages. The estrogen responsive tissues within the human female receive the unnatural horse estrogen message. The human females' body was not designed to receive horse specific estrogen message content. Recall that Uzzi Reis MD OB/GYN, author of **Natural Hormone Balance for Women**, says it very well. He asks, "Are you a horse? Do you eat hay? Then why take horse estrogen?"

Part of the female steroid tone derives from estrogen. Each estrogen has a different shape that determines its message content. When this natural shape is altered, the message content changes. Over twenty different types of natural estrogen occur in plants and animals. Also add in the unnatural environmental contaminants - the estrogen mimics. The estrogen mimics pummel most owners with inappropriate message content (adrenal chapter). An imbalanced message content caused by the wrong types and amounts of estrogen delivers a confused message to estrogen dependent tissues. The precise shape of natural estrogen has been altered which diminishes health. Properly proportioned amounts of human estrogens convey a precise message to the target cells that prove necessary to maintain health.

Hormone replacement strategies that contain abnormal progesterone substitutes further compromise steroid tone. Only one real progesterone molecule occurs naturally. The precise shape of the real progesterone molecule contains the message content needed for true health. Altered or synthetic progesterone lowers steroid tone further by interfering with the biosynthesis of other steroid hormones. Compounding the health problems concerns the fact that other steroids require progesterone as their building block. Progesterone substitutes retard this process. The process becomes retarded when progesterone substitutes fool enzyme machines that need real progesterone to build other steroids. Unfortunately, the altered shape of synthetic progesterone cannot serve as a building block for other needed body steroids.

Natural progesterone cannot be patented and therefore it lacks profit potential for its manufacture by pharmaceutical companies. Complications occur with the use of progesterone substitutes. They always have side effects (a different shape changes the message content). This fact alone leads to imbalances in steroid tone. Progesterone proves necessary for building many other steroid hormones that are needed within the body. These other steroids elevate steroid tone and a healthy body manifests.

An analogy given by the late progesterone expert, Dr. John Lee MD, states that progesterone provides the basic 'chassis' for many other steroid designs. Dr. Lee points out that the progesterone substitute situation is like auto manufactures that use a common chassis for multiple car types. A failure to construct the chassis properly during the assembly process halts the remainder of automobile assembly at different points. Where this occurs depends on where the defective chassis lesion occurs. This leads to a marked slowing in finishing out different automobile types at the auto factory.

Similar to automobile assembly, abnormal progesterone substitutes can jam the steroid assembly process in female ovaries and adrenals. The 'assembly lines' are jammed within the enzymatic machinery of the cells because synthetic progesterone has an altered shape. The altered shape is close enough to get into the assembly line (enzyme machine) but not close enough to build from. No new steroids can be built because the substitute steroid is not the correct shape to be processed into other urgently needed steroids. However, it is close enough in shape to natural progesterone to bind to the enzymatic machinery. Once these substitutes engage within the enzymatic machines, they compete with the small amount of natural progesterone for the manufacture of other steroids.

Steroid mismatch, quantified in severity by a diminished steroid tone, leads to a poor quality of life. This is the first part of a complex problem. Part of the solution involves obtaining an accurate steroid hormone profile. The twenty-four hour urine test, which is quantitative and qualitative, proves as a start for addressing where one stands in his/her steroid tone.

The unfortunate female that continues to take abnormal hormone messengers often feels lousy while on an accelerated path to old age, as well. One of the central problems with altered mixtures of steroids (prescription estrogens and progesterone substitutes) concerns the fact that they interfere with and diminish the androgen component of steroid tone. The lower steroid tone that results puts the female in androgen steroid deficiency. The androgen message content is needed to rejuvenate her cells, remains available. Really a deficiency in the androgen message content allows insufficient DNA programs to respond in regard to cellular maintenance and rejuvenation activities

Also frightening, concerns the growing practices of well meaning physicians prescribing the known liver toxin, methyl testosterone. Again, this is not true testosterone and therefore its side effect profile, if read will scare most readers. Scientific fact: Methyl testosterone usage carries the risk of peliosis hepatitis (blood filled liver cysts) and liver tumor development. For these reasons, other countries have long ago outlawed its use.

The adrenals and gonads perform independent tasks for the maintenance of steroid tone. Adrenals have unique hormone products that will be discussed in detail here. This will be followed by a discussion of the adrenal contribution to the androgen class of steroids (build up and maintenance) by its synthesis of DHEA. The adrenal contribution to steroid tone depends on the health of these glands. This is the first determinant of steroid tone and the adrenal component of this will be reviewed first.

Manufacture sites for the different components of Steroid Tone

Adrenal component:
  DHEA
  Cortisol (normal levels only)
  Estrogens (normal levels only)
  Androstenedione
  Aldosterone
  Progesterone

Gonad component:
  Estrogens (normal levels only)
  Progesterone
  Testosterone
  Androstenedione

Each of the above steroids contains precise message content needed by cells in order to expend energy efficiently. Any of the above steroids causes problems when excessive or deficient. The emphasis on excessive cortisol and estrogen above only serves as a reminder for the frequentness of their abnormal increase in standard clinical practice. When correctly proportioned, the cells receive the message to spend energy wisely, which allows for youthfulness.

There are six determinants of steroid tone. As was stated previously, five of the six the owner has control over. This subsection is divided into six parts for each of these determinants.

Steroid Tone

First Determinant - Health of Adrenals and Gonads

The adrenals and gonads contribute to steroid tone by their unique contributions and overlapped contributions. This subsection will explain:
  1. **How chronic stress lowers the adrenal contribution to steroid tone**
  2. **Steroid tone from adrenals and gonads depends on the adrenal manufacture of aldosterone.**
  3. **Types of adrenal androgens manufactured compared to the gonads**

4. **Overlap between estrogen and progesterone produced in the adrenals and gonads**
5. **Introductory remarks about powerful androgens manufactured in the ovaries and testes.**

The contribution of the adrenal gland to steroid tone will be the first consideration in this subsection. The adrenals part of the first determinant of steroid tone is a good place to start the discussion. It concerns the effect of chronic stress on steroid output of the adrenals.

Chronic Stress, Adrenals, and Steroid Tone

Survival is the primary role of the adrenal glands. Survival of chronic stress comes with a high price on steroid tone. Physiologically, just standing up is stressful. The change in gravitational force is tremendous when going from sitting to standing. Without concerted interplay between cortisol and adrenaline, this would not be possible. Cortisol, secreted by the adrenal cortex, puts blood vessels in a responsive state each morning before waking up. Adrenaline, made by the inner part of the adrenal, also increases when one is upright or stressed. The body design allows for a certain average level of cortisol manufacture. The body design can handle occasional stress, as well, without detrimental effects.

The human body needs about 20-25mg/day of cortisol for the maintenance of high steroid tone. Orally this translates to about 40mg/day because of the liver first pass effect that deactivates cortisol. A cortisol deficiency results in a fall in blood pressure followed then by unconsciousness. Sufficient adrenal output of cortisol facilitates correcting a falling blood sugar, as well. Therefore cortisol deficient owners often present with fatigue, hypoglycemia, sugar cravings and low blood pressure.

Recall, the more insulin secreted, the higher the amount of cortisol needed to counteract insulin's message directing the liver to remove sugar molecules out of the blood stream. Remember, abnormal insulin need arises usually after Growth Hormone secretion falls. This in turn leads to the consequent fall off of IGF-1 as well (the body's major insulin for the cells beyond the liver).

This primary defect sets the stage for more insulin need (insulin resistance). These unhealthy bodies survive during the between-meals-state from the more violent means of elevating blood fuel (**Dr. Herb Joiner-Bey's** term). Cortisol proves the major player in these bodies. Epinephrine and glucagon fail to deliver message content without enough cortisol messages preceding them, because cortisol directs the DNA programs to manufacture each of their receptors. **This fact explains why cortisol deficiency presents with low blood pressure and hypoglycemia**.

Cortisol also serves to tone down hyper-vigilance of the immune system. In health, this results in the prevention of inappropriate activation against body tissues manifesting as autoimmune disease and allergies.

However, when the secretion of cortisol rises higher than normal, the body directs energy away from cellular maintenance to accommodate the stress reaction whether real or imagined. Deferred maintenance occurs when the body temporarily lowers steroid tone to survive a perceived threat. The human body can handle occasional deferred maintenance. Survival of a perceived threat by the body redirects body energy into fuel release (catabolic) and out of rejuvenation pathways (anabolic).

The job of steroid hormones is to reroute body energy as the situation merits. When a chronic survival situation occurs, more cortisol (catabolic) and less androgen (anabolic) release and steroid tone therefore decreases.

Deferred maintenance in a car proves similar. An owner can get away without an oil change once in awhile. However, when the body perceives one stress after another, the aging process begins. There must be adequate time for ongoing repair and cellular maintenance activities.

The stress response can become complicated with the discussion of the numerous physiological particulars and associated hormone cascades and feedback loops. Summarize mentally when the body perceives a survival threat, time is essential to maximize physical energy. The body is smart enough to know that an 'oil change, cellular garbage removal, spark plugs changes, etc.' are poor uses of energy when survival is the issue. However, if this threat becomes chronic, then deferred maintenance delivers consequences to the physical body.

Mantra: Hormones carry the messages that direct energy expenditure. For this reason, cortisol production increases drastically when stress occurs. High cortisol production directs energy away from rejuvenation activities and into maximum energy for physical strength and alertness so the body can survive the perceived stress. Beyond the stress response, there is an additional adrenal steroid hormone, aldosterone. Aldosterone proves important to the overall strength of certain cell types. In many ways, the aldosterone level functions as the supreme determiner of steroid tone.

Aldosterone – Maintenance of Steroid Tone

The adrenal glands respond to a narrow control range of salt and water balance that is largely controlled by the amount of aldosterone message content. The adrenal cortex secretes aldosterone within the glomerulosa layer. Potassium level, stress, and angiotensin type two are the three determiners for the amount of aldosterone that the adrenal gland releases.

The secretion of aldosterone directs three main events directed by its instruction of various cell DNA programs (genes):

1. Increased sodium retention relative to potassium removal from the body.
2. Increased cellular charge (increased power to the cell force field) of cardiac and brain cells
3. Increased steroid biosynthesis within the adrenals and gonads.

All the different steroid manufacture rates within the body depend on adequate aldosterone levels. Shared roles exist for the adrenals and gonads in relation to their steroid production roles. Steroid production rates within both of these glands will determine steroid tone. Conversely, they prove different in their unique steroid products that each produce.

Most aldosterone manufacture takes place in the adrenal glands. Remember, the amount of aldosterone produced determines how much of the other body steroids occur. When aldosterone production goes well, the benefit of increased steroid tone occurs. However, when aldosterone production goes poorly, the liability of decreased steroid tone (adrenal chapter) occurs.

Androgens – Contribution to Steroid Tone

The adrenals and gonads share in the manufacture of androgen steroids (the builders and maintenance stimulators). By far the major androgen manufactured within the adrenal is DHEA. This overlap of androgen production between the adrenals and gonads forms a backup system for the maintenance of steroid tone. Health wise, it proves advantageous to have both glands helping in the production of steroid tone. High steroid tone promotes these activities in an efficient and youthful manner. However, in a culture that takes female ovaries on a regular basis, the backup system is better than nothing.

The contribution of DHEA to steroid tone begins to rise at age 7 and peaks around age 25. This level then proceeds to decline throughout life and reach about 10% of peak levels in the last year of life. Notice: the prime of life coincides with DHEA being the most plentiful steroid hormone (see below for why this is important).

DHEA levels decline more quickly in people with high insulin states. Recall, high insulin release rates during the fasting state requires an increased cortisol message to counteract the message of insulin to lower the blood sugar too far. Increased cortisol need directs the adrenals to manufacture more cortisol. Generalize: high stress causes the DHEA levels to fall in order to accommodate the increase in cortisol biosynthesis rate. It has been known for over 80 years that chronic stress leads to anabolism (DHEA) sacrificing itself to maintain catabolism (cortisol) secretion within the adrenals. Cortisol and DHEA are manufactured from cholesterol stores within the adrenal.

There are several different types of androgens made in the body. DHEA is only one of several. Important point: DHEA provides the foundation for continued health and this is why its peak levels coincide with the prime of life.

A mind twist now occurs: Each body tissue has its own preferred androgen that maximizes its anabolic response. The source of each cell's preferred androgen has recently shocked the scientific community. However, clinical medicine seems to be the last to know and continues to ignore what science has revealed. Hence many patients still receive inferior hormone prescriptions (see intracrinology explained below). Summarize for now that when cells receive their preferred androgen, they invest appropriately in repair and rejuvenation. When directions come from their preferred androgen, the different body parts will remain vigorous and vital.

The revolutionary scientific understanding called intracrinology continues to radically alter previous steroid assumptions. Dr. Fernand Labrie pioneered this concept. Basically, he was the first to realize that most anabolic repair in the body occurs in a sex neutral fashion. In other words, either releasing estrogen or testosterone into the blood causes a sexual attitude. However, hidden from view is the beautiful life giving process of peripheral conversion (intracrinology).

Comprehending this concept allows one to see the wisdom of the healthy body secreting more DHEA into the blood stream compared to any other body steroid. Previously, scientists dismissed it as weak because they failed to appreciate that although it initially releases into the blood stream as weak DHEA, it eventually converts within many cells of the body into powerful steroids. Importantly, the powerful steroid conversion within the target cell hides because before it leaves, after delivering message content to the genes in that cell, it becomes a specific inactive metabolite. For this reason, only the physician who routinely checks 24-hour urine results will see the adequacy of these important metabolites. In addition, the androgen adequacy of the skin, brain, organs, muscles, bones, joints can be ferreted out in a general way.

These types of inquiries add predictive accuracy. Total body androgen exposure quantitation requires competency of what these important metabolites mean. Investigating, whether a patient has them or not ensures safer prescribing practices.

Lung tissue seems to prefer DHEA (anabolic message) for rejuvenation that is balanced with the right amount of cortisol (catabolic message). Blood vessels seem to respond in rejuvenation with a preference for DHEA and only small amounts of cortisol as the counter balance message. Muscle cells seem to prefer testosterone for maximal activation in rejuvenation and growth. Skin benefits maximally from dihydrotestosterone (DHT). The heart needs balanced input from testosterone, thyroid, cortisol, and DHEA for continued vitality. The brain, while healthy, concentrates DHEA at five to six times the plasma level of this anabolic steroid. This fact has led some researchers to declare DHEA the youth hormone. It is more accurate to say DHEA is one of the youth hormones and qualify it within the concept of balance. Owners can only have steroid balance when their steroid tone is high.

Progesterone and Estrogen – Contributions in Men and Women to Steroid Tone

Adrenal glands make progesterone and estrogen. Adrenal production of these hormones can become very important in a woman's menopausal years. Menopause creates a drastic reduction of ovary activity for steroid production. This source for these hormones is important throughout life for men. Men need the message content of these hormones for their steroid tone, just like women, but in lesser amounts. Healthy adrenals supply men and women with adequate amounts of these steroids.

Obese male and female owners convert excessive testosterone into estrogen within their fat cells. Zinc deficiencies rev up this process by activating aromatase activity. Aromatase is the enzyme that converts testosterone into estrogen. Breast enlargement in these male owners commonly proves as a consequence of this phenomenon.

Gonads - Steroid Tone

Optimal steroid tone is realized when adrenal glands and gonads remain healthy. Alternatively, health can be regained if these glands have been damaged with an accurate real hormone replacement program. A real hormone replacement program requires an accurate *hormone report card* before the physician can advise an owner in the continuum from health to diminished function. Part of the *hormone report card* involves an assessment of *steroid tone*. This is best ascertained by a well-run twenty-four hour urine test.

Both the six links in the ovary system and the adrenal system need to be intact for healthful *steroid tone* to come from the gonads and adrenals. The adrenals can help failing gonads. Function of either system needs to be determined by an accurate assessment of *steroid tone*. Sometimes supplementation is necessary for the owner with failing glands for their rejuvenation program. This program will help these owners heal from the effects of low *steroid tone* (see ovary, testicle and adrenal chapters).

This subsection leads up to all six determinants of *steroid tone*. Recall that five of six of these determinants are additional considerations, which can allow healing to occur without chronically prescribing hormone replacement. Low *steroid tone* often requires the help of a knowledgeable physician to remedy it. It helps to again separate for emphasis the contributions of the adrenals and gonads (ovaries or testes) to overall *steroid tone*.

Adrenal component of steroid tone:	Gonad component:
DHEA	Estrogens
Cortisol (normal amounts only)	Progesterone
Cortisol diminishes tone in excess	Testosterone
Androstenedione	Androstenedione
Progesterone	
Estrogen	
Aldosterone	

Note cortisol is mentioned twice to emphasize that its excess powerfully diminishes steroid tone.

A scientific assessment of the adrenals and ovaries steroid output is the first determinant of steroid tone. The other five determinants have a moderating influence on the initial steroid tone (discussed in above and below subsections). Testes work with adrenal glands promoting steroid tone. The only difference between ovaries and testes, as far as their steroid production roles, concerns their relative proportions of the different gonad derived steroids produced.

The secretion proportions of estrogen and progesterone are higher in the ovaries and testosterone and androstenedione are lower in women compared to men. The opposite proportions exist in men. When testes cells are healthy, these glands will activate (see secretogogues below) contributing to a higher steroid tone. However, injured testes generate lower steroid tone because of the consequent diminished contribution of important steroids. Similarly, inured or weakened ovaries contribute deficiently towards steroid tone.

These cases need to have the six links in the testes or ovary system chain of health assessed (see ovary and testes chapters). Sometimes the assessment leads the physician to recommend real hormone replacement therapy. In other cases the four other determinants of steroid tone, that an owner controls, can be corrected (explained below). Nutrition of the glands describes one factor that powerfully influences steroid tone and remains under owner control.

Nutritional Adequacy and Steroid Tone

Unhealthy, physical signs occur in people who eat processed foods. Puffy, bloated faces, sagging skin, and loss of muscular definition exemplify the nutritional deficiencies processed food causes. Fast food restaurants provide an excellent place to make these clinical observations.

Before steroid replacement knowledge developed, unless you were an Asian who imbibed in good quality ginseng, less androgen would be manufactured with each passing year. Less androgen manufacturing, leads to lower steroid tone and the consequent ungraceful decent into old age.

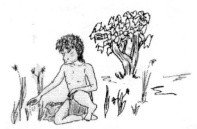

Poor nutrition causes gonad and adrenal cells to possess a decreased ability to free up cholesterol and move it inside the mitochondria. The mitochondrion (plural is mitochondria) is the site within the gonads or adrenal glands cells where cholesterol converts into early steroid precursors. Cholesterol needs to move into mitochondria before the first step of steroid manufacture occurs.

Once cholesterol moves inside the mitochondria it converts into the various early steroid hormone precursors. After several simple conversions, the end product within the mitochondria is pregnenolone, the starting point precursor steroid that proves necessary to build all other steroids. Importantly, after pregnenolone forms inside the mitochondria from cholesterol, it undergoes conversion into other steroids outside the mitochondria. Unfortunately, this internal conversion from cholesterol to pregnenolone proves more difficult as the owner ages.

There are four reasons the conversion of cholesterol to pregnenolone develops a roadblock with age:

1. **Aldosterone content within becomes diminished secondary to a processed food diet (see below).**
2. **Necessary vitamins and cofactors for biosynthetic reactions of these conversions diminish.**
3. **Cholesterol content diminishes within the adrenals and gonads (statin drugs?)**
4. **The common method of taking pregnenolone supplements has possible detrimental side effects.**

This fourth additional point needs emphasis before proceeding with the remedies for the other three causes of diminished steroid biosynthesis. This additional factor exposes many short sighted and half thought out approaches to steroid replacement. Pregnenolone supplementation can partially bypass the need for these mitochondria first step reactions.

However, the side effect of taking pregnenolone as a supplement for waning steroid production is that it contains cortisol-like message content of its own. Increased cortisol message content is warranted in certain clinical situations. However, in most situations, when it is within one's blood stream after oral ingestion, it will contribute to decreased overall steroid tone.

Recall, steroid tone becomes negatively influenced when cortisol message content rises above a very low threshold. In the normal state, pregnenolone never enters the blood stream in increased amounts. Normally, it converts within the adrenals and gonads into other steroids.

To counter act these problems, pay attention to the first three nutritional factors of adrenal and gonad support. The first of the three nutritional factors affecting the health of these glands involves the owner's history of diet preference. This determines the aldosterone level of most owners. Aldosterone levels respond to either a 'real food' diet or a 'processed food' diet. As aging proceeds, eating processed foods leads to an eventual depletion of one's mineral balance.

Around middle age owner's bodies become deficient in mineral balance through the chronic ingestion of processed foods. Processed foods have the wrong mineral proportions. The right mineral proportions prove necessary for high steroid tone. Real foods (unprocessed and natural) will have a much higher proportion of potassium and magnesium content. In addition, real food sodium content is lower than processed food.

The opposite situation of mineral balance exists in owners who arrive at middle age with a history of a preference for processed foods (dead food). This food type is diminished in its potassium and magnesium content from food processing (see mineral table). Processed foods usually have high amounts of sodium added. Many middle-aged owners, who eat processed foods, prematurely suffer the consequences of a decline in their steroid tone.

The central steroid defect from a chronic 'dead food' diet is diminished aldosterone production required for normal blood pressure.

One group of bodies still tries to produce appropriate aldosterone in this chronic situation of a dead food diet, but high blood pressure predictably results. Recall, the dead (processed) food diet is high in sodium and low in potassium. However, the human body was designed to ingest the reverse of mineral proportions, which the processed food diet provides. For example, sodium retention beyond healthful amounts causes fluid retention, which causes elevated blood pressure.

Another group of owners' bodies sense inappropriate sodium content and reduce aldosterone levels to compensate. However, the price paid by these owners' involves their diminished steroid synthesis rates as a consequence from diminished aldosterone levels. Visualize the painful choice that each body type discerns only because they receive dead food.

Fortunately, the owner who takes an active role in the procurement of a real food diet (section three) enjoys an advantage.

In contrast, the 'dead food' (processed) diet accelerates the path to an old body in two major ways. First, diminished aldosterone or elevated blood pressures are the choices given to the body that feeds on dead food. When a body chooses the lower aldosterone route, steroid tone suffers and the owner ages faster. Conversely, when a body chooses to maintain steroid tone by keeping aldosterone elevated in the presence of a processed food diet, the blood pressure elevates. When the blood pressure elevates the owner again becomes older by a failure to honor the second principle of health, avoiding hardening processes.

    The second reason that the steroid production rate begins to fall with advancing age concerns the deficiency in vitamins and cofactors. Vitamins and cofactors prove necessary for the manufacture of many different steroids. These prove as additional nutritional dependent factors that effect steroid tone. Enzymatic machinery must be in good working order to allow efficient steroid biosynthesis. Individual enzymes (cellular machines) need specific trace minerals and cofactors in order to perform in the creation of the different steroids. Only when steroids are manufactured at appropriate rates can steroid tone be high.

    An analogy is the automobile that has a full tank of gas, but all the oil is drained out. In addition, the spark plugs and carburetor are missing. Missing components are like the cofactor and vitamins steroid producing enzymes (machines) need to make the necessary steroids. When there is a cofactor deficiency, steroid production diminishes. When steroid production diminishes steroid tone falls.

    A partial list of vitamins required for the manufacture of steroids is vitamin A, pantothenic acid, folate, most of the B vitamins, and vitamin C. The adrenal gland has the highest tissue concentration of vitamin C in the body under healthful conditions. This fact might provide a clue as to why vitamin C is so important in the owners continued survival for the prevention and surviving the stress of illness. The stress of surviving an illness requires an increase in steroid production. The need for vitamin C goes up with stress and illness.

    The accessories, in the car engine analogy, lends itself to understanding the reason that dietary attention and discretion become so important as owners navigate their search for health and happiness. Youth can survive for a while without the critical nutrients needed by cellular machinery. However, youthfulness that endures cannot. 'Father time' is there to observe old cellular parts struggling to work beyond their normal life span without molecular replacement parts. The body can only acquire new molecular parts through dietary intake of the molecules needed (section three).

In addition, food processing destroys important nutrients required for the proper function of enzymes. There are at least five B vitamins contained in whole grains that decrease by half within one week of grinding it into flour (half life = time for half to be gone). Oxidation of these unstable and bulky molecules occurs after the grinding process.

Before growing, in the natural state, vitamins are positioned precisely within the seeds molecular architecture to confer stability. However, when grains or seeds are ground into flour this process destroys the protection provided by its architectural framework. This consequence occurs because the grinding process exposes these unstable molecules to the oxidative forces. Oxidative forces (heat, air and sunlight), in turn, diminish their nutritional value.

Oxidation also takes place in vitamin-fortified foods exposed to heat, air and sunlight for the same reasons. Just because manufactures add vitamins to the box or can doesn't mean they are still intact when the owner ingests it. In contrast, real food still contains vitamins and minerals that the creator intended.

Vitamin supplements are more stable, but absorption characteristics differ widely from brand to brand. Vitamins and vitamin-fortified foods are deficient in some of the vitamins that are removed when food is processed. For example, folate, pantothenic acid, and lipoic acid are especially susceptible during food processing. Compounding the deficiency problem is the fact that many vitamin fortified foods and supplements are deficient in these three vitamins!

When one of these is missing it is as if there is a malicious conspiracy within the food industry to make owners weak and old. The weakest link in a chemical reaction sequence will stop a body process. In a pantothenic acid deficiency, carbohydrate and fat combustion greatly curtails. With a lipoic acid deficiency, carbohydrate can only convert to lactic acid that builds up in the tissues and is evidenced as sore and achy muscles. Adrenal and gonad tissues need tremendous amounts of fuel for energy. Therefore, when these vitamins become deficient steroid tone diminishes.

Additional trace minerals are needed within the adrenals and gonads for maintenance of steroid tone. For example, minerals like zinc and magnesium need adequate stomach acid for absorption. Many western owners are prescribed medicines that block acid production. These owners could therefore become deficient in many of these critically needed minerals despite a healthy diet.

A diet containing sufficient organic and unprocessed whole grains, vegetables, eggs, fish, meats, nuts and fruit promote steroid tone. A real food diet promotes steroid tone by the fact that it contains the proper proportions of minerals and vitamins to promote the health of steroid producing glands (other body tissues as well).

Many plants also contain antioxidant (anti-rust) molecules that confer particular benefits to specific tissues. Examples include lycopene found in tomatoes for prostate health, bioflavonoids found in berries for blood vessel health, acanthocyanadin found in bilberry for retina health, silymarin found in the milk thistle for liver health. Carelessness in how these foods are processed can destroy much of the anti-oxidant content and hence their potential benefits.

The lower the antioxidants in the diet, the more the need for anabolic steroids to direct increased repair. Increased repair is necessary when diminished protection exist from the oxidants. When oxidant damage occurs, elevated steroid tone becomes necessary to compensate for the increased injury rate. Think about the fact that all football players need a very high steroid tone to compensate for the increased injury rate that playing their sport entails.

Increased steroid tone compensates for the increased injury rate because when steroid tone stays high, anabolism remains high. Obviously, possessing both high steroid tone and optimal nutrition allows the best health possible. In order to maximize the intended benefits of sufficient steroid tone, purchase only quality supplements or real foods that comes from fresh organic sources.

When certain tribes throughout the world are studied, it is observed that they enjoy remarkably good health and greater freedom from the ravages of chronic disease. These tribes share a common denominator of a diet high in plants that have high progesterone or progesterone precursors. Some of the plants known to contain relatively high amounts of progesterone or progesterone precursors are: pomegranates, European mistletoe berries, panax ginseng, Mexican wild yams and halotorrhea floribunda.

Environmental Toxins and Steroid Tone

Many toxins exert their effect on adrenal and gonad health. Environmental affects on steroid tone (hormone mimics subsection) increase the estrogen-like message content in an owner's body. Increased estrogen message content creates problems in anabolic balance and in estrogen responsive tissues that include men's prostates. Many of these mimics and toxins prove far reaching in their ability to disrupt the ideal natural hormone message content. Natural hormone message content imbalances and this negatively affects steroid tone. Effective measures exists that limit exposure to environmental toxins, which diminish steroid tone. By limiting exposure to these toxins one can restore the message content provided by anabolic steroids.

Several lifestyle practices limit toxin exposure to steroid producing glands. First, limit exposure to hormone mimics. Consume organically grown food whenever possible. The food supply describes how most of the hormone mimics invade an owner's body. Clean water consumption avoids many of the hormone mimics. Stay away from golf courses because of the heavy use of hormone mimic-like molecules. Second, education about toxins in the home is important. Avoid the counter-productive stress of being paranoid; just try to reduce chemical exposure within reason. Third, with increased public awareness campaigns about the consequences of continued industrial, agricultural, and food distributors practices that allow this problem to perpetuate, things will change for the better.

Genetic Inheritance and Steroid Tone

Genetic predisposition toward weakness or strength forms a component of steroid tone. Some owners have strong adrenals and gonads that increase their advantage for creating steroids. If the increased steroids are of sufficient quality then a longevity advantage follows through as an increase in steroid tone. Some owners are born with weak adrenals and/or gonads. The weakened glands do not supply steroids sufficiently. Following the advice of the other five determinants of this subsection will help make things right.

The cornerstone to coaching a borderline functional owner in adrenal and gonads health concerns an accurate steroid report card. Only with an accurate assessment will there be any hope of correctly replacing steroids that begin to wane around middle age. An accurate assessment contains a blood analysis for certain hormones and a twenty-four hour urine test for steroids. These values are the baseline for later treatment and inquiry.

Genetic inheritance knowledge is useful in that it helps the owner understand potential weakness. Genetic weakness predisposes owners for disease. Awareness about personal genetics allows ways to pay special attention to weak links that are carried on

DNA programs. Family history falls into this realm of consideration. Hormone assessment increases accuracy of the current situation.

Steroid tone has a genetic component, although the genetic component is a mind twist to understand. There are two different angles to consider regarding genetics and steroid tone. First, concerns the fact about the consequences that result from diminished steroids instructing one's genes. **Realize, the DNA provides nothing until the right hormone arrives.** Without sufficient steroid message content instructing the genes they fail to activate. Each time a gene fails to activate it means that the protein for which it codes proves insufficient.

Each protein insufficiency added on top of the other translates into the typical middle age feeling that something has changed. Second, gene activation variability results from poor quality in regard to the proportions of the different steroids produced. This fact describes the competition between anabolism and catabolism. It acknowledges that in the end, good health requires a balance between these two extremes of message content. Finally, remember that both of these genetic variability's are worsened by the other five-lifestyle redeemable habits discussed in this subsection.

Some family lines produce extremely strong bodies because they produce a superior steroid tone. Other genetic lines produce less vital strength in the adrenals and gonads. Vitality wanes when gonads and adrenals begin to fail in their production of rhythmical and adequate steroid messages to the cells. This process describes a falling steroid tone.

Realize the role genetics plays in many common degenerative diseases is often sensationalized in the effort to market what is for sale within the complex. However, in the vast majority of cases, the quality of steroid message instructing the genes commands primacy over the genetic inheritance. Much genetic vulnerability can be overcome by lifestyle modification.

In addition, with careful assessment, many genetically predisposed owners with low steroid tone can be helped by supplementations with real steroids in the correct physiological doses. Unfortunately, the science that empowers owners to actively improve their genetic vulnerabilities collides with the more lucrative approaches offered by the complex. Sensationalism aside, improvement in steroid tone empowers owners to avoid genetic weakness from manifesting.

Emotional Energies and Steroid Tone

The overall emotional quality delivers a powerful effect on steroid tone. Positive emotional experience communicates to steroid producing glands to increase the steroid tone mixture output (section six). In contrast, negative emotions influence steroid glands to believe survival is the issue. When the body perceives a survival threat, either real or imagined, stress steroids increase and rejuvenation steroids decrease. As a consequence, when chronic negative emotions occur, this mechanism lowers steroid tone.

America is a stressful place to live in many respects. Deadlines, job insecurities, modern life complexities, noise pollution, environmental pollution, and electromagnetic pollution all take their toll on the human body. The body experiences these emotional stresses energetically by the changes in the informational substances that the glands secrete. The stress response informational substances include cortisol. Cortisol levels increasing causes the relative proportion of its message content among other steroids to increase as well. This proportional change lowers steroid tone.

Specific dynamics occur in the way cortisol opposes androgens and the energies that direct this process. The dominant emotional energy determines how the body spends available energy. The hormone messages that secretes result from, in part, the different emotional energies. In this way the different types of emotions have a profound effect on energy usage patterns.

Studies have shown male teammates' testosterone increases immediately before a competition and remains elevated during the event. Studies also show that the teammates testosterone will remain elevated when the game is over, only if they win. This fact provides contrast between the negative emotions of losing and the positive emotions of winning. The outcome of the event not only affects the quality of emotions, but the quality of steroid tone. Studies have also shown chronically depressed owners have lower DHEA levels than aged matched controls that are not depressed.

That the quality of emotions affects overall steroid tone can be understood in a general way. The adrenals have the choice of making more DHEA or more cortisol. Positive emotional experiences usually allow DHEA levels to remain adequate. Positive emotions translate into the body as a low stress situation.

When the body perceives a low stress situation, more energy channels into rejuvenation activities. However, bodies that perceive survival threats contained in the negative emotions, release more cortisol. The body has limited energy. Hormone messages direct energy expenditure. The stress response channels energy expenditure by the types of hormones that it summons.

When negative emotions cause stress hormones to increase, the energy channels into catabolic pathways. Recall, catabolic pathways consume body structure for increased fuel availability within the blood stream. The survival response also involves the inhibition of rejuvenation activities. Increased fuel availability brought on by stress describes a primitive design feature.

Remember, modern stress differs from primitive stress, which usually involved a physical challenge. Physical challenges need extra fuel to maximize strength. However, modern mental stress requires no physical response. This explains how the modern day result of this design feature, in a setting of chronic negative emotions, increases the catabolic direction of energy while decreasing its anabolic component. Here, the cortisol message content increases and the androgen message content decreases.

DHEA is one of the body's main androgens. All androgens convey a general cellular message that says to invest adequate cellular energy into rejuvenation and infrastructure investment. Alternatively, as previously stated, cortisol, because it is catabolic, directs cells to put on hold cellular rejuvenation and infrastructure investment. However, negative emotions direct a powerful message channeling energy into catabolism by increasing cortisol.

Only optimal cortisol conveys a harmonious and less dramatic message. However, high cortisol amounts excrete, when the body perceives a survival threat. This directs energy toward survival pathways. Survival pathways are necessary in mounting a strong physical response at the expense of cellular maintenance and rejuvenation. For these reasons, emotional energy powerfully effects steroid tone.

Take home point: Excess cortisol has the ability to direct energy away from youth maintenance activities. The message content from high cortisol levels directs energy toward survival. For this reason, some scientific circles have called the chronic elevation of cortisol the 'death hormone'.

This title refers to chronic deference of cellular maintenance activities when cortisol chronically elevates. This accelerates wear and tear changes because less anabolic (repair) message content exists. One of the seven deterrents (principles) to wear and tear changes (old age) involves having adequate message content to rejuvenate. Message content to rejuvenate comes from the anabolic steroids. The hormones giveth and the hormones taketh away. When anabolic steroids balance with the catabolic steroids, steroid tone remains high and health can continue.

As a general rule, the faster the metabolic rate in body tissue, the more vulnerable it becomes to deferred maintenance activities. High metabolic rate tissues, like brain and heart tissue, consequently become more vulnerable with decreased steroid tone. The overall quality of the mixture determines high or low steroid tone. High steroid tone quantifies the tendency for percentages of different steroids in the blood stream to approach optimal.

High steroid tone directs the body to invest appropriate energy in repair of the wear and tear changes inherent in life activities. At the same time, high steroid tone directs appropriate rest intervals and is synonymous with the balance of message content between anabolic and catabolic steroid hormones. Optimal steroid tone needs to occur if youthfulness and healing are to occur. Pertinent to this subsection: The quality of emotions has a powerful effect on the consequent steroid tone.

That emotions effect steroid tone proves as an essential concept to combat the ravages of life and emerge as an owner who ages gracefully and lives life fully. The fact that positive emotions promote high steroid tone means that appropriate levels occur for testosterone, DHEA, androstenedione, and progesterone relative to the total amounts of cortisol-like substances within the blood stream. The balance between opposing steroids makes the health difference.

The human body needs re-building activities followed by rest periods. All building and the owner become the stiff body builder and/or the aggressive personality types. When energy channels to the extremes of a body builder physique or the aggressive personality type, too much unhealthy anabolism takes place. Cortisol induces appropriated cellular rest periods in the healthy state. Balance needs to occur between rest and adequate periods of androgen secretion. Emotional energy either facilitates or upsets this balance.

The physical stress of vigorous exercise causes the temporary elevation of cortisol that directs energy toward maximal strength activities. This means cellular maintenance decreases. The difference between exercise stress and emotional stress concerns the fact that physical exercise increases testosterone as well as cortisol when emotions allow it. When the emotions allow it, testosterone remains elevated after exercising and cortisol levels decrease.

During the stress of physical exercise there is no need for extra insulin because the increased blood sugar, directed by cortisol, is appropriately consumed by physical exercise. **In addition,**

healthy owners, while exercising, maintain their blood fuel with sufficient Growth Hormone release. The more Growth Hormone released, the higher the IGF-1 and the more protein is protected from combusting to satisfy fuel needs at the mercy of cortisol. Recall, these two facts allow for both diminished cortisol and insulin need. Also recall, thyroid hormone adequacy determines the amount of Growth Hormone manufactured in the pituitary. Something to think about the next time a physician counsels that low normal thyroid is fine.

In marked contrast, with emotional stress, excessive cortisol secretes into the blood stream. The elevated blood sugars that cortisol causes, prevent Growth Hormone release. The message of cortisol is completely different in the absence of the testosterone message. The message difference results more from the increased insulin required and the lack of testosterone when mental stress occurs. Making matters worse, part of the stress response involves increased prolactin release, which also powerfully inhibits testosterone release.

It is important to emphasize that part of the stress response concerns the soaring cortisol secretion relative to other steroids. Chronic stressful emotions raise cortisol levels relative to other androgens. This accelerates wear and tear within cells because cortisol redirects cellular energy during chronic stress or emergency situations. The body response to an emergency situation is always the same, whether it is real or imagined. The body directs energy out of rejuvenation and into increasing fuel availability, which is derived from dismantling body structures (protein, fat, and carbohydrate).

As was previously stated, the more metabolically active the body tissue, the more vulnerable it becomes to deferred maintenance activities. The brain has one of the highest metabolic rates within the body. **Therefore, chronic emotional stress has the potential to contribute to the rate of brain aging quickly.** The brain ages more quickly because energy chronically directs into survival pathways. When survival pathways activate, rejuvenation (repair and maintenance) activities inactivate. These changes become physically manifested in diminished cell membrane integrity, aging intracellular factories, and enzymatic machinery. There also arises the increased tendency for oxidized fats and proteins to build up inside cells. As oxidized fats accumulate, they condense into waste known as lipofuscin. Clinically, the aging brain manifests in a slower reaction time and progressive memory impairment for new events and concepts (the 'Red neck' idea).

The dominant hormone message often reflects the dominant emotional energy. Positive emotions of love, forgiveness, joy, hope, and contentment convey to the body that all is well. The body naturally produces a steroid consistent with that emotional state. Conversely, negative emotions of hate, anger, fear, and sadness direct an increase in the production of stress hormones. Beyond the effects of emotions on steroid tone are factors that increase the presence of the rejuvenation-type steroids. Scientists call such factors secretogogues.

Secretogogues and Steroid Tone

Secretogogues enhance the output of the rejuvenation message content contained within the steroid class called androgens. Androgen message content increases when secretogogues increase. Examples of secretogogues are regular exercise and certain plants like panax ginseng.

Counterbalances to stress are the practices that promote secretion of the strength promoting and rejuvenation steroid hormones (DHEA, testosterone, and progesterone). Secretogogues promote these secretions. Given adequate nutritional support and adequate adrenal and gonad health, certain practices promote optimal secretion of body building steroids and promote elevated steroid tone. Without some of the three criteria of adequate nutritional support, adrenal and gonad health being present there cannot be an adequate response to a secretogogue. Secretogogues can't pull strength hormones out of a dying gland. The shriveling gland affects other functions.

An analogy for this involves the similarities between factories and cells. Old gonads and adrenals are like an order arriving at a factory and the condition of the factory is found in disrepair. The disrepair is evidenced by aged factory support structures (organelles) and aged machinery (enzymes) that have worn out and fallen apart. Very little of this order can be acted upon (hormone creation) because of these conditions.

Before the factory can respond to the order, it needs to be remodeled and upgraded in its infrastructure and machinery. The adrenal and gonad 'factories' prove similar in that they need the proper infrastructure investment provided by adequate molecular replacement parts and the right hormones (message content) for direction. Sedentary owners send the wrong message content (hormones) and their 'factories' tend toward disrepair. This fact explains the root of the saying, 'use it or lose it'. Exercise proves as a secretogogue directing cells to receive improved message content and hence invest in rejuvenation.

Owners with poor steroid tone hate to exercise. Only some of this feeling result from long standing habits that produced an attitude. Part of the problem lies in the fact that sedentary owners have a diminished secretogogue influence in their lives. Also a significant biochemical component occurs for this aversion.

Poor steroid tone predictably occurs when the physical condition deteriorates. As a consequence, out of shape owners' body cells encounter steroid mixtures that reflect poor physical exercise habits. In this way, sedentary lifestyles accelerate the aging rate.

Conversely, a well-trained athlete possesses sufficient types and amounts of steroids that reflect high steroid tone. Highly trained and physically fit cells of an athlete receive steroid messages that direct cellular energy into maintenance and rejuvenation. Realize, their genes activate efficiently because their cells receive the proper message to invest in rejuvenation. In this way, to the highly trained athlete, regular exercise acts as the secretogogue stimulant for anabolic steroid production.

Take home point: chronic stress of modern life makes matters worse by encouraging cells to invest energy foolishly, which accelerates wear and tear on the body. Stress reroutes life-sustaining energy into survival mode. When poor exercise habits are added to the daily routine, deterioration becomes more aggressive in assaulting the body form. The higher the stress in life, the more need to counter balance with secretogogues. Exercise is a reliable secretogogue. Owners in the middle of modern life stress need to exercise.

Unhealthy owners need to know that their body wants to heal. However, their body needs the correct informational message to do so. Higher steroid tone carries the information needed to heal the body. Optimal steroid tone doesn't return over night. It involves a gradual process just like becoming unhealthy proceeds as a gradual process. Understanding that with the passage of time, vigor and vitality will increase as the owner persists in improving the quality of informational messages that his/her cells receive. The secretogogues, like exercise, help owners begin healing. Their cells begin to receive improved information from higher steroid tone that exercise provides.

The secretogogues increase the amount of energy available for cellular rejuvenation and infrastructure redevelopment. These restorative activities increase because steroid tone increases. Owners committed to their recovery program notice positive changes every time they look in the mirror and in the improvement in the way that they feel as the months go by. Recovery doesn't have to be expensive or complicated. Recovery can start today with a commitment to understanding the nutritional needs and the emotional environment that gives and takes energy from the owners life. The body begins to heal with improved nutritional quality and through a daily walk, stretch and breath exercises.

The ability of exercise to increase steroid tone crosses over into its effect on emotional energy as well. Positive emotions confer an energetic rhythm to cells by facilitating improved quality of informational substances that course through the blood stream (section six). The emotional energy of happiness, joy, laughter, self-love, and forgiveness are all ways to increase the rate of healing. Exercise adds positive emotional energy to an owner's life. This fact describes an effect beyond its secretogogue influence.

Owners are asked to remember the last time they experienced happiness and what it felt like. This provides instruction for remembering what the cells felt via the informational substances. Happiness energy directs reflective release of the appropriate informational substance that communicates to the cells that all is well. This message allows the cell to harmoniously interact with maximum efficiency and aliveness.

CHAPTER NINE

Four Misunderstood Steroids

The *four misunderstood steroids* are thyroid hormone, vitamin A, vitamin D, and aldosterone. Many in the scientific community will now protest. First, they will protest this point because in a peripheral way, aldosterone and vitamin D are already considered steroids. However, they are grouped together here because they possess under emphasized steroid-like power to regulate the DNA program of cells. Second, thyroid hormones and vitamin A are generally not classified as steroids.

However, thyroid hormones and vitamin A are among the most powerful hormones, which include the steroids, in that the quality of the entire group's presence determines the activity of the genetic program. Like steroids, thyroid hormones and vitamin A directly bind DNA and carry message content by virtue of their precise shape induced vibration. All of the misunderstood steroid-like hormones regulate cell DNA by the amount of their presence or absence. Because the fate of the body depends on how well these four hormones release; they will be briefly described.

Steroid-like Properties of Aldosterone

Aldosterone is the first misunderstood steroid hormone to be considered. Currently a narrowness of thought exists with regards to the impact of aldosterone on certain cells. Many physicians think in terms of water and salt balance only when they consider aldosterone. Aldosterone influences certain cell types in their ability to increase cell membrane charge. Maintenance of an optimal cell charge only takes place when there is adequate instruction from aldosterone and thyroid hormones. These two hormones instruct certain genes to activate that increase the force field (cell membrane charge or cell voltage).

The higher a cell's voltage the more work it is capable of performing. In the maximal function of cardiac and nerve cells this proves particularly important. Important concept to emphasize: The stronger the force fields created by a cell type, the more work it is capable of performing (see sections 3 and 5). A more powerful electrical charge also provides added protection from inappropriate penetration of harmful ions (excess calcium). This is important for the continued operation of a nerve cell (section 6).

One of the seven indicators of aging within involves diminished cellular charge (cell voltage). Lastly, aldosterone plays a fundamental role in the instructional activation of gonadal and adrenal DNA. The DNA programs of these glands that activate in this way, allows increased steroid manufacture rates.

Recall, certain medications, supposedly called angiotensin converting enzyme (ACE) inhibitors, lower blood pressure by poisoning the message delivery system of aldosterone release by the adrenal gland. Currently a debate exists concerning the exact mechanism of how these prescription drugs works (section one). Aldosterone diminished message delivery describes the mechanism physicians are given.

Recall blood pressure lowers through several other but under reported mechanisms (sections one, the adrenal and kidney chapters). For the purpose of the current discussion, only the aldosterone lowering message mechanism remains pertinent because of its secret side effect.

Very few doctors are educated about the importance of aldosterone in stimulating the adrenals and gonads in their steroid production roles. Lower aldosterone message content arriving at the heart and nerve cells also diminishes the ability of these cells to increase their force fields to the strength required for maximum function (section five). Diminished force fields within nerve and heart cells lead to progressive disabilities in these cells performance (*low cell voltage syndrome*).

Circumstances arise where aldosterone production must be suppressed. When physicians become aware of the importance of aldosterone, they will understand the appropriate times and methods for accomplishing this. They will also avoid reducing aldosterone production when suppression proves inappropriate.

> This narrowness of learning that occurs in medical educations provides one example of how well informed patients can help curious physicians understand what science has revealed. Alternative methods for natural ways to heal high blood pressure are more fully discussed in section one. The current medical system controls the behavior of physicians through a mixture of three things.

First, acceleration in busy work takes away from a doctor's time and desire for new learning. Second, people that become 'certified experts' are often the ones who learn early on to keep their mouth shut when they stumble upon scientific inconsistencies while being indoctrinated with the official view of medical treatment strategies. How convenient to hide this proven technique from public consideration. Third, the medical legal rule of the 'standard of care' must not be violated. Any deviation from the sanctified approach will alienate a physician into a legal battle with the complex. Again, hidden from public view, the medical board often castigates physicians that fail to adhere to even the scientifically invalid dictums. The medical industrial's viewpoint has profit to consider. The best protection that an outspoken physician has is to design ways to make it painful for these authorities if they choose to obstruct what science knows.

This being said, never under estimate the power contained in even one man's life when he lives it properly. Like ripples in a pond spreading forever outward, so it is when at the grass roots, people begin to create ways for their physicians to again practice and learn different ways that lead to healing.

Steroid-like Properties of Thyroid Hormone

The thyroid hormone, like the steroids and vitamin A, shares the unique ability to penetrate through many body chambers and barriers. It also shares the powerful ability to reach and direct the DNA programs of cells. This powerful ability instructs which genes under its influence turn on and off. The only other hormones that are this powerful are the steroids and vitamin A.

Fragmenting this small group of hormones, which instruct the DNA programs, leads to their interdependent roles to be misunderstood. Alternatively, it would be more scientifically consistent to group thyroid, vitamin A, and the steroids together into an umbrella class which denotes their special powers to instruct gene activity. Hormones that instruct DNA programs (genes) behave conceptually in a 'steroid like' manner even though molecularly they derive from a different class.

This improved grouping would then lend itself to a definition of steroid-like tone. Steroid-like tone describes a complete assessment of the message content, which directly reaches the DNA of cells. Deficiencies of vitamin A and thyroid message content lead to receptor problems with the other mainstream steroids. The expanded role that thyroid message content plays within cells will be explained in the thyroid chapter. Unfortunately, the role of the thyroid is largely disconnected from other steroids and vitamin A within the clinical setting. This unfortunate mindset causes the larger group, of which thyroid is a hormone member, to be misunderstood.

Vitamin D and its Steroid-like Properties

Vitamin D is misunderstood as a steroid because its role of instructing the DNA of the cell is downplayed. A more complete assessment of steroid tone would include this in the evaluation. This steroid's measurement is not commonly available in the twenty-four hour urine test. Vitamin D precursor is made within the skin from cholesterol when sunlight strikes it. At the level of the kidney, the final decision is made about activating the precursor or degrading it for removal in urine. The kidney makes this decision based on how much calcium is available within the blood stream.

Vitamin D instructs different DNA programs of the cells in how to interact with calcium. When too much vitamin D becomes available within the cells, they take in excessive calcium. Too much calcium causes the consequences of brittle bones, soft tissue calcification, kidney stones, and mineral imbalance. In addition, magnesium deficiencies exacerbate calcium imbalance. On the opposite extreme, too little vitamin D causes loss of calcium. Keeping these facts in mind elucidates why blindly adding active vitamin D to milk may be inappropriate.

Vitamin A and its Steroid like Properties

By its name, vitamin A is immediately misunderstood. Unlike most other vitamins, vitamin A contains message content by virtue of its molecular shape (just like vitamin D). In contrast, all other vitamins (except vitamin D) simply facilitate bodily chemical reactions. Cognizance here, allows one to see that both vitamins A and D act in the body as hormones and not just vitamins.

In addition, vitamin A has the ability to go anywhere within the body and deliver message content to the DNA program of a cell. Realize, vitamin A behaves within the body more consistently as a hormone. Also realize it proves necessary for the steroids and thyroid hormones to function properly because it proves crucial to their binding specific genes properly. Without proper gene binding it does little good to have the proper amounts and timing of steroids and thyroid hormones reaching one's 70 trillion cells.

In contrast, by calling it a vitamin, a tendency arises to hit an intellectual roadblock that needs to be crossed in order to appreciate the consequences of this molecule's deficiency or excess. Only, a real food diet (section three) supplies ample vitamin A. Here, little tendency exists to develop deficiency of this important substance.

Vitamin A must be obtained in the diet and can become toxic, at high levels, because excess amplifies its instructional content of cellular DNA beyond healthful parameters. The only way to overdose on vitamin A is to take high dosage supplements (above 50,000 IU a day) for over three months. Too much vitamin A causes thinning hair, dry and scaly skin, bone spur formation, and brittle bones.

Vitamin A deficiency leads to diminished functional abilities of cells that coat the body (skin and cornea) and cells that line body cavities (the gastrointestinal tract and lungs). Conditions like ichthyosis vulgaris are caused by a vitamin A deficiency. Skin cancers are promoted by this deficiency as well.

Unfortunately, little encouragement occurs from physicians for decreasing cancer risks through ingesting adequate vitamin A. Adequate adrenal function depends on vitamin A to instruct adrenal cell DNA activation programs. In the healthful state, the liver is filled with vitamin A and releases it as needed.

Vitamin A is actually a complex of similar vitamins that promote cell maturity. Immature cells form a central property of cancer cells. Adequate vitamin A complex intake is a cornerstone for the prevention of cancer. Almost all cells contain DNA programs that are responsive to message content of vitamin A complex.

Some vitamin A derivatives occur in plant seeds. These prevent cell division until they are removed when the right conditions occur. For example the right conditions occur when the planting technique is correct. Likewise, within the body, Vitamin A message content seems to be involved in preventing the cells from undergoing rampant cell division. Unfortunately, this fact is almost entirely ignored by mainstream cancer specialist in attempting to stop cancer cell division (tumor growth).

Finally, low normal thyroid function causes feeble livers. These livers consequently possess a diminished ability to digest dietary vitamin A contained in the form of carotene. Carotene is the form of vitamin found in the diet. One carotene needs to split in half to make two vitamins A molecules. Making matters worse concerns the fact that vitamin A sufficiency forms one determinant of thyroid hormones' ability to activate certain genes. Visualize the vicious cycle that occurs simply because very few physicians counsel their patients about these interdependent relationships.

This section was included to help science become more consistent in its regard for the role of the *four misunderstood steroids*. In the chapters that follow insight will develop about these four misunderstood steroids. In the next chapter, the message content of the thyroid hormone and the reasons malfunction of this gland often continues to be missed in the clinical setting will be explained. In addition, methods of healing from this problem will be addressed.

CHAPTER TEN

THYROID GLAND

As discussed earlier, the amount of thyroid message content determines how hot the power plants (mitochondria) flame will burn within the cells. Thyroid hormones also determine the sufficiency of the important membrane pumps (Na/K ATPase) occurring within the 70 trillion body cells. In addition, the amount of T3 (active thyroid hormone) arriving within the pituitary determines how much Growth Hormone this gland manufactures.

This last point again illustrates the interdependence of different body hormones for health to continue. It also provides a clue that maybe high normal thyroid function is desirable for those who desire to slow down the aging process. One of the reasons low thyroid functioning patients age so quickly involves their markedly diminished ability to make Growth Hormone. Recall, Growth Hormone adequacy powerfully determines defense of body protein levels while one is fasting or exercising. However, mainstream medical physicians are often not taught about this important consequence to health when its levels decline.

For healing purposes terms like metabolism and respiratory quotient will be side stepped in favor of understanding why a hot burning cellular 'power plant flame' is desirable. Standard thyroid tests used today are often falsely reassuring. Understanding and considering the variables, involves how thyroid hormones function at the cellular level. The idea here is to avoid being misled into a prescription for anti-depressants or cholesterol lowering drugs when the true culprit is low thyroid function.

The first part of this chapter reviews some of the general variables of thyroid function. Later in the chapter these variables will be organized into the seven links of health chain for optimal thyroid gland function. All seven links need to be discussed along with the confounding variables if the medical inquiry is to be trusted as accurate.

There are many variables not routinely considered in today's office setting. Hence, many owners remain on an accelerated path to an old body because one or more scientifically valid variables interfered with the accuracy of their test results.

Envision a wimpy, feeble furnace that heats a home with worn out components and blocked air filters. No matter how much the fuel mixture increases or air is added to the room, until someone repairs the worn out parts and cleans the air intake the furnace will always burn poorly. When the furnace burns inefficiently, the home remains cold.

This analogy describes what owners with low thyroid function experience within their many trillions of cellular power plants. Their cells have adequate fuel, usually to excess, but their power plant flame is so weak it can't burn any hotter. Thyroid hormone delivers informational direction, at the cell level, to the DNA programs. With adequate thyroid hormone, come the instructions that direct the DNA program to spend energy on the repair of the mitochondria (power plant components). Without continuous repair and rejuvenation within the mitochondria, the ability to combust fuel and create energy packets compromises. The cell needs these energy packets to perform useful work and to charge up its membranes to maximum voltage.

Almost all cell types depend on an adequate thyroid message. Thyroid message content generates energy for cell work and heat maintenance (except in the brain, lymphatics, spleen, and testes). Part of the thyroid message instructs the DNA of the cells to make appropriate power plant (mitochondria) investments. This includes new structural rejuvenation projects in the form of new mitochondrial structural proteins and enzyme machines.

One example concerns the ongoing need for the specialized structural power plant fats, cardiolipin. Power plant fats form an integral part of the mitochondria structural architecture. Some cell types contain up to 2000 mitochondria (power plants) in each cell. All the mitochondria in the body combust a common fuel derived from carbohydrate, protein, or fat, called acetate. Acetate is the only fuel type that combusts in the presence of adequate oxygen within the mitochondria. Acetate is the simplest fatty acid.

In order to burn protein, the liver must change it into carbohydrate (a process known as gluconeogenesis). In turn, all carbohydrate before it can be combusted within the power plant must be converted into acetate. In the end the power plants can only burn one type of fuel, acetate. Acetate derives from all three-food groups only with the proper vitamins and cofactors presence (chapter one) to convert them to acetate.

Remember, acetate is the simplest fatty acid. It is important to emphasize the fact that aerobic metabolism involves fatty acid combustion only. How many thyroid-like problems arise solely from nutritional deficiencies that prevent the three raw fuels conversion into acetate (see nutritional deficiency caused disease section one)?

Even though the brain does not need thyroid message content to stoke its furnace to capacity, it does need the help of thyroid for generation of an adequate cellular force field and waste removal. The ability of thyroid hormone to improve the cellular 'force field' is enhanced by adequate aldosterone. Both of these hormones are from the steroid-like class in that they penetrate deep into the cell and provide their message directly to the DNA. When thyroid hormone message content delivery occurs, the activated DNA leads to protein synthesis.

Recall one additional type of protein synthesis, which thyroid message content directs: Its sufficient presence increases the number of mineral pump machines that generate the electrical charge (cell voltage) within the cell membrane (see section 3). This process describes an addition to DNA activated protein synthesis of improved mitochondria structural components for most other cells, mentioned above. The number of these mineral pumps is also a major determinant of caloric expenditure. Another clue for how reassuring patients in the low normal range of thyroid function may not be valid.

In summary, the thyroid hormone tells the DNA of the cell to switch on synthesis of programs that maximize the mitochondria performance and integrity. In nerve and cardiac cells adequate thyroid along with aldosterone, are fundamental in powering up the cell membrane charge (section five) to maximal potential. The thyroid has steroid-like powers. It sets the stage for the capability of the cells in regards to the generation of energy for work and heat.

Like the steroids and vitamin A, thyroid directly determines whether certain DNA programs activate or silence within a cell. Within the whole group, each of these hormones specific shape conveys different vibratory induced message content to specific DNA segments. Consequently, the proportions between each hormone type within this powerful group determine what the genetic program accomplishes at any given time.

Inefficient cellular furnaces also prove inferior for the incineration of the ever-generated cellular trash. This fact probably explains how the condition of myxedema accumulates within the skin of untreated hypothyroid patients. Myxedema denotes puffy bloating of the skin and occurs in severe cases of low thyroid function. Just below the front part of the knee is one common area of accumulation. These cells clog with accumulating cellular trash that normally burns within the cellular furnace.

In contrast, owners that have too much thyroid are similar to a furnace that burns too hot. When the cell power plant burns too hot, the cell has to throw in the 'furniture and house structural components' (doors and flooring). These structural components become necessary because normal fuel delivery channels alone can't meet the needs of the furnace. By this mechanism, untreated high thyroid leads to marked weakness and body wasting. Too much thyroid depletes the structural integrity of the cell in order to keep the cellular power plant stoked.

The thyroid gland itself depends on message content from the pituitary gland, which instructs it to produce its product, thyroid hormones (T3 and T4). The thyroid gland also needs the pituitary derived message content to maintain its proper size. Nutritionally, the thyroid needs quantities of the amino acid tyrosine and a continuous supply of iodine. The thyroid then needs the ability to release adequate thyroid hormone daily. Once the thyroid hormone releases, in order for it to be fully activated, it needs a precise removal of one of its iodines out of a total of 4 on a single thyroid hormone molecule. Unless the correct iodine disengages, the thyroid message becomes lost. Certain mineral deficiencies lead to inactive enzyme machines whose sole task involves the removal of the correct iodine. Many owners run into trouble here. They have defective activation mechanisms in operation.

Iodine deficiency and iodine excess inhibit thyroid gland function. Various drugs hamper the ability of the body to take the right iodine off. When certain medications do this they make the owner functionally hypothyroid. Instead of removing the precise iodine that confers the most active form of thyroid hormone, because a different iodine disengages and it becomes worthless.

Almost all thyroid released from the gland has 4 iodines per hormone molecule (T4). Recall, the most active form only occurs after a specific iodine disengages, with the help of these select few enzyme machines, the deiodinases. This conversion creates what doctors like to call T3. Realize, if any other iodine comes off of the 4 iodine containing precursor hormone version molecule, then worthless rubble occurs. When rubble occurs instead of the active form of thyroid hormone (T3), cells lack appropriate direction within their thyroid dependent DNA programs.

Selenium deficiency decreases the ability for activation of thyroid with four iodine atoms (T4) to T3 within the brain and placenta. When these organs are unable to activate thyroid to its more active form, T3, they each receive decreased message content. Decreased message content in the brain from T3 will lead to diminished ability of the nerve cells to charge their membranes.

This type of deficiency causes two consequences. First, the nerve will have diminished ability to perform work (easy fatigue and mental slowness). Second, the nerve will possess diminished ability to protect itself from harmful ions that are waiting to get inside and bind inside the nerve cell's delicate contents. Unfortunately, western trained physician often fail to counsel owners about these facts (Salpolsky).

Acute and chronic illness, trauma, cancer, kidney failure, and myocardial infarction can lead to faulty iodine removal. Scientists like to call this inactive form, reverse T3. When the wrong iodine disengages, reverse T3 forms. Reverse T3 has no biological activity (no message content). Consequently, measurement of a 24-hour urine test for T3, and reverse T3 is the most accurate way to assess thyroid adequacy at the tissue level. T3 is eight times more powerful, in message content, than the initially released T4. T3 cellular levels therefore prove very important to overall health.

Stress decreases thyroid gland stimulation because it causes diminished TSH release from the pituitary. In these cases, the doctor can measure a normal pituitary hormone message (TSH) directed at the thyroid gland. In addition, acute stress causes the sudden increase in free thyroid hormone but when chronic stress occurs thyroid function eventually diminishes (explained below). When thyroid function diminishes, the cells' receive decreased thyroid message. Unfortunately, the measurement of a TSH only, constitutes the emerging standard of care for thyroid inquiry. For the above reasons, when stress increases this value proves misleading.

Many additional perturbations occur that alter the effectiveness of thyroid message content at multiple levels from stress. Stress also increases secretion of acute phase reactant proteins into the blood stream. In general, the acute phase reactants proteins enhance survival ability in the setting of combat like stress (physical stress). However, with mental stress they can cause problems. The acute phase reactant proteins include complement, C-reactive protein, fibrinogen, and interferon. Pertinent here, as mentioned earlier, interferon further suppresses thyroid activity during times of stress. Consequently, normal TSH levels can be misleading when increased interferon releases during stress.

Also for reasons that will be explained shortly, the pain or anxiety of the blood draw can temporarily increase free values of thyroid hormone. Lastly, cortisol levels that increase during stress also suppress thyroid gland activity by suppressing the master gland, the pituitary. For this reason, the stress induced suppression of the pituitary, spuriously decreases the commonly tracked TSH.

This all makes sense when one thinks about repairing the power plants when the body perceives an emergency (stress). Repair activity becomes a low priority when survival message content occurs. The body cannot discern the difference between real or imagined stress. The physiological response to mental and physical stress is initially the same. For the reasons mentioned above, stressed owners, by nature of body design, tend to be hypothyroid even though their lab tests come back normal.

Some common clinical signs of low thyroid function are:

1. **Hair coarsens, prematurely grays, and becomes sparse.**
2. **Skin dries out and yellows**
3. **Voice becomes husky and low**
4. **Thinking slows**
5. **Memory worsens**
6. **Cholesterol increases in the blood stream**
7. **Armpit temperature before getting out of bed is less than 97.6 degrees (basal temperature)**
8. **Bowel movements tend towards constipation**
9. **Lateral edges of the eyebrows are missing.**
10. **EKG voltage tends to be diminished**
11. **Cold intolerance compared to the normal population.**

Other symptoms additionally surface as a consequence of turning down the power plant flame within the cells. Consistently low body temperature provides a good clinical marker of those owners who have tissue level thyroid resistance, but may have normal thyroid levels of T4, T3, and reverse T3. Often peripheral thyroid resistance syndromes result from vitamin A deficiency. This vitamin (hormone) proves necessary throughout the body in helping the thyroid DNA receptors activate. Additionally, zinc deficiencies can prevent the proper activation of DNA programs (zinc finger malfunction).

Some people have normal levels of thyroid parameters measured by even the best testing methods available. They may still have a thyroid problem. An association exists for both attention deficit and hyperactivity disorder with this type of thyroid resistance (vitamin A, selenium and zinc deficiency all cause this problem). Thyroid resistance means that thyroid levels are normal, but the receptors for receiving thyroid message content are somehow diminished in their performance. One of the consequences of diminished thyroid message content within a developing brain is attention deficit disorder. This evidence suggests that the thyroid plays a role in normal brain development. How many of these owners really suffer from vitamin A, zinc or selenium deficiency?

Lastly, the thyroid can be inhibited by the food ingested. Certain foods contain thyroid-inhibiting substances that are found in foods from the Brassicacae family of vegetables - rutabagas, cabbage, and turnips. All of them have been documented to inhibit thyroid function.

Lony elucidated the importance of this. She was a 25-year old who developed swelling in her thyroid area. Standard testing showed her thyroid function to be diminished. The specialist involved with her care was unaware that certain foods consumed in excess can produce this swelling. This particular patient loved large helpings of rutabagas, cabbage, and turnips. When this patient discontinued this practice, her neck swelling subsided. Despite this, her specialist is still found to be advocating her need for continued medical therapy.

This subsection was about general considerations for what the thyroid does and needs. In the next section the general considerations are organized into the seven levels of where the thyroid system can fail. The seven levels are best conceptualized in their interdependence by seven links in a chain. When the weakest link fails the system fails. Science is present to do a better job of inquiry as to the true status of thyroid message content reaching cellular DNA programs.

Seven links in the Thyroid Chain of Health

First Link - Hypothalamus

The hypothalamus releases TRH (thyroid releasing hormone) when stimulated by three different mechanisms - lowered amounts of T4 and T3 (active thyroid hormones) in the circulation, cold weather, and adrenaline (epinephrine). One of the jobs of the thyroid is to provide the mechanism for warmth. Cold weather increases the need for heat production. The adrenals release adrenaline when body temperature begins to fall.

Adrenaline also helps raise body temperature by stimulating fat to enter the blood stream. The fat liberated heads for the trillions of cellular power plants. When adrenaline reaches the hypothalamus it begins the first step of raising the body temperature. Adrenaline within the hypothalamus stimulates the first link in the thyroid chain, the release of TRH. The TRH released will then go directly to the pituitary. When TRH arrives in the pituitary, its message stimulates this gland to release TSH (thyroid stimulating hormone). This is the second link of the thyroid chain. Before discussing the second link of the thyroid chain it is worth mentioning the processes that inhibit the first link.

The natural inhibitory factors of the first link (TRH release) are high circulating levels of T4 and T3. A certain class of blood pressure and prostate shrinking medications called alpha-blockers also inhibits this first link. When this medication is prescribed, the clinical signs for the hypothyroid state should be rigorously followed. When the first link experiences inhibition, these owners will suffer the consequences of diminished thyroid message content instructing their DNA program.

In contrast, the natural control of the hypothalamus involves both increased T3 and T4 and this will decrease first link activity. No need exists to stimulate the chain with seven links into activation if enough active thyroid message content already occurs within the body. However, in the case of the alpha-blocker medications, the first link is fooled by the medicine itself. If this medication proves necessary, thyroid supplementation should be considered at the first sign of inadequacy.

Second Link - Pituitary

Link two in the thyroid chain of health is the pituitary gland. The pituitary gland is often called the master hormone gland. It has some control over how the many endocrine glands grow and perform their task of making specific hormones. The glands that the pituitary has some control over are the gonads, the thyroid, the adrenals, the parathyroid, and the endocrine aspect of the liver, the pancreas, and the kidneys. The general theme of the how much the pituitary stimulates a hormone-producing gland is a controlled process.

The first general control occurs by how much of one or more of the hormones manufactured in that gland are sensed within the blood stream that reaches the pituitary. The second general control, at the level of the pituitary, occurs through other modifying molecules that augment or inhibit pituitary secretion. Conceptually, secretion modification either helps the pituitary 'listen' or 'ignore' what the hypothalamus (first link) directs by TRH release.

When the pituitary receives the message from the first link, it arrives in the form of TRH. The pituitary response to TRH may vary. Certain powerful competing forces arise within the pituitary gland itself. The summation of these competing messages will determine whether or not the pituitary 'listens' to what the TRH released by the hypothalamus instructs. The competing messages must be summarized at the level of the pituitary, which either enhances or inhibits the pituitary response (listening ability or deafening ability). The summation of these competing messages, at link two, determine whether the pituitary listens to the message or ignores it.

Factors that enhance the pituitary's ability to listen involve high estrogen states and the diminished activity of link five, the de-iodinases. The enhancement of the link two responses in the presence of estrogen demonstrates how ovary status and thyroid interrelate. Hot flashes during early menopause are caused by the wide fluctuation of estrogen levels. Hot flashes either lessen or intensify by this thyroid and estrogen interdependence.

In contrast, inhibitors of pituitary responsiveness to TRH message content are the hormone somatostatin, dopamine, and other dopamine agonist like bromocriptine. High cortisol levels caused by stress will also lower the pituitary response to TRH. All of these molecules inhibit the pituitary from releasing TSH even when normal levels of TRH instruct it to do so. Notice, the above situations provide additional examples for how over reliance on a TSH test result can mislead.

When stressed, part of the stress response inhibits link two in the thyroid function chain. This makes more sense when one understands the simultaneous stimulation of link four. Link four, is discussed below, but briefly here, it involves the level (link) where thyroid travels within the blood stream. When cortisol levels increase in the blood stream, thyroid hormone displaces from its carrier protein. The freed thyroid hormone content (increased free T3 and free T4), in the blood stream, increases and then exits into the numerous cells.

When thyroid hormone levels increase inside cells, the effect is that the cells immediately begin stoking the power plant flame for energy production. At first, this seems like a contradictory action of cortisol message content to different levels within the thyroid function chain. It resolves when one remembers that the body was designed to survive physical stresses.

Stress affects multiple levels of the thyroid system chain of health. The first level that stress interferes with is the pituitary gland (second link). The creator did not design the body to be mentally stressed day in and day out from modern life. The body was designed to handle short burst of stress - like running from death.

The design of the body, when stress occurs, involves maximizing an increase in physical energy quickly. This is accomplished by the quick displacement of thyroid hormone off its carrier protein within the blood stream. This displacement allows a burst of thyroid hormone to enter the cells. The surge of thyroid hormone stimulates the mitochondria in the cells (through DNA program activation) to produce more energy. The ability to do this comes with a price: The body has turned off the pituitary (link two). This means the other links, below level two, deplete quickly.

When physical stress is the issue, the body is smart enough to know that the manufacture of more thyroid hormone is a waste of energy in the short run. However modern stress proves different in that the time course can become chronic. This situation explains how chronic stress eventually inhibits the level of thyroid hormone within the blood stream. Eventually the thyroid hormone becomes depleted from cortisol inhibiting effects on the pituitary gland. When stress inhibits the pituitary link, the successive other links eventually run out of thyroid hormone.

In order to better understand how the common testing of the second link (the TSH level) can fool the doctor when stress occurs, the fourth link needs to be mentioned out of turn. The fourth link, the blood stream amount of thyroid hormones, depends on all prior links. In the short run, the stress reaction triggers the carrier protein, the fourth link, to dump massive amounts of thyroid. However, cortisol inhibits the prior links, including the pituitary. The higher links inhibition diminishes the release of more thyroid hormone for further body use. By this mechanism, chronic stress eventually depletes what was available within the blood steam before stress occurred.

Chronic stress provides one clinical situation where the physician can be fooled with a normal TSH result. The result may be normal, but the following links are not. When prior links fail to function properly, numerous cells lack adequate thyroid message content within their DNA programs. When the DNA programs fail to receive these important messages, cells fail to spend energy on thyroid directed rejuvenation. Adequate rejuvenation, at the cell level, is partly the responsibility of thyroid message content. For this and other reasons, the best assessments for this is the armpit temperature before arising and a twenty-four hour urine test for output of thyroid hormones.

Third Link - Thyroid

The thyroid gland is the third link in the chain in regard to power plant function and cell membrane charge within the trillions of body cells. Ideally, the thyroid manufactures adequate thyroid hormone when directed by the pituitary. Like the pituitary, there are many competing messages within the thyroid that either interfere or enhance the thyroid gland's ability to 'listen' to the pituitary message. Healthy thyroid glands that listen to pituitary cause adequate amounts of thyroid hormone release into the blood stream. Unfortunately, exacerbating the opposite of this fact concerns that stress will diminish the pituitary directed TSH amount released even when the thyroid is becoming 'deaf' to its message (see link two).

Many physicians remain unaware that excess iodine in the diet poisons thyroid gland function. Thyroid function will decrease with too much iodized salt in the diet. This fact allows an effective and simple treatment for an overactive thyroid gland. Other thyroid gland inhibitory substances that can be found in food are nitrates, thiocyanates, perchlorate, lithium, and possibly fluoride.

At the level of the thyroid, the potential exists that an owner's antibodies will attack their own thyroid tissue when their adrenals become weak and unable to retain normal immune function. Adrenal status improvement forms an early indicator in the disease process that can potentially save the thyroid from total destruction. William McKenzie Jefferies, MD, in his book *Safe Uses of Cortisol,* explains the 'how to' parameters very well. This education is about adrenal dysfunction and its role in this type of thyroid gland disease.

The thyroid gland link affects the ability to have healthy cellular power plant flames and maximally charged cells. As was previously mentioned, certain edible plants, in excessive doses, poison this gland's ability to perform these tasks. The Brasasciae family that includes broccoli, cabbage, turnips, and cauliflower are some of them. Realize, only large and frequent amounts produce a wounded thyroid gland (goiter) but it does happen.

Fourth Link – Blood Stream

All blood stream transport parameters comprise the fourth link in the chain of thyroid health. The blood stream provides the transport mechanism for healthy cellular power plants and maximally charged cells. The body requires adequate amounts of thyroid hormone transported in the blood stream by the cells at all times.

The major thyroid transport parameters are:
1. **The amount of thyroid carrier protein within the transport system**
2. **The blood stream; the amount of substances within the transport system which desire to displace thyroid off its carrier protein**
3. **The rate of thyroid release into the transport system**
4. **The rate of thyroid hormone destruction by the liver that constantly removes thyroid from the transport system**
5. **The ability of the cells to suck thyroid out of the transport system**
6. **The proportion of 'dead thyroid' hormone within the transport system.**

The thyroid gland is like a faucet dumping more thyroid hormone into the blood stream and the cells are constantly removing it. This sucking action promotes the idea that the cells act like a 'drain' removing thyroid hormone that the thyroid gland dumps into the blood stream. The amount of thyroid hormone in the blood stream that binds to its carrier protein (thyroid binding globulin or TBG) retards the ability of the cells to suck out thyroid hormone. The amount of thyroid hormone in the blood stream is where modern medicine stops looking. It usually ignores links five through seven.

The amount of thyroid in the blood stream is an estimated value when a laboratory measures it. The blood sample measurement of thyroid hormone contained in the blood stream provides an estimate before drain-off mechanisms deliver it to the cellular DNA programs. The carrier proteins are large enough to escape the ability of the drains to suck various hormones out of the blood stream. Thyroid hormone can bind to its carrier protein and resist the drain sucking it out of the system.

The liver comprises the first big drain that sucks thyroid hormone out of the blood stream. Healthy livers possess more power to suck the small amount of free thyroid hormone out of the blood stream. Only free thyroid hormone, not bound to a carrier protein, can enter the cells. The rate at which the liver can suck out thyroid forms a powerful deterrent for available thyroid hormone to the other cells. Important point: Only the free level of thyroid hormone can be sucked out of the blood stream by the liver.

A healthy liver deactivates many hormones more quickly, including thyroid. In the case of thyroid hormone, when it freely circulates, little ability exists to prevent the liver sucking action. This process competes with its ability to deliver its message content to other cells. The creator countered this problem by designing various carrier proteins that bind their hormones tightly while in transit within the blood stream. 99.9% of thyroid hormone binds to its carrier protein.

Certain factors will raise or lower the amount of free thyroid hormones in transit in the blood stream. When the blood stream fails to have adequate carrier proteins for thyroid, in order to keep the same level of hormone in the blood stream, the thyroid has to increase its production rate. When the drain (liver) is more effective at the removal rate, there has to be a greater faucet flow (the gland secretion rate) to keep the transport system levels the same. In these cases, their thyroid gland has to work harder to keep blood levels adequate

Certain drugs induce a larger liver drain (faster liver metabolic rate) for hormones like thyroid. A larger liver drain is synonymous with a faster removal rate. Some of them are phenytoin for seizure disorders, rifampin an antibiotic for tuberculosis, and carbamazepine a psychiatric medicine. These medications exert this effect because they increase certain enzymatic machinery within liver cells.

The amount of carrier protein in the blood stream creates another competing force to thyroid drain off by the liver and other cells. The higher the carrier protein levels, the better the prevention of various drains sucking out thyroid hormone. By avoiding the liver enzymatic machinery, the cells are also limited in their ability to remove thyroid hormone. Chronically high levels of thyroid hormone and estrogen promote an increase in carrier protein levels. These facts describe a double edge sword in that these high levels help keep the liver drain at bay, but also retard the drain leading into the tissues (cellular DNA level). The consequence here is that the amount of thyroid, in the blood stream, becomes less available to the cells. Despite the cells having less access to normal amounts of thyroid, the blood test will look deceptively good during acute stress (see above and below discussion).

Women who take birth control pills can have signs of low thyroid function despite normal blood tests. This side effect results from high estrogen message content that stimulates an increased production rate of the carrier proteins. Common blood test will measure a normal value of thyroid hormones, but they do not routinely measure the level of carrier protein in the blood stream. Remember, the amount of carrier protein for thyroid hormones directly competes with the ability of cells to access thyroid hormone for their DNA programs. Increased thyroid hormones or estrogen levels that persist cause the levels of thyroid binding protein to increase. When binding of thyroid hormone increases, the hormone has trouble releasing into the tissues because it remains trapped within the blood stream. Thyroid bound to high levels of carrier protein traps it in the blood stream. Unless thyroid hormone can deliver message content to the level of the DNA program, in trillions of cells, a normal level in the blood stream does little good.

Certain factors lead to a decreased level of thyroid carrier protein levels. These factors lead to the opposite situation results: The liver can drain off the thyroid hormone produced more quickly making the thyroid work harder. At the same time, the other body cells can access the thyroid hormone more easily while a higher level remains free. The thyroid gland needs to make more thyroid hormone per day to keep blood levels in the normal range. Carrier protein levels decrease when androgen steroid hormones levels increase, chronic illness occurs (chronic stress), and in starvation conditions.

Certain agents within the blood stream (fourth link) are able to displace thyroid hormone off of its carrier protein. Certain acute physical situations occur in life where the body suddenly needs massive amounts of thyroid in the tissues. Mental stress and certain medications can inappropriately elevate free thyroid by dumping it off its carrier protein. Regardless of how thyroid gets displaced, these situations can make blood test measurements appear normal when they are not. The inappropriate displacement of thyroid hormone off its carrier protein will reverberate all the way down to the cells DNA program.

Situations, in addition to stress, which displace thyroid hormone off its carrier protein, are: aspirin, phenytoin, phenylbutazone, diazepam, and increased blood heparin. These situations acutely make thyroid hormone more available to liver drain off as well as the tissues drain. For example, heparin

increases the amount of free fatty acids secondary to its activating lipoprotein lipase. Lipoprotein lipase activation causes the increase of fatty acids in the blood stream. Increased fatty acids in the blood stream, in turn, displace thyroid hormones off their carrier protein, TBG.

This mechanism is also used by cortisol and epinephrine to increase fatty acid levels caused by stress. This leads to thyroid hormone displacement, as well. Stress hormones cause a sudden increase in free fatty acid levels in the blood stream. By this mechanism, heparin and stress both displace thyroid off its carrier protein making it more available to the drains. Here again, the common medical inquiry fails to consider whether the test results are altered towards normal because of the above described factors.

The amount of 'dead' thyroid versus active thyroid hormone in the blood stream must be considered. Illness can rapidly raise the amount of dead thyroid hormone in the blood stream. Scientist call the dead thyroid hormone, reverse T3. Clinically, the thyroid can be making its hormone properly, but some other process can 'kill off' message content by deactivating it. Unless physicians routinely check this in their chronically ill patients, they will miss opportunities for healing a problem caused by a low thyroid hormone level.

Link Five – Enzyme Machines & Selenium

'Enzyme machines' exist that amplify the message content of the thyroid hormone, T4, initially released into the blood stream. These machines, the de-iodinases, comprise link five in the thyroid chain of healthy cellular power plants and maximal cell charge abilities. The presence of adequate selenium proves necessary for these machines to function. Selenium deficiency will prevent the important body enzyme machine, de-iodinase, from activating thyroid to full power. Scientists denote this activation as conversion of T4 to T3. T3 is eight times more powerful for telling DNA programs what to do. For any amount of thyroid, this conversion amplifies the message content by a factor of eight.

Link Six – DNA Receptor

The DNA receptor that the T4 and T3 binds to around the DNA are link six in the chain of healthy cellular power plants and maximally charged cells within the body. Like other steroid-like hormones, thyroid hormones are interdependent on other steroid-like hormones for the completeness and integrity of their receptors. Steroid-like hormones and thyroid hormones cannot activate DNA programs without adequate functional receptors at the level of the target cell. For example, often, there needs to be adequate vitamin A and cortisol message content or the thyroid hormone fails to have completed receptors.

When the thyroid receptors at the DNA level are incomplete, the thyroid hormone's message content delivery proves impossible. This is known as peripheral thyroid resistance. When peripheral thyroid resistance occurs, blood tests can be within normal for thyroid parameters, but these people are far from well. They have all or many clinical signs of diminished thyroid function.

In this situation an astute physician who notices the clinical signs of hypothyroidism, but normal blood values will cautiously try supplementation strategies. These strategies are worthwhile when armpit temperatures remain consistently low. He/she will also make an inquiry into the levels of vitamin A and cortisol.

All prior links in the system can function perfectly, but if link six is defective, these owners will present like any low thyroid function owner. Their blood values can all be normal. At the level of the cell DNA program, where it matters, the ability to receive message content impairs because the receptor is incomplete. Often the culprit is insufficient vitamin A or cortisol levels. These two hormones are needed in order to direct the DNA to finish the manufacture of the thyroid receptor. These patients are best diagnosed by a twenty-four hour urine test for steroids and thyroid hormones. The vitamin A status can be surmised by a lab test or by physical signs (unhealthy skin for age).

Link Seven – Receptor Formation

Some of the thyroid hormone message content directs receptor formation for 'lesser' hormones message to be heard. These types of hormone receptors formed are vulnerable to an inappropriate attack by the immune system. This is link seven in the chain of thyroid health. The hierarchy of hormones subsection will make the seventh link in the system of thyroid health more comprehensible.

Recall, steroid-like hormones are the only hormones that directly activate or silence the genes. Thyroid hormone is a member of this group. Part of the consequence of its gene activation message, results in the manufacture of specific types of protein composed receptors.

Some of the DNA programs activated by thyroid involve specific proteins that organize into receptors for the 'lesser' hormones. These lower level hormones depend on adequate thyroid message content for the manufacture of their receptors. Without their receptors presence, it does little good to have these other hormones arrive. Hormones cannot deliver message content without their receptors being present. Many diseases arise because of receptor formation deficiency or receptor destruction. Asthma is sometimes caused by this defect in the receptors needed by epinephrine to keep the airways open.

For example, some thyroid message content directs specific genes into the manufacture of cell membrane receptors (composed of proteins) for the recognition of adrenaline (epinephrine) in the lungs. In some owners, their adrenals fail to keep their immune system from attacking these types of receptors. By this mechanism, in some types of asthmatic patients, adrenaline receptors lining their lung airways (bronchioles) are inappropriately destroyed by their immune system. This process describes an example of a level seven problem with thyroid function. This level does not involve the part of thyroid message devoted to power plant flame improvement in the cells. It also does not involve the membrane pumps that generate cell voltage. It involves other parts of the thyroid message that direct different DNA programs to manufacture adrenaline receptors.

The discussion about the seven links in the chain of thyroid system health elucidates how the common thyroid clinical inquiry often proves incomplete. Some of the popular blood tests can be inaccurate. Sometimes the twenty-four hour urine test can be deceptively normal. It is valuable to consider the stress level operating in an owner's life. Lastly, the medications and foods that are ingested can have dramatic effects on thyroid message content. For these reasons, the clinical signs of low thyroid function are often the most accurate. Section seven will review the best testing parameters within the context of the *hundred thousand mile* physical exam.

Cutting edge scientific thought: Food allergies cause IgG antibodies and these cause Graves's disease and Hashimoto's thyroiditis. Sometimes simply identifying the offending food and eliminating it from the diet leads to improvement. This mechanism is best documented in scientific literature concerning gluten antibodies (see bibliography).

CHAPTER ELEVEN

TESTES

An ailing physician almost one hundred years ago stumbled on the central role that the testicles play in the maintenance of health. He had been suffering from progressive deterioration of his musculoskeletal structures and depression. Out of desperation, he acted on a scientific inkling that the testes were somehow related to youth. He received the world's first testicle transplant from a cadaver. Anti-rejection techniques were not understood back then, but while the transplanted testicle was still functional, he noted dramatic improvements of his mental outlook and physical abilities. He also noted a dramatic improvement in his muscle contours and size. In addition, his arthritic symptoms lessened considerably. Lastly, he noticed both an increased zest for life and a heightened vitality in his physical stamina.

About the same time, across the Atlantic Ocean, one of the first endocrinologists, Albert Lamond MD was conducting autopsies on the testicles of extremely long-lived men. He also researched male prowess and abilities of his living subjects. He noted consistently that testicular health was a predictor of the health of the man. In addition, to his research on testicles, he was one of the first physicians who prescribed extracts from the different endocrine glands. These extracts included the thyroid, pancreas, ovary, testes, adrenals, and occasionally the pituitary. He became world famous for his success at reversing some of the effects of aging.

Eugene Shippen MD, in his book ***Testosterone Syndrome***, writes "I have never seen an older male patient in excellent mental and physical health whose testosterone levels were not well within the normal levels." A fair share of men's testosterone is made in their testicles.

What the complex sells often skirts around central hormonal considerations that predictably begin to decline at the onset of middle age. Testosterone decline often manifests in men as decreased libido, loss of skeletal mass, loss of muscle mass that produces sagging and less taut skin (especially on the face and arms), loss of liver function, loss of kidney function, joint and diffuse body aches, loss of confidence, decreased concentration ability, memory deficiencies, hot flashes, and progressive fatigue. In addition to these symptoms, there is also the tendency for increased body fat. As testosterone falls the fat synthesis message of insulin becomes more powerful.

None of these symptoms are surprising when one understands testosterone's importance to health. The powerful role that steroid-like hormones play centers on their ability to switch off or on the DNA programs (genes). Testosterone is a steroid-like hormone. Its shape is such that when it binds to DNA, its message directs cellular energy toward infrastructure investment and rejuvenation

Consequently, a lowered testosterone level creates a deficiency in cellular rejuvenation message content. When less rejuvenation message content occurs, the DNA programs fail to activate at the youthful level. Without rejuvenation activities occurring, the wear and tear of aging begins. On average aging begins in middle-aged men and continues for the remainder of their lives. Eventually the man begins to have a 'worn down by life look'.

Unfortunately, the science that verifies these facts presents in a disorganized and disjointed format. Without an organized presentation, many physicians remain unaware of the relationship between the degenerative processes and the decline in the male hormone, testosterone. In addition, the emphasis and presentation in medical schools often fail to educate physicians in these congruous facts.

However, the holism of these facts relates a strong correlation with physical and mental decline to the fall in testosterone. A fall in testosterone is often remedied by simple replacement therapies or lifestyle changes. These programs can be used to prevent and/or reverse the decline into an old body physique (see steroid tone).

In order to decide where one stands between normal and deficient testicle function, there needs to be a competent and thorough inquiry into steroid hormone status. The common standard of care is often superficial and as a consequence misses opportunities for healing. The testes evaluation is similar to the adrenals and ovaries so far as the links in the chain to consider before ruling out testicle dysfunction.

Six Links in the Chain of Testicle Health

There are six links in the chain that need to be intact or clinical testicle dysfunction will manifest.

1. **Hypothalamus**
2. **Pituitary**
3. **Testes**
4. **Blood stream transport parameters**
5. **Peripheral conversion to estrogen before it delivers the testosterone message**
6. **DNA receptor completeness - Very little known about this in the mainstream textbooks and therefore beyond the scope of this manual**

The reason these are all mentioned together is that many well-meaning physicians miss one or more of these levels in their workup considerations and because of this miss opportunities to heal. Unfortunately, there is a popular tendency to prescribe abnormal testosterone substitutes in lieu of the real hormone. Similar to hormone replacement for women, these patented substances contain altered message content because their shape has been changed. The message content of steroids resides inherent in their exact shape. A change in the shape alters the message content that the DNA receives. Clinically, these changes manifest as side effects.

One common example results from the chronic ingestion of the abnormal hormone replacement, methyl-testosterone, which is given to men and women. One side effect concerns the increased tendency to develop bloody cysts in their livers (peliosis hepatis). This is not known to occur with natural testosterone. One other caution, some testosterone injection preparations contain a deliberate contaminant, mercury. The mercury contaminant is under the hidden code name, thimerosal, in the inert ingredients. This is a known liver and neuron toxin.

Before discussion of the six ways to break the links in the chain of the testosterone message occurs, these pit falls need to be addressed. Awareness of the side effects of contamination and substitution will help to prevent another problem from developing. Be cautious about taking prescribed hormones.

First Link – Hypothalamus

The first link in the testicle system of health is the hypothalamus at the center of the brain. The decisions of the hypothalamus facilitate or inhibit all other links in the testicular chain of health. When the first link activates it secretes GRH (gonadotrophic releasing hormone). The amount of GRH released in men and women is determined by estrogen content. This means that the amount of body estrogen inversely determines the activity level of the hypothalamus (first link).

Trouble lies in the fact that there are many environmental estrogens in the food supply (estrogen mimics). Increased estrogen from the food supply can fool the hypothalamus to believe the body has all the sex hormones it needs. For this reason the sperm count of men has fallen worldwide.

The increased environmental estrogen makes its way inside the body. The increased estrogen message content that results, tells the hypothalamus there is enough testicle steroid production. The estrogen content in men and women determines the hypothalamus activity for stimulating the gonads to increase their steroid production. One determiner of steroid production rates concerns the estrogen content reaching the hypothalamus, as body design assumes when estrogen reaches a certain level, the other steroids are at a certain level as well. This is erroneous with environmental estrogens. They increase estrogen message content reaching the hypothalamus without increasing the other gonad steroids. For men, a diminished first link activity reverberates all the way down the testicle chain of health. Testicles need informational direction from the previous links. When this stimulatory information diminishes the testosterone dependent sperm production rate falls off. Like the other endocrine glands, without information the testicles begin to shrivel. For these reasons, the precautions listed earlier in the adrenal chapter are applicable to men as well.

Second Link - Pituitary

The second link in the chain to testicle health is the pituitary gland that hangs off the underside of the brain. Several competing hormone messages within the pituitary occur that either facilitate or harm the ability of the pituitary to activate the next link in the chain. The next link is the testicles. Like the second link in the thyroid chain of health, these hormonal factors either facilitate the pituitary's ability to 'listen' or 'turn a' deaf ear to the message content of the hypothalamus when it releases GRH.

In addition, when stress levels increase, the release of another hormone within the pituitary causes testicle activity to suppress (see below). Furthermore, when stressed, the hormones that stimulate the testes are suppressed by the elevation of cortisol. Cortisol elevation at the level of the pituitary suppresses the release of follicle stimulating hormone (FSH) and leuteinizing hormone

(LH). The testicles need these two hormones that the pituitary manufactures and releases for growth and production of their testicle products.

Simultaneously, with cortisol increases, an additional hormone releases in the stress response, prolactin. Prolactin is also manufactured in the pituitary. When prolactin exceeds normal levels, the gonads (ovaries or testicles) are further inhibited. In the case of the male, their testicles are inhibited when prolactin levels increase from chronic stress. Chronic stress diminishes the size of the testicles. The size of the testicles decreases with the decrease of steroid production at the direction of the prolactin message content.

When steroid production decreases the rate of sperm production decreases. If this is the suspected problem, a serum prolactin level is in order. A twenty-four hour urine test for cortisol and its metabolites is also helpful in establishing the cause of diminished testicle function. Other causes of prolactin elevation that have the same side effects are serotonin re-uptake inhibitors prescribed frequently as antidepressant medications (or anything that raises brain serotonin levels) and decreased thyroid function because thyroid-releasing hormone (TRH) is also a powerful stimulator of prolactin release from the pituitary.

Recall, in both women with high blood estrogen levels that commonly occur in women taking birth control pills and excessive exposure to hormone mimics also elevate prolactin levels. Prolactin levels elevate because higher estrogen levels tells the body it is pregnant. Conversely, lower estrogen levels stimulate the pituitary to release LH and FSH because the hypothalamus and pituitary are sensitive to estrogen levels.

Link Three – Testicle Level of Function and Directions

The informational directions received determine the testes level of function. If they receive both growth factors (LH and FSH) and nutritional molecular building parts (section three) the production of sperm and steroid hormones tend to be adequate. However, if testicles receive primarily prolactin message content there tends to be inhibition of their function resulting from the effects of the first two links of the testicle health chain

At the testicle level, there is an additional powerful hormone, aldosterone that determines the ability of the testicles to make steroids. Aldosterone is manufactured in the adrenal glands. Steroid production is stimulated and enhanced by aldosterone levels. It is the steroid hormone responsible for beginning the manufacture of steroids from the raw material, cholesterol. Without sufficient aldosterone message content the testicle has difficulty in starting the steroid manufacture process. Factors that increase aldosterone levels (high potassium, ACTH and Angiotensin II) will also lead to increased steroid production in the testicles. Increased steroid production in the testes leads to increased message content reaching the cells to invest available energy in rejuvenation. Conversely, factors that diminish aldosterone levels will cripple the testicles ability to manufacture steroids (low potassium diets, certain blood pressure medication). Consequently, the third link of testicle health, the testicles themselves, depends on proper message content from the adrenals and pituitary.

Some owners that arrive at middle age after eating a processed food diet can no longer handle normal aldosterone levels without a simultaneous increase in their blood pressure. The crux of their blood pressure problem is not aldosterone, but the chronic ingestion of reversed ratio minerals content, which deviate from body design. When the mineral content of food reverses, the body will eventually develop health problems around middle age.

Middle age is often accompanied by a breakdown of the body's ability to deal with years of ingesting a reversed mineral content diet. In the case of the testicles these owners, if they are going to continue to have adequate testosterone, will tend to have high blood pressure. If the body decreases aldosterone production to help keep blood pressure normal, the testosterone level will fall. Certain medications prescribed to treat blood pressure have the potential to lower testosterone because they also lower aldosterone production rates (chapter three).

Blood pressure problems with aldosterone are avoidable when the owner consumes a diet with proper mineral proportions. Real food contains the proper mineral proportions. Processed food (dead food) contains the wrong mineral proportions. The potassium and magnesium content generally deplete during food processing. In addition, processed food tends to have large amounts of sodium added to prolong its shelf life. This combination can poison the testicles around middle age. They are not receiving enough aldosterone, which decreases in order to lower blood pressure.

The body was designed for at least three times the intake of potassium compared to sodium. When mineral consumption occurs in these designed proportions there is no problem when aldosterone levels elevate. Blood pressure elevates on the reversed mineral proportions diet (processed food) because of the side effect of fluid retention. This occurs because of the incompatible reversed mineral ratios contained in the processed food diet. Rather than just educate physicians and owners about this simple consequence of a processed food diet, owners are given blood pressure prescription medication.

Around middle age some testicles turn down their production rate of testosterone because aldosterone elevation, while on a processed food diet, will elevate blood pressure. Alternatively, some men are prescribed blood pressure lowering medications, the ACE inhibitors, which lower steroid production rates. The steroid production rates in both cases decrease from the testicles receiving diminished aldosterone message content.

On the other extreme are male owners who continue to make adequate testosterone while consuming a dead food diet. These individuals experience increased blood pressure around middle age. The blood pressure elevates with increased aldosterone on a processed food diet due to the altered mineral content. The altered mineral content contains increased sodium but diminished potassium and magnesium. These reversed mineral proportions directly conflict with general body design. Chronically altered mineral intake will cause sodium to be conserved as well as water. This combination elevates blood pressure.

Recall the dominant mineral in a body chamber powerfully attracts water. Outside the cells, the extracellular space that includes the blood stream, sodium is the dominant mineral by far. However, inside the cells, the intracellular space, potassium and magnesium are the dominant minerals. Visualize the 'tug of war' for where water goes when sodium is dominant after years of ingesting reversed minerals (see mineral table). Simple fact: excessive water in the blood stream pumps up the pressure! Making matters worse, stress hormones promote sodium retention while encouraging potassium and magnesium loss!

There is an important but uncommon exception to this general pattern. Some owners manufacture the hormone atrial natruretic peptide (ANP) at high levels. ANP is a powerful peptide hormone made within the heart. High rates for this hormone's manufacture and if it is not destroyed before it reaches the kidney, it can override the desire of aldosterone to conserve sodium and water and blood pressure remains normal. Although these owners have an override system that allows for increased aldosterone despite a processed food diet, they will be unhealthy in other ways. Their lack of health is explained in section five.

Both the testicle and high blood pressure problems are completely avoidable when an owner adheres to a real food diet (section three). A real food diet proves naturally high in potassium and magnesium and low in sodium. A real food diet is consistent with the way the human body was designed to interact with mineral proportions. The mineral proportions in food affect powerful hormone systems. Altered mineral proportions disrupt the testicle system.

Link Four – Blood Stream Transport

The blood stream transport level of testosterone is often the only link in the chain that receives inquiry. European studies have shown that the majority of certain steroids transport in the red blood cells. The other way that steroids transport concerns carrier proteins. Only a very small amount of steroids exists free within the liquid phase of blood. Higher carrier protein levels, for a particular steroid, lower its free amount within the serum. This fact describes a similar concept that occurs with thyroid hormone in that it is a double-edged sword. On one edge a higher carrier protein level impedes the rate of the liver sucking the various steroids out of the blood stream. On the other edge, it impedes the cells ability to suck them out, as well.

The new fact is that the steroids are transported in the red blood cells themselves. The amount of steroids transported in the red blood cells is the larger proportion of the total amount in transport in the blood stream. The amount of steroids and carrier protein in the red blood cells is not routinely measured. This means a blood value from different owners could mean different things entirely. The higher the estrogen or thyroid levels, then the higher the carrier protein level will be. These two hormones direct the liver to increase production of carrier proteins. As a consequence, for the same total serum levels that occur in two different patients there could be an entirely different risk for testosterone deficiency. For example, an owner with a very high carrier protein levels could be extremely deficient at the DNA level in his cells. If he is unfortunate enough to receive only a total serum level and not have the carrier protein level included, he will be misdiagnosed if the carrier protein level remains higher than normal.

Until an accurate and routine laboratory test becomes available for the red blood cell contribution of steroid transport, physicians and owners will have to wait. It is likely that the flexibility of red blood cells powerfully determines how readily a steroid, like testosterone, can enter cells at the capillary level.

Recall, at the capillary level, red blood cells must traverse a vessel that is smaller so compression is involved. Similarly, the mechanical squeezing (flexibility) of all red blood cells is largely ignored as far its contribution to the rate of oxygen delivery to the cells. This same red cell flexibility factor is again ignored for steroid delivery (chapter two) rates at the capillary level into the cells themselves. These problems with the accuracy of blood measurements of steroids lend further credence to the value of a twenty-four hour urine test for steroids, their metabolites and thyroid hormones output. Someday there will be additional measurement in the blood stream that includes a more accurate assessment of these variables.

Link Five – Peripheral Conversion of Testosterone to Estrogen

The prevention of the peripheral conversion of testosterone to estrogen describes the fifth link. Healthy male owners convert very little testosterone to estrogen. The testicles make the majority of testosterone, which does little good for the cells if it converts to estrogen before it can deliver its message content to the DNA programs in the cells.

When testosterone converts to estrogen before it can deliver message content, a powerful unraveling of the male form begins. The male form can only be maintained when the proper proportion between estrogen and testosterone exists. Certain factors alter the optimal ratio around middle age. Until these factors are effectively mitigated, supplementation or the manufacture of testosterone in the testicles will do little good. In these cases it preferentially converts to estrogen. The higher estrogen within the male body has powerful repercussions on not only the male form, but also the testicles themselves (see first link).

Three common factors that increase the conversion rate of testosterone to estrogen are increased body fat, zinc deficiency, and methyl donor deficiency. Minimizing each of these three will allow testosterone to increase. When testosterone increases, the cells receive the message to increase rejuvenation. When rejuvenation increases, cells increase their infrastructure development activities. Adequate infrastructure redevelopment reflects in the mirror as an improved physique.

Increased body fat creates a vicious cycle of increased estrogen. Fat cells contain an enzyme called aromatase that converts testosterone to estrogen. The more fat, the more aromatase increases that converts testosterone to estrogen. Increased estrogen perpetuates an increased body fat in the male in the same way as a female.

Some well-meaning physicians prescribe testosterone for middle-aged patients and obtain poor results. Until aromatase activity diminishes, testosterone supplementation proves counter productive. Often these males are cranky, irritable and develop breast tissue. An estrogen level, especially estrone, from a blood sample or a twenty-four hour urine test should be included in the hormone evaluation for men.

There are two possible methods for side stepping aromatase activity. The first involves sticking to a low carbohydrate diet that will decrease insulin and reduce fat production. Once fat levels have decreased, testosterone supplementation may be effective. The second method to consider involves prescribing dihydrotestosterone (DHT), which cannot be converted to estrogen as readily and is ten times more powerful than regular testosterone.

The conventional dogma says to keep DHT away from the male scalp. This form of testosterone is said to create male pattern baldness when it reaches high levels in the scalp tissue. A cream is best for this reason and can be applied to the penis, abdomen and breast areas.

If the conventional dogma were completely true why would DHT promote hair growth everywhere else? Insight is gained when one examines an ignored detail about hair loss preventers, like Propecia. Physicians are taught that Propecia, (finasteride), works by inhibiting 5-alpha reductase, the enzyme that converts testosterone to DHT. What remains ignored is the additional fact that this same enzyme inhibits the inactivation of cortisol. Correcting the DHT and cortisol imbalance is more likely to explain some of the benefits of finasteride medication. In fact many twenty-four hour urine results taken from viral, full head of hair and healthy elderly men show high DHT, cortisol and DHEA levels.

DHT will tend to support prostate growth. In the estrogen dominant male, DHT will probably contribute to an enlarged prostate. Higher estrogen creates more DHT receptors in the prostate. Estrogen is also felt to have a direct growth promoting effect in prostate tissue, as well.

Increased estrogen causes prostate changes that are unique. It has been known for almost 20 years that estrogen stimulates the prostate to undergo cystic metaplasia (abnormal cell division) and hypertrophy (enlarge). The physician who routinely checks 24-hour urine test results before prescribing hormones will quickly notice that men with prostate problems tend to have the highest estrone levels (about 80-90% of the time).

Suspicion also occurs in men with full heads of hair. Estrone maintains the hair line to some degree and it seems to be high in about 90% of the full headed hair males after 50 years old or so. In all cases, estrogen levels need to be monitored. It is also important to follow serial PSA values (monthly for the first four months and then every six months) when there is any doubt. In the case of the middle aged male, there is always doubt.

There are two methods for decreasing the activity of the aromatase enzyme. First, normal amounts of zinc inhibit aromatase activity. The highest concentration of zinc is found in oysters. This may explain why oysters have long been associated with aphrodisiac activity. Second, keep the methyl donor system healthy. The methyl donor system is healthy when there are sufficient methyl groups for the DNA stabilizing, hormone creating, and hormone deactivating system (section three).

Recall the body needs a methyl group at the rate of one billion times a second. When owners continue to eat processed food, they will eventually become methyl deficient. Some of these methyl deficient bodies will take a methyl off of testosterone with the help of the enzyme aromatase. When this happens testosterone converts into estrogen.

Nutritional deficiencies can disable the hormone system by multiple mechanisms (section three). Before discussing nutritional building blocks that make up the body form, a hormone pecking order needs to be established. By understanding the hierarchy of hormones in the body, owners become less gullible to the agenda of the complex.

CHAPTER TWELVE

Hierarchy of Hormones - Informational Substances

Before proceeding with this book, it helps to have a concise grouping of how the different hormones can be separated into a successive hierarchy. The hierarchy between the different hormones concerns their degree of influence and length of action when compared to one another. There are four basic groups of successive levels of influence on how the body spends energy. Hormones direct cell energy usage. The more powerful the hormone group, the more central it is in where energy directs when it arrives.

It helps to elucidate the common error of how mainstream medicine often focuses on the 'lesser' hormones. The lesser hormones get the press coverage while the more powerful hormones are only peripherally addressed. By taking this approach to chronic disease treatment strategies, symptom control is all that is possible. Symptom control medical approaches always produce side effects and have nothing to do with healing. By adding back the hormone hierarchy these errors become easy to expose.

Grouping the different informational substances (hormones) into four groups will help in understanding the interdependent relationship of the many various hormones. Also, many chronic degenerative diseases will begin to have healing solutions.

Common degenerative diseases more amenable to healing once the hormone hierarchy is addressed are: adrenal gland caused asthma, rheumatoid arthritis, systemic lupus, fibromyalgia, osteoarthritis, adult onset diabetes, obesity, some neurodegenerative diseases, some cases of heart disease, ulcerative colitis, Crohn disease, some liver diseases, some kidney diseases, some cases of senility, and muscle wasting diseases. Section three will also bolster the success rate for treating some of these diseases by adding in the all important food allergy consideration and work up.

All of these diseases have an increased likelihood of a solution when the clinician attends to these diseases' treatment in a logical progression from the most powerful hormone imbalances down to the weakest. When supplementation strategies are needed, real hormones are used because only they contain accurate message content. The body was designed for real hormone message content. Mantra: whenever the altered shaped of the hormone substitutes are given in place of real hormones, side effects likely follow. Life is vibrational and consistently communicates in this fashion via the hormones. The vibration depends on the shape of the molecules of life. Shape changes allow a patent, but the message content changes. Simple science discussed here but not commonly taught in a way that physicians can understand.

The four groups in the hierarchy of hormones are:

Group 1 - the supreme commanders of body energy

This powerful group of hormones directly switches off and on different DNA programs (genes). The DNA programs activated in a cell determine the activity of the cell and the degree of repair (rejuvenation). The activity and state of repair determine the usefulness of the cell. When cells are given good informational direction from the level one hormone class, they will be productive and healthy. The thyroid hormones, all steroids, and vitamin A comprise the level one hormone class. Logically, the quality of the mixture and amount of level one hormones reaching the over one hundred trillion cells forms a central determinant of health. An owner's health is powerfully influenced because these hormones all contain message content that instructs the DNA (genes) program activity.

The level one hormone class (steroids, vitamin A and thyroid hormones) comprises the only hormones powerful enough to directly interact and instruct cellular genetic material (the DNA). Quality of the proportional mixture between these hormones determines the highest level of energy expenditure. At this primary level these hormones quality of presence determines whether a cell uses available energy efficiently or not. This class of hormone has access to every body chamber (the skin chapter). All healthy owners predictably have high quality message content amongst the level one hormone class. Conversely, unhealthy owners predictably have lousy hormone quality as part of their aging process. These owners will continue to age prematurely, until someone helps these owners regain more optimal message content.

Group 2 – the amino acid chain

All hormones message content is about directing cellular expendable energy, likewise with the level two hormones. Level two hormones deliver a message when they bind to a cell surface receptor (their own unique type) or they bind a receptor inside the target cell. The level two hormones are only able to influence cell energy expenditure on existing cell structures and enzymatic machinery activity. They are not able to direct DNA programs in the manufacture of new cell structures or new enzymatic machinery. Only a level one hormone is powerful enough to accomplish this.

Insulin and glucagon provide examples of level two hormones. Like other level two hormones, they consist of a specific sequence of amino acids that twist around in three-dimensional space. The shape of these specific sequences and resulting twist contains precise message content. Insulin and glucagon are also an example of level two hormones that contain opposite message content. The message content difference between insulin and glucagon directs the target cell to spend energy in the opposite way.

Consistent with other level two hormones, each can only affect existing cellular enzymatic machines or structural content. Insulin turns off the enzyme machines that glucagon turns on. Likewise, the message content of glucagon turns off what insulin turns on. Each of these opposing hormones has enzyme machines that they activate. The direction of energy within a cell determines which enzymes are quiet or active. Hormones direct which way energy moves in a cell. Catabolism versus anabolism describes an example of opposite energy movement.

The liver cells prove instructive as an example for the opposite energy direction between the message content of insulin and glucagon. Insulin directs liver cell energy into fuel storage (anabolism). Fuel is stored in various locations, but insulin stimulates the liver in the manufacture of glycogen, triglycerides, cholesterol, LDL cholesterol and VLDL cholesterol.

Insulin also inhibits the liver from turning amino acids into sugar and fat. The more insulin in the body, the more these activities occur within the liver. Conversely, glucagon directs the liver to release stored fuel and curtails new cholesterol and triglyceride manufacture (catabolic effect). It also stimulates the liver contained enzymatic machines to make sugar from available amino acids (gluconeogenesis).

Some level two hormones are further endowed with the ability to leave a 'last will and directive' before being chewed up into their component parts by intracellular machinery. Intracellular machinery eventually dismantles the level two hormones. This ability describes an intermediate step. The last will and directive of some level two hormones occurs between activating their receptor and being dismantled. The last will and directives are additional messages to the cell created by level two hormones activating level four hormones. These messages exist for a limited time. During that time, the level two hormones affect which level four hormone precursors a cell will receive message content from (Sears).

Insulin and glucagon provide good examples of how a hormone's presence determines which level four hormone precursors are formed. Also consistent is the fact that level four hormones precursors, stimulated by insulin, have the opposite effect on cell energy, when mature, as the direction that glucagon level four hormones impart (see group 4 below).

Group 3 – the subservient hormones

The level three hormones are composed of single amino acids, which have been structurally modified or are from short chains of amino acids. These hormones depend on directives of the higher hormones 'stage setting'. The level one and two hormones set the stage for structural integrity and enzyme machinery contained in a cell. The stage setting is centrally determined by the level one type hormones at the DNA level. In turn, the level two hormones determine the activity of the setting, the enzymes. The level three hormones channel blood and fuel to the cells. However, the level three hormones depend on level one type hormones for directing the manufacture of their receptors. Without enough level three-hormone receptors being made, many chronic diseases begin (like asthma from epinephrine receptor deficiency). Finally, the level four hormones can only affect the 'props'inside the cell (explained below).

Biogenic amines, cytokines, and endothelin all belong to the level three classes of hormones. Dietary deficiencies can effect development and manufacture of these hormones. Many different vitamins prove important for biogenic amine's manufacture. In general, the level three hormones have an effect on the caliber of blood vessels and properties of the cells in these vessels in a certain area of the body.

Which level three hormones (muscle chapter) delivers message content in a certain blood vessel, determines much about the oxygen availability, nutrient delivery, waste removal, stickiness and leakiness of that vessel's wall, its clotting tendency, and immune cell behavior.

Group 4 – local acting, subservient hormones

These hormones exist for seconds, only long enough to deliver message content to nearby cells. Within seconds of their release they are deactivated. It is helpful to regard these hormones as only having an influence for both the duration and as far as the sound of their 'voice' will travel. This is in contrast to the other three levels of hormones that can travel more extensively in delivering their message content.

Some of the level four hormones, like nitric oxide gas, have powerful penetration abilities through body barriers. Although nitric oxide has powerful penetrating abilities, its message content delivery ability is limited due to its rapid deactivation. This short lifespan diminishes the distance of influence of nitric oxide's message content.

Other level four hormones, like the ecosanoids (hormonal fats) that include prostaglandins, leukotrienes, and lipoxin are also limited by their short life spans. The ecosanoids come from essential fatty acids (hormonal fat precursors). These include linoleic, linolenic, and arachidonic acid. All three of these essential fatty acids can only be obtained in the diet. The type of diet determines which level two hormones message content will predominate.

Recall, an example of the opposing possibilities of level two hormones and how they determine what level four hormones are possible occurs between insulin and glucagon. The opposite message content contained between glucagon and insulin has a powerful influence on which level four precursor hormones are possible. High carbohydrate diets tend to promote the pro-inflammatory hormonal fat precursors to line many cells.

By this mechanism, certain low carbohydrate and high protein/fat diets promote anti-inflammatory hormonal fat precursors (section three). The type of level two hormones limits the possibilities for which level four hormone precursors line numerous cells. Those hormonal fat precursors that line the surface of cells determine the likelihood of developing or preventing some malicious chronic degenerative diseases. Some diseases effected by the presence or the absences of hormonal fat precursors are cancer, heart disease, arthritis, depression, fatigue and immunodeficiency syndromes.

There are three principles about the ecosanoids (hormonal fats) that are important. First, only green plants can make two out of three of these hormonal fat precursors called the essential fatty acids. Animals like salmon that live in the wild eat plankton and therefore contain significant amounts of these two plant manufactured essential fatty acids. In contrast, farmed, grain-fed animals are raised without these essential fatty acids presence (Weil, 2001).

The green plant manufactured essential fatty acids are linolenic and linoleic acid. Free-range chicken eggs are also good sources for these plants derived essential fatty acids. In addition, wild game such as elk and deer are also sources for these two essential fatty acids. These are good sources for essential fatty acids because of the high content of green plants in these animals diet. Green plants are the source of the anti-inflammatory fatty acids, linolenic and linoleic acids. Non-green roots and grains are more likely to contain the pro-inflammatory arachidonic acid. Store bought chicken, meat and eggs, because the animals are grain fed, will be higher in the arachidonic acid type.

Second, eating all the right essential fatty acids can still output the wrong hormonal fats. Recall, these fats are subservient to the more powerful higher hormones. Level two hormones like insulin and glucagon determine which hormone fat precursors become created from essential fatty acids in the diet. The essential fatty acids in the diet are the raw material created for precursor hormonal fats. As a consequence, the balance of message content between insulin and glucagon predetermine which precursors are created.

Third, hormonal fat precursors are ideally contained on all the cell surfaces. When released, these hormones have a limited area of influence because of their short lifespan. Scientists denote this shortened hormone lifespan by the term paracrine. Paracrine hormones can only deliver message content in their immediate area of release. All level four hormones are paracrine in nature. The level four hormones are only released when triggered by higher hormones. Sub-optimal hormonal fat message content has a powerful influence on several chronic diseases.

The hormonal fats are so important that many powerful medications work by poisoning their ability to be produced. Some medications that work by poisoning hormonal fats are aspirin and related non-steroidal anti-inflammatory medications, cortisone derivatives, and the newer cox 2 inhibitors. These symptom control approaches have consequences to the balance of fine tuning abilities occurring in cells. All of these redirect body energy. With an understanding of hormonal fats and how to optimize their function, one can work with their body and begin healing.

Nitric oxide has a powerful ability to lower blood pressure and is also within this fourth class of hormones. It can only briefly increase blood delivery into its local area. This is how the medication Viagra works and why all the warnings about it lowering blood pressure are given. This medicine, by a circuitous route, allows nitric oxide increases and this follows into enhanced blood flow to the penis. This natural blood flow regulator requires the presence of the nutritional co-factors arginine, riboflavin, tetrahydrobiopterin, and thiol for its biosynthesis. Thiol is contained in garlic and onions. Tetrahydrobiopterin derives from folate. How many hypertensive and impotent owners originate simply from these nutritional deficiencies?

Be aware of the hierarchy of different hormone groups and what dietary factors are required for them to be produced. Owners who have optimal balance at each level are in good health. Conversely, a lowered quality of informational content occurring at any of the successive levels or dietary deficiencies leads to health consequences. The science exists to help owners receive better hormones and good nutrition. In the next section the owner will begin to understand how the different molecular parts assimilate into the body and how deficiencies lead to breakdown processes.

SECTION THREE

SECTION THREE..*251*

    PRINCIPLE FOUR: YOU ARE WHAT YOU SUPPLY AND
    ABSORB..252

CHAPTER THIRTEEN 254

    DIGESTION 254

CHAPTER FOURTEEN 310

    PANCREAS..310

CHAPTER FIFTEEN...323

    AVOID THE TORTURE CHAMBER DIET 323

PRINCIPLE FOUR: YOU ARE WHAT YOU SUPPLY AND ABSORB

Many owners become unhealthy only because they fail to understand what their body's need. For example, bodies that receive the nutrition they need stop craving the next feeding event. A major component of obesity perpetration resides in **the hungry cell syndrome**. The *hungry cell syndrome* results when the wrong hormones release and this abnormally shunts excessive nutrition into storage (fat). The consequent deficient fuel delivery causes the other body cells to remain hungry.

Owners that understand this fact can maintain a focus on ways to realign their hormones' message content (see previous section discussion). Similarly, insight into what good nutrition entails and how it happens further facilitates healing the middle-aged body.

This section consists of three chapters. The first concerns the understanding of what food is and how the body assimilates it into the body structure. It also includes a trip down the digestive tract. In the following chapter, the horomes that influence the pancreas are discussed. The third chapter facilitates the application of basic nutritional knowledge and empowers the unhealthy owner to successfully shed fat and/or rebuild body structure.

Still other unhealthy bodies exist on the emaciated extreme of poor health. Likewise for them, nutritional understandings pave the way for healing their absorption dilemmas. **Recall, the other extreme of unhealthy bodies, the obese body, also suffers from a wasting disease, loss of body protein, but its loss remains hidden amongst the fat.** However, in both extremes, until someone explains to them how to regain their functional tissue through both better nutrition and hormone realignment their wasting disease will continue.

This section emphasizes the maintenance and rebuilding of the body's functional components through attention on what the body needs to absorb. The prevention of body breakdown occurs because only functional digestive tracts maximize the absorption of nutrients. In addition, the owner needs to make good nutritional decisions or there will be insufficient supplies of these important building blocks (replacement molecules) arriving for their digestive tract to absorb.

Reactions of life use up molecular parts quickly. Consequently, a continual need for new sources of quality molecular parts exists throughout life. Molecular replacement parts serve; in making body structure, as fuel, maintain cellular electrical charge, as hormones, as metabolically active proteins, and as facilitators of enzyme machine activities.

Structures that are alive, cells, require a constant supply of quality molecular replacement parts because the process of life degrades molecules. This chapter explains how these molecular replacement parts are obtained and assimilated. When replacement parts assimilate, the rejuvenation program continues.

Conversely, inadequate molecular replacement parts leads to an old and flabby or shriveled body. The pursuit of longevity concerns how to obtain and assimilate quality molecular replacement parts, the third principle of longevity. Quality parts are necessary to prevent the old body manifestation that results from the accumulation of worn out parts. Bodies with worn out parts contain hungry cells that desire new molecular replacement parts. Unfortunately, the obvious consequences of inadequate molecular replacement parts or a deficiency in their quality fails to be comprehended by many owners. Often this disconnection results from scientific communications being explained in an abstract manner.

It deserves overall emphasis that each cell type needs a continuous supply of specific molecular replacement parts. These molecular replacement parts are needed in specific amounts and sufficient quality to maintain healthy cell function. The processed food diet is deficient in regenerative replacement parts. Deficiency, excess or inferior quality interferes with health. Obesity and emaciation describe manifestations of diminished health. Less well appreciated concerns the realization that both of these extremes result, in part, from the *hungry cell syndrome*.

When the digestive tract fails, health consequences ensue such as:

- Cellular trash accumulation
- Loss of cellular integrity (old and worn out molecular parts)
- Deficient molecular parts needed to manufacture adequate informational substances (hormones and neurotransmitters)
- Inadequate cellular charge (mineral imbalance)
- A progressive deficiency in the ability to maintain cellular energy requirements (vitamin deficiencies, rust and poor quality fuel intake)
- Deficient amounts of the many different types of metabolically active proteins that allow the cell to burn calories while it performs the work of living

CHAPTER THIRTEEN

DIGESTION

The Body is Analogous to a Temple that is Alive

The ongoing assimilation of molecular replacement parts is similar to the non-living building world. In each case, fundamental building components, each with specific roles, create the overall whole (wire, bricks, two by fours, windows, light sockets, trusses, etc.). These components have the potential, when assembled correctly and proportionally, to become an elaborate temple. Multiply the architectural complexity of the ongoing body molecular parts replacement program. Throughout life this replacement program proves necessary for healthy structure and function.

The body can be thought of as a dynamic, living temple that will, in time, wear out its constituent molecular parts as it pulsates with the energies of life. Wear and tear creates the accumulation of defective molecular structural components and enzyme machines. The body temple requires precise maintenance of its internal structure and energy flow parameters. It can only obtain these parts from other temples (living things). However, less appreciated concerns the fact that these other temples must be precisely dismantled or rubbish instead of replacement parts results. The precise dismantling of these temples describes the process referred to as digestion.

Healthy owners have digestive systems that assimilate their continuously needed replacement parts into their body. Availability of sufficient parts results from precise dismantling of other temples in the digestive tract. The absorption of these molecular building blocks and fuel sources (to power the 'intra-temple electronics') occurs in a rhythmic fashion. After absorption of these parts, they reassemble into complex components (cell structure or enzymes) or combust as fuel in the cellular power plants (mitochondria).

The reactions of life diminish when the digestive tract malfunctions in its ability to precisely dismantle a molecular building block. The lack of replacement parts leads to many chronic degenerative diseases. Chronic degenerative diseases have a component of causality in the *hungry cell syndrome*. Obesity and body emaciation provide two examples of chronic degenerative disease.

The hungry cell syndrome results from:
- Poor nutritional choices (empty calories)
- Improper dismantling ability, within the digestive tract, for critical molecular components, which the cells need to replace their worn out structural components or old enzyme machines
- Poor quality communication between digestive cells secondary to imbalanced hormone tone
- Injury to various digestive chambers and structures
- Once nutrients assimilate into the body, the wrong hormones occur with the consequence being that the liver converts excessive nutrients into fat (section two)

Hungry body cells turn up the appetite centers' volume. These owners are constantly in the *torture chamber* of desire for the next feeding event. The *torture chamber* always wins until they are taught how to feed their cells with what they need. Well-fed body cells do not cry out for more food. The processed food diet perpetrates the *hungry cell syndrome*. The *hungry cell syndrome* propagates when molecular replacement parts become deficient.

Digestive Tracts and Molecular Supply Lines

All too often the nutritional integrity of cells is superficially addressed. This simple omission causes many owners aging rate to accelerate. The disassembly of protein, carbohydrate, and fats relies on numerous digestive juices. These juices must occur in a specific sequence and be of a sufficient amount. Protein disassembly provides a prototypical example from the three different food groups that can facilitate comprehension of problems with the dismantling process - digestion.

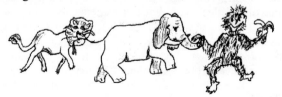

Proteins are comprised of twenty different molecular shapes (amino acids linked end to end). Each amino acid type has a different shape and contains unique chemical qualities. The order of sequence of amino acid connection and the proportions of different amino acids determine the resulting properties of a protein.

It helps to visualize twenty different miniature animals as analogous to the twenty different amino acids that make up all proteins. Different animals occur in various sequences and numbers as they line up. The average number of amino acids strung together in a protein equals 500. This allows a mental picture of the average protein molecule. This chain would have so many tigers, so many elephants, etc. The specific order of these shapes and the amount of each type confers a unique chain (twenty different building block shapes, corresponding to twenty different amino acids that link together to form a protein). In order to build this chain, the body can only obtain the different lions, tigers, and bears from properly dismantled (digested) other chains (protein meals). In order to build new necklaces, a tiger separates as a whole tiger and not a half of a tiger and half of an elephant. If this occurs, the building block potential of the different shapes reduces to rubbish.

The body can produce only twelve of the different amino acid types. It cannot manufacture the other eight. When the body manufactures its own amino acids it depletes essential ones that must be obtained in the diet. For this reason, the best situation occurs when an owner consumes proper proportions and amounts of all twenty amino acid types.

The healthy digestive tract, when presented with these chains (proteins), starts methodically dismantling them. Realize, the proteins must be precisely disassembled or useful replacement parts cannot be absorbed. When amino acids absorb, they can be used for building new proteins (chains).

The unique order and amounts of different amino acids confer specific qualities and abilities for each protein. Some proteins contain many sulfurous amino acids. Other proteins have extra nitrogen. Still other proteins have extra acid content. The overall amino acid order and content determines protein function.

Some proteins are used for structural integrity (cell membrane, organelles, hair, bone, ligaments, etc.). Some serve as transport vehicles in the bloodstream for critical minerals, steroids, and gases (calcium, testosterone, and oxygen respectively provide such examples). Other proteins function as cellular machines (enzymes). Still others form into the many different types of informational substances (insulin, glucagon, and IGF-1).

The body requires a continuous supply of quality building blocks (amino acids) in order to maintain availability of different protein types. Amino acid building blocks need to be structurally intact when absorbed. The digestive process fails unless the consumed protein meals dismantle precisely into their component amino acids.

Molecular Replacement Parts Require Precision Dismantling

The public is led to believe digestion is analogous to food that grinds up in a blender. The perpetrated story implies that this slurry sucks up into the bloodstream and dissipates among the different body cells for use. The temple analogy exposes this gross simplification.

If a building explodes, rubbish results because little salvage ability remains in the way of reusable structural components (intact doors, windows, trusses, flooring, appliances, etc.). In order to have any reusable structural components derived from a temple, a precise dismantling process needs to occur. No reusable building components persist without precision dismantling occurring first. Similarly, the human body digestive process needs to be orderly and precise in its ability to dismantle the various food building blocks, nutrients, vitamins, and chemical reaction facilitators (cofactors).

Shrink down to the size of a molecular glass ship. In this glass ship visualize an imaginary trip through the digestive tube. The trip down the digestive tract from mouth to anus involves passage through multiple chambers. Each chamber concerns a specific digestive process that needs to occur before movement to the next chamber becomes appropriate. These processes occur all along a healthy digestive tube.

The digestion that follows each meal needs to be orderly and precise. This process dismantles the food consumed into its building block molecular components. Next, these molecular components absorb into the body at specific sites along the tube. Once these different molecular replacement parts absorb into the cells lining the tube, they eventually secrete into the blood stream. Here, they distribute to different body cells and reassemble into new temple components or burn up as fuel. Realize disease and old age results when the supply of these necessary replacement molecular parts becomes scarce.

Overall schema: Only with adequate molecular supply lines, adequate workforce, optimal workforce environment, integrated communication with the salvage team and sufficient enzymatic machines will appropriate cellular rejuvenation occur. Successful assimilation leads to new cellular structural repairs, new transport vehicles, new cellular factories, new informational substances, and adequate cellular trash removal. Without adequate cellular rejuvenation all the cells are forced to make due with old cellular machines (enzymes). Also, cellular trash accumulates. The cellular factory components age because they work long after their useful life spans.

The Task at Hand for the Digestive Tube

The accomplishments of a healthy digestive system after a meal is best understood when the different components of that meal are isolated. These isolated components need to be discussed in regards to their unique contribution and their particular dilemma before body assimilation occurs. The dismantling of protein was already reviewed above. Some of the other meal components of disassembly are discussed below. A trip down the tube in the glass ship follows in the next chapter after review on these basics of digestion.

How to Dismantle Carbohydrates

Carbohydrates break down into sugar and comprise the quickest food group to be absorbed. Almost 100% of sugar absorbs within a healthy owners digestive tract at the rate of 120 grams an hour (about 500 calories). Fat absorbs the slowest and protein assimilates a little quicker than fat.

For this reason, hunger returns more quickly following carbohydrate meals. However, there is an additional reason that this fuel type causes more hunger: Carbohydrate intake also obligates more insulin release.

Recall from section two, exaggerated insulin release becomes necessary in overweight owners because some other glandular process has failed. In these owners, insulin processes a larger proportion of the elevated blood sugar after IGF-1 falls following carbohydrate intake. As insulin increases, there are grave additional consequences in the stimulation of eating behavior and the fat making machinery (see section two).

Mentally summarize that increased insulin arriving within the liver instructs it to hog excessive nutrition and convert it into cholesterol and fat. Meanwhile, the fall off of IGF-1 means that the cells outside of liver and fat have less ability to feed on the nutrition within the blood stream. Visualize the 'tug of war' between the relative amounts of IGF-1 versus insulin determining where fuel flows within the body.

Recall, middle-aged bodies suffer from less IGF-1 and consequently need excessive insulin to stay alive between meals. Consequently, excessive carbohydrate consumption promotes an unstable blood sugar (excessive insulin requires excessive counter regulatory hormones). For this reasons, excessive consumption of carbohydrate increases insulin to unhealthful levels. High insulin levels and high carbohydrate consumption create a vicious cycle between the insulin-induced obsession for food and the consumption of carbohydrates. As insulin levels rise, weight gain occurs. **Insulin is the most powerful of all growth factors for fat.** The failure to counsel trapped owners about this fact leads to unnecessary suffering in the western world today.

Carbohydrate, whether it is complex (bread, potatoes, pasta, or grains) or simple (fruit, sugar, corn syrup, honey) break down into one or more of the simple sugars (glucose, fructose or galactose). Intestinal absorption of sugar is independent of insulin level.

Insulin levels need to rise after the intestines absorb sugar and dump it into the blood stream. Realize, the amount of insulin needed becomes proportional to the sugar load absorbed and the severity of the IGF-1 deficit. Healthy owners have many times the IGF-1 compared to insulin within their blood streams. Consequently, they need much less insulin to uptake sugar fuel into the body cells outside the liver and fat.

Conversely, unhealthy owners need extra insulin because their IGF-1 levels have fallen (one cause of insulin resistance). Actually, increased insulin need more accurately describes insulin resistance at a root level. The hungry body cells beyond the liver desperately need excessive insulin as a fuel nozzle since IGF-1 proves insufficient.

Recall, whatever the insulin secretion rate the liver always receives the highest insulin message content because of its relationship to the pancreas secreting insulin into the portal vein that heads straight into this organ. Unfortunately, before any insulin escapes the liver trap, excessive amounts of it need to arrive within the liver and this increases the fat maker message. As was explained in section two, the abnormality of insulin arriving and instructing increased liver removal of fuel while the blood fuel falls (fasting, exercising, or between meals) requires excessive counter regulatory hormone release to prevent death. This excess in turn violently instructs the liver to urgently dismantle protein for fuel generation. This typical middle-aged scenario explains increased fat while muscles and organs hide their shriveling amongst the fat. It also explains the decrease in metabolism typical for middle age.

Key concept: Only by excessive insulin releasing into the portal vein, can some of it make it beyond the liver (visualize the 200,000 pure insulin receptors per liver cell) in an attempt to bring total fuel nozzle hormone levels up to deliver sufficient fuel to the hungry body cells beyond the liver.

More perspective is added when one realizes that the 70kg individual contains only about six grams of sugar within his/her entire blood stream. Now visualize a meal containing 20 grams of dietary carbohydrate. Recall, it can absorb into the blood stream at the rate of two grams a minute. One unit of insulin removes about five grams of sugar from the blood stream. So the entire 20 grams absorbs and summons about four units of insulin to promptly return the blood sugar down to normal. Too fast or too slow leads to health effects (explained in the liver chapter). The point to consider here, for now, regards the small amount of total sugar within the blood stream and the fact that many modern junk meals contain over 200-300 grams of sugar. Think about the tremendous load that this places on the body just to maintain blood sugar balance.

The greater the total body potassium deficit, the more insulin needed to process a given amount of sugar intake.

The insulin resistance problem compounds when carbohydrate consumption takes place without potassium. Processed food diets contain less potassium relative to carbohydrate content. Conversely, real food diets (natural and un-adulterated foods) contain high potassium relative to carbohydrate content (see mineral table). When owners pay attention to this, tolerance for carbohydrates increases. Sufficient potassium needs to be present to lower the insulin requirement for the amount of carbohydrates consumed. Potassium proves crucial to take sugar out of the blood stream.

As was previously mentioned, only real food contains sufficient potassium with carbohydrate. This causes processed food to contain reversed mineral proportions compared to body design. Altered minerals within some middle-aged owners' bodies cause **low cell voltage syndrome**. *Low cell voltage syndrome* manifests as weakness and fatigue. Until these owners receive counseling on how to correct their mineral imbalances they will continue to grow old at a rapid rate (section 5).

Ignoring this simple fact about potassium-depleted foods prevents understanding another cause of **insulin resistance**. Insulin resistance means that more insulin needs to be secreted for the carbohydrate load ingested to return the blood sugar to normal. The blood sugar returns to normal with less insulin when sufficient potassium remains available. One potassium molecule with the help of insulin or IGF-1 moves one sugar molecule out of the blood stream.

Potassium deficiencies create a big component of health issues that begin in middle age. The degenerative processes that begin with potassium deficiencies in middle age often contribute to obesity, abnormal cholesterol profile, decreased steroid tone, high blood pressure, nervous irritability, diabetes, protein deficiency and decreased energy levels (see section five and six). For these reasons, middle age disease can sometimes be avoided when the digestive relationship between potassium intake and carbohydrate intake is realized and acted upon.

A Few More Words on How to Dismantle a Protein

As was mentioned above, the various amounts and sequences (the chain) of 20 different amino acids make up the different protein types. Nutritional value ceases, for building block purposes, when the digestive tract fails to precisely dismantle protein molecules. Precision dismantling proves as a prerequisite for obtaining the continuous supply of amino acids needed for ongoing rejuvenation projects.

Additional concerns arise if consumed proteins partially digest (fragments that contain three or more amino acids). The absorption of amino acid sequences three or more long has the potential to activate the immune system. This fact forms the basis for how food allergies start in infants fed foreign proteins before their digestive tracts develop a sufficient barrier. When an undeveloped digestive tract cannot digest protein completely, it will leak the partially digested protein fragments into the blood stream. Once these protein fragments float in the blood stream they will activate the immune system of an infant. When the immune system activates an allergic response becomes possible. Activation occurs when it 'sees' the same sequence again from the ingestion of the same food. The immune response occurs and manifest as food allergy.

Partial digestion and absorption of protein fragments can be a powerful immune system activator against the body, autoimmunity. Autoimmunity means that the body's immune system attacks its own body structure. One cause of autoimmune disease occurs when certain processes injure the integrity of the tube of the digestive system. When the tube integrity deteriorates it will leak undigested fragments that normally do not penetrate until they are completely broken down. Examples of diseases that contain a component of food allergy within their etiology are rheumatoid arthritis, systemic lupus, multiple sclerosis, colitis, psoriasis, asthma, ankylosing spondylitis and some thyroid diseases. Some clinicians call this **'leaky gut syndrome.'**

Alternatively, and just as insidious, concerns those owners who suffer from insufficient stomach acid secretion. Jonathan Wright, MD pioneered the concept and work up for owners that develop food allergies only because the primary trigger towards complete protein digestion depends on sufficient stomach acid secretion (explained later).

Visualize the mechanics of leaky gut: Defects occurring on the inner protective layer of the digestive tube facilitate leaky gut syndrome. Glycosaminoglycans (GAG) compose this innermost protective layer. As this layer continually forms in the digestive tube and degrades, it creates mucus overlying the new GAG layer. Some scientists call the GAG layer the matrix. In fact, through out the different linings of the body such as the skin, the respiratory tract, the inner lining of the blood vessels, the GAG layer forms a protective barrier in these areas. In addition, it is this architectural support meshwork (GAG) that inflates cells, forms cartilage and connects cells together. All of these are formed by GAG. Paradoxically, mainstream medicine often fails to discuss or consider this important layer in the maintenance of health. This is folly because as GAG diminishes so does these owners' health.

In order for doctors to appreciate all these facts about GAG, they need to know all the many alias names that it goes by within the literature. Some of them are: cell coat, mucopolysaccharides, basal lamina, ground substance, and it serves as a component of the cytoskeleton, matrix and cartilage.

Since GAG formation is so important to one's overall health, pertinent connecting facts for what determines its formation rate are in order. The amount of IGF-1 determines a particular body local's amount of GAG formation rate. Many physicians remain unaware of this fact because the vocabulary uniting this association has been changed. The older literature described IGF-1 as sulfation factor.

Sulfation describes the critical step in the formation of GAG building blocks, composed of either galactosamine or glucosamine, where sulfate adds to them. As long as sufficient IGF-1 (sulfation factor) instructs the locals listed above then adequate GAG forms.

Realize GAG cannot form properly without sufficient sulfation on each glucosamine and galactosamine.

The addition of sulfate powerfully sucks in water because of its strong electrical charge. The more adequate the water content, in a body area, the less shrinkage. It is important to emphasize that the addition of sulfate creates a strong electrical charge. The electrical charge sufficiency proves particularly important in barrier areas like the digestion tube.

Mentally summarize that it is largely the sufficiency of GAG content in the body that opposes the forces of gravity, which desires to squish cells flat. Only with the presence of sufficient highly charged GAG will the ability to impede shrinkage through the prevention of water loss occur. Only high electrical charge resists the forces imposed by gravity. Shrinkage occurs from drying out and has been recognized since antiquity to be fundamental to the aging process. Visualize old bodies as possessing inadequate electrical charge in their various body chambers and hence they shrivel and dehydrate.

Remember, IGF-1 levels depend on adequate Growth Hormone release, a healthy liver and adequate androgen telling the liver to make IGF-1. In addition, sufficient pituitary manufacture of Growth Hormone depends on adequate thyroid hormones levels. For this reason, if any of the above four basic requirements fail health suffers. The above hormonal and glandular interdependencies prove as bedrock for longevity (pay attention here).

Nerd corner

A similar vocabulary change preceded the old name of IGF-1 being called sulfation factor. This name change helps to propagate yet another 'disconnect' in physicians minds regarding IGF-1's important role in sugar metabolism. This older name calls IGF-1, the nonsuppressible insulin like activity of the blood. The old name sheds light on IGF-1's important role in sugar metabolism. The new name helps to instill fear of the same molecule being a growth factor for cancer cells. Never mind the fact that all healthy people have high levels of IGF-1. Change the name and you can better manipulate how physicians think.

Another powerful 'disconnect' results from the fact that insulin amounts, in almost all medical textbooks, are measured in microunits or micromoles. However, IGF-1 is measured in nanograms. This helps to perpetuate the concealment of the fact that IGF-1 occurs at levels many times greater than insulin. Finally, for now, exercise normally causes insulin levels to fall towards zero. The highest pure IGF-1 receptor concentration is located in the muscles! If more physicians were aware of these facts they would begin asking why the body design would do this. The next step would be economic disaster for the medical industrial complex.

Normally, the digestion process disassembles larger molecules that would activate the immune system. The immune system activates against foreign sequences of protein. Viruses, bacteria, fungus, and partially digested proteins in food contain foreign protein. The body circumvents protein meals containing foreign protein amino acid sequences by dismantling these proteins into their constituent amino acids. Individual amino acids are too small to activate the immune system. These small building block molecular parts, (amino acids) transport in the blood stream to different cells. Once inside the cells, gene activity directs how the individual amino acids arrange into new proteins. In this way, amino acid molecular parts organize to create complex structures (proteins) in the cells and thus avoid immune systems activation in the blood stream.

A Component of Old Age Results from Old Proteins

Old age or chronic disease occurs when the integrity of the individual proteins begin to breakdown. It helps to think of it as the animals that make up the imaginary chain as they become deformed, acquire worn down edges, or attach to debris. The diminished ability to replace proteins as they break down and wear out defines a crucial process of aging. Poor nutritional absorption that results from lack of efficiency in the digestive tract or misguided protein choices cause decline in protein dependent cellular rejuvenation.

The face of someone old and decrepit results, in part, from his or her lost protein integrity. At the molecular level this is nothing more than damaged individual amino acids, which alter the overall effected protein structure and function. The functions of protein encompass their role in cellular support. Support functions are compromised when the underlying protein shape becomes deranged. Deranged proteins have a diminished ability to perform other functions like work and trash removal. These faces, at a molecular level, have accumulated cellular garbage, poor informational substance message content, decreased cellular electrical charge, and accumulated cell rust.

All owners will head this way more quickly without proper nutrition motivation. Better daily nutrition choices that impact cell regeneration and healing provides a place to start. For this reason, optimal digestive juices and operative digestive structures encompass integral parts of healing. Also realize new protein synthesis requires specific gene activation. All genes code for specific proteins. For this reason, the genes provide nothing until the right hormone arrives. (section 2)

Surprises about Where Protein Comes From

Approximately 50% of digested protein comes from the meal content; 25% from proteins within the digestive juices that digest themselves after they perform their roles; and 25% comes from sloughed cells that line the intestinal tube that are also digested. The intestinal tube lining cells have a life span of only 3-5 days. They are sloughed into the tube much like how a snake sheds its skin. In turn, digestive juices dismantle them into their original building blocks. These molecular parts recycle into other cell rejuvenation programs.

The individual amino acids comprise the interchangeable molecular building parts of proteins. As long as a building block (amino acid, fatty acid, vitamin or cofactor) remains structurally intact it is free to be used or recycled into any cell synthesis or rejuvenation project again and again.

The ability of an amino acid to interchange terminates when its structure becomes damaged. Replacement of a molecular part only becomes necessary once wear and tear weakens molecular function. In healthy owners, their cells constantly dismantle damaged proteins and efficiently replace them with new proteins.

Healthy bodies contain the sufficient ability to supply the much-needed molecular replacement parts. Adequate replacement parts facilitate efficient cellular trash removal systems and adequate informational substance content. Fat is another molecular building part that the body requires for structural integrity.

Some Important Facts about Fat and a Few More That Mysteriously Have Been Kept a Secret

Four Important Roles for Body Fat (lipids):
1. Cell structure and water retention (simple fats and cholesterol)
2. Hormone precursors
3. Fuel
4. Brain fats keep nerve cells happy

Specialized lipids (fats), fatty acids, triglycerides, and cholesterol make up the basic structural fats of the body. These building parts are often used as covering for trillions of cell membranes. These occur as part of the cell covering structure (plasma membrane) and organelles (cell factories). These structural fats integrate between varying combinations of interspersed proteins. Both the simple structural fats and the more complex, specialized structural fats compose membranes. The complex group contains lipids with extra molecular parts like phosphate or choline. Ultra-specialized fats contribute additional properties to body function by their role in specialized cells and organelles.

Beautiful skin demonstrates the importance of structural fat. Fat polishes the surface and prevents shriveling by retaining water. Prevention of cellular water loss describes a major function of fat. Inadequate fat content, in type or amount, causes or accelerates water loss. Shriveling and cellular inefficiency occur when water content decreases.

Hormone precursors

Certain lipids (fats) behave as informational substances. These can be thought of as hormonal fats and derive from the essential fatty acids. The body cannot produce essential fatty acids. They must be acquired through dietary sources and absorbed by the digestive tract.

Essential fatty acids transform into message carriers (hormones). Hormonal fats have their own message content contained in their precise shape. Hormonal fats promote information exchange between neighboring cells. Scientists call these types of hormonal messengers the ecosanoids. Availability of essential fatty acids, which the body needs to make certain hormonal fats play a role in the prevention of heart disease, arthritis, and inappropriate immune activation.

Ecosanoids can be further divided into three groups: prostaglandins, leukotrienes, and lipoxin. All of these ecosanoids derive from arachidonic acid, linoleic acid, or linolenic acid-the only known essential fatty acids. Dietary choices and the higher level hormones circulating in the body determine what type of essential fatty acid eventually develop into hormones in cells (See *Entering the Zone* by Barry Sears).

Consume fats that lead to a prevalence in anti-inflammatory, heart disease preventing, and immune system optimizing types of message content. Sources for these types of essential fatty acids are found in cold-water fish, borage oil, wild game meats, chicken eggs fed greens, evening primrose oil, algae and vegetables.

In order to have good message content, there needs to be the right higher hormones. Only when there is more glucagon and less insulin hormones will there be the proper direction for the good precursor hormonal fats to be manufactured from the dietary derived essential fatty acids (see *Entering the Zone* by Barry Sears or the hierarchy of hormones in section two).

Some owners consume diets that lead to the promotion of heart disease, inappropriate activation of the immune system, and inflammation producing fatty acids (informational substance precursors). These disease exacerbating hormonal fat precursors occur on cell surfaces when insulin predominates. The partially hydrogenated fats (Tran fats) also contribute to this process. Some body processes will activate inappropriate message content when the disease promoting types of fatty acids make up an owner's cell membranes. They promote the above diseases because they contain inappropriate message content.

Fat as Fuel

The third role of fat in the body is to serve as fuel. Per gram of weight, fat provides triple the energy content of protein, and double the energy content of carbohydrate. However, only optimal hormone content (message content) permits accessibility of this excellent fuel source to the cells for caloric needs. Which hormone dominates the message content determines the fat access availability for fuel needs. For this reason, if the wrong hormones dominate message content then the fat cell content becomes off limits as fuel. This condition, and all the complications to other body systems, traps the body in obesity (see chapter four).

Fat as an Insulator

The fourth role of fat concerns the electrical circuitry of the central nervous system. These electrical insulator types of fats possess unique types of components that provide for the maintenance of proper nerve conduction and health. **The fact that the human brain has more fat weight than nerve cell weight illustrates this point.**

Plant Leaves Provide the First Clue that Lipids are Cool

The ordinary plant leaf demonstrates the water conservation role of fat in the cells. The leaf endures hours of hot sunshine without crinkling or wilting under normal conditions. Leaves possess the right amount of molecular surface structure to retard moisture loss. The leaves are rich in lipid-derived wax. Wax is just slightly modified fat. The fat that lines the surface of the body's cells provides similar water conservation properties in the skin cells. Oils float on the surface of water and provide a vapor barrier against water loss.

The lipid lining of the cells serves to keep cells from shriveling up. A shriveled group of skin cells manifests, to the naked eye as wrinkles. For this reason, inadequate cell membrane lipid, in types and amounts, provides one mechanism that leads to wrinkled cells.

The faces of owners who adhere to a low fat diet acquire deep creases between the inferior lateral margins of their nose extending downward towards the edge of their mouth. Later, more wrinkles crease these faces. Inadequate fat content accelerates water loss that causes these changes.

The Successful Dietary Fat is Bad Misinformation Campaign

Lipid (fat) has been given a bad name by the medical industrial establishment. For many years, people have fallen victim to disjointed information. This happens when the dogma for sale and literature dispensed by the sanctioned scientific community is sensationalized.

Availability of information has a profound influence on the practice patterns of medical practitioners today. Some have encountered the medical opinions of doctors like Bernstein, Atkins, Schwarzbein, and others. Their unique viewpoints led this author to a curiosity about what scientific knowledge had been ignored.

Scientific knowledge is often ignored in a profit driven health care system because it is less profitable to make it available for review by physicians and owners.

For example, there is a big difference between diet derived fat versus liver synthesized fat. Owners who acquire fat from too much diet derived healthy types of fat have a lower health risk than owners who gain fat from liver manufactured sources. Fifty years ago, medical research documented that liver manufactured fat was hard compared to many dietary sources of fat.

The liver will only manufacture fat if it receives the informational message to do so. The hormone that directs the liver to make carbohydrate into fat is insulin. The two types of pH neutral fat are triglyceride and cholesterol.

Remember, insulin and IGF-1 comprises the only fuel nozzle hormones (IGF-2 excluded for now in order to simplify). When the 'nozzle' correctly inserts, the food groups can be taken up out of the blood stream and into the cellular fuel tanks.

Carbohydrates abnormally sequester towards the liver when not enough IGF-1 occurs in the blood stream to help insulin. IGF-1 is the other fuel nozzle hormone. Visualize the competition between IGF-1 and insulin arising from the differences of their anatomical secretion pathway. In addition, the higher the carbohydrate consumption, the more insulin needed to process the sugar load when IGF-1 levels begin to fall around middle age. For this reason, higher insulin levels cause more message content to pummel the liver and direct it to make carbohydrates into fat (cholesterol and triglycerides).

Normally, almost no insulin is needed in the fasting, exercising and between meal states. The normal situation occurs because IGF-1 instead of insulin serves as the fuel nozzle in these states and prevents hungry cells. Realize, unhealthy bodies that need insulin (a fuel nozzle) to stay alive while between meals or exercising suffer additional damage from the need for excessive counter regulatory hormones.

The 'tug of war' between the blood sugar elevating hormones and insulin within their liver creates unstable blood sugar consequences. The excessive needs for the counter regulatory hormones save them from death. Mentally summarize that higher insulin content within the blood stream causes a higher 'volume' directed at the appetite center of the brain. The volume control of the appetite center responds to unstable blood sugars.

Compounding the fuel deficit, concerns the fact that the higher the blood insulin content, the more "locks" placed on access to stored body fat for energy mobilization. The body is smart and consistent. The overall message content of insulin within the body concerns itself with the storage of fuels. The body stores fuel as fat and to a limited extent as glycogen (slightly more than one pound is the upper limit of storage ability throughout the entire body!).

For this reason, the owner's upper limit of insulin secreting out of their pancreas limits the amount of body fat possible. The greater the pancreas production rate of insulin, the more weight gain tendency when dietary indiscretion occurs. For this reason, body insulin deficient exposure rates limit fat accumulation. Conversely, some owner's pancreas gland proves extremely capable and they gain weight abnormally well when their IGF-1 falls.

Good Reasons to Fear the Insulin-Directed Manufacture of Fat

When insulin directs the liver to manufacture fat, it is called LDL cholesterol (the bad cholesterol). This type of cholesterol does damage by accumulating in the blood vessels. LDL cholesterol accumulates in the macrophages that line the arteries. Recall, the often-omitted detail about carbohydrate induced cholesterol and triglyceride complexes originating from insulin's direction within the liver: These fats are hard. This property occurs because when the liver turns carbohydrate into LDL cholesterol it makes it into butter like fat! However, when owners eat butter when it arrives at the liver, if it has sufficient B vitamins, the fat component turns into olive oil! Until one grasps this mind twist the complex will successfully persuade them that fat is bad and carbohydrate is preferred!

Simply because of body storage design, higher manufacture rates of LDL cholesterol, increase the likelihood that this type of fat and cholesterol will accumulate within the arteries. This becomes a likely process in those owners who tend toward high blood insulin levels. Often, these owners eat high carbohydrate diets, possess mineral imbalances, produce suboptimal thyroid hormones and/or are stressed. The maintenance or return of health requires that these facts be addressed.

Macrophage collection of LDL cholesterol problems can show up in laboratory test as increased LDL cholesterol and/or as an elevated triglyceride level. For clarity this text will mostly refer to LDL and the reader needs to remember about the triglycerides. In the next few subsections it will be explained why the macrophage cells, being stuffed full of LDL cholesterol, create a problem for blood vessels.

Macrophages Stuff Themselves on LDL Cholesterol

Some owners have a big drain off of LDL cholesterol out of the blood stream and into their fat cells. Their blood fats (LDL cholesterol) stay down even when they eat insulin-producing foods. Not all owners are insulin sensitive. Owners who can eat carbohydrates without retaining fat in the belly area (spare tire of middle age) demonstrate this. Usually the explanation concerns the fact that these owners have a higher IGF-1 level, which means they need less insulin to process a sugar load. Still other owners indulge in high carbohydrate diets, but have a genetically superior sized 'drain ' (fat cells) once LDL cholesterol dumps from their liver into the blood stream. These owners will become fat, but their abdominal fat cells are so proficient at the removal of liver manufactured fat that the serum levels of LDL cholesterol remain normal.

However, most middle-aged owners are insulin sensitive and will follow the increased insulin message into two health problem areas: For most owners health problems occur in the form of progressive obesity and additional elevation of LDL cholesterol (and triglycerides) in the blood stream. Important point: A portion of the LDL cholesterol and triglyceride insidiously collects in the macrophages that line the blood vessels. Visualize the problem here: These owners do not have a sufficient sized 'drain' off into their fat cells.

The 'drain' describes the exit rate of LDL out of the blood stream and into the fat cells compared to the rate of liver output of LDL production. Deficiencies of either or both vitamin A and thyroid hormone will cause an additional exaggeration of the slow down in the removal of blood fat.

In a certain proportion of these insulin sensitive owners the chronic increased carbohydrate load, falling IGF-1 levels, sedentary lifestyle, mineral imbalance and their body size combine to exhaust the ability of their pancreases to make enough insulin. At this point, the blood sugar starts to rise. Scientists call this situation adult onset diabetes (90% of all diabetic victims). Conversely, some owner's pancreases manage to manufacture and secrete all the insulin needed to keep their blood sugars normal. However, both of these groups go on to develop heart disease because high insulin levels cause their blood vessel disease problem (see the liver chapter).

271

Why the Body Needs Cholesterol Supplied Through the Diet

Cholesterol is just a type of pH neutral fat. The other main type of pH neutral fat is triglyceride. The body needs to make storage and structural fat pH neutral to avoid ionic imbalances. This explains why it remains desirable to liberate fatty acids only as they are needed for fuel.

Each type of cell requires a certain amount of cholesterol for its structural integrity. Cholesterol content in a cell is meticulously regulated to prevent destructive cellular health consequences. Cholesterol provides the building block molecule from which all steroids are made. In addition, the same enzyme that makes cholesterol, HMG Co A reductase, also makes Co enzyme Q 10 and dolichols (the molecule that holds muscle cells together when tension occurs). Unfortunately, because the popular statin drugs poison this enzyme they also curtail all three processes (see inflammation and heart disease in section six).

Liver manufactured fat is always packaged with cholesterol and specific proteins before being dumped into the blood stream. Once the cells have absorbed their maximum load of cholesterol, there becomes little metabolic opportunity for liver secreted cholesterol. The amount of cholesterol secreted as LDL by the liver increases with rising insulin levels.

Remember the body is smart and consistent. LDL manufacture, under insulin's direction, possesses a design that optimizes storage. Insulin is the fuel storage hormone within the liver. Physicians are not taught to think about this simple consequence of excess insulin exposure. The metabolically slow fat cells then become responsible for removing LDL cholesterol piece by piece with the help of lipoprotein lipase. Lipoprotein lipase needs heparin as a cofactor for activation. Mast cells secrete Heparin.

The Big Difference between Liver Manufactured Fat and Dietary Fat is a Secret

Triglyceride is always packaged with varying amounts of cholesterol. Technically both cholesterol and triglyceride are the body's main pH neutral fat types. Triglyceride and cholesterol need to associate with protein in order to float in the blood stream. Consequently, the variable that determines fat availability to the metabolically hungry cells concerns the construction types of carrier proteins.

An important difference exists between carrier proteins occurring between the livers manufactured fat and fat derived from the diet. Diet derived fat has less potential to accumulate in blood vessel walls because the carrier protein of dietary fat contains a protein package that has less potential to plug up a vessel.

Where fat originates provides the crucial difference between transport packages. When fat-cholesterol-protein complexes originate in the digestive tract following a meal, the metabolically hungry cells easily absorb them. Remember, insulin is the fuel storage hormone. When insulin directs the liver to make cholesterol-fat-protein complexes, they are designed for storage and not immediate fuel needs. One more way the body proves smart and consistent.

Mantra: The intended design of the insulin message content concerns itself with fuel storage in the body. The majority of fuel storage occurs as fat. Normal amounts of diet derived fat form complexes that are rapidly assimilated by the metabolically hungry cells (skeletal muscle, cardiac muscle, kidney, etc.). In contrast, liver manufactured fat is designed to form complexes that are not readily cleared from the blood stream except by fat and macrophage cells.

For this reason, insulin directed fat-cholesterol-protein complexes are less able to serve as fuel. In other words, they are designed at the direction of insulin, the fuel storage hormone. Again, the body is smart and consistent. The consistent message of insulin causes greater amounts of stored fuel (glycogen and fat). The insulin directed fat-cholesterol-protein complexes are designed with fuel storage in mind.

The Unique Way Fat Absorbs from the Diet Illuminates the fallacy of the 'Fat is Bad Campaign'

A physiologic fact clarifies the lack of stickiness of diet-derived fat on vessel walls. Dietary fat and cholesterol absorb via the lymphatics, which differs from all other nutrients. This means that lymph vessels receive the highest vessel concentration exposure of dietary cholesterol and fat. Yet, atherosclerosis (the growth of fat within vessels) of lymphatic vessels is unheard of. This truth occurs despite the fact that hemodynamically (the flow of fluid within a vessel) lymph fluid moves in a sluggish manner compared to blood flow within the arteries. Hence, if there were anything sticky about diet derived fat, it would be more pronounced in the sluggish lymph vessels.

The difference between the types of cholesterol-fat package that blood vessel walls encounter compared to the cholesterol-fat-package that lymphatic vessels transport following a fatty meal explains this fact. This difference explains the true cause for the majority of heart disease: Excess insulin. The insulin directed and liver manufactured cholesterol-fat packages collect in blood vessel walls within the macrophages. Anatomically, the lymphatic vessels are not exposed to insulin directed and liver manufactured cholesterol-fat packages. They are only exposed to diet derived cholesterol-fat packages that do not deposit along lymph vessel walls.

If only medical schools taught that **the body is smart and consistent**. Insulin directed fat and cholesterol particles are constructed with storage in mind. Long-term storage sites for these types of particles are found in the liver, blood vessel macrophages, and fat cells. Conversely, diet derived fat and cholesterol particles, the chylomicrons, contain a design that readily allows removal by the body cells and they are stored short term or used as fuel.

Remember, even though lymph vessels are sluggish in flow characteristics and exposed to very high levels of diet-derived fat and cholesterol, they do not plug up. Anatomically the small intestine delivers fat and cholesterol into the lymph vessels following a meal. The protective factor for lymphatic vessels involves the fact that they have no exposure to liver manufactured cholesterol-fat-protein complexes (LDL). Intestinal lymphatic vessels eventually drain into the left neck area, the thoracic duct. In this location the fatty parts of digestion dump into the blood stream.

In contrast, other products of digestion such as protein, carbohydrates, minerals, and vitamins, etc., dump directly from the intestinal cells into the portal vein. The portal vein collects all blood and nutrition (except fat and cholesterol) from the digestive tract and takes it straight to the liver.

Consequently, the blood vessels clog up whenever insulin levels rise to the point of directing the liver in excessive manufacture of the sticky type of cholesterol-fat packages (LDL cholesterol). This is sticky because it is taken up by the macrophages that line blood vessels. Macrophages are immune system scavenger cells that under well-fed circumstances bed down on blood vessel linings and stuff themselves with LDL cholesterol

By this mechanism, when the liver creates excessive fat-protein-cholesterol complexes (LDL cholesterol), they often incorporate into macrophages in abnormal amounts. Excessively stuffed macrophages with LDL cholesterol grow and grow. Year after year they continue to accumulate LDL cholesterol and eventually form giant cells called foam cells. Foam cells are the earliest lesions recognized by scientist as the beginning of heart disease.

Some of the places that macrophages bed down and become foam cells occur in the coronary arteries, hearing apparatus, kidney vessels, peripheral leg vessels, and retina. These tissues prefer fat for fuel. The LDL cholesterol accumulation trouble compounds within a sedentary owner.

High insulin levels in sedentary owners allow LDL cholesterol to continuously collect in the macrophages. These cells permit fat to collect due to lack of exercise. After many years, this vicious cycle allows fatty streaks to grow enough to block blood flow. Blood flow can suddenly worsen in these narrowed areas when other factors promote blood clots to form. When severe enough, the constriction causes cell death to cells that are beyond the blockage.

The other common mechanism for the sudden loss of blood flow is vessel spasms in the narrow area. These two climaxes are the typical scenario for the number one killer of Americans past middle age, heart disease. The earlier available information on this subject has been disjointed and fragmented.

Take home point: High insulin producing bodies manufacture more fat and cholesterol. Insulin directed cholesterol-fat packages are designed for storage depots. These packages designed for the storage depots of the body are slow to drain off out of the blood stream. In addition, these individuals suffer further risk for this type of heart disease when they are living sedentary lifestyles and have unmanaged stress (see stress subsection, chapter four), contain

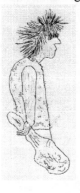

mineral imbalances, suffer a fall in IGF-1 levels and/or consume high insulin promoting diets. All five of these risk factors increase insulin levels. Increased risk arises from the increased tendency for macrophages to ingest more LDL cholesterol than is healthy.

The relationship between high insulin levels because of falling IGF-1 levels, high stress levels, reversed minerals ratios diet, high carbohydrate intake and sedentary lifestyles are the crux of the problem for the majority of all heart disease victims. The other risk factors for heart disease development accelerate this primary

disease producing mechanism in the blood vessels. Rather than focus on the hopeless mantra about some owners genetics, empowerment comes from a focus on how dietary and lifestyle changes prevent the problem.

Some owners have a greater tendency for heart disease based on primitive survival strategies. A survival advantage was obtained in prehistoric times when a body could store fat in times of plenty in order to survive periods of famine. Consequently, owners who made more insulin possessed a survival advantage. Back then the food supply was unpredictable so there was no accumulation of blood vessel fat.

However, the modern day food supply continues uninterrupted in supply to these same survival equipped insulin producing machines. Add in the greatly increased insulin requirement that becomes necessary to handle a chronic processed food diet. This fact arises secondary to this popular diet's diminished potassium content. Today, these same survival equipped owners are now fat producing machines.

An owner still has the ability to turn off his/her fat making machine. The liver fat making machine turns off by consistently choosing a low insulin requiring diet, obtaining ample potassium, minimizing sodium, doing aerobic exercise, correcting the other fat promoting hormones, and stress management (as suggested in earlier chapters). Instead of helping owners understand this, they are led down the erroneous path of what is for sale by the complex.

Unfortunately for the average owner little incentive exists to share (publish and sensationalize) this basic scientific understanding. The 'fat is bad campaign' contains largely hype that allows the relationship between insulin and blood vessel disease to remain a secret. Knowledge about the insulin secret jeopardizes the more lucrative approaches for treating blood vessel disease.

However, the lucrative approaches contain side effects and toxicities that if commonly known would create even more reluctance for these symptom control methods. Symptom control, so prevalent within the mainstream paradigm, has nothing to do with healing. Passive owners are stuck with symptom control and all its unfavorable side effects. However, what about those owners who possess the focus to commit to a path of healing?

The Weak Spot in the Complex's Campaign against Dietary Fat

The 'fat is bad' media campaign has a weak spot. Simply by monitoring their cholesterol profile while on a high good fat/protein and low carbohydrate diet exposes the weak spot. This dietary approach directly contrasts with the official campaign against fat and in favor of a high carbohydrate diet.

The owners, who try a high protein/fat and low carbohydrate diet for three months or more while they defer judgment, will likely see several improved health benefits. At the end of this time period, each owner should assess the improved mental clarity that occurs because less 'brain fog' occurs: Hypoglycemia induced by high carbohydrate diets has stopped.

They will also notice a decreased appetite due to the fall of insulin levels. This allows less brain appetite center stimulation for the next feeding event. In addition, there will be consistent weight loss because of lowered insulin levels. This in turn, frees the 'locks' on the body's access to fat stores. Finally, a dramatic improvement in the cholesterol profile occurs due to less insulin message content instructing the liver to make carbohydrates into LDL cholesterol.

Attention to thyroid function, adequate androgen output from the adrenals and gonads (testis or ovary), optimal cortisol output, and IGF-1 levels also prove important for normal fat parameters to occur. Also, aerobic exercise should be optimized enough for the muscles, skeleton, and cardiovascular system to be utilized to full capacity. These changes transform an owner onto the longevity track of life.

The high protein/good fat and low carbohydrate diet becomes less controversial when reviewing the epidemiological studies that have noted the absence of heart disease in cultures that consume a low carbohydrate, but high fat/protein diets. Eskimos exemplify this fact. Eskimos also exemplify the relative safety of obesity acquired through over indulgence in fat intake. Many Eskimos are obese because of the arctic climate. The type of fat Eskimos make is opposite to liver manufactured fat that arises from a high carbohydrate diet. However, when these same Eskimo peoples begin to adhere to a high carbohydrate diet, after about 20 years they develop heart disease at rates similar to their western contemporaries (Atkins 1999).

This correlates with the relative absence of heart disease in America until the 1900's. Up until this time, the general population survived on a high fat and protein diet (chicken, meat, eggs, and beans). The carbohydrates that were available were unprocessed and hence contained sufficient potassium content. Remember, when the potassium content is high, the need for insulin diminishes. After the turn of the century, as processed sugar and cereals became available, the 20-year rule began to tick. This epidemiological tool measures the time between a change in cultural behavior and a public health effect. By the 1920's heart disease had become an epidemic in America. (*Atkins, 1999*)

On the Other Hand: Chemically Reactive Fats in the Diet Cause Heart Disease

The consumption of unhealthy fats is not allowed in high fat diets if one wishes to be free of blood vessel disease. The people of the world free of heart disease, while they indulge in a high fat and low carbohydrate diets, are not the ones that consume high amounts of chemically reactive fats. Chemically reactive fats have the scientific name, partially hydrogenated vegetable fats (Tran fats). This distinction about good fat and bad fat is often overlooked and leads to confusion in the minds of clinicians as well as owners in regard to the safety of high fat diets. Diets made up of real fats are safe while diets made up of large quantities of chemically reactive fats are not. Chemically reactive fats contribute to oxidation (rust) in the blood vessels.

The chemically reactive fat groups are chemically altered polyunsaturated fats. The chemical process of hydrogenation has altered them. The hydrogenation process causes a twisting deformation that denotes an unnatural occurrence compared to real fats. Numerous baked goods, margarines, breads, snacks, and chips have altered fats added to them.

The hydrogenation process provides one example where altered fats add firmness to the product. These polyunsaturated fats are chemically altered and become more twisted when they stack together. Fats in the body need to be stacked together in the cellular membranes (the lipid bi-layer). The twisted configurations of chemically altered fat means they form awkward fat conglomerates (irregularities) that line the cell membrane.

Endothelial cells fit together like tiles on the interior blood vessel lining. These cells, like all cells, have a cell membrane made up of fat interspersed with proteins. The polyunsaturated partially hydrogenated fats are also chemically reactive with many oxidizing agents that may be in the blood stream (aluminum, fluoride, oxygen radicals, carbon monoxide, ozone and other smog components, etc.).

When these fats oxidize, they promote 'Velcro' formations on the inside wall of the blood vessel. This formation summons the macrophages to lay down a temporary patch job that sometimes fails to be repaired. Making matters worse, when LDL cholesterol is high, these macrophages collect fat and eventually grow into foam cells.

Consequently, a component of blood vessel health depends on whether the inner lining layer (the tiles) of the blood vessel wall composes itself with the chemically altered polyunsaturated fats (hydrogenated fats) or healthy fats. The diet determines this content. Diets consisting of fast food fats, margarine, fried foods, baked goods, and commercial breads will add twisted fats to the lining layers of that owner's blood vessels. In contrast, diets that contain real fats promote surfaces in the blood vessel, which are composed of the less chemically reactive fats (real fat).

Picture two beautiful flowerbeds planted side by side. In one, short stocky stems grow and in the other fragile, slender stems grow. The contrast between the two types of stems allows an analogy that elucidates the body fat type composition problem.

Short stocky stems are analogous to blood vessel friendly fats (olive oils, fish oils and canola oils). They are more durable. Good fats lining one's arteries only become possible when the owner makes appropriate diet choices when consuming fats. However, fragile long stems are analogous to chemically altered polyunsaturated fats (found in junk food, processed food, and fast food). They are more vulnerable to numerous oxidizing agents that occur in the blood stream.

Visualize a dog (oxidizing agent) that sequentially runs around in each type of flowerbed. The short stocky stems sustain less damage because of the differences in structural characteristics between the two types of flowerbeds. The oxidative vulnerability in the blood vessels is analogous to what happens in the blood vessel lining cells when unhealthy fat is eaten. The vulnerability of blood vessel lining cells to trampling by the "dogs" being unleashed in the blood stream is determined by the composition of the "stems."

In a dirty environment where air pollution, water pollution, and food contaminants prevail, the blood vessel lining cells are overexposed to oxidizing agents (rust producers). The rust producers are analogous to the dog running around in the flowerbed. Real fats versus altered fats are analogous to the durability of the stems in the flowerbed. The more chemically reactive (altered) the fats become, the more they create rust (Velcro formations). In contrast, the more the lining cells in the blood vessels compose themselves with real fats, the more durable they become when confronting oxidizing agents.

This consideration gradates the relative risk of different types of dietary fat and their potential to produce disease. The amount of abdominal fat serves as a clinical marker for diet and/or lifestyle that leads to higher insulin levels. Men who have a greater abdominal measurement than hip measurement evidence high insulin levels. Women who are greater than 80% their waist compared to hip measurement evidence high insulin as well. Until insulin levels become optimal, by diet and lifestyle changes, health deteriorates.

In addition, the higher the oxidant exposure load that operates on a daily basis, the more important it becomes to minimize consumption of the chemically reactive fats. Owners who are chronically exposed to air pollution, water impurities (fluoridation), and impurities in their food will have an increased rate at which their chemically reactive fats oxidize. Chemically reactive fats oxidize when exposed to harmful pollutants. Improving dietary fat choices and avoiding environmental 'rust' producers allow healing.

Liver Manufactured Fat Clogs Blood Vessels

It has been known for years that LDL cholesterol synthesis rates are controlled by the balance between the levels of insulin and glucagon. The insulin message tells the liver enzyme, HMG CoA reductase, to make sugar into cholesterol. Conversely, the glucagon message instructs the liver to stop making cholesterol by inhibition of this same enzyme. Glucagon also stimulates the release of fuels into the blood stream. For this reason, healthy, active people with a higher glucagon level will have lower cholesterol levels.

Unfortunately, glucagon will not help people who are sedentary and obese because glucagon stimulates the dumping of fuel into the blood stream from the liver. In chronically sedentary types, the extra fuel stimulates the release of insulin, eventually. This effect provides an example of the weight and counterweight system that keeps opposing hormones in balance. People who sit around all day, but eat the right diet initially promote the release of glucagon. However, they lose the benefits of glucagon when insulin needs to be secreted to manage the extra fuel that glucagon directed to be made and secreted into the blood stream.

Extra insulin need arises because sedentary owners have little use for increased fuel in the blood stream that glucagon directs. However, if owners on glucagon promoting diets were to exercise, they would use the extra fuel and need less insulin. Lower insulin relative to glucagon signifies that the liver enzyme, HMG CoA reductase, will stay less active and hence less cholesterol is manufactured. When this happens, the serum cholesterol level decreases.

Owners have a choice about taking toxic medication to lower their cholesterol or to heal. Medication often becomes unnecessary if they begin a program that helps their liver to work properly. Practices that raise glucagon and lower insulin keep cholesterol within the healthy range for the vast majority of owners. A high protein/good fat, low carbohydrate diet promotes the optimal ratio between insulin and glucagon. The proper balance of these two hormones is difficult for sedentary owners because of the eventual need for increased insulin (see above).

Additional Hormones Beyond the Diet, But Influence Digested Foods to Deposit as Fat

Most owners who take active steps in daily exercise and dietary decisions will notice a dramatic fall in their blood cholesterol: Their glucagon and insulin ratio have been favorably altered. But in order to really maximize one's healing, adequate message content from other body hormones are also important - androgen (from adrenals and gonads), estrogens, thyroid hormone, IGF-1, and cortisol. When these correctly proportion blood fat-cholesterol-protein complexes become even more favorable.

These considerations can be assessed (except for IGF-1) through a complete 24-hour urine test that includes a quantitative and qualitative analysis of what hormone levels are manufactured. Healthy owners have optimal amounts of critical steroid, each type's respective metabolites and thyroid hormones that pass into their urine over a twenty-four hour period.

In contrast, unhealthy owners pass sub-optimal amounts of critical androgen steroid hormones and possibly excessive amounts of estrogen and stress steroids. If thyroid function is inadequate, the urine is often the most reliable way to detect the deficiency. These hormone considerations become important when lifestyle and dietary modification fail to improve the cholesterol profile.

The need for a twenty-four hour urine collection illustrates what science has revealed versus what is practiced. Hormone levels can fluctuate widely in the blood stream. Some hormones have life spans measured in seconds. Most have life spans measured in minutes. When a blood sample is taken, the amount of hormone measured in that sample reflects that bloods

informational content at the instant the venous sample was drawn. This method provides an accurate measurement only if the hormones in question are relatively stable in the blood stream.

However, most hormones vary widely throughout the day in the blood stream. The many different informational substances convey a precise message to the body cells. Obviously, different activities of daily living obligate the release of different hormones that communicate to cells on how to spend their energy. For this reason, each of the varied life situations requires different informational direction of the body energy quotient.

For examples: the hormone levels and types during stress, pleasurable activity, fasting, romance, feeding, rest or post exercise will predictably be different. Realize different activities and emotional states require a change in the blood stream information. Only with changes in the blood stream informational content can energy redirect into the appropriate form required for that state. Visualize the ongoing dance of anabolism versus catabolism. Healthy people stay in balance and unhealthy people do not.

An accurate method to assess hormone tone and pressure incorporates the basic scientific understanding that over a typical twenty-four hours an average amount of hormone output will occur. An average day in one's life causes typical nutrition, stress, romance, fatigue, exercise and rest. As a consequence, the sufficiency of the body's most powerful hormones and their consequent metabolites that need to direct these states spill into the urine.

Urine hormone measurements are useful only when the hormone of interest exits the body via the kidney. This is true for thyroid and steroid hormones. Critical point: this method includes measurement of the different metabolites of these most important body hormones. Metabolites instruct the steroid savvy doctor whether the patient's hormones move in good directions or more harmful direction. Remember, these hormones with the addition of vitamin A directly determine which genes turn off and on. The quality of gene activity determines the sufficiency of body protein content. Adequate protein in turn provides metabolism. Health depends on a sufficient metabolic ability.

Urine collected over a typical day can more accurately measure the types and amounts of hormones present. Also currently, urine provides the only way to check the all-important metabolites as well. Finally, the technology used to measure hormones in the urine involves the more sophisticated and accurate method, Gas chromatography mass spectrometry (GC mass spec).

For example, one change of simple hydrogen's orientation can be discerned with this technique. Pertinent to this technique involves that it can separate out the 10-fold potency difference between testosterone and dihydrotestosterone. The difference in potency depends on the orientation of the number 5-position hydrogen. Unfortunately, saliva and serum testing cannot accurately discern this important difference. Compounding the weakness of using serum and saliva concerns the emerging realization about the suspect accuracy of the technology on which it is based. These methods utilize antibodies. Accepted accuracy is plus or minus 20%! Recently several scientific inquiries into the accuracy for multiple assays using this technology found the majority of them to be even more inaccurate than the modest standard stated above! Because of these findings several studies have recommended that women and prepubescent children not rely on these popular methods of hormone measurement for testosterone. Add in the blip in time, during sample collection, which both tests rely on, as well, and one begins to see weakness in the current standard of care.

The question now rings out: If this is true then why doesn't my doctor know about it? The answer involves the additional disturbing detail that the scientists of the world are all discussing the emerging science of intracrinology. Here scientists now recognize that weak precursor steroid hormones within cells turn into powerful hormones, like testosterone, and then instruct the genes. This means that proteins are made based on the sufficiency of the precursor pool of steroids circulating in the blood stream.

However, most shocking concerns the realizations that before these powerful, created within the cell, steroid hormones leave the genes they convert into metabolites. This fact blares out about the inadequacy of steroid testing using saliva and serum because total body testosterone exposure cannot be discerned with these two favorite approaches. The reason is that these darlings of the medical establishment fail to measure the all-important metabolites (see side bar below for the rest of the answer).

Finally, realize that most of the larger hormones composed of amino acid sequences (peptides or proteins) do not reliably pass in the urine relative to body exposure levels. For this reason, this class of hormones must be measured in the blood stream. Insulin, glucagon, IGF-1, and some of the larger pituitary and hypothalamic hormones provide examples of this class. The overall point being, if a more accurate method for the assessment of hormone status exists, patients have the right to know about this option

.

Physician's Sidebar

Many physicians are unaware that they are victims of an education that has removed some basic scientific understanding that conflict with profit. There have been numerous instances where a patient brings in a well-run twenty-four hour urine analysis only to be scoffed at by their conventionally trained, but limited second opinion physician. Owners are advised to have a little fun with these types of practitioners. Ask them to explain all the big words that describe the different breakdown products of certain hormones as a start to this fun adventure. A good physician at this point will admit that he doesn't understand the results and will look into it. Unfortunately, many physicians that are confronted with what they do not understand habitually resort to attempts to discredit approaches that inquire above their education level. When one confronts the later type of practitioner, it may be time to begin thinking about a new doctor.

Fluids and Electrolytes

Fluids and electrolytes describe the water and minerals that make up the various body juices. Digestive juices additionally contain enzymatic machines that are specific to each digestive chamber where food presents. The mineral component of juices and body processes that have an effect on the adequacy of digestive juices will be covered in this subsection.

Good health remains possible when adequate juices secrete and absorb at the proper time during the digestive process. The digestive system requires the appropriate quality and quantity of digestive juices or degenerative processes occur. These degenerative processes rob the body of vitality when the quality of mineral content contained in the digestive juices deranges.

Each adult consumes about two quarts of fluid every day. In addition to this fluid intake, the digestive tube itself secretes an additional seven quarts into the meal contents. The digestive tube needs to secrete various digestive juices in order to assimilate the various molecular parts contained in one day's food intake.

Ideally, the seven additional quarts of digestive juices secreted each day occur in properly proportioned amounts. These different digestive juices secrete into the tube as various chemical reaction concoctions that contain molecular 'machines' designed to dismantle different food types. In the end, the bowel movement contains less than 1 cup of water. Amazingly, the typical digestive tube encounters two and a half gallons of fluid every day. When the digestive tube remains healthy it reabsorbs not only most of these fluids, but also usable molecular parts.

The Amount of Digestive Juices Secreted in the Tube

Daily ingested fluid: >2 quarts

Daily secreted juices into the digestive tube from the various digestive-lining cells: >7 quarts

Salivary glands >1.5 quarts

Stomach secretions >2.5 quarts

Gallbladder secretions >.5 quart

Pancreas secretions >1.5 quarts

Intestinal secretions >1.5 quarts

Total fluid load daily passed into the digestive tube is >9 quarts

Total reabsorbed fluids daily farther down the tube on average is 8.8 quarts or diarrhea manifests.

Jejunum 5.5 quarts reabsorbed
Ileum 2.0 quarts reabsorbed
Colon 1.3 quarts reabsorbed

The mineral content of the digestive juices and meal form a determinant for the ability of the body to reabsorb the fluid in the digestive tube before it arrives at the rectum. Diarrhea results from too much fluid. Constipation results from too little fluid reaching the rectum. Fiber and certain minerals keep water in the tube. Consequently, the ingestion of these substances promotes loose stools.

Certain minerals or substances pull water with them as they move down their concentration gradient. Scientists call this process osmosis. Osmosis describes a way for predicting which direction water will move. Substances that pull water with them as they move into different body chambers are called osmotically active. These types of substances are actively involved in the digestive tube, intestinal cells, kidney filtration system, etc. When these substances move from one body chamber to the next they to pull water with them.

When healthy, the act of absorbing the molecular building parts contained in a meal pulls water back out of the digestive tube. As a consequence, bowel movements of healthy owners do not contain excessive osmotically active material and therefore, their stool contains little water. For this reason, deficiency or excess in osmotically active bowel contents leads to constipation and diarrhea respectively.

Indigestible fiber has a weak osmotic effect. This allows sufficient water to stay in the bowel movement and facilitate regularity. Sources of indigestible fiber are vegetables, fruits, seeds, and psyllium husks. Some minerals incompletely or poorly absorb so they osmotically retain water. Examples of poorly absorbed salts are the salts of magnesium. Examples of osmotically active minerals or substances are vitamin c, and some antacids.

Part of the task of efficient digestion involves adequate mineral absorption. Minerals usually present to the digestive tract in the form of a salt. A salt signifies that positive and negatively charged minerals occur together. The positively charged mineral of the salt is more important and is always named first. Examples of commonly ingested salts are ferrous sulfate, calcium citrate, magnesium oxide, potassium chloride, and sodium chloride. When a salt absorbs into the body from the digestive tract it pulls water with it. However, when a salt fails to absorb in the digestive tract it will retain water within the tube. This fact explains why some mineral salts have a laxative effect.

Calcium and iron are important minerals. The salt they hook on to (the negative half) will determine how readily they absorb into the body.

Most owners are aware of the importance of obtaining adequate calcium and iron. Often times, this opinion results from an effective media campaign. However, the more important a mineral is to body processes; the more potential it has to harm body tissues if the mineral fails to be carefully regulated. Calcium and iron illustrate the importance of mineral control within the body tissues.

Calcium Can Help or Kill Cells

Calcium intake requirements are on the mind of most owners. Calcium plays an important role in the maintenance of adequate bone mass. Many owners ingest some form of calcium salt on a daily basis. Unfortunately, there has been very little attention given to taking too much calcium when certain factors exist. Calcium intake, in these cases, can accelerate the aging process.

Calcium is controlled and channeled in the tissues of the body by an elaborate regulatory system of hormones. Calcium content must be narrowly channeled. Therefore, an elaborate system of calcium regulatory hormones becomes necessary.

Calcium can be better understood when one realizes that all the body's 70 trillion cells operate as miniature batteries. Maintaining a concentration difference between calcium and magnesium charges the cells. Calcium is pumped outside the cell while magnesium is pumped inside the cell. Calcium occurs at high concentrations in the fluid around the cell because of this pumping around the membrane (a ratio of 12,000:1). Magnesium maintains a relatively high concentration inside the cell.

Adequate cellular energetics (adequate ATP formation) maintains this electrical gradient between these two opposing minerals. A similar gradient occurs between sodium outside the cell and potassium inside the cell. Cells constantly drain this gradient between these opposing minerals. The energy released from drawing down the gradient is used for cell work. Energy released by the draining process is like any activated battery. In the case of cells, the energetic gradient is constantly drawn upon and used to live. Simultaneously, the healthy cell constantly recharges the gradient difference by utilizing ATP derived from the cell power plants (mitochondria).

Sufficient ATP recharges the membrane gradient between these opposing minerals. Specific mineral pumps maintain the concentrations differences of these minerals around the membrane. Mineral pumps are located in the membrane and require ATP to power them. Recall the amount of mineral pumps and hence cell voltage depends on thyroid hormone adequacy. For these reasons, the more mineral pumps and the better the mineral balance, the higher the cell voltage possible.

Higher voltage, like in any battery means more work is possible. This chain of connectedness logically extends to the bottom line of the higher the concentration differences, about the membrane, between the opposing minerals, the higher the amount of energy available for the cells.

The differences in concentration between calcium and magnesium about a cell's membrane allow the performance of useful cellular work. The concentration gradient also prevents harmful ions from penetrating the cell and causing damage within. Healthy cells are able to generate large concentration gradients between calcium and magnesium and also between sodium and potassium. They achieve this concentration gradient by having highly functional mineral ion pumps in their membrane (like sodium/potassium ATPase). These pumps exchange opposing minerals against their concentration gradient. **This battery charging process occurs in all the body's 70 trillion cells.**

The large concentration difference between opposing minerals around the membrane creates electrical potential. The energy contained in the membrane drains down to perform cellular work. The same principle applies to any battery when it provides the mechanism for donating energy to power a toy. Also, both types of batteries (the cell and the toy battery) require a way to recharge that prevents depletion.

All batteries, whether living or manufactured, need to keep their mineral content within carefully gated channels. When the channels are circumvented battery corrosion results. Likewise calcium needs to be channeled into and out of cells by carefully regulated channels. The cell performs work when calcium enters through specific channels. The pumping of calcium outside the cell and magnesium inside the cell requires ATP energy. Sufficient ATP allows the cell membrane to recharge as it depletes.

However, if calcium penetrates inside the cells inappropriately (outside the gated channels), it harms intracellular structures (molecular corrosion). Once inappropriate calcium penetrates inside a cell it is difficult to remove it. As owners age, inappropriate calcium sneaks in and chemically reacts with delicate intracellular structures. If enough calcium gets inside a cell, the mitochondria begin to sequester it. Eventually extra calcium causes the mitochondria to swell and weaken. Weakened mitochondria become less capable in their role as a power plant facility (ATP generation). Later, inappropriate entry of calcium into a cell irreversibly deactivates enzymes.

Conversely, when calcium enters a cell through the appropriate channels (gate), it does not have a destructive effect on the cell. The movements of calcium, through these channels and down its concentration gradient releases electrical energy that the cells use to perform the work of living. In contrast, processes that accelerate inappropriate calcium accumulation in the cell accelerate aging.

Calcium's concentration within different parts of the body is elaborately contained by a complex interrelated group of hormones. These different hormones occur at diverse entrance and exit sites for calcium throughout the body. Situations that overwhelm or disrupt these regulators of channeling calcium safely through and in the tissues can cause cellular harm.

Some of the calcium regulatory hormones and proteins are worth mentioning. Calcitonin hormone opposes parathyroid hormone. Androgen hormones opposes cortisol hormone. Active vitamin D hormone opposes inactive vitamin D. Blood albumin content opposes the freely dissolved blood calcium.

Recall the antique weight scale with a weight and a counter weight. This provides an analogy to a hormone being secreted and the fact that there will always be a counter-regulatory hormone (counter weight). The counter weight hormone always attempts to balance the response. Hormonal imbalance leads to disease due to the breakdown in the balance between the opposing hormones. Loss of balance between the opposing hormones "tips the scale" out of the optimal equilibrium. The loss of hormonal balance within, tips energy usage into unbalanced pathways that lead to wear and tear. Wear and tear manifest in the tissue that receives message content from the out of balance hormonal state.

Body tissue wear and tear all too often results from poor quality message content. Poor quality message content, in turn, results from sub-optimal hormone mixtures. This leads to a disorganized cellular direction on how to spend energy wisely. The balance between the different opposing calcium controlling hormones determines where calcium channels. There needs to be a balance between regulatory and counter-regulatory calcium hormones or tissue injury becomes possible. Inappropriate calcium can enter a cell and injure its delicate intracellular contents (sections five and six).

Certain Minerals Opposition Charges the Cell Battery

The body's system of chemical reactions sustains life. Often times these reactions are powered by the concentration gradient between opposing minerals around the cell membrane. Certain opposing minerals create electrical membrane potential between these minerals. The cell membranes accomplish this difference in mineral concentration by specialized pumps located within its membrane. Each type of membrane pump powers itself by the energy contained within the ATP molecule. ATP availability determines the ability of a cell to recharge its membrane. The better a cell recharges its membrane, the more energy available for cellular work.

One of the main caloric expenditures of the body involves energy used by these various mineral pumps. They are present throughout all cells in the body. Consistent with this fact, large amounts of ATP are necessary to charge the differential between these opposing minerals against their concentration gradient. The more ATP manufactured and used, the more calories burned. Combustion of calories creates ATP within the mitochondria. In turn, a major share of the ATP created powers the membrane pumps that create the huge concentration differences between opposing minerals. Remember, the concentration buildup of these opposing minerals can be used in the performance of cellular work.

Magnesium in high concentrations in the cell opposes the high concentration of calcium outside the cell. This allows an electrical gradient that the cell can harness to function optimally for that cell types purpose. This process proves similar for how a car battery discharges in the wiring of the electrical system to power many gadgets. Likewise, the cell "battery" (the cell membrane) powers the activities of life.

However, the cell membrane requires a constant energy to resupply power for maintaining the gradient between calcium and magnesium (also between sodium and potassium). This is also similar to a car battery that needs to be recharged while the auto burns fuel. Remember, the combustion of protein, fat, and sugar occurs only after processing into combustible derivative called acetate. Acetate is the simplest fatty acid.

When acetate is exposed to oxygen within the power plant (the mitochondria) of the cell, some of the energy released stores as ATP. The energy contained in ATP can then be used to recharge the cell membrane by powering the mineral pumps. This describes the process that continually occurs throughout life in the trillions of cellular batteries contained within the body. Energy is contained in the membranes and is created by the concentration differences between these four minerals.

Calcium better be happy once it absorbs into the body

Healthy cells avoid unnecessary oxidation from inappropriate escape of un-channeled calcium inside the cell. Potential trouble always lurks inside the body if calcium is allowed to bind to an anion (the negatively charged molecules within any cellular protein) that precipitates (forms a solid).

Calcium always forms the positive part of any salt that it forms. Some salts of calcium prefer to stay in solid form and do not dissolve well in body fluids. Calcium salts outside of bone and teeth tissue are of the dissolvable variety in a healthy body. Even under the best of circumstances, cells confront numerous potential precipitate formers (in-dissolvable salts). Failure to constantly flush these from body tissues allows solid salts of calcium to form. Common clinical examples of this process are found in kidney stones, osteoarthritis, bone spurs, and calcium deposits in soft tissues and blood vessels.

Excessive dietary intake of phosphates and oxalates can lead to acceleration of these solids deposition in the tissues. An increase in water consumption helps the body clear these substances. Of special note, soda pop (diet and regular) contains high amounts of phosphate. Unfortunately, there is a price to pay for clearing it through the urine: Each phosphate molecule cleared from the blood stream requires an obligatory loss of one calcium molecule. Soda pop contains phosphate, but lacks calcium.

As a consequence, in order to remove excess phosphate, there needs to be calcium removed from somewhere else in the body! If consumption becomes chronic (as in the case of the habitual soda pop user) the bone calcium leaches out of the bones to allow phosphate removal. This shows up clinically on x-ray as premature loss of bone mineral content (osteopenia and eventually osteoporosis).

Energetic situations occur that allow inappropriate calcium into the cell. These are also a concern. These situations are more destructive to the most metabolically active cells (nerve, heart, kidney, etc.). For example, Dr. Salpolsky from Stanford University has documented the metabolic consequences of low blood sugar in the hippocampus (an area of the brain involved in learning and memory).

Low blood sugar in the brain leads to low energy in these nerve cells. The 'force field' diminishes and a consequent massive in flux of calcium can occur. This vulnerability stems from the fact that the brain cells, under most circumstances, can only utilize sugar for their raw fuel needs. However, most other cells readily utilize protein and fat for alternative raw fuel. Recall all body cells must convert these three raw fuels into acetate before it becomes refined fuel.

Unfortunately, this raw fuel restriction makes brain tissue more vulnerable to low blood sugar. In turn, low energy in a nerve cell, caused by low sugar availability in this situation, allows the massive influx of calcium. It is the massive influx of calcium that irreversibly harms intracellular contents. In these cases, calcium harms cells because the low energy content within the cell membrane allows it to penetrate the cell through inappropriate methods. **The vulnerability of cells in low energy states can be visualized by imagining the star ship Enterprise in an attempt to**

ward off the attack of missiles. The star ship Enterprise does this by powering up its force field. This is similar to what any cell in the body must constantly perform in order to keep out inappropriate ions like calcium.

Every cell must power up energetically against the influx of calcium (and other harmful ions) through inappropriate channels. Calcium can be an 'intracellular missile'. That is, when it penetrates the cell outside of the appropriate channels (the membrane pumps), it forms solid complexes with cell components.

Other states of cellular energetic depletion occur in situations where the blood or oxygen supplies compromise (drowning or cardiac arrest) or if vulnerable tissue excite beyond its energetic capacity to maintain adequate cellular membrane energy (seizure). All of these mechanisms injure cells because they allow the depletion of the cell membrane's electrical charge (the force field). When the 'force field' depletes, a massive influx of inappropriate calcium enters the cell. Excess levels of calcium react destructively with intracellular components. (*Sapolosky, 1992*)

Calcium's energetic opponent, magnesium, doesn't need the same strict regulatory control within the body. Magnesium doesn't seem to form solids in the tissues, but forms soluble complexes (those that dissolve in body fluids). This difference in behavior, between calcium's chemical reactive properties contrasted to magnesium's, helps explain why the presence of calcium becomes necessarily layered with hormonal protection systems and backup protection systems.

Dietary factors can affect the availability of calcium within the body. Different body minerals, which include calcium, are necessary to power up the trillions of cell batteries. The cell batteries are used for the reactions of life and to defend the cell from outside the cell's hostile ions. For now, recognize, calcium can be hostile when the body fails to properly regulate its presence (section five).

Iron: Life Giver or Testicle Taker

Good health requires functional glands. Recall the genes provide nothing until the right hormone arrives. In the male, one of the main glands that offer message content to help repair and regenerate is the testicle. Unfortunately, excessive iron accumulation within the testicle poisons its functional ability.

Fortunately, the body contains elaborate hormonal systems and back up systems that are designed to prevent the entry of excessive iron into the body. In addition to the testicles, the heart, pancreas and tongue are all sites of excessive iron accumulation. Scientists call the early stages of this disorder, hemosiderosis and later, the more advanced form, hemochromatosis.

Iron is a lot like calcium: The access of iron to various tissues must be precisely regulated by the digestive tract. Iron must be carefully utilized within the hemoglobin molecules of red blood cells to carry molecular oxygen to the tissues.

However, if the multifaceted protective mechanisms of the body fail to prevent excess iron in certain body cells, tissue destruction occurs. Testicles become particularly vulnerable when iron control systems breakdown. For these reasons, iron needs to be heavily regulated toward balance in the healthy state.

Men lose about .6mg per day of iron and women lose about twice this amount during their menstrual cycle years. Normally, a body will carefully attempt to match iron absorption rates to loss rates in order to maintain iron balance. Phytic acid, phosphates, and oxalates in the diet bind iron in the digestive tube into solid complexes. However, the excess presence of these types of substances can prevent adequate absorption of iron into the body tissues that need it.

The body needs small amounts of trace minerals. These include iron, zinc, manganese, cadmium, selenium, copper, and nickel. All of these trace minerals need adequate stomach acid to be absorbed. The stomach's mineral power pump performance requires adequate acid to function. The creator designed a power pump in the stomach that exchanges the trace minerals for one acid proton ($H+$).

The power pump maintains adequate trace mineral absorption. Acid deficiency can potentially compromise trace mineral absorption. Adequate stomach acid also facilitates the less absorbable form of iron ($Fe+3$) to complex with vitamin C. Only when Fe 3+ is chemically reacted upon will it form the more absorbable form ($Fe+2$). It is only the Fe 2+ form of iron that carries oxygen when associated with hemoglobin in the red blood cells. Inadequate stomach acid causes vitamin C to be in its inactive form.

Adequate stomach acid allows iron absorption in the stomach-lining cell. Once iron is inside this cell, a protein, ferritin, designed with iron safety considerations carefully sequesters it. The gut lining cells have a lifespan of only 2-5 days. The body must decide whether it needs this iron or not. If the answer is negative, the iron sloughs off (when the cell dies) into the digestive tube where it passes in the next bowel movement. This mechanism provides the first body defense against iron overload that prevents tissue injury.

Nerd corner

The fact that the stress response leads to blood vessel inflammation, when it becomes chronic, involves the fact that certain inflammatory proteins release. C-reactive protein is only one of several of these types of proteins released within the stress response. Collectively these proteins are known as the acute phase reactants. Other acute phase reactants include: fibrinogen, complement, interferon, haptoglobin, ferritin, and ceruloplasmin. The increase of these protein types within the blood stream, in a setting of physical stress, makes sense.

The physical stress of combat or running from a large animal requires the increased activity of the immune system, blood clotting and remanufacture of new blood cell components. Each of the above acute phase reactants contributes to this overall scheme for surviving physical trauma. However, in the setting of chronic mental stress when these acute phase reactants also increase there becomes the increased tendency for blood vessel inflammation. Type A personalities provide one example of how some owners find themselves always in survival mode (the stress response).

The above cause and effect relationship of the acute phase reactants and chronic stress develops a more comprehensive picture. An elevated C-reactive protein develops only one small part of the overall picture of blood vessel inflammation process. Other specific acute phase reactants like ferritin and fibrinogen contribute directly to blood vessel inflammation.

Healing type-A personality individuals' blood vessels becomes possible when they understand the bigger connection of the scientific facts. Rather than falling for the complex's tactics of creating hopelessness about the cruel hand that genetics has dealt so take your cholesterol lowering prescription, healing becomes possible. Healing occurs when a type-A personality is provided insight into the importance of increasing positive emotions and the physical activity level while decreasing the stressful behaviors. As chronic stress tendencies resolve, the acute phase reactants decrease.

The relationship to increased acute phase reactants and a tendency to retain excessive iron may better explain one healing effect of chelation therapy. The chelating agent, EDTA, removes iron. Many heart and blood vessel diseased owners were long ago noted to have elevated ferritin levels. Iron excess is emerging as a new risk factor for blood vessel disease. The higher the serum ferritin levels the higher the iron in the body. As the chelation treatments progress their ferritin levels begin to fall. Could it be that one of the benefits of chelation therapy is that it reduces excess iron and therefore allows the blood vessel to begin healing? Tying

> together the type A personality, high serum ferritin and the possible benefit from chelation begins to help one think outside the box of the standard but fragmented way for discussing heart disease.

The next layer of body protection from iron is found in the transport protein, transferritin that orchestrates delivery into the various iron storage depots. If iron accumulates to high levels, these storage depots become injured first. The body protects itself from additional iron storage damage by increasing the transferritin level in the blood stream. Transferritin levels are sometimes used to measure the risk of this storage problem. Common storage sites of tissue injury resulting from iron excess are: pancreas damage, cirrhosis, hepatic cancer, and gonad injury. Iron overload also presents with a tanning effect that result from its deposits in the skin.

In addition, there is the emerging evidence that excess iron levels directly injure blood vessels. One likely mechanism for increased iron entry into the body is the type A personality type who is always in survival mode (the stress response). The stress response unleashes the primitive adaptation acute phase reactants. Ferritin is an acute phase reactant. Its increased presence provides a mechanism for why stressed owners (type A personality types) may accumulate more iron than is healthy. (see box)

Common nutrients and minerals need to be present in the diet for the availability of adequate molecular parts. The common hormone influences on what happens to these raw foods and minerals, once they are absorbed into the body, was discussed. The following discussion centers on how the different digestive juices dismantle the molecular building parts themselves. The body constantly needs reusable molecular components for regeneration and fuel. When raw food dismantles with precision there will be reusable components available for absorption.

A TRIP DOWN THE DIGESTIVE TUBE

With the completion of what is ideally contained in the diet, it is time for an imaginary trip down the digestive tube. Imagine shrinking down to the size of a single cholesterol molecule and hopping aboard an indigestible glass ship. The final destination will be the toilet bowel. The trip begins within a bite of food that contains proteins, carbohydrate, fats, vitamins, and minerals. A spinach and squash quiche would contain most of these.

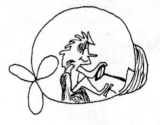

The first thing most travelers notice would be the roughness of the ride beginning in the mouth. In the mouth chewing up and down occurs along with the salivary juices that secrete into this one bite of food. The juices squirt out from various chambers of the digestive tube and contain precision food dismantling machines (enzymes). All of the digestive juices from each chamber prove very adept at disassembling the architectural framework of the different foods into their building block components.

The mouth is the first digestive chemical reaction chamber. In the mouth, the salivary juices contain enzymes. The salivary secreted digestive enzymes begin the dismantling of fat and carbohydrates contained in each bite of food.

The first juices secreted in the mouth contain molecular machines (enzymes) capable of breaking carbohydrates down into their simple sugars. Additional enzyme machines dismantle fats into free fatty acids. The disassembly of carbohydrates occurs rapidly. The rate of disassembling fats, by these first machines, occurs rather slowly.

All human digestible carbohydrate breaks down into the simple sugars; glucose, fructose, or galactose. Common examples of indigestible carbohydrate occurring in nature are wood and various plant fibers (lettuce). Simple sugars start to become available for absorption starting in the mouth.

In contrast, fat disassembly occurs as a much slower digestive break down process. One fat molecule is called a triglyceride molecule. One triglyceride molecule is made from three fatty acid molecules joined together by a single glycerol molecule. The act of digestion frees three fatty acids and one glycerol per triglyceride molecule. These dismantle in the process of digestion. Fat cannot absorb until it breaks down into these component parts.

Understanding What Fat is When it is Swallowed

The type of fat swallowed in the bite full of food is important. There are many different types of fatty acids found in nature. Different types of food break down into their own unique fatty acids. Before disassembling fat, the bite of foods fatty acid content has combined with glycerol. Each glycerol can connect to three fatty acids. The combination of three fatty acid types connects to one glycerol, which makes each type of fat (triglyceride). The combination of the different types of fatty acids makes up the fat content type in a particular food. Scientists call some fatty acids essential because the body cannot manufacture them. These essential fatty acids have powerful effects on the way blood vessels respond to injury, tissue inflammation, and the immune system response to various stimuli. By this mechanism, an imbalance of essential fatty acids could tip the scales towards disease.

Fatty acids can be two carbons (acetate) to twenty-four carbons long. In this world, each carbon binds four times to the same or to different elements at a time. Each carbon atom is always bound to something four times. If two of these bonds bind twice to another carbon in the fatty acid chain, scientists call this an unsaturated fatty acid. If the double bond occurs only one time within a given fatty acid it is called mono-unsaturated. If the double bond occurs more than one time in a fatty acid it is called polyunsaturated. The more unsaturated (the more times carbon binds twice to another carbon) in a fatty acid, two things occur.

First the fatty acid twists up in a bulky way making it more likely to be liquid at room temperature. Visualize this as the difference in gathering wood for a campfire when it is all bent and twisted versus the straight sticks. The twisted sticks are cumbersome and awkward. They don't stack well like straight sticks. Polyunsaturated fatty acids don't stack well. Because they do not stack well, they are liquid at room temperature.

Second, whenever a double bond occurs more than twice within a fatty acid, it confers a reactivity to rust promoters that may be in the blood stream. If the fatty acid is mono-saturated it reacts less readily to rust promoters than the poly-unsaturated varieties. For this reason, the type of fatty acid content present, in the bite of food, determines stability or reactivity.

Returning to the Voyage Down the Digestive Tube

Back in the glass ship; note that up to 30% of the fat and a slight majority of carbohydrates in this bite of food digests from just the contact with the saliva containing digestive machines (enzymes). Farther down the tube, different digestive machines release from the pancreatic secretions. These secretions aggressively continue to dismantle the remaining complex carbohydrates and fat molecules contained in this food.

Suddenly, a violent lurch forward occurs and the tiny glass ship moves into the esophagus, traveling at about four centimeters a second toward the stomach. Swallowing coordinates so that when the food and salivary juices reach the upper stomach valve it opens and permits smooth passage to the acid bath chamber.

Acid Bath Chamber

The stomach constitutes the second digestive chemical reaction chamber. In a healthy stomach miracles occur. Special cells deep within tunnel like pits open into the inside of the stomach. These special cells lining the numerous tunnels that exit on the stomach surface are called parietal cells. The parietal cells make and secrete stomach acid. A very good reason explains why these cells lay hidden beneath the inner surface of the stomach underneath the further protection of stomach mucus: The acid these cells secrete is so powerful that it would digest the acid producing cells themselves. Looking out of the glass ship in the stomach chamber, one would see that beneath the mucus layer there are numerous small pits that are poke-a-doted all along the middle area stomach lining. From these pits, acid juices would be flowing out from their source deep below.

The second type of stomach cell, chief cells, occurs deep down inside these tunnels, as well. These tunnels also open on the inner stomach surface. The chief cells specialize in the production of one model of protein disassembly machine. The originally secreted version of this enzyme machine for protein disassembly, pepsinogen, remain inactive until its 'wrapper' gets pulled off, whereupon scientists call it pepsin. The wrapper is composed of an amino acid chain that conceals the active part of this protein disassembly machine. To pull the wrapper off of pepsinogen requires that adequate acid be present or inactive factory product ends up lying around in the stomach doing nothing.

Adequate acid also needs to be present to provide working conditions that this model of protein dismantler requires. Further down the tube the enzymatic machines require the opposite working conditions. These enzyme machines need basic pH (alkaline) to activate. As soon as the food leaves the stomach there must be adequate alkaline juices flowing out of the pancreas or the next group of digestive machines will not activate. Different digestive chambers require different pH balance to activate the enzyme machines pertinent to that chamber. Some owners get into trouble because they have not been counseled on ensuring the proper pH balance for the chamber activities in question. In the stomach the pH needs to be sufficiently acid or the digestive enzyme machines will not activate.

Adequate stomach acid also protects owners from the passage of intact bacteria, viruses, fungi, and various digestible protein toxins. It protects because acid destroys these potential invaders. Some toxins do not adequately digest within the digestive tract. Inadequate digestion (disassembly of foreign toxins) can lead to food poisoning. For these reasons, acid content creates an important first line defense against opportunistic pathogens. These pathogens wait for the chance to enter a body. Very few microorganisms can survive the acid bath in the stomach. This sterilizes the contents entering the small intestine under normal circumstances. If a microorganism makes it into the small intestine, it confronts many more noxious surprises.

Important point: Acid is needed for three things. First, acid destroys pathogens. Second, acid signals the stomach-esophagus valve to close tightly preventing heartburn. Third, acid needs to be present in sufficient amounts to stimulate the pancreas when the food exits the stomach. Only when the pancreas receives adequate acid stimulus will it vigorously release alkali and other powerful digestive machines that it manufactures.

Various informational substances (hormones) secrete into the blood stream and into the digestive tube at specific sites as food travels toward the rectum. The stomach chamber involves the first digestive chamber where hormones play a role in the strength of these types of secretions. The message content of the hormone, gastrin, stimulates histamine. Histamine stimulates acid release. In a healthy stomach, the informational content released coordinates efficient dismantling and absorption of nutrients in a meal by the acid and enzyme secretion.

A cornerstone principle for healthy digestion concerns the ability to secrete adequate stomach acid. Paradoxically, many owners suffer from heartburn symptoms because they have a stomach acid deficiency (Wright). Additional owners suffer acid indigestion symptoms because they do not make enough protective mucus (see further discussion in this chapter). Until these situations are identified, which process (acid over production, deficient acid production or deficient mucus production or both) these owners' health will suffer.

James Privitera, MD, author of *Silent Clots*, says it very well. "I don't know any body process that improves with age. Telling patients that as they age their stomach improves its acid output is inconsistent with this fact." Dr. Privitera realizes that acid deficiency or mucous deficiency often predates indigestion problems.

The minority of heartburn patients makes too much acid. In these cases, their stomach problems become amenable to the expensive acid suppressors available. However, many patients are incorrectly diagnosed with acid over production when the real problem causing their heartburn results from acid under-production. Weak acid accessing the esophagus can still burn a hole and cause painful irritations. Acid does not belong in this anatomical area. Suppressing weak acid output damages other digestive processes. (*Wright and Gaby, 1998*)

The stimulus for the stomach-esophagus valve to shut tightly is the presence of adequate acid in the stomach contents. Without adequate acid to stimulate the tight closure of this valve, heartburn symptoms occur when a patient lies down with a full stomach. Physicians denote this condition as gastro-esophageal-reflux disease (GERD). The mechanism often involves acid under production, with consequent reflux backward through an inappropriately relaxed stomach valve. This process occurs in many heartburn sufferers. However, there are a few patients who have incompetent stomach valves for other reasons (hiatal hernia).

Another consequence of inadequate stomach acid secretion concerns the diminished pancreas stimulus to secrete its juices. The pancreas needs adequate acid to stimulate release of digestive and acid neutralizing juices. Without an adequate pancreatic stimulus, further protein and fat dismantling and absorption become compromised. This manifests clinically as patients who habitually avoid high protein meals because of the digestive difficulties that follow.

In addition, acid deficient output diminishes digestion and absorption of critical minerals. Calcium, magnesium, iron, copper, zinc, and nickel all require acid in order for the operation of the 'one for one' acid exchange pump. The mineral exchange pump that the stomach is responsible for allows the absorption of the above needed minerals. These types of mineral absorption pumps need acid (H+) to exchange for each trace mineral absorbed.

Remember, adequate acid production provides powerful protection from the dirty outside world of microorganisms seeking access to the internal anatomy. Fortunately, there are powerful alternatives available to the standard prescriptions used to suppress acid production in the treatment of heartburn. Healing involves soothing the inflamed tissue (esophagus, stomach, or duodenum). In the cases of stomach inflammation, there is likely a diminished mucus production.

Mucous production depends on the presence of high quality hormonal fats (essential fatty acid derived) and adequate IGF-1 levels. The non-steroidal anti-inflammatory medications, like aspirin, poison the hormonal fats. This causes a decrease in mucous production and an increase in stomach vulnerability towards irritation and erosion.

Owners with diminished IGF-1 (in the older literature called sulfation factor) lack the stimulus to form mucous properly. Stomach mucous is formed from GAG (glycosaminoglycans). Sulfation describes the critical step in GAG formation from the building blocks galactosamine and glucosamine where sulfate adds on. Adequate sulfate is required to keep mucous fully functional (slimy).

It is the adequate interplay between IGF-1 and the hormonal fats (prostaglandins) that determine whether sufficient mucous production occurs. Rather than educate physicians and patients about these basic interrelationships they receive educational emphasis that grooms them into thinking in a scientifically fragmented manner. Fragmented thought occurs when basic scientific relationships are eviscerated from the medical textbooks or they are discussed in a circuitous manner.

Fortunately, certain plants possess the ability to calm and soothe irritated digestive tissues by creating mucous. They are not commonly acknowledged because they are affordable and effective. Licorice root proves very effective in soothing inflamed gastrointestinal tissues. Unprocessed licorice root can raise blood pressure by prolonging the influence of fluid retaining hormones made by the adrenals. Consequently, this fraction of licorice root needs to be removed. This process is known as de-glycerrhization. Enzymatic Therapy Co. makes an excellent form of this root in a powdered form (DGL licorice).

If an owner takes this processed form when the next attack occurs, relief will be minutes away. The heartburn relief will occur without altering the gastrointestinal physiology. Licorice root powder creates thick mucous when swallowed with small amounts of water. This mucous is like the protective mucous made naturally by the stomach and protects against digestive acids. Unlike acid suppression pharmaceuticals, de-glycerrhized licorice root has no side effects and allows irritated tissues to heal.

After adequate healing of the inflamed tissues occurs, the next step can be undertaken. A holistically trained physician needs to supervise the next step because certain stomach conditions contraindicate this approach. The next step involves the supplementation of stomach acid with meals. The goal is to restore adequate acid to the digestive process in order to make nutrient digestion more effective.

Deficient acid producers are often deficient in secretion of the first protein-dismantling machines called pepsin. For this reason, it is beneficial to take a supplement that contains both acid and pepsin. The product label will say pepsinogen denoting the inactive form. When combined with water and acid it will be activated to pepsin. With successful acid and pepsinogen supplementation, patients notice an increased tolerance for high protein meals. For example, the increased ability to digest larger portions of steak, fish, and chicken, etc.

Typically, acid supplementation should be done during consumption of a protein meal. Adequate fluid should be swallowed with the hydrochloric acid pills, as well. The best dose per pill contains approximately 600mg of hydrochloric acid. The dose per mid-meal should be increased by one pill until a warm feeling is noticed. This sensation denotes that the correct dose of acid supplement has been exceeded by one pill. If this sensation occurs, with the next meal decrease the dosage by one pill. If acid deficiency involves part of the digestive problem, supplementation will lead to feelings of increased well being following protein meals.

Alternatively, consuming alcohol with meals enhances the digestive process through the stimulation of acid output. Caffeine has been documented to stimulate acid secretion as well. However, some of these fluids destroy the mucus lining that protects the stomach from digesting itself. Examples of substances that disrupt the integrity of this mucous barrier are excess alcohol, vinegar, bile salts, and aspirin-like drugs (ibuprofen, aspirin, indomethacin, etc.).

The discussion of the hormones and nervous control of acid secretion can be complicated. Both of these acid producing mechanisms pathways converge on histamine, which increases when the vagus nerve activates and from the hormone, gastrin. Histamine directly causes the acid producing cells to release acid into the stomach. Blockers of histamine release (Tagamet, Zantac, and Pepsin) are commonly used to decrease acid release. Alternatively, the more powerful proton pump inhibitors (Prilosec and Prevacid) act by their ability to poison the acid producing cells in the stomach.

In summary, there are three main determinants of stomach function: the adequacy of acid production, the quality of the mucus layer which protects the stomach lining from digesting itself, and the quality of the enzyme machines which release when sufficient acid presents. Looking out from the glass ship into this stomach, all three of these processes occur in an orderly fashion.

The next stop in the glass ship occurs upon exiting the stomach through the pyloric valve. Immediately outside the stomach two drains that enter the small intestines are noticed. One drain comes from the gallbladder. The other drain comes from the pancreas. Food trickles out of the stomach valve. This causes each drain to gush with its own characteristic juice and mix with the partially digested food.

Pancreatic Juices and What They Need to Perform

The pancreas requires adequate stomach acid to stimulate it to release its stored juices. Pancreatic juices contain two basic components. The first component contains the acid neutralizing juice. It is needed because this chambers enzymatic machinery works only in an alkaline environment (the opposite of an acid environment). These digestive machines operate in the third digestive chamber, the small intestine. While the partially digested meal contents seep from the stomach, the pancreas secretes its juices. Pancreatic juices contain bicarbonate that reacts with the acid forming carbon dioxide gas and water. A healthy pancreas secretes more bicarbonate than there is acid present. The second component of pancreatic secretions, its digestive machines, requires an alkaline environment for proper function.

The second component of the pancreatic juice contains unique pancreatic enzymatic machines. Their design further dismantles fats, proteins, and, to a lesser degree, the few remaining complex carbohydrates. These juices comprise only part of the whole complement of digestive juices in the third chemical reaction chamber. The first chemical reaction chamber is in the mouth and the second in the stomach. Each of the chemical reaction chambers requires different work environments (acid or basic). The different work environments are necessary for the enzymatic machines secreted in that compartment to become fully functional.

Just like in the stomach, the enzymatic machines released within this digestive chamber, the duodenum, release with their 'packages' wrapped around them. The enzyme machinery floats around idly and is useless until their wrapper is removed. The wrappers in this chamber are composed of amino acid chains that cover the active site of these additional protein disassembly machines. The inactivity precaution before secretion prevents the pancreas from digesting itself. The intestinal digestive chamber activation of this type of enzyme machinery depends on the cells lining the intestinal tube.

The cells that line the intestinal tube contain an unwrapping enzymatic machine. This particular machine activates only one of the pancreatic-produced enzymes. Scientists call this particular, pancreas secreted, enzymatic machine trypsinogen while its still in the wrapper and trypsin when it unwraps. Enzyme machines produced in the intestinal lining cells unwrap trypsinogen to trypsin. The intestinal lining cells protect themselves from digestion by their own layer of mucous. Trypsin, once freed, 'unwraps' all the other pancreatic digestive machines contained in 'wrappers'. Important point: Once trypsin has been freed, it begins to digest any protein that is not concealed behind the protective mucous barrier.

The Intestinal Chamber

The intestinal chamber is the third chemical reaction chamber. It receives chemical concoctions from the gallbladder and pancreas that dump into its proximal portion. The three different successive areas of this chamber reabsorb the majority of the secretions that occur higher up in the digestive tube. These chambers are the duodenum, the jejunum, and the ileum. The cells lining the intestinal tube look like shag carpet. One strand of carpet is composed of millions of intestinal lining cells called villous. Millions of strands make up the shag carpet and provide maximal absorptive contact with the digested food.

The intestinal lining is called the brush border where the digestive building blocks (amino acids, simple sugars, various fatty acids, vitamins, nucleic acids and minerals) absorb into the body. Each type of molecular building component absorbs at specific sites along this digestive chamber. Like the stomach, the cells lining the small intestine tube protect themselves from digestion by a mucous layer. Each specific molecular part (amino acids, sugars, various fatty acids, minerals, and vitamins) relies on a specific transport method through this mucous layer. If a molecular part cannot successfully cross through this mucous barrier, it cannot assimilate.

The short life span of the digestive lining cells (the brush border) illustrates how body molecular parts are recycled and reused interchangeably. The recycling arises because these cell types continuously slough off into the digestive tube every two to five days. A snake sheds its skin in a similar fashion, but here it occurs from the inside of the tube. When these cells are sloughed off, they dismantle (are digested) into their molecular building parts. These mix with the food content contained in the digestive juices. These molecular parts then reabsorb by the digestive tract to be used somewhere else. Interchangeability of a molecular part ends only when it becomes damaged. Secretion of dead cells and the eventual re-absorption of the remaining useful molecular building blocks illustrate the interchangeability of the molecular parts that enters and leaves the tube. The interchangeability of molecular parts is an important concept.

Millions of recycled molecular parts move around the body. These same molecular parts build themselves into a structure that later dismantles into its molecular building parts only to again recycle into yet another molecular structure. This occurs constantly at different locations throughout the body. The end to the interchangeability of molecular body parts arises only when they become damaged. Replacement of the damaged molecular parts explains why a continuous supply of new and high quality molecular parts must become available through the diet and digestive assimilation.

In summary, the stomach allows seepage of its contents out of the pyloric valve and into the small intestine. Vigorous pancreatic contractions release sufficient acid neutralizing bicarbonate. Bicarbonate release occurs in excess of the acid present to produce the opposite (alkaline fluid) work environment. An alkaline pH optimizes the simultaneous release and activation of the unique pancreatic digestive machines. The pancreatic digestive machines are designed to work best in an alkaline environment. In the small intestine chamber the final dismantling process of fats, protein, carbohydrate and the genetic material building blocks occurs. The third digestive chamber also contains the sites where these molecular building blocks absorb into the body.

The Gallbladder Secretion

The gallbladder secretes juice out of the second hole in the proximal duodenum. Fat in the meal forces the gallbladder secretion to be a simultaneous secretion out of the second drain hole. Fats need additional molecular concoctions in the intestinal chemical reaction chamber in order to be dismantled. The gallbladder secretion solves the problem of fat floating on water. The meal content floats in copious digestive juices that are water based. They do not mix well with fat. The gallbladder secretes salts and acids that will break oil into tiny droplets. This process explains how the dairy industry makes the fat in commercially available milk stay dissolved in the milk. These substances are called emulsifying agents. The gallbladder secretes emulsifying agents made from acids of cholesterol and the break down of hemoglobin salts. In specific ratios, these substances raise the fat absorption from 50% without a gallbladder to 95% with a gallbladder.

The entire contents of the gallbladder secrete into the upper small intestine (duodenum) and are reabsorbed at the end of the small intestine (the ileum). After being reabsorbed, they quickly re-secrete into the gallbladder at such a rate that they recycle 6-8 times per day.

Nutritionally - The Owner is Only as Good as What He/She Absorbs

The healthy owner accomplishes the orderly uptake of different nutritional building blocks. Uptake becomes possible and occurs as individual parts become available to the brush border cells. Billions of brush border cells line the small intestine tube. In this digestive chamber, the quality of juices that come out of the pancreas and the gallbladder significantly effect how the body absorbs nutrients. This process also concerns the health of the brush border cells and their associated protective mucus.

The small intestine handles more than nine quarts of fluid per day. By the time meal remnants reach the large intestine (colon) only 1-2 liters of fluid remain. By the time they leave the colon in the bowel movement, less than one cup of the original nine quarts passes in the feces.

Digestion involves the secretion and re-absorption of large amounts of water. The content of the fluid changes considerably as the food moves down the digestive tube. These changes facilitate the dismantling tasks that need to occur. The fluid, salt, and even the enzymatic machinery parts largely reabsorb and recycle again and again.

The voyage down the small intestine in the glass ship has seen almost all the nutrients absorb that the meal contained. The meal remnants contain mostly indigestible fibers and friendly bacteria that comprise 50% of stool weight. Only small amounts of fat and protein still remain in the stool. The glass ship arrives at the passageway to the next digestive chamber, the cecum. The next digestive chamber is the large intestine (colon).

Health Cannot Occur Without a Happy Colon

The colon (large intestine) comprises the fourth chemical reaction chamber for the nutritional remnants still in the meal. In addition to finishing the digestive process, the colon is one of six organs that take out the trash (see Taking Out the Trash section). Constipated people do not take out their colon trash very well. On the opposite extreme, are those owners who suffer from chronic diarrhea. Chronic diarrhea means that the body discards important minerals, water, nutrients, and vitamins with the trash. On top of this backdrop of colon tasks concerns the unique requirements of the healthy colon being colonized by helpful bacteria.

The large intestine requires certain bacterial colonies to assist it in performing its many biological functions. If the right bacteria live in this chamber, good things happen. The right bacteria (mostly acidophilus and bifidus bacteria) re-acidify the meal remnants again. The meal remnants are all that is left of the meal that has finally made its way to the colon.

It is very important to overall body health that the colon contains ample friendly bacteria. These bacteria produce many B-vitamins and vitamin K. The colon-inhabiting bacteria feed the colon lining cells by changing indigestible fiber into carbohydrate. Second and more importantly, these bacteria change some of this carbohydrates into the short-chained fatty acids that are particularly nutritious for the needs of the colon lining cells.

If one of the colon functions fails health consequences occur. It is worthwhile to consider some of these imbalances and the simple ways an owner can return to balance. The first imbalance concerns the colon's role as one of the organs responsible for preventing the fifth path to an old body, taking out the trash. It is important to identify the role of the colon in this path to longevity. The fifth path is about taking out the cellular trash that accumulates daily as the cells perform the work of living.

When certain conditions exist, the colon becomes compromised in its ability to perform its necessary trash removal task. The first compromise involves the wrong bacteria or amounts inhabiting the colon chamber. The second arises from trash removal problems that occur when the colon contents become fiber deficient. This prevents helpful bacteria from being able to create butyrate for the colon lining cells nutritional needs. Butyrate is a short chain fatty acid that colon cells prefer for energy (Bland). Third concerns the water retention role that fiber plays in keeping bowel movements soft. Fourth involves the chronic retention of feces or constipation that encourages the formation of toxins (putrefaction). Putrefaction results in the re-absorption of some of these poisons back into the body.

The last compromise concerns yeast organisms over growing in the colon chamber. Decreased acidity encourages yeast overgrowth. Sufficient colon acidity depends on adequate amounts of acid-producing bacteria. Whenever an owner takes antibiotics, the risk arises that these friendly bacteria will die. Friendly bacteria also die from chronic consumption of chlorinated water. When friendly bacteria die, the acidity of the colon decreases and this encourages yeast overgrowth. This allows the release of more toxins into the system. A careful, laboratory performed stool analysis can identify most of these common problems.

All of the trash removal problems are made worse when certain hormones become deficient in the colon. The primary hormones for colon health are thyroid, cortisol, IGF-1, and vitamin A. When any of these become deficient, colon health suffers.

Low thyroid function manifests as chronic constipation because thyroid message encourages energy production in the colon cells. Only through sufficient energy creation can the colon motility and activity be normal.

Cortisol deficiency leads to colon inflammation and mucus abnormalities. Therefore, colitis is very responsive to cortisol medication. Often these patients have a thyroid problem as well.

Nerd corner

Decreased IGF-1 levels lead to a decrease in the protective layer of glycosaminoglycans occurring throughout the body. The glycosaminoglycan layer protects the cells that line the body cavities (respiratory tract, gastrointestinal tract), blood vessels, the matrix that inflates and holds cells together within the body and the body surfaces ability to hold water and prevent shriveling (skin and organs). The IGF-1 level determines the adequacy of this protective layer in the colon. The consequence, within the colon, of the glycosaminoglycan layer becoming deficient concerns an increased propensity for toxic molecules to leak into the body. The increased toxic load further burdens the liver (see liver chapter).

Many physicians remain unaware of these important roles of IGF-1. Part of this results from the numerous different names given to IGF-1. In order to connect the overall effect of IGF-1 within the body a physician would need to know the other names for IGF-1 within the medical literature: nonsuppressible insulin like activity of the blood, sulfation factor, and somatomedin C. They would also

---

need to know that IGF-1 levels depend on a healthy liver, adequate androgen (DHEA and testosterone) and sufficient Growth Hormone release. The sulfation factor nomenclature describes the fact that sufficient amounts of this hormone are needed to create the highly charged GAG (glycosaminoglycans) that form in the above-described areas within the body. Sufficient amounts of GAG in the above areas allow sufficient barriers to protect body tissues. Deficient GAG in the colon sets up the conditions for leaky gut and colon inflammatory diseases. Deficient GAG in the blood vessels increases the overall injury rate to the underlying lipid bilayer. Deficient GAG within the cells and around the cells causes a diminution of these electrically charged meshworks that hold water in the body. When water content decreases the shrinkage into old age begins.

Vitamin A makes cells grow up. Cancer is a problem of cells not growing up. Some cancer cells do not grow up solely because they are deficient in vitamin A. Sufficient vitamin A is necessary to instruct DNA programs. Vitamin A is particularly important in the same cell types for which the glycosaminoglycan layer forms a barrier. Signs of vitamin A deficiency show up most obviously on the skin. Examples of this include roughened skin, pigmentation spots, and fine wrinkles. When these are present the same tendency exists in the colon.

For these reasons, colon cancer risk can be lowered by adequate vitamin A intake. Vitamin A is found in high levels in carrots, squash and avocados.

The last chapter only skimmed the liver's role in whether one is healthy or aged. Follow the fuel and one will understand many middle-aged diseases. Obesity, heart disease and diabetes, in their common forms begin in the liver. The liver determines what happens to fuel following a meal and between meals. Many middle-aged associated diseases begin because the liver misappropriates fuel. Section four will discuss the important role the liver plays in what happens to absorbed nutrients. The next chapter paves the way for understanding the discrepancy between what science knows contrasted to what is taught about the importance of balance of the hormone message content instructing the liver on whether to store or release fuel. The pancrease because it plays a pivotal role in instructing the liver in both energy storage and release is the topic of the next chapter.

CHAPTER FOURTEEN

PANCREAS

The Hormones that Prevent the Pancreas from Killing

As was previously discussed, the exocrine part of the pancreas secretes digestive juices. This chapter reviews the additional important pancreatic secretion known as the hormonal pancreas (the endocrine portion). Most of the time dietary habits determine which type of hormones the pancreas secretes. Realize, the type of hormones that the pancreas chooses to secrete has a powerful effect on what the liver will do with the fuel supply (sugar, fat and protein).

For example, insulin message dominance leads to one extreme of liver activities involving fuel supply. Insulin that the pancreas secretes, directs the liver to store carbohydrate in the form of glycogen (the minority form of stored body fuel). When the capacity of the liver to store carbohydrate as glycogen becomes filled (100 grams), insulin directs the liver to manufacture the rest of the carbohydrate into LDL fat molecules. LDL fat is designed as a transport package destined for the major fuel storage sites.

Eventually, some of the newly liver synthesized LDL cholesterol releases into the blood stream. For this reason, the high production rate of these types of fats can show up as an increased LDL cholesterol or triglyceride level. From the blood stream, the LDL cholesterol moves into the fat storage areas of the body (blood vessel macrophage cells and belly fat). Recall from chapter one that the rate of this disposal determines the measured LDL cholesterol value in the blood stream but nothing about how engorged the macrophages, lining the arteries, become. This fact explains why fifty percent of heart attack victims had normal cholesterol levels.

In contrast, the other extreme of hormonal direction from the pancreas to the liver occurs when diet and life style direct the pancreas to release glucagon message content into the portal vein that leads straight into the liver. The glucagon message directs the liver to dump its stored sugar and fatty acids into the blood stream. These molecules are readily accessible sources of raw fuel used to power the cell factories. Therefore, the glucagon message contains opposite liver intended information relative to that of the insulin message. When glucagon predominates, fuels are released into the blood stream from the liver for use as fuel in the cellular power plants. In addition, the glucagon message stimulates the liver conversion of amino acids into more sugar (a catabolic effect).

For these reasons, it is important to consider the balance of message content that the liver receives for how it is directed to deal with raw fuel (sugar, fat and protein). Whether fuel is stored or released is determined by this basic pipeline of information flowing from the pancreas into the liver. When balanced informational content occurs, the pancreas secretes optimal amounts of the opposing hormones insulin and glucagon. Sadly, failure to understand this dynamic 'tug of war' between these opposing informational substances leads to unnecessary prescriptions, surgical procedures, and disease complications.

Healthy owners use almost all their pancreas secreted insulin and glucagon instructing their liver on how to handle fuel. Ninety percent of the glucagon hormone secreted by the pancreas is used in the liver. The glucagon message directs the liver to release stored sugar (as glucose) and fat (as fatty acids) into the blood stream. In addition, the message of glucagon stimulates the liver to manufacture more sugar from amino acids made available to the liver (a catabolic effect). Recall, amino acids are used to build protein. Protein adequacy powerfully determines the metabolic ability of a cell.

Also contained in the message content of glucagon is the cessation of the liver synthesis of cholesterol. The glucagon message content accomplishes this by instructing the inactivation of the enzyme HMG CoA reductase in the liver. This is the same enzyme that most cholesterol lowering drugs inhibit as well. Perhaps some owners prefer knowing how message content works before committing to potentially toxic medication (see inflammation and heart disease subsection in section six). Lastly, the glucagon message content inhibits further synthesis of fat in the liver. Overall, the glucagon message instructs the liver to maximize fuel delivery into the blood stream. Efficiency here, allows more fuel uptake in the 60 trillion or so additional cellular power plants.

In contrast, insulin delivers the opposite message to the liver. Healthy owners use up eighty percent of their insulin message content on it instructing the liver to store fuel (a blood sugar lowering event). Fuel is stored as fat (unlimited) and a small amount of glycogen (100 grams in the liver and 400 grams in the muscles). The insulin message in the liver can be summarized as: stop the manufacture of amino acids into sugar, suck the sugar out of the blood stream and sequester it in the form of glycogen within the liver, and when the capacity to store sugar is filled (about 100 grams in the liver) it then directs the liver to manufacture extra sugar into LDL cholesterol.

For this reason, increased insulin arriving within the liver causes a higher LDL cholesterol manufacture rate through its direction to activate the enzyme, HMG CoA reductase, which manufactures cholesterol in the liver. Simultaneously, insulin directs conversion of the extra sugar into fat in the liver (saturated fat type triglyceride). Recall three fatty acids join one glycerol molecule to form the pH neutral triglyceride. Both triglyceride and cholesterol are really just the body's clever way of maintaining fat in a pH neutral manner until fuel is actually needed. Excessive fatty acids obviously create a pH problem.

Next, the newly manufactured fat and cholesterol molecules manufactured in the liver combine with specific proteins to form LDL particles. These specific proteins contained in LDL cholesterol allow it to be water soluble for transport in the blood stream. LDL particles are secreted from the liver into the blood stream. These particles are destined for the storage depots within the fat cells that line the belly and macrophage cells that line arteries.

As an aside, substances such as caffeine stimulate pancreatic secretion of both insulin and glucagon at the same time. Here the more powerful effect is glucagon as evidenced by a slight increase in the blood sugar level. As a consequence, owners who suffer with a damaged pancreas, such as in insulin deficient type diabetic, should take particular note of this caffeine-induced effect. Excessive blood sugar increase occurs because as the caffeine arrives at the pancreas there is no ability to increase insulin. Consequently, in the insulin deficient diabetic, when glucagon becomes unopposed by insulin, it promotes blood sugar increases! When was the last time anyone heard about a conventionally trained physician warning their diabetic patients about this problem?

Actually, there are a total of four hormones, including glucagon, that counter the effects of insulin within the liver. When one or more of these counter regulatory hormones fail, it leads to unnecessary suffering and disease complications. Many cases of hypoglycemia, poorly controlled diabetes, muscle wasting, and other chronic degenerative diseases result from a failure to comprehend the 'weight and the counter weights' of hormones that affect liver fuel direction parameters. When the liver physiology becomes unbalanced, an altered response to insulin occurs.

Insulin's message content desires to direct the liver to suck every sugar molecule out of the blood stream (an energy storage event). Unfortunately, when the counter response to a high insulin levels at the level of the liver becomes deficient, a dangerously low blood sugar can result. By this mechanism, countless owners suffer from 'roller coaster' blood sugar levels brought about by imbalances in their ability to mount an effective counter response to excessive insulin.

Four main counter response hormones occur that the body needs in order to keep insulin effects balanced. Each one has advantages and disadvantages. Glucagon was earlier introduced and the other three will be compared for how they counter insulin's blood sugar lowering abilities within the liver.

Insulin serves as the weight in the antique weight scale analogy. For health to occur, it takes all four other 'counterweights' in effective amounts to rebalance the 'weight scale'. The weight scale balances when two processes occur. First, there needs to be an appropriate amount of sugar and fat in the blood stream created by adequate amounts of the four counter regulatory hormones. Second, the need for the presence of adequate insulin-like growth factor type one (IGF-1) is necessary. Unfortunately, very few physicians realize that IGF-1 facilitates entry of these fuels into the cellular power plants outside the liver and fat storage cells.

The counterbalancing hormones that oppose the action of insulin are glucagon, cortisol, adrenaline, and growth hormone. Many poorly controlled diabetic conditions arise from failure to consider the status of the counter regulatory hormones (liver chapter). Other countless owners are misdiagnosed with mood disorders, seizures, depression, and even hypochondria when aberrations in the counter response hormones are the true culprit. Fortunately, if these owners better understand this often ignored interplay between these opposing hormonal forces then healing becomes possible.

Cortisol as a Counter Regulatory Hormone to Insulin

Above and beyond the opposing message content between glucagon and insulin are the other counter regulatory hormones. Recall, cortisol is a level one hormone secreted by the adrenals. It contains powerful message content directed at liver cell DNA programs (genes). One example for the consequence of insufficient cortisol directed DNA programs activation in the liver, involves the diminished ability of the liver to recognize the glucagon message.

Sadly, this important fact is often skirted around in the medical textbooks. In these textbooks, in a disorganized and fragmented way, there is an acknowledgment that cortisol is necessary for the liver to respond to the glucagon message. However, its clinical significance fails to be comprehended: The consequence of cortisol deficiency is that the liver cannot recognize the glucagon message content without enough of it to direct the manufacture of glucagon receptors through DNA program activation.

Unfortunately, in most middle-aged bodies, cortisol is expected to be the heavy weight that opposes insulin's blood sugar lowering effects (reason explained below). Recall, the adrenal glands make cortisol. For this reason, many owners who suffer from weakened adrenal function also experience brain 'fog' symptoms thirty minutes to three hours following a carbohydrate meal. Recall, carbohydrate intake increases the need for more insulin secretion from the pancreas. There then needs to be an adequate ability to manufacture and release increased cortisol from the adrenal to counter the increased insulin's desire to lower the blood sugar level below optimal.

Adrenal deficient owners experience low blood sugar because a high carbohydrate diet necessitates an increased insulin release. Diminished cortisol release ability means that an ineffective counter weight occurs and this promotes hypoglycemia. In addition, cortisol also directs other liver cell DNA programs in the manufacture of the enzyme, glycogen synthase. As a consequence, insufficient cortisol also causes deficient glycogen storage, which predisposes these owner types to even more hypoglycemia events. Overall point: Unless adequate counter regulatory hormones effectively counter the increased insulin release, the blood sugar will fall. Realize, in most middle aged owners, cortisol is the main counter regulatory hormone to insulin's blood sugar lowering effects.

For example, after growth hormone levels fall off around middle age, cortisol becomes the primary hormone to counter the insulin message within the liver. One of the ways cortisol counters the insulin message is by instructing liver cells DNA programs (genes). Recall the previous example that cortisol instructs liver cell DNA programs in the manufacture of the glucagon receptors necessary for the liver to respond to glucagon. Recall, as well, the pancreas releases glucagon during times of low blood sugar. However, unless the glucagon encounters its specific receptor within the liver it proves worthless to counter a falling blood sugar.

Unfortunately, many owners continue to suffer from low blood sugar because no one evaluates their adrenals' ability to increase cortisol production in the presence of high insulin levels.

Adrenaline as a Counter Regulatory Hormone to Insulin

Adrenaline (epinephrine) saves lives when the adrenal glands' ability to release sufficient cortisol diminishes. Unfortunately, adrenaline message content also depends on cortisol to direct the liver DNA programs (genes) to manufacture its receptors. Most of the time, adrenaline needs to serve as a counter hormone to insulin only when something goes wrong and the blood sugar falls too low. In non-diabetics this occurs when they consume a high carbohydrate diet and insufficient cortisol secretion ability manifests. Many of these owners avoid death but suffer profound anxiety and irrational behavior secondary to excessive adrenaline causing these side effects.

Realize excessive adrenaline release to counter a drop in blood sugar, causes the side effects of pounding heart rate, anxiety, and sweating palms (the symptoms of shock). Many unsuspecting owners that love to binge out on carbohydrates develop these wide swings in blood sugar and fail to understand the anxiety like symptoms that follow. These symptoms result from the blood sugar falling and then being rescued from death by a massive outpouring of adrenaline.

Nutritional adequacy is the concern of the fourth principle. Some unfortunate owners have weak adrenals and therefore poor cortisol production. The problem magnifies when the additional disaster of poor nutrition occurs. In addition, some of these owners suffer increased risk for seizure disorders because their blood sugar fall father than most (section six).

Actually, both cortisol and thyroid hormones are needed to manufacture a mature adrenaline receptor. Like cortisol, thyroid hormone is also a level one-type hormone. Thyroid message content is also needed to direct liver cell DNA programs in the synthesis of part of the adrenaline receptor (thyroid chapter). As a consequence, deficiency or excess in these interrelated hormones cause a sub-optimal human experience. The sub-optimal experience occurs because the mature adrenaline receptor manufacturing process requires direction by both of these level one-type hormones.

William B. Ferril, M. D.

Growth Hormone is the Most Misunderstood of the Counter Response Hormones to Insulin

The most misunderstood and neglected role of the counter response hormones to insulin is Growth Hormone (GH). This neglect occurs because its name leads owners down an erroneous mental image path. Growth hormone's protein conservation message delivered to the liver explains where its name originates. Protein conservation is a pre-requisite for growth to occur. Growth Hormone outside of the liver, other than its stimulatory effect on cartilage cell growth, has few direct effects on other tissues.

However, within the liver, one direct effect concerns its ability to act like modified glucagon at the level of the liver with two important exceptions. First, involves the fact that unlike glucagon, Growth Hormone directs powerful protein sparing effects (anabolic). Importantly, Growth Hormone in the liver inhibits the conversion of amino acids into sugar (promotes positive nitrogen balance). The second difference from glucagon involves the fact that GH directs the liver to release a special hormone called insulin-like growth factor type 1 (IGF-1). Like glucagon, it stimulates the release of sugar stored as liver glycogen into the blood stream. Also like glucagon it stimulates the liver to release stored fats into the blood stream as fatty acids for fuel.

Insulin-like growth factor type 1 (IGF-1) can only release following Growth Hormone's presence. Confusion arises from the fact that the affects of IGF-1 message content, directly opposes the initial fuel release effects of Growth Hormone (its diabetogenic effect). Many fail to appreciate that IGF-1 release occurs simultaneously to the Growth Hormone directed liver release of sugar and fat into the blood stream. Normally this tandem of events stabilizes the blood sugar rise that GH initially causes.

Understanding the overall effect caused by the sequential release of growth hormone followed by IGF-1, allows one to appreciate a beautiful hormonal cascade operating in healthy owners. The more IGF-1 released, the less insulin needed. In fact, older medical physiology textbooks acknowledged this fact but called IGF-1 the non-suppressible insulin like activity of the blood stream. They further asserted that it makes up 93% of the insulin like activity of the blood stream! What happened to this knowledge? Who removed it?

Growth Hormone stimulates the release of fat and carbohydrates from liver stores into the blood stream. The second part of the effect involves the simultaneous release, from the liver, of adequate insulin-like growth factor (IGF-1) into the blood stream. The IGF-1 hormone in the peripheral tissues (blood stream) behaves very much like insulin does in the liver and body fat cells. For this reason, the body needs less insulin when the liver secretes adequate IGF-1. Ideally, adequate growth hormone stimulates sufficient IGF-1 release into the blood stream and the peripheral tissues, like muscle, are facilitated to procure fuel (carbohydrate and fat). This process describes the insulin-like effect of IGF-1.

Sufficient release of IGF-1 negates the initial increase in blood sugar and blood fat caused by the presence of Growth Hormone's message to the liver. Mechanistically IGF-1 behaves like insulin in the peripheral tissues. IGF-1's presence instructs the peripheral tissues to take up the fuel released by Growth Hormones presence. In fact the highest pure IGF-1 receptor concentration occurs in muscle.

Unfortunately, many clinicians fail to appreciate this sequential arrangement that operates in the healthy population. Both IGF-1 and insulin bind to the same cell receptors to varying degrees. This makes sense when one realizes their similar message content in regards to their providing instruction to different cells within the body to take up fuel out of the blood stream (a *fuel nozzle effect*).

Important point: Different cell types have different affinities for IGF-1 and insulin, and different cell receptor concentrations for each. For example, the liver and fat cells have the highest amount of pure insulin receptors of any other cell. There are about 200,000 insulin receptors per fat or liver cell. Here, insulin persuasively directs these tissues to store fuel. Importantly, IGF-1 has one thousandth the binding affinity of insulin to fat cells.

In contrast, the IGF-1 receptors are found throughout most of the rest of the body cell types. Recall, IGF-1 blood levels, in healthy owners, occur at levels one hundred times that of insulin levels. This fact explains why many disease processes have their origins in a falling IGF-1 level (*hungry cell syndrome*). When the IGF-1 level falls, insulin needs to be secreted in abnormal amounts (commonly called insulin resistance). Increased insulin inflicts health consequences that increased IGF-1 does not share.

A major advantage of adequate IGF-1 to that of higher insulin is that insulin levels determine the amount of body fat. Fat is the major stored fuel type because there is a limited ability to store sugar as glycogen. Total body storage capacity for glycogen is about 500 grams (about 2200 calories). About one hundred grams are stored in the liver and the other four hundred grams are stored in the muscles.

Unfortunately, sedentary and well-fed owners have little opportunity to draw down these stored forms of sugar. In addition, processed food often proves potassium deficient. Sufficient potassium proves necessary before glycogen manufacture occurs. This detail explains, yet another mechanism for how these owners abnormally upregulate LDL cholesterol synthesis rates because this pathway does not require potassium. By these mechanisms, the more sedentary and well fed the owner, the more carbohydrates channel into the fat and cholesterol making machinery within the liver. Remember, insulin directed pathways are designed with fuel storage in mind. The major fuel storage sites occur in arterial macrophages and the fat cells.

In contrast, when an owner is healthy most of his insulin production is used at the level of the liver following a meal (a blood sugar rising event). In addition, less insulin is needed when there is the increased presence of IGF-1 because it also facilitates the removal of sugar from the blood stream (the cells outside of the liver and fat). Remember, IGF-1 once secreted into the blood stream hangs around for along time helping out as a fuel nozzle.

Unlike insulin, which has a major effect on the liver and fat cells' ability to remove sugar out of the blood stream, IGF-1 exerts its effect in the periphery cells (muscles, bones, joints and organs). IGF-1 competes with insulin as to where nutrition is sucked. Visualize the tug of war for where fuel channels. Higher IGF-1 favors increased nutrition procurement for muscle, bone, joints and organs cells. Conversely, higher insulin levels favor the uptake of nutrition out of the blood stream by liver and fat cells (*hungry cell syndrome*).

Recall the two major stimuli for Growth Hormone release: The GH releasing stimulus results from fasting and intense exercise. Both of these conditions produce a decrease in blood level fuel. This decrease causes an initial rise in growth hormone that initially directs the liver to release IGF-1, sugar, and fat into the blood stream. In turn, the released IGF-1 acts like insulin in facilitating peripheral uptake of the released fuel from the liver. In this way, the healthy body has a mechanism for ensuring that appropriate amounts of fuel are in the blood stream between meals and when physical exertion draws down the blood fuel.

Exercise has a powerful contributory effect on the amount of Growth Hormone released and hence, IGF-1 levels. This release does much the same thing in the periphery that insulin does in the liver and fat storage cells. However, low blood sugar effects are prevented because growth hormone also directs the liver to dump sugar into the blood stream while the liver is releasing IGF-1. The design of IGF-1 facilitates the peripheral cells uptake of fuel out of the blood stream that, in these cases, growth hormone started. However, when Growth Hormone production falls off and consequently IGF-1 as well, the need for increased insulin production intensifies. In these unhealthy situations, insulin is forced to pick up the slack in the periphery (muscles and organs). This defect describes one of the mechanisms for insulin resistance (liver chapter) occurring in metabolic syndrome (Syndrome X).

Normally, increased IGF-1 levels occur for the opposite reasons of increased insulin levels. For example, the increase in IGF-1 in the exercising or fasting state (a blood sugar falling event) facilitates cellular uptake of the Growth Hormone stimulated liver released sugar and fat into the blood stream. However, the fuel storage status in the liver depends on enough insulin directing the liver to suck up nutrition for storage purposes following a meal (a blood sugar rising event). As a consequence, without sufficient insulin, insufficient stored fuel to release occurs when GH directs the release of fuel and IGF-1 from the liver.

In contrast, the healthy body balances the blood fuel supply following meals and between meals. Both insulin and IGF-1 remove nutrients from the blood stream following meals (a blood sugar rising event). Normally, insulin predominantly directs nutrients into the storage pathways that occur in the liver and fat cells. Conversely, IGF-1 directs nutrients into the vast majority of other cell types. The healthy body having at least one hundred times more IGF-1 than insulin in the blood stream evidences this fact. In addition, normally between meals IGF-1 serves as the fuel nozzle.

Unfortunately, increased insulin becomes necessary to shore up lagging Growth Hormone caused diminished IGF-1 output. There are three subtle, but dangerous consequences to a body that relies on increased insulin production. First, the stimulation of the appetite center leads to an increased tendency to gain weight. Second, increased insulin stimulates the liver in the manufacture of excessive LDL cholesterol. Third, there is increased reliance on cortisol, glucagon and adrenaline to keep the blood sugar elevated, between meals, when Growth Hormone levels fall.

One consequence of normalizing blood sugar levels between meals with elevated cortisol, glucagon and epinephrine is a loss in protein conservation ability. Recall, only Growth Hormone defends body protein when fasting. Less body protein leads to shrinking muscle mass and organ size. These are some of the major characteristics of the onset of aging.

Growth Hormone release occurs from regular exercise, low normal blood sugars, glucagon, the low secretion rate of serotonin in the hypothalamus, and when the hypothalamus neurons secrete dopamine. There are other details, but if one keeps these five determinants in mind it encourages making better choices.

The above discussion gives a mechanistic explanation for why couch potatoes tend to develop insulin resistance. Increased insulin resistance will eventually exhaust the genetically determined ability of the pancreas to increase insulin production. When this happens, it exhausts the pancreas beyond its genetically determined capability manifesting in adult onset diabetes.

Making things worse is the fact that when GH secretion rates fall the protein content in the body decreases proportionally. GH is a fundamental requirement for the conservation of body protein between meals. Without adequate GH between meals the body increases the secretion rate of cortisol, glucagons, and epinephrine in order to maintain blood sugar levels. All three of these will activate the liver machinery that converts protein stores into sugar (gluconeogenesis). For this reason, these unfortunate owners suffer from a wasting disease hiding amongst their fat (chapter four).

The other extreme of health contains highly trained athletes who secrete high levels of IGF-1 secondary to increased growth hormone secretion. Increased growth hormone secretion occurs because exercise increases fuel delivery requirements. GH is one of the main hormones that raise the liver secretion rate of fuel into the blood stream and body protein content is spared from breakdown. In contrast, the other three fuel increasing hormones, cortisol, epinephrine, and glucagon make protein fair game.

Another benefit of high IGF-1 levels is that less insulin is required. The highly trained athlete needs very little insulin for efficient fuel delivery into exercising muscle cells because of his/her high IGF-1 levels. In fact, insulin levels fall towards zero during exercise in well-trained athletes for this reason. Also by this mechanism exercise lowers LDL cholesterol levels. In other words, decreased need for insulin results in a lessened stimulus to manufacture LDL cholesterol in the liver.

It has long ago been known that Growth Hormone levels decline with age. A sedentary life style accelerates this decline. Conversely, regular exercise increases IGF-1 levels secondary to increased Growth Hormone release.

These facts unite several health consequences of insulin resistance into a common thread of causality. There is sequential decline of growth hormone and IGF-1 levels with certain diets and lifestyles, with aging. The decline of these two hormones explains some of the insulin resistance occurring with advancing age and sedentary lifestyle. It also explains how regular exercise remedies insulin resistance by raising growth hormone and IGF-1 levels.

Applying this association could save owners the unnecessary complications of diabetes and the acceleration of their aging rate. Lastly, the fall in Growth Hormone levels brought about by a sedentary lifestyle explains why muscle and organ mass are lost. Growth Hormone conserves protein content. For this reason, unless owners have processes operating in their lives that encourage GH secretion, they will lose protein. Unfortunately, more than protein loss occurs when patients' doctors fail to have time for adequate study of the above listed valid hormonal considerations.

Some physicians are now committed to breaking free of the complex's 'shackles'. One movement, 'Keep It Simple', has origins in Seattle, Washington. The basic tenant is that a large proportion of health care expenditure goes to paperwork and time devoted to feeding the government and insurance bureaucracy. Physicians that participate in this movement have decided that good health care is facilitated when these interests are eviscerated from their workday. They no longer recognize insurance or government programs and as a consequence reduce the cost of an office visit per minute. In addition, they are freed intellectually to study and learn about the latest scientific paradigms.

Greater momentum would be realized if more owners understood the consequences to their doctor's ability to continue learning as long as they continue to jumps through bureaucratic hoops. Valuable energy expenditures in these wasteful pursuits leads inevitably to less time for one to follow their curiosity hunches to their logical conclusion.

A clear insight into the consequences of a medical system run by the profit interests of the complex is analogous to junk food. Although junk food tastes like food, it will harm the body if it is continually ingested. Owners are continually bombarded by clever methods of advertisement that encourage consumption of these injurious ingredients. Most owners know that these junk foods are harmful, but everyone else does it and they feel better. Slowly but surely more owners have become aware that environmentally contaminated foods, which are full of chemicals, toxins, and hormone mimics, will injure body functions. The food industry complex still touts the latest clever come on, but there are less gullible owners with each passing year.

The strategies of the profit driven health care system are becoming suspect. Many astute owners have cultivated an awareness of the need of the medical industrial complex to sensationalize what is for sale. Profit driven healthcare will remain partial to the expensive and symptom control medicine because there is no incentive and in some cases a disincentive to discuss the holism of what science has revealed.

Inexpensive solutions to health problems hurt profit margins that, when lowered, the tax that the government collects diminishes. Healing is bad for the economy and the government's ability to collect money.

Movements like 'Keep It Simple,' are a start to allow some physicians' time to rediscover their passion for healing. They have begun to discuss among themselves radical new ideas that are more consistent with the scientific evidence that has been revealed.

In many cases, the bond among physicians is stronger than the pigeonholes of the complex hierarchy. Good things are happening and many brave patients can be thanked for the help they have provided in stimulating doctors to learn. Patients often bring fresh ideas because they have had less brain washing history. Physicians often become vulnerable to narrow thinking because of their extended educations funded by the complex. Fortunately, many still possess the spark of curiosity that led them to their life's work. These are the physicians who are able to listen with an open mind about successful encounters for patients with alternative healing modalities. Alternative methods for healing begin to make mechanistic sense when some of the old scientific truths are re-included in the analysis. This can occur when the holism (commonly eviscerated from mainstream medical educations) of scientific revelation reunites with the pieces of disjointed medical thought so prevalent in the complex today.

One of the new paradigms developing concerns the hormones that promote lean body mass versus the hormones that encourage the liver to hog excessive nutrition. Unfortunately, when the liver becomes the nutritional hog of the body most other body cells remain hungry (*hungry cell syndrome*). Making matters worse concerns the fact that the vast majority of nutrients hogged by the liver become fat that is destined for the storage depots (fat and macrophages). Owners who suffer this fate can be thought of as living within the *torture chamber of desire* for the next feeding event. Thankfully, healing transpires when ways to exit the *torture chamber* are explored. In the next chapter, the ways out of the *torture chamber* will be examined.

Cutting edge scientific thought: Certain cases of insulin dependant diabetes (type I) are caused by gluten induced IgG antibodies. Avoiding this food type has reversed some cases of diabetes if caught before total islet cell burnout occurs (see bibliography).

CHAPTER FIFTEEN

AVOID THE
TORTURE CHAMBER DIET

Lack of attention to the consequences from abnormal hormone levels occurs with the complex endorsed diet. Abnormal hormones create abnormal urges in its adherent's feeding behavior. Abnormal hormones exaggerate feeding obsessions.

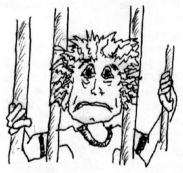

The torture chamber effect describes the feeding obsessions that result from this official diet. As long as the American public believes in the diet, endorsed by the complex, there will be continued economic need from the complications of obesity. Examples of these complications are: high blood pressure, diabetes, and heart disease. The dishonesty in the complex endorsed diet easily exposes itself when some basic but missing facts return to the analysis.

A narrow band of truth occurs in the complex endorsed diet but it concerns only one type of physique. The physique for which the complex endorsed diet works occurs in an athlete or adolescent who already exists at his/her ideal weight and/or peak performance. Peak performing athletes attain optimal weight and have achieved optimal physical fitness. Through training, genetics, and/or age, they have the right balance of hormones.

Owners at ideal weight and physical fitness levels have properly proportioned hormone message content. This allows the proper appetite stimulation and exercise motivation to continue. They can handle increased carbohydrate intake that necessitates only a slight increase in insulin production because they have high IGF-1 levels. They tolerate slight increases in insulin because their lifestyles and/or genetics allow a sufficient amount of IGF-1 counter hormone. Important point to consider here: The counter hormone

IGF-1, successfully counter weights the fat building message of insulin.

However, as middle age approaches, most owners are not endowed with superior amounts of androgen (section two) and Growth Hormone, which are necessary for high IGF-1 production rates and release to continue. Unfortunately, there has been little acknowledgment of basic scientific facts about the relationship of dietary choices and hormone consequences to feeding behavior. Some notable exceptions are found in the diet plans of Drs. Atkin's, Schwarzbein and Sears. Even fewer acknowledgments occur about the circular trap that feeding behavior dictates the consequence of which hormones secrete. This explains the vicious and circular trap overweight owners find themselves in, despite earnest attempts to diet.

When obese owners adhere to the complex endorsed diet's tenants, powerful hormones release. These stimulate a preoccupation with the next feeding and a decreased ability to shed fat. It is a travesty to withhold acknowledgment that the complex endorsed diet creates a virtual *torture chamber* of emotional desires in the owner who expends effort to make positive health changes when his/her attempts to change are doomed. Unfavorable hormones within destine them for eventual defeat. For this simple reason, weight loss efforts become hopeless until they obtain guidance about changing their hormones for the better.

Dr. Atkins was one of the first American physicians to recognize the powerful role that hormones play in feeding behavior. He did this by reviewing what was known about the hormone, insulin, in basic medical physiology textbooks. He studied cultures that do not have high rates of obesity and obesity related diseases. Dr. Atkins first began to apply what was known over thirty years ago about hormone levels and consequent feeding behavior.

He correctly reasoned that insulin levels that are allowed to reach higher than optimum levels act as a powerful appetite stimulant. This creates an obsessive preoccupation for the next feeding event. He understood that insulin has a dramatic effect on the ability of the body to manufacture fat. He also understood how insulin prevents the body from accessing fat reserves.

Health benefits from lowering insulin levels are receiving renewed interest. Lowered insulin levels will decrease the stimulation in the appetite center of the brain and also increase the ability to use fat for energy. Obesity is on the increase in America and it can rarely be curtailed without an improvement in feeding behavior hormones.

It is important to extend the important work of doctors like Atkins, Bernstein, Sears, and Schwarzbein. Their immense contributions allow consideration of the other obesity related hormones (chapter four). Briefly, the other hormones, in addition to insulin, that need to be normalized before weight loss occurs are cortisol, androgens, estrogen, IGF-1, epinephrine, and thyroid. Attention to the rebalancing of these hormones provides an extension of these authorities work and a magnification of the weight loss possible.

In addition, the importance of real food versus processed food also needs to be added into the plan. Real foods provide the mineral nutrition necessary for maximum avoidance of the complications from obesity related disease. The real food component of successful dieting explains why the opposite approach to dieting has some success. These diets for which Dean Ornish and Nathaniel Pritikin are most famous, do a better job about expressing the importance of real food in place of processed food. However, these diets fail their adherents because of the high insulin that results from the high carbohydrate content contained in these diets. In the end both diet camps on the extremes have some success, but each fails in maximizing success by ignoring either the hormones or the importance of real food.

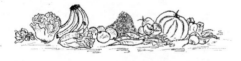

Consuming real food (from the garden, off the tree, organic eggs, fresh fish, fresh chicken and meats that have not been canned or salted) helps avoid ingredients that are easily missed in the high protein diet. High protein dieters need to take care not to consume high protein sources from processed food. Processed food is any food that comes in a box, bag or a can. The requirement of putting food into a box, bag or a can necessitates adding unbalanced minerals like sodium, which deviate from body design.

The diet that has the least success in the long haul is the ADA diet. The ADA diet takes the worst features from both diet extremes. It advises consumption of 50-60% of total daily calories from carbohydrate. Carbohydrate consumption in this proportion of total daily calories condemns the obese owners into a life within the vicious *torture chamber* cycle. Weight gain consequences occur because carbohydrates obligate a rise in insulin levels. The *torture chamber* also involves a degree of other hormone imbalances.

Do the math: An owner that needs 2000 calories a day and that adheres to this diet would obtain about 250 grams of carbohydrate a day if the 50% yardstick is used. Remember that normally the entire amount of sugar contained in the blood stream is about 6 grams. Add in the fact that the body can absorb dietary sugar at the rate of 2 grams a minute.

Making matters worse, over weight owners almost always have decreased IGF-1 (less than 150ng/ml) so they already need excessive insulin to process a sugar load. Excessive insulin spilling out of the pancreas confronts 200,000 pure insulin receptors per liver cell before a small fraction makes it beyond to serve as a fuel nozzle. This means the liver sucks up more of the sugar than the other body cells because it receives the most fuel nozzle hormones. Most of this sugar converts into fat and cholesterol because this is the major way the liver stores energy. This stuff is then packaged into LDL cholesterol and the liver secretes this into the blood stream. It is curious to this author that the mainstream textbooks fail to unite the above simple cause and effect relationships.

A discussion of the additional hormones involved in obesity brings up a concept that Dr. Atkins calls **metabolic resistance**. Metabolic resistance describes those women for whom the low carbohydrate diet proves slow to effect weight loss. However, this author feels that the high protein diet approach fails to acknowledge that many of these women need the added benefit of androgen (DHEA and testosterone).

Androgen deficiency explains some of the cause for this phenomenon quite well, as it is androgens that oppose fat gain. Fat gain opposition occurs because androgens provide message content to the liver to increase IGF-1 production. Visualize that more IGF-1 secreted competes with the insulin within the liver as to where fuel ends up, as fat or in the metabolically hungry cells, like muscles and organs. Fat gain accentuates in some female owners because they have less androgen compared to men. The removal of the ovaries and the onset of the menopause can exacerbate androgen deficiency. Consideration of the 24-hour urine test for steroid production will identify this type of metabolic resistance caused problem.

Once androgens are attended to, in as safe a way as possible, these metabolically stymied female owners need to understand how to encourage increased Growth Hormone release. Exercise and fasting will stimulate the capable pituitary's release of Growth Hormone. Recall, sufficient thyroid hormones within the pituitary direct the adequate manufacture of Growth Hormone. For this reason accurate thyroid function assessment proves important for any weight loss program.

An additional cause of **metabolic resistance** concerns the increased production rate of the stress hormone, cortisol. High cortisol and/or its metabolites levels in the urine identify other owners who have trouble with weight loss despite strict adherence to low carbohydrate diets. Most physicians miss this common fact because they fail to obtain 24-hour urine test for cortisol and its metabolites. In fact, often times the typical Syndrome X owner really suffers from an overactive stress response that leads to, in middle age, insulin resistance, high blood pressure, premature heart disease and obesity (see inflammation and heart disease in the heart chapter).

High stress will increase cortisol release. Increased cortisol in a setting of mental stress will elevate blood sugar inappropriately (encourages gluconeogenesis) and it will only come down with exercise or increased insulin secretion. It is the increased insulin secretion brought on by stress occurring in a sedentary lifestyle that leads to obesity. The intensity of the problem often magnifies because many weight gain prone owner's adrenal glands prove particularly adept at cortisol production when they feel stress. Also, chronic excessive gluconeogenesis (protein catabolism) slowly destroys these owners metabolism because protein adequacy determines caloric expenditure potential.

Often times, obese owners make more cortisol with the same amount of life stress compared to a non-obese owner. Increased cortisol causes an inappropriate increase in blood fuel that has nowhere to go in a sedentary owner until insulin releases. Only exercise and stress management will provide a way to stop this hormone cycle in the torture chamber.

Remember, thyroid hormone levels need to be carefully evaluated. The thyroid gland determines the rate at which calories can be burned in the cell power plants (see thyroid chapter and chapter four). As mentioned above, it also powerfully determines how much Growth Hormone the pituitary manufactures. This dependency explains, in part, why thyroid hormone deficiency owners age so quickly: Recall, Growth Hormone provides the only defense of body protein content during fasting or exercising states. Adequate defense of protein allows a healthy metabolism to continue into middle age and beyond. Adequate metabolism allows the body to better participate in the life experience.

Estrogen levels, when high, as occurs in pregnancy and birth control pill usage, exacerbates the obesity problem in some female owners. Environmental estrogen problems can occur in men and women (see hormone mimics). High estrogen levels stimulate Growth Hormone release, but inhibit IGF-1 release. This aberration leads to insulin resistance because less IGF-1 becomes available to help insulin with fuel uptake by the cells outside of the liver and fat. Consequently, increased insulin becomes necessary to bring the blood fuel level back to normal. The higher the insulin level, the more liver fat making machinery is stimulated to make fat and cholesterol. More fat then becomes available for storage sites in the liver, arteries, and fat cells.

Recall, the placenta rescues most pregnant women's high estrogen state by increasing the secretion of human placental lactogen, which increases its IGF-1 production to 2-3 times normal blood levels. However, the high estrogen states of women on estrogen prescriptions do not have a placenta to correct the fall of IGF-1. High estrogen levels cause a fall of IGF-1 and these owners' liver make more fats from the high insulin needed to correct the deficit. Note that it is the high cortisol levels of the pregnant state that are thought to cause insulin resistance (see cortisol discussion as to why this is so).

Epinephrine release is an extension of the stress response. Like cortisol it contains message content that instructs the liver to elevate fuel in the blood stream. When mental stress occurs there becomes little need for the extra fuel in the blood stream. Eventually, insulin needs to be released to normalize excess blood sugar caused by mental stress's inappropriate elevation of the blood fuel. Increased insulin leads to an increased fat making message in liver and fat cells.

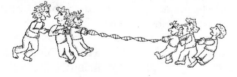

A 'tug of war' exists between the hormones that help shed fat and the hormones that make fat. It is worthwhile to assess whether these interrelating hormones occur in excess, deficiency, or are present in the optimal amounts needed for a healthy body.

Thin people who eat as much as they want are not always fine specimens of raging androgen production. Deficiency in muscle mass usually provides a clue that increased androgen may not be the reason for their perpetual thinness. Emaciated skinniness in the presence of increased caloric intake can be due to poor digestive absorption of critical nutrients. Still other owners become unable to manufacture extra insulin in a setting of increased carbohydrate intake. They never develop diagnosable diabetes because their pancreas limps along with just enough insulin and liver IGF-1 output to keep it from spilling over into the urine (see liver chapter).

All of the Popular Diets Today Miss Vital Consideration for Weight Loss (Each has Part of the Puzzle, But Not the Whole Picture)

Two different extremes in diet philosophy have been introduced. Each has a part of the puzzle that will help shed fat. Each also contains an impediment to weight loss. The best science in each diet's approach needs incorporation, while avoiding its downside.

High protein and fat with low carbohydrate diet plans are incomplete in their effectiveness because they do not emphasize the importance for obtaining the right mineral ratios. Their incompleteness sheds light on how some of the other diets have a weight loss effect. Some other diets have a weight loss effect because they inadvertently partially address mineral balance. The omission of mineral balance creates the hormone imbalances (higher insulin) that the high protein diet philosophy attempts to avoid. Mineral imbalance will occur any time processed food dominates in the diet.

On the up side, the high protein diet leads to lower insulin levels. In contrast, the upside of the fresh and raw food dieters is that they contain properly proportioned minerals that will better help with hormone balance. On the downside these diets contain higher carbohydrate so the insulin need becomes higher. **Higher insulin levels prove counter-productive to any diet effort.** Mineral intake balance is important to decrease the obesity hormones initially.

The Body's Mineral Design Conservation Features are Obsolete in Face of the Processed Food Diet

The human body was designed for a natural mineral ratios intake. This would be a minimum of three to one ratio for potassium compared to sodium. In addition, there should be sufficient magnesium to counter calcium. **Unfortunately, the sodium and potassium intake ratio more than reverses when one adheres to a processed food diet.** Magnesium intake is commonly deficient as well.

In prehistoric times a survival advantage occurred for anyone who could retain sodium. Natural food is relatively deficient in sodium content compared to potassium. When one eats natural food (real food) the potassium to sodium mineral ratio is greater than three to one. **However, processed food has a drastically altered mineral content. Processed food diets have greatly diminished potassium and magnesium content. At the same time a processed food diet has a greatly increased amounts of sodium added to preserve the shelf life of the product. This combination causes a chronic imbalance between potassium and sodium (see mineral table).**

The same owner types that once, in prehistoric times, had a survival advantage now have a disadvantage if a processed diet is chronically consumed. These owners retain sodium inappropriately and have reversed mineral content included in the processed food diet (see mineral table). Around middle age owners on a processed food diet will develop a whole range of health consequences. This indulgence causes six obesity related health consequences. **Realize the owners who predispose to health consequences from the high sodium and low potassium diet were the genetically superior human design machines of prehistoric times. However, in modern times, as long as they adhere to a processed food diet, they remain on a rapid self-destruct program.**

Six Different Ways Obesity Propagates Secondary to the Mineral Imbalance occurring around Middle Age:

7. **Insulin resistance**
8. **Increased fat and cholesterol synthesis in the liver**
9. **Loss of protein content**
10. **Decreased steroid biosynthesis to keep blood pressure normal**
11. **Slower metabolic rate**
12. **Stress exacerbates the mineral imbalance and weight gain**

All six of these factors need to be circumvented if one desires an effective weight loss rate. If one optimizes all seven hormones (section two) that lead to obesity and corrects their mineral imbalance, their diet plan becomes more complete because they now apply the best from the different diets available. Concurrently they also omit obsolete components of these other diets in light of new scientific understanding. These are important if one really wants to know what makes them fat. When owners know what makes them fat they can progress. After all, becoming aware is part of healing.

Chronic Mineral Imbalanced Diets Cause One Type of Insulin Resistance

The chronic consumption of a mineral imbalanced diet will lead to the need for increased insulin secretion. Increased insulin becomes necessary because insulin needs sufficient potassium to deliver sugar into the cells. One potassium ion helps carry one sugar molecule out of the blood stream and into a cell.

The chronic ingestion of reversed ratios between potassium and sodium leads to a decreased availability of potassium for insulin directed sugar removal out of the blood stream. The delay of the blood lowering effect of insulin leads the pancreas to secrete more insulin eventually.

The delay of potassium availability occurs after many years of consuming reversed mineral ratios. The blood stream amount of potassium contains only 2% of body potassium. The other 98% of potassium resides in the cells. It is the potassium in the cells that sacrifices itself to keep the smaller potassium pool constant in the blood stream.

Owners that eat processed foods will inevitably deplete their total potassium. The potassium in the blood stream can be thought of as the 2% 'tank' of potassium content. It is the very last tank to deplete. Unfortunately, the standard blood test performed at the doctor's office measures the serum component in the blood stream only. Realize the blood stream value will only change after the larger tank severely depletes. The larger tank, containing 98% of potassium resides inside the numerous cells. Cells, including red blood cells, will sacrifice their potassium content in order to keep the blood levels in the normal range.

Herein reveals the deception occurring in America today: Physicians wrongly reassure their patients about the potassium levels in their blood stream while they have not inquired about the status of the larger tank. Failure to consider the consequences that ensue when the body becomes chronically deprived of the correct ratios between potassium and sodium intake leads to chronic degenerative diseases. Insulin resistance related disease is only one of several consequences of diminished potassium compared to sodium content.

Examples of chronic degenerative diseases that have a component of causality as a consequence of imbalanced potassium to sodium intake are: adult onset diabetes, high blood pressure, high cholesterol, and obesity, fatigue, and anxiety syndromes.

Insulin resistance can eventually progress into adult onset diabetes (liver chapter). The accompanying signs of obesity, high blood pressure and an abnormal cholesterol profile often associate with adult onset diabetes. The mineral balance between potassium and sodium dramatically affects all four of these processes. Misery propagates when this important relationship remains ignored.

One type of insulin resistance is caused by a chronic imbalance between potassium and sodium intake. As the mineral imbalance increases more insulin secretes to normalize sugar intake because most cells require potassium to bring sugar aboard. For each sugar transported, into most cell types, requires one potassium ion. The trouble arises from the fact that the cells donate their potassium to the blood stream when potassium occurs in scarce supply. Unfortunately, the needed potassium donation occurs by sacrificing the potassium content of body cells (98% tank of body potassium).

The pancreas senses that the blood sugar remains elevated and more insulin eventually releases, as the cells sacrifice potassium the blood sugar eventually normalizes. Important but often overlooked point to ponder: Potassium deficiency inhibits insulin release and this causes blood sugar-lowering delays, but eventually the cells sacrifice potassium and more insulin releases. These details explain some cases of postprandial elevated blood sugar problems (diabetic glucose tolerance curves).

Insulin resistance describes the increased amount of insulin needed to do the same job for a specific sugar load. When an owner's pancreas exhausts in its ability to produce additional insulin, then adult onset diabetes results and blood sugar begins to rise. However, many people's pancreases prove able to keep making more and more insulin and therefore they do not develop diabetes. Unfortunately, the high insulin levels make both of these types of owners obese and to have abnormal cholesterol production rates. The only difference between these two types of owners concerns that in one the pancreas reaches exhaustion and consequently the blood sugar rises.

In both types the high insulin levels promote the blood vessels sequestering fat. The ability of insulin to lower the blood sugar depends on sufficient potassium. Less potassium availability delays the ability of insulin to lower the blood sugar level.

Eventually more potassium leeches out of the cells and the pancreas senses this delay and more insulin eventually secretes. The immediate consequence occurs within the body cells that sacrificed their potassium content, which insulin needs to work. For example, cells need potassium to charge up their voltage and to stabilize proteins.

Visualize excessive insulin allowing more meal nutrition to be hogged within the liver. Recall, the anatomy of insulin secretion allows the liver to receive the majority of its message content before even a small amount makes it beyond the liver's 200,000 pure insulin receptors per liver cell.

The end result is that the peripheral cells receive less nutrition. They need adequate potassium to bring sugar aboard. In contrast, the liver uptakes a higher amount of sugar and processes it into more fat and cholesterol than is healthy because potassium is not needed by the liver when it converts sugar into fat. However, in order for the liver to store sugar as glycogen there needs to be a fixed amount of potassium available. Again the potassium deficiency changes the balance from the way that healthy livers store energy.

Blood vessels get fat and people get fat when the fat maker message is present. Insulin always delivers the fat maker message. If there is no insulin, there is no fat. With high insulin there will be more body fat. The potassium deficiency of middle age is one cause of insulin resistance.

Increased Cholesterol and Fat Synthesis in the Liver

Increasing message content in the liver to make more cholesterol and fat occurs when insulin resistance develops. Cholesterol and fat are made from the sugar that does not enter other cells because of diminished potassium content. Diminished potassium content impedes the ability of the peripheral cells, like muscle cells, to uptake carbohydrate nutrition.Consequently, in these cases the increased blood sugar becomes more liver accessible. The liver does not need potassium to suck sugar out of the blood stream and begin making fat and cholesterol. All the liver needs are adequate message content from insulin to begin sucking out the blood sugar. However, the liver still needs adequate potassium, like other cells to store sugar as glycogen.

Remember, glycogen storage requires fixed amounts of potassium to sugar. Without adequate potassium the liver is only able to make cholesterol and fat. Making matters worse, the increased availability of sugar in the liver and the excessive insulin message required here accelerate the liver manufacture rate of cholesterol and fat particles. These in turn are later processed into LDL cholesterol. Increased levels of LDL (high cholesterol and triglyceride content) cholesterol provide a hallmark of high insulin states. This mechanism explains the potassium deficient diet's contribution to this problem.

In the insulin resistant state, at the level of the liver, the low carbohydrate diet can fail to protect the owner because no one has counseled them about their potassium deficiency. Potassium deficiency will lead to increased insulin production (insulin resistance) even on a low carbohydrate diet. If these owners restore total potassium content (it often takes 3 to 6 months), their insulin needs will drop dramatically over time.

Consider the many owners on diuretic pills to control their high blood pressure. High potassium intake pulls water into the cells and out of the blood stream (a blood pressure lowering effect). Conversely, high sodium pulls water into the blood stream (a blood pressure elevating effect). Diuretics unfortunately pull potassium along with sodium out of the body. This last fact explains the insulin resistance, worsening cholesterol, and more difficult hypertension problem that eventually ensues for owners chronically ingesting these prescriptions.

Many owners on low carbohydrate diets do not correct their potassium deficiency and this alone causes an increase in their insulin levels. The increased insulin levels direct the liver to produce greater amounts of LDL cholesterol from the little carbohydrate consumed. When LDL cholesterol levels increase there becomes an increased risk for blood vessel disease and obesity. The increased insulin level directs both of these disease processes.

However, when an owner increases their potassium content they will be able to tolerate more carbohydrates without abnormal increases in their insulin levels. Obese owners are warned to initially curtail carbohydrates dramatically to decrease the appetite center activation that insulin directs. Eventually, the more normal the weight becomes the more carbohydrates from real food allowed.

The reason adequate potassium content in the body figures so importantly for controlling cholesterol concerns two factors. First, it enhances its ability to help normalize blood sugar with less insulin. Less insulin means less fat and cholesterol synthesis in the liver. Recall, the liver is a faithful servant that does as the message directs. Second, sufficient potassium is needed before the liver can store sugar as glycogen. Alternatively, diminished potassium availability stimulates that the liver removed sugar convert into cholesterol and fat.

The tug of war between glucagon and insulin in the liver was previously discussed. The low carbohydrate diet, in the presence of adequate body potassium, allows more glucagon message content. More glucagon message content will, in physically active owners, curtail fat and cholesterol synthesis. This explains why owners on high protein and fat diets with low carbohydrate intake have decreased cholesterol levels.

Realize the fact that one needs adequate potassium for their body to hold onto protein. This fact has been known by science for over fifty years. Remember decreased protein content causes shrinking muscles, organs, skin, and bones. In addition, proteins comprise the metabolically active (they burn calories) constituent of the body.

Mineral Imbalanced Diets Lead to the Loss of Body Protein

Owners that arrive at middle age with a history of consuming processed food diets will experience chronic protein depletion in their tissues. These bodies sacrifice cellular proteins in order to obtain sufficient potassium for the blood stream. This process takes many years to manifest. Even though their protein depletes at a slow rate, eventually these middle-aged victims begin to look typical. Usually it manifests as an increased middle area from fat accumulation and smaller muscles in the limbs and chest areas. The protein depletion also shrinks the size of their organs.

The protein depletion process occurs because potassium in the cells stabilizes the protein content. When a cell loses potassium the protein content will decrease. Little muscles, little organs, and shriveled skin result from mineral imbalanced diets because processed food contains an altered mineral content.

Less body protein translates to decreased cell function in the affected cells and less need for cell energy. Less energy equates to fewer calories needed before weight gain occurs. Less energy also means less ability to participate in what life has to offer. The cycle of obesity breaks when a middle-aged owner begins to understand how to regain mineral balance. The first step of this process involves a commitment to real food diets that restore mineral intake in their proper proportions (see mineral table).

Mineral Deficient Diets Reduce Steroid Production to Have Normal Blood Pressure

The body, which chronically feeds on altered mineral ratios, faces a difficult choice in middle age: It can try to maintain steroid production, but the side effect is an increase in blood pressure. Alternately, some bodies decrease steroid manufacture, but blood pressure normalizes.

Owners that eat a real food diet can secrete optimal amounts of aldosterone without raising blood pressure because they consume the right ratios of minerals. Conversely, owners that eat processed foods consume mineral ratios that destroy body functions. These altered minerals eventually strain the ability to keep an appropriate mineral balance.

The altered mineral balance causes the middle age problem in both cases. Some bodies increase blood pressure to continue manufacturing adequate steroids that depends on adequate aldosterone production in the adrenal (see below). Other bodies diminish aldosterone production, but have a normal blood pressure. Although these owner's bodies have normal blood pressure they will age more quickly because of their lowered steroid production rates. Lowered steroid production rates mean that there will be less rejuvenation message content. Less rejuvenation message content leads to the accumulation of wear and tear changes in these bodies. The more wear and tear changes accumulate the older that body looks and feels.

Aldosterone gives the message to the adrenals and gonads to increase steroid production. Owners do not tolerate increased aldosterone levels with mineral imbalances between potassium and sodium. Potassium and sodium imbalanced owners will conserve excess fluid when aldosterone levels elevate. Excess fluid leads to blood pressure elevation.

Mineral Imbalances Lead to a Slower Metabolism

The diminished protein content slows the metabolic rate. Protein content comprises the active metabolic fraction (the part that burns calories) of body tissue. Proteins, like enzymes and mineral pumps, consume energy and therefore metabolize calories. Metabolism also slows with mineral imbalance because there is less electrical potential across mineral depleted cell membranes. Here, mineral imbalance slows metabolism because it diminishes cellular charge (the cell voltage). The majority of energy expenditure in the body, at rest, concerns recharging its trillions of cell membranes (the cells' voltage). Visualize 70 trillion body cells as miniature batteries. These can only recharge adequately when the right mineral ratios oppose one another.

Each cell uses the cell membrane charge energy to sustain life. Less membrane energy content occurs when the minerals alter from their optimal proportion. This is similar to what would happen to a car battery that had its mineral content altered. As the car battery membrane's mineral concentration alters so does its ability to perform useful work. Car batteries function better when the manufacture adds in the proper mineral proportions between the membranes. This fact is a prerequisite before maximal charge can occur. So it is with body cells, before they can charge optimally the right mineral proportions need to be available.

The food industry is not cognizant of this basic body design feature. Magnesium and potassium deplete in food from processing it. Next large amounts of sodium combine into processed food in order to retard spoilage. This formula of altered mineral ratios dumps into cells year after year (see mineral table). Around middle age feeble cell batteries lead to weakness, fatigue, diminished calories burned and weight gain (*the low cell voltage syndrome*).

Stress Exacerbates Mineral Imbalance

Mental stress increases insulin need. Recall, the stress response elevates the blood sugar. This feature of the stress response was designed to survive physical stress but with mental stress the fuel has nowhere to go. The pancreas eventually senses the elevated blood sugar and insulin is released into the portal vein.

Increased insulin leads to an increased fat making message content. However, there is an additional way that chronic stress makes fat. It concerns the extra potassium loss that cortisol causes. Cortisol increases during the stress response.

Increased cortisol causes increased sodium retention and increased potassium loss. This aldosterone like effect of cortisol occurs because at high levels cortisol will create message content similar to aldosterone in its sodium retentive effects. Sodium retention and potassium wasting are not a problem with normal levels of cortisol. Cortisol at normal levels is weak in its message content to retain sodium and excrete potassium.

Surgeons are well aware of this fact. The body cannot survive the stress of surgery unless there is a massive output of cortisol from the adrenal glands. The increased cortisol excretion rate depletes potassium. For this reason, surgeons routinely give intravenous potassium postoperatively because the owner's body will secrete increased cortisol in order to survive the stress of surgery.

The increased potassium in the IV prevents a precipitous fall in body potassium. With mineral balance in mind the real food diet that allows this is contrasted with the processed food diet.

Two Diets on Opposite Extremes in Mineral Content

Real food is high in potassium and magnesium, unprocessed and low in sodium (see mineral table for specifics).

Fresh vegetables	Fresh fruit
Eggs	Fresh meat, chicken and fish
Low salt cheese	Brown sugar
Unprocessed rice	Unprocessed grains
Unprocessed nuts	Unprocessed beans (dry or fresh)
Potatoes	Avocados

Processed food is high in sodium content, but low in both magnesium and potassium

- Anything that comes in a box
- Anything that comes in a can
- Anything from a fast food restaurant
- Anything that has more sodium content than potassium content
- Some frozen foods have sodium added
- Store bought bread, with a few exceptions
- Condiments (catsup, soy sauce, salad dressing, steak sauce, and pickles)

A general goal is to obtain over four thousand milligrams of potassium, less than one thousand milligrams of sodium, over three hundred milligrams of magnesium and about five hundred milligrams of calcium a day.

A word of caution becomes necessary for those owners that are already overweight. Overweight owners need further dietary restriction within the real foods that are high in carbohydrate content. Even though some foods are real foods, when an owner is already overweight, the high carbohydrate foods need to be further restricted. Carbohydrate curtailment allows insulin needs to drop.

A lowered insulin need is the primary move for exiting the *torture chamber*. Once one moves outside the *torture chamber*, they can begin to lose weight. Weight loss accelerates when both the carbohydrate intake and the mineral imbalanced components are corrected.

As a normal weight approaches, there will be increased tolerance for more carbohydrate. Every owner's physiology differs and needs the counsel of a competent physician for sustained weight loss to occur. A good place to start involves the almost complete elimination of carbohydrate contained real food and all processed foods. The high carbohydrate containing real foods are potatoes, rice, beans, grains, brown sugar, honey, and pasta. Following this initial approach will counter the IGF-1 deficit occurring in obesity by creating less insulin-produced side effects. Once the target weight, mineral balance, and hormone balance are achieved, some carbohydrates, from real food sources can be allowed. Again, each owner's physiology is unique. The counsel of a competent physician is necessary.

As a general guide keep carbohydrates consumption below 100 grams a day. Very few middle aged and Syndrome X types can consume more than this much carbohydrate a day without gaining weight and seeing their blood fats worsen.

Summary of the Weight Loss Considerations:

- Optimal hormone levels for insulin, cortisol, androgens, estrogen, thyroid, epinephrine, and IGF-1
- An exercise program to counteract cortisol and increase Growth Hormone
- Stress management
- Real foods diet that provides a balanced mineral intake
- Correct nutritional deficiencies (see nutritional deficiency in section one)

Case History (Application of Weight Loss Principles)

Philip was a forty-three year old professional that began to notice weight gain over the last several years. His weight gain occurred despite a vigorous work out schedule that was often one hour long for each session. Workouts included runs in the mountains; strenuous uphill climbs, and prolonged mountain bike rides. Despite his commitment to fitness training, he continued to notice a slow, but progressive 'fat tire' around his midsection. He attempted to follow the ADA diet and was always hungry. Food was constantly on his mind. He was in the torture chamber. Hormones drove his excessive feeding behavior.

Eventually Philip came across some high protein diet type books and figured it would not hurt to give this contrary advice a try. In these books it was explained how to get insulin levels down and how this would greatly diminish the preoccupation with the next feeding event.

Through my counsel, Philip eventually went on to learn about several other hormones that affect feeding behavior and the tendency to gain weight. He also began to understand the hefty contribution of insulin to his high cholesterol level. To Philip's credit he exercised regularly, which increased his testosterone production and secretion from the gonads. Testosterone counteracts the desire of insulin to make fat by raising IGF-1 production. He came to understand that even with regular exercise, middle age leads to a tendency for decreased testosterone production.

Philip began to understand how increased carbohydrates consumption increases his insulin secretion that eventually tips the scale, in the setting of falling testosterone, for increased fat manufacture. The middle-aged body tolerates less carbohydrate because IGF-1 levels have fallen consequent to a fall in testosterone levels (note: DHEA is also important here).

Marked genetic variability occurs for how much insulin one needs to stimulate the liver into excessive production of LDL cholesterol. When LDL and/or triglyceride levels elevate, as a general rule, then suspect high insulin as the culprit. Remember that diminished thyroid function, specific nutritional deficiencies and very rare genetic defects can cause the same abnormalities of increased blood fat of this type. Strict adherence to a low carbohydrate diet will dramatically lower LDL cholesterol in most people. The status of other hormones (thyroid, androgen, cortisol, IGF-1, estrogens, and adrenaline) importantly affects any weight loss effort. Finally, mineral balance and its influence on insulin levels need to be optimized if weight and cholesterol normalization is to be realized.

Individuals with high testosterone (athletes, young adult males, and body builders) can tolerate a higher carbohydrate intake. Likewise, an owner with mineral balance between sodium and potassium can handle more carbohydrate intake. In both cases, these owners need less insulin to move sugar into their cells. Less insulin correlates with a diminished fat manufacture rate.

It is the high testosterone and Growth Hormone, with consequent IGF-1 increases, combination occurring in youth that allows a decreased insulin equirement. The increased Growth Hormone levels increase IGF-1 release, which facilitates sugar uptake out of the blood stream without the fat manufacture message content contained in the insulin hormone.

Once fat begins to accumulate the body hormones must change in order to return to a trim physique. This summarizes what happened to Philip before he realized this fundamental fact in the attainment of a more youthful physique again.

When an owner achieves his/her optimal weight, some increased (tailored to activity level) carbohydrate intake becomes allowed. Owners like Philip need to understand that by decreasing their insulin and cutting back on carbohydrates, they will decrease the stimulation of their appetite center in the brain.

As owners head into middle age they destine themselves to failure if they adhere to the ADA diet. Failure usually manifests as a slow, but steady increase in abdominal obesity measured from one year to the next. **The *torture chamber* always wins until a hormonal harmony facilitates weight loss again.**

Knowledge provides power to take action in the destiny of one's physique. This happened in Philip's case as he applied basic hormone knowledge his 'middle aged physique' began to rejuvenate to a closer version of his youth. He also noted a dramatic decrease of total cholesterol and LDL cholesterol (triglycerides). This means that Philip will have to watch carbohydrates more closely than others because a return to unfavorable cholesterol will always result if insulin levels again increase.

This dramatic improvement in Philip's LDL cholesterol and triglycerides occurred despite his eating four eggs with extra cheese every morning for breakfast. This effect explains the ability of the high protein and fat diet to raise glucagon while lowering insulin. The change in the hormone ratio will turn down the rate of liver synthesized cholesterol.

Philip received an added weight loss advantage by regularly engaging in aerobic exercise that of course burns calories but also stimulates the gonads to manufacture and release increased androgens. The ratio between glucagon and insulin will improve with regular exercise. Glucagon turns off cholesterol synthesis in the liver and increases fuel in the blood stream. However, increased fuel release caused by the glucagon message, without a corresponding adequate exercise program, eventually requires more insulin. Viewed in this way, it becomes clearer why regular exercise proves as one of the biochemical advantages for prolonged health.

Later in the workup process, I noted high stress operating in his life. Prolonged stress depletes adrenal glands and affects the quality of the adrenal secretion. It does this by increasing cortisol release rates that directs energy away from cellular rejuvenation and into survival pathways. In addition, when stress is prolonged it shifts away from the optimal ratio between DHEA (an adrenal androgen with testosterone-like activity) and cortisol production (decreased quality of the adrenal secretion).

More cortisol and less DHEA production result from the chronic stress response. Making matters worse, increased cortisol is one of the hormones that direct the gonads to manufacture and release (by a circuitous pathway) less androgen. The increased amount of cortisol also directs the liver to dump sugar into the blood stream. Unfortunately, modern stress is usually mental in nature. Remember, this extra sugar cannot be used without physical activity. When this sedentary stress occurs, insulin releases to bring the blood sugar back down to normal.

When stress becomes the operational emotion there needs to be consideration about the message content to raise blood sugar even when no carbohydrates are eaten. Now this discussion flips things on their head. As cortisol increases, the reoccurring body theme that the hormones need balance comes into play. The only difference here concerns the fact that stress creates a situation where cortisol is the weight that needs the counter weight of insulin to put the breaks on the increase in blood sugar. This fact provides another mechanism for creating a torture chamber within if prolonged stress occurs.

The fact that cortisol raises blood sugar makes sense teleologically when one remembers the advantage of increased blood fuel in physical survival situations. Prehistorically, when a human ran from the jaws of some large animal, a rapid rise in blood sugar conferred a survival advantage by increasing the physical strength. Ample fuel in the blood stream facilitates muscle fuel delivery. However, the problem today occurs because many stresses are psychological (mental). The predominance of psychological stress means that no flight ever comes. Here, the stress molecules circulate and direct valuable energy inappropriately. **One of the inappropriate consequences of mental stress concerns the increased blood sugar that it causes.**

The final point about Philip was the hardest part for him to realize. Mineral imbalance in middle age plays a substantial role in fat production. Little recognition occurs between the connection for mineral balance and fat reduction. This information remains missing from many diets offered today (see above mineral balance discussion).

Philip eventually began to appreciate the many similarities between car batteries and his cells. He began to realize that he would not alter the intended mineral composition of a car battery any more than he would his trillions of cells. This relationship helped him to understand that unless he took in mineral ratios similar to body design, his many cell batteries would deplete. When minerals are consumed in the proper design ratios the cell batteries can charge. Only a body that has fully charged cell batteries can sufficiently liberate enough potassium into the blood stream to help sugar enter cells. Adequate potassium lowers insulin requirements dramatically. The mineral determinant is the fifth determinant of how much insulin a body needs to normalize its blood sugar. All five determinants were eventually improved in Philip's life.

In summary, the five basic determinants of insulin requirements are:
1. Carbohydrate load
2. Mental stress load
3. Exercise level
4. IGF-1 levels (dependent on both Growth Hormone and androgen levels). Excessive estrogen can also decrease IGF-1 despite Growth Hormone and total androgen levels being normal or high.
5. Mineral ratios of intake within the diet.

When these five basic determinants become optimal an owner will have a normal insulin level. Other factors exist (see earlier discussion on hormones), but these make up the central players of the fat manufacture rate potential in a body. They need to be reconciled first and the other factors can be worked on later.

This entire section has been about how the body assimilates molecular replacement parts. Additionally, it continued the discussion of how the healthy body directs these parts appropriately while the unhealthy body does not. This section also touched on the important role of certain organ systems in allowing the ever-accumulating body trash to exit. The colon discussion began this important topic. In the next section, four additional organ systems will be reviewed that also contribute to the body's ability to eliminate waste.

SECTION FOUR

SECTION FOUR *344*

    PRINCIPLE FIVE: TAKING OUT THE TRASH WATER345

CHAPTER SIXTEEN 348

    KIDNEYS 348

CHAPTER SEVENTEEN 374

    LUNGS 374

CHAPTER EIGHTEEN 399

    SKIN 399

CHAPTER NINETEEN 418

    LIVER   418

PRINCIPLE FIVE: TAKING OUT THE TRASH WATER

Some people collect trash in their yards, houses, and cars. Grime is everywhere. So it is with certain owner's cells that collect

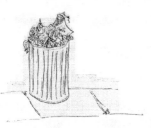

trash water within their body tissues and chambers. These cells cry out for someone to please take out the garbage. Dirty cells lose functional ability. The most powerful trash remover, water, needs the help of certain body organ systems. These organ systems filter out the trash water or recycle it after being purified.

The trash collectors of the body, filters and purifying plants, fall under the domain of six organ systems; the lungs, kidneys, liver, skin, colon, and immune system. A common factor occurs, besides water, which determines the functional ability of the six trash removal organs. All six of these organs need adequate thyroid message content. Recall, the thyroid message is among the most powerful hormone class, the level one-type hormones. Only these most powerful hormones directly instruct these organ types' cellular DNA programs (genes).

Thyroid message content facilitates infrastructure development activities in the cells of these six organ systems. Failure to recognize this central determinant for trash removal systems has significant health consequences. All six of these organ systems need adequate thyroid message content to function. For this reason and others, inadequate thyroid message content results in prematurely old bodies. This fact underscores the relationship between the fifth and third (optimal informational message content) principles of healthful longevity.

Diminished thyroid function in these six trash removal organ manifests:
1. Within the lungs as decreased ability to increase oxygen delivery under physical stress. Thyroid hormone, in lung tissue, forms a determinate for the lung's ability to respond to increasing adrenaline message content.
2. Within the kidneys the thyroid level determines infrastructure investment activities of kidney cells. This keeps the kidney tissue from succumbing to filtration

pressures, which desire to inflict harm on the delicate epithelium, which lines the functional unit of kidney, the nephron.

3. The liver cells depend on thyroid message content to direct the investment in the rejuvenation of the liver cell.

4. When thyroid message content falls at the level of the skin cell, there are many deleterious changes that ensue that include:

   a. Dryness, scales, the puffiness of myxedema, and yellow discoloration

   b. Hair thins with additional premature grayness and brittleness.

5. When these clinical signs occur in the skin, the less obvious role of the skin in trash removal also diminishes

6. Low thyroid at the level of the colon manifests clinically as chronic constipation that causes backward absorption of many putrefaction molecules. These leaking back into the body can eventually overwhelm the ability of the liver to detoxify them and they can spill into the general circulation.

7. In the immune system, diminished thyroid message content decreases the ability of immune type cells to consume (phagocytize) unwanted cells (cancer, bacteria, virus', and debris).

Failure to take out the trash, which continuously generates within the cells, can lead to some chronic degenerative diseases such as certain types of arthritis, tumor growths, degenerative skin changes, diminished organ function, and some of the mental deterioration syndromes.

The body has an ongoing problem caused by the toxic waste that spews out of its trillions of cellular factories. Owners who practice habits that improve waste removal strategies enjoy an advantage in the maintenance of their physical health. Alternatively, owners who stuff their cells with waste begin to look like they feel.

Waste products build up in the cells, around the cells, and in the blood stream. External sources of trash add to the internally generated accumulations and increase the overall waste removal burden. Examples of these external trash generators are the increased air pollutants, water pollutants, food adulterants, and toxicities from prescription drug breakdown products.

A useful metaphor that addresses trash accumulation is found in the rivers, deltas, and lakes of the earth. Only when the river that feeds the deltas and lakes remains clean, can downstream entities stay pristine. When factories dump waste into streams and rivers, not only the river becomes polluted. The downstream deltas and lakes suffer contamination as well.

The ongoing problem of cellular trash removal has many of the same challenges. Pristine mountain lakes prove similar to young cells in the non-polluted state. The wilderness river deltas with their delicate ecosystems that depend on clean water are like the spaces between the cells (the interstitial space). The rivers receive both the clean and the polluted tributary waters. River purity and blood stream purity become compromised when 'factories' dump toxins into them. The actions of life create waste that constantly dumps into the blood stream.

Unlike the physical world of rivers, deltas, and lakes, the body has elaborate cleansing systems built into the waterway system. These elaborate cleansing systems remove toxins and purify wastewater. The ability to remove the ever-generating waste depends on the health of these six organ systems.

Unhealthy cells, much like polluted lakes, accumulate trash water, secondary to a failure of these trash removal systems. This process also describes what happens to water that surrounds cells and fluids in the waterways (plasma, lymph, and cerebral spinal fluid). Failure of the trash removal systems in the cells, around the cells, and in the blood stream causes trash water accumulation. Many health problems arise simply because no one helps these owners heal their six trash removal organ systems.

Body composition normally contains (approximately) 67% water. Generous supplies of clean water bathe tissues. Adequate clean water allows the toxins to flush away. Ongoing trash removal enlivens continued health. However, some owners accumulate trash water because the capacity of their trash removal systems suffers decline. Each of the six trash removal organ systems has unique contributions and abilities. An interrelationship occurs between these sanitation and recycling facilities.

This new principle describes where the cellular trash comes from and how the body design disposes of it. The different types of cellular trash and where they originate will be considered. Kidneys are the first trash removal organs that will be discussed. Some other functions of the kidneys, maintenance and health are also included.

CHAPTER SIXTEEN

KIDNEYS

The kidneys filter the fluids that pass through the blood stream. They decide what to keep and what to discard when the blood passes through its filters. The kidney comprises one of the main trash collectors for the small and electrically charged 'dust' particles. Electrically charged 'atomic dust' particles result from food combustion. When food metabolizes certain charged particles evolve as byproducts and become the waste of the cellular factories. This process describes one type of cellular waste that discharges into the waterways (the blood stream and lymphatics).

These charged particles include acids generated in the process of the combustion of carbohydrate, fat, and some proteins. The lungs remove the majority of acid produced as a consequence of these combustion processes. However, the kidney provides the only place where certain types of acids can exit. Consequently, diminished kidney function causes these types of acids to accumulate in tissue (all the different types of body structure).

Amount of acid in tissue plays a role in determining:
1. **How well the enzymatic machinery functions.**
2. **The vulnerability of the cellular architecture.**
3. **The energetic charge of the cellular battery (cell voltage)**
4. **The ability to generate energy.**

For example, the kidney filters two different types of 'atomic dust' particles that need to be carefully regulated. The first concerns the acid content, hydrogen protons ($H+$ protons). The second regards the fact that the kidney carefully attempts to regulate the body's mineral concentrations. The four main minerals that are regulated are sodium, potassium, magnesium, and calcium.

Diseases like high blood pressure often result after the kidney's fail in their mineral balance efforts. Unfortunately, this truism fails to be fully comprehended in the clinical setting. However, after one identifies the reason that the kidney inappropriately wastes or conserves a specific mineral, healing can begin (explained below).

The kidneys accomplish elimination and conservation through elaborate workstations along the nephron (the functional unit of the kidney). At rest, the kidney receives 25% of the blood flow in the body. Every 24 hours it filters over 180 liters out of the blood. After processing, it ends up on average returning 179liters of this fluid back into the blood stream. Realize, the 180 liters of filtrate squeezed out of the blood each day contains vital minerals, sugar, amino acids, fatty acids, and hormones along with the trash needing to be removed. It is the kidney's job to constantly decide what waste is and what needs to be conserved.

Cellular Discharge of Organic Acids and the Solution is the Responsibility of the Kidneys

The first part of the kidney's trash removal role concerns the importance of acid removal. Acid content describes the amount of positively charged hydrogen protons separated, in space, from their negatively charged halves. All acids have hydrogen as their positively charged half, but can have numerous negatively charged halves. The ease with which the positive (hydrogen proton) separates from the negative half in a fluid determines the strength of the acid.

The more these dissociations occur the stronger the acid. The molecular qualities of the negative half determine the separation tendency. Weaker acids separate less readily from their positive and negative halves.

Remember, the amount of acid content in living tissue determines its energetic capabilities, the functional abilities of the enzymatic machinery, and whether components dissolve or solidify in that tissue. For these reasons, good health becomes impossible without the right acid content in the different tissues.

Different body chambers require specific acid content for their optimum function. The stomach requires adequate acid production as a prerequisite to turn on its secreted enzymatic machinery to full capacity. After the food exits the stomach and trickles into the duodenum, the opposite conditions occur.

This next chamber needs an alkaline environment, the opposite of an acidic one. These conditions depend on the release of the acid neutralizing juices delivered from the pancreas. This only becomes possible when the pancreas manufactures sufficient alkaline juice and secretes it into the duodenum chamber (the initial part of the intestine beyond the stomach). Here, the enzymatic machinery, designed to finish what the stomach started, requires a much higher alkalinity (the opposite of acid) for optimal function.

Note pure water is pH neutral at 7. Chemists denote the strength of an acid as a number less than 7. The lower the number the stronger the acid will be. Similarly, they denote alkaline by numbers greater than 7. Also similar is the fact that the strongest alkaline solution possible is 14. Realize that different body chambers require a different pH for optimal function. For example the much publicized blood pH of 7.4 is hyped up but the acidic skin of 5.5 is often ignored.

An additional ignored example concerns that a little further down the digestive tract in the colon, the food remnants must be again sufficiently acidified or yeast over growth occurs. Take home point; none of these chamber's specific acid level requirements can be maintained without the kidney faithfully regulating certain types of body acid content.

The kidney allows other tissues to maintain the right amount of organic acid content similar to the catalyst that allows the right electrical charge to occur. The right electrical charge keeps life energy unfolding. It is the job of the kidney to either excrete or conserve certain acids that it constantly filters.

Understanding the basic chemistry of opposing ions (charged mineral halves that are either positive or negative) proves important for comprehending the role of the kidneys for taking out trash. The molecular physical world involves opposing molecular forces. All molecules are composed of atoms that are drawn together by these forces seeking relative stability once united. Some atoms have more strength than others.

Chemists measure this by the electronegativity of an element relative to all other elements. There are 106 elements. The stronger the electronegativity of an atomic element, the more force these elements possess to gather negative charges. Negative charges are gathered by the stronger elements from the electrons they steal from the weaker electronegative elements. Equal numbers of positive (protons) as compared to negative (electrons) charges exist in the universe.

Chemistry involves the study of combinations of the atomic elements that occur. Also the science of chemistry involves an interest in the energy contained within these associations and in the energy released when they break apart. The natural world (the physical world of nonliving things) moves in the direction of more stable molecular arrangements.

In the process of achieving more stable molecular arrangements these changing molecules give off energy much like a battery that runs down. This process describes the fundamental law of entropy. The science of Physics denotes this as the third law of thermodynamics.

Interestingly, living things somehow violate the basic law of entropy because living things trap energy into usable packets after combusting food with oxygen (ATP formation). In turn, the energy liberated from the breakdown of ATP into ADP is used to build complex molecular machines, power the energy needs of cell factories and membranes, drive complex chemical reactions that sustain life and manufacture complex architectural structures at the cellular level.

Realize, life energy somehow moves simple molecular arrangements in the opposite direction and creates more complexity (section six). The life process of complex molecular creation is not possible without a strict control of the acid and mineral content in the fluids which baths cells. It is the kidney's job to ensure that certain acids and most minerals content remain optimal.

As was previously mentioned, the process of cellular combustion of foodstuffs generates large amounts of acid. Having just the right amount of acid ensures that the biological molecules stay in the right configuration. The right amount of acid around allows the molecules to possess the right electrical charge consistent with optimal function. Remember, different body chambers have their own optimum level of acid content that creates the most efficient work environment for the enzymatic machines designed for that chamber.

Bottom line; the body requires that the right amount of hydrogen protons be in a certain body fluid. These protons are sufficiently distanced from their negatively charged half, and this creates the electrical milieu that will optimize other local molecular charges. Consequently, acid excess or deficiency in tissue leads to energetic, electrical, molecular, and structural aberrations.

The kidney removes one type of trash that constantly forms called organic acid. The organic acids constantly discharge from the cells into the blood stream. One of the kidney's roles regards its ability to excrete organic acids.

A requirement exists beyond the need for the right amount of acid to be present. It concerns the need for the proper amounts of essential minerals (calcium, magnesium, sodium, potassium, chloride, bicarbonate, and others). The proper amount of these minerals becomes impossible when the kidneys fail to excrete the excess minerals and conserve the deficient minerals.

When the right acid and mineral requirements occur an optimal electrical environment evolves throughout the remainder of the body for each cell type. In addition, optimal minerals and acid harmonizes the multiple electrical charges of the bulky molecules (proteins, phospholipids, mucopolysaccharides, and nucleic acids). Without ongoing competent conservation of scarce minerals and removal of excessive ones the electrical milieu disintegrates. Simply, the kidney removes excess organic acid and mineral trash.

The right electrical charge occurs with balanced acid and mineral content. The kidney needs to remove the organic acids that cellular factories constantly generate and ensure that the proper balance of essential minerals occurs. The minerals continually exit or accumulate. The kidney sorts out what needs to excrete and what needs to be conserved. The ability to perform this task forms a determinant of the overall health.

Two main types of acid occur in the body, gaseous acid (carbon dioxide) and organic acids. More carbon dioxide creation occurs than does organic acid. Much of the acid generated from the cellular factories exits through the lungs as carbon dioxide except organic acids, which need to exit through the kidney.

Lactic acid provides one example of an organic acid that is not removed by the kidney. Instead it requires processing in the liver. Alternatively, examples of organic acids created by the reactions of living cells are acids of sulfate, phosphate, nitrate, carbonate, and ammonia. These waste acids generate from the cellular factories up stream and are mostly removed by kidney filtration processes. In addition, most ammonia needs to be converted into urea (four ammonias per molecule) in the liver before the kidney excretes it into the urine (see liver chapter).

Mineral Balance and Other Organs that Help the Kidney

Each human kidney is composed of 1.3 million complex and vibrating filter machines. Scientists call these filters, a nephron. The term nephron describes the functional unit of the kidney. At rest 25% of all the blood volume circulates through the kidney. Before the blood can leave the kidney it must pass through the filters contained in the nephrons, the glomerulus. Healthy kidneys know what the body needs and what the body needs to through away.

The kidney in cooperation with the lungs removes the majority of acid generated in the body and serve as a primary regulator of its mineral content. Healthy owners maintain stable amounts of the essential minerals and acid content that proves unique for each cell type.

Two main things need to happen if the total concentration of these minerals is to remain at optimal levels (sodium, chlorine, potassium, calcium, magnesium, bicarbonate and phosphorous). First, there needs to be an adequate intake in the diet and a digestive tract capable of absorbing what is offered (section 3). Second, the right amount of message content needs to be delivered to the kidney that instructs excretion or conservation of minerals. In living things, how much and which hormones arrive at the tissue in question determines the message content. When these two processes occur the owner remains in mineral balance.

Some other organ systems interrelate to the kidney in the task of acid and mineral balance. As was previously mentioned, the lungs are responsible for removing the gaseous acids generated in cellular factories. However, lungs are minimal players in regard to mineral balance.

Two other organ systems, the colon and skin, help the kidney with mineral balance. They contribute to the maintenance of mineral balance when adequate supplies are present. Some backup overlap exists between the trash water removal organs. *In all cases, of acid and mineral balance, these organ systems need the help of the most powerful medicine of all, water.*

Mineral Balance – Proportions of Minerals in the Diet

The most common diseases that originate in the kidney result from the chronic ingestion of imbalanced minerals in the diet. The typical situation involves one in which an owner eats predominately processed food. Unfortunately, these food groups possess a drastically altered mineral content from their natural state. Only real food contains the natural proportions of minerals that the body needs. As was previously mentioned many times, food processing diminishes magnesium and potassium content and increases sodium content.

Now it is time to apply the already mentioned facts about natural food containing the right mineral content in the context of the kidney. Real (natural) foods are: fresh vegetables, fruits, meats, chicken, fish, and grains, beans, and seeds before they are processed. These foods all contain excellent mineral ratio content and when fresh, are high in potassium and low in sodium. In contrast, processed food comes in a box, can, and bakery bag or is served at a fast food restaurant. Food processing removes potassium and magnesium while it adds sodium (see mineral table in section one).

Green colored foods or seeds are also high in magnesium. Magnesium and potassium deficiency arise because Americans consume large amounts of processed foods. Consequently, owners who subsist on processed foods develop mineral imbalance caused diseases. More pertinent to the trash water removal functions concerns how altered mineral intake eventually curtails the ability of the kidney to remove excess minerals. Minerals in excess comprise a form of kidney trash. Certain situations arise when one mineral becomes deficient and other minerals occur in excess. The processed food diet favors this scenario.

Many prescription drugs become chronically necessary because clinicians ignore sub-optimal mineral intake inherent in the typical American diet. Altered mineral intake patterns result in many types of high blood pressure problems, fluid retention, bodily wasting syndromes, and many different syndromes of mineral excess and/or deficiencies.

Mineral Balance depends on the Quality of the Message Content

In the kidneys, as in the other organs, a recurring theme occurs: The quality of the message content forms a central determinant for the functional ability in that target organ. The quality of the message content determines how the kidney directs its energy expenditure.

The science that unites these two vital concepts (message content and minerals) is well developed. The trouble begins in the clinical setting from the fractured medical thought among the specialties. As medicine becomes increasingly ultra -specialized a trend toward disjointed and incomplete reasoning arises. It propagates in the absence of the light of holism for what science has revealed.

Holism often leads to healing. Many times healing from disease becomes a matter of understanding where the imbalance began. Imbalanced acid and minerals lead to extra trash water and high blood pressure. Healing from high blood pressure provides a good example for the importance of scientific holism.

When the Trash Removal Systems in the Kidneys Fail High Blood Pressure can Result

Ideally, at the onset of the first clues that an owner heads toward mineral excesses or deficiencies caused diseases like; high blood pressure, arthritis, or fluid imbalance the trash water would be thoroughly evaluated. Trash water evaluations include attention directed at the quality of the hormone message and mineral content arriving in the kidney.

Early diagnosis of high blood pressure is easy to heal when the mineral deficiency is quickly identified and corrected. In most cases, high blood pressure involves chronic potassium deficiency and sodium excess. This imbalance causes damage to the kidneys with the passage of time. Kidney damage itself then contributes to further elevate the blood pressure. Remember, low potassium diets damage kidney function (hypokalemic nephropathy).

Before kidney function becomes permanently damaged the correction of the potassium and sodium imbalance will heal the problem. This fact provides an example where symptom control medicine leads to the consequence of needing a permanent prescription. Here, the kidneys sustained damage because symptom control medications were administered rather than a diet that included balanced mineral content.

Symptom control medicine usually affects a disease symptom by poisoning some enzymatic process. Recall the earlier example of poisoning an enzymatic process that concerns the common prescription class called the angiotensin converting enzyme inhibitors (ACE inhibitors). ACE inhibitors are commonly prescribed for high blood pressure control. ACE activates angiotensin 1 to angiotensin 2.

Unfortunately, when one targets the kidney content of this enzyme machine, it proves impossible to spare poisoning the same enzyme machines found in other parts of the body. Two additional locations for this enzyme are the lungs and testes. In the lungs ACE controls inflammation. In the testis ACE promotes adequate steroid synthesis, like testosterone.

In some cases this may be the only way to lower blood pressure to a safe level. However, in the majority of cases, safer ways exist to cure or prevent high blood pressure. Actually one of the main beneficial effects of this type of blood pressure medication, the ACE inhibitors, concerns their ability to help conserve body potassium content. If owners were counseled on this fact to begin with, before kidney damage became permanent, they could then attempt a real food diet (section three).

Most high blood pressure problems are the result of the kidney failing to remove trash. Blood pressure can be lowered to safe levels if one addresses the cause of the accumulating trash water. Rather than poison an enzyme to bring blood pressure down, consider the four common kidney derived causes of blood pressure elevation: insulin excess, magnesium deficiency, inadequate potassium intake relative to sodium intake and cortisol and/or aldosterone excess. In each case the ability of the kidney to remove trash water compromises. When trash water accumulates in the pipes the pressure elevates.

These causes can be traced back to being at least partially the result of hormone message content mismatch. This results in the wrong hormones being delivered to the kidney and this misdirects it on how to spend its energy. Additionally, the deficiency or excess minerals cause high blood pressure because the kidney fails to remove trash properly. The kidney responds to whichever hormones deliver it message content. Message content determines how the kidney directs energy expenditure.

Also, a two way street exists in that the kidney can send out appropriate or inappropriate message content to distant tissues via the secretion of its own informational substances (hormones). The types and amounts of hormones (informational substances) that the kidney excretes determine whether it proves helpful or exacerbating for an existing imbalance.

A holistic approach to blood pressure control includes an assessment regarding hormone tone (the quality of informational substances). It also includes attention to the importance of mineral balance. The science exists for an accurate assessment of the major hormones and minerals within an owner. It is time to implement what science knows so that healing opportunities are not missed.

Blood pressure elevations can begin in the kidneys with dysfunction of the trash removal of minerals. High blood pressure can be thought of as a consequence of the kidney failing to take out its share of waste. Effort needs to be spent detecting common aberrations of insulin excess, magnesium deficiency, potassium imbalance, and excess cortisol and/or aldosterone. Some owners prefer this approach before committing to symptom control medicine.

Insulin Caused High Blood Pressure

Often blood pressure lowers when owners commit to a diet·
that reduces the need for insulin since the counter response to insulin
is largely cortisol. Cortisol has powerful fluid retaining side effects
when it rises above low levels. Recall the antique weight scale and
picture that the more insulin one has to secrete (the more
carbohydrate or sedentary stress, the more insulin), the greater the
needs for larger counter weight, cortisol. The body needs more
cortisol to oppose the desire of insulin to suck every sugar molecule
from the blood stream. Especially in unhealthy people (explained in
section two), cortisol is one of the main counter weights to insulin,
but because cortisol elevation promotes fluid retention it can elevate
blood pressure.

Insulin authorities like Bernstein and Atkins feel that insulin
has a direct effect on the kidney that promotes blood pressure
elevation. To really know how insulin interacts with the kidney
further research is needed.

Already mentioned earlier concerns Stanford researcher, Dr.
Gerald Reaven, who coined the term Syndrome X that describes
insulin excess owners who have high blood pressure, amongst other
pathologies. Syndrome X also includes symptoms of owners who
are on an accelerated path toward heart disease. These owners seem
to have an excessive oxidation (rusting phenomena) rate in their
tissues. Insulin excess is felt to be one of the main aberrations that
allow Syndrome X to work its body destruction (chapter three).
Syndrome X starts with high insulin and eventually leads on into
fluid and sodium retention.

Excess fluid and sodium retention become trash water that
the kidney should remove. Some authorities feel that insulin excess
is responsible for half of all high blood pressure states. A lowered
carbohydrate intake will decrease the need for insulin. When high
insulin causes high blood pressure then attention here is warranted.

Magnesium Deficiency Caused High Blood Pressure

Another group of high blood pressure patients can be helped
by high quality magnesium supplementation. Magnesium is a
powerful smooth muscle relaxant. Smooth muscles are plentiful in
the arteries.

Magnesium supplements occur as salts that contain a
positive and negative half that separate when dissolved in water.
Like acids, salts in the body fluids in the right amounts create the

357

proper electrical milieu that allows life processes to continue. They charge the system.

The similarity between a salt and an acid is that both are made with a positive and a negative half. However, with acid hydrogen always occupies the positive half. In contrast, salts contain different types of positively charged halves. Usually these are minerals, but never only hydrogen as the positive half. Both acids and salts can have the same types of negatively charged halves. When a salt contains the same negative half as an acid it's called the salt of an acid. Lastly, minerals are always on the positive half. Magnesium is a mineral.

The body charges trillions of different cells electrically (the voltage) by the manipulation of the potential differences between the various minerals across a membrane. On opposite sides of the membranes the concentration differences between the salts and acid content creates potential energy (voltage). The cells constantly draw upon the potential energy contained in these membranes for the reactions of life. At the same time, the mitochondria continually recharge the membrane's energy content by supplying continuous ATP (adenosine triphosphate) to the membrane pumps. It is the energy released from the cleavage of ATP into ADP (adenosine diphosphate) that powers the membrane pumps in the trillions of body cells. Bottom line; these mineral differences are constantly being recreated to prevent membrane energy depletion.

Remember, the process is similar in the car battery that always needs to be recharged when the motor consumes fuel. Likewise, when the cell burns fuel it creates ATP in the mitochondria that it uses to constantly power the membranes. The membranes re-power from the mineral pumps contained within it that exchange magnesium for calcium. Other pumps exchange sodium for potassium. Recall, as well, the membrane pumps amounts on almost all of the body's 70 trillion cells is determined by the adequacy of thyroid message content. Consequently, owners that suffer from thyroid hormone deficiency also suffer from low voltages in their cells (sections two and five).

The electrical power contained in cell membranes is created by the difference in concentrations across the membrane of the various minerals. Excessive minerals behave as trash because they alter the proper proportion from those that reflect the balanced opposing minerals state. Mineral deficiencies can also alter the proper proportion between opposing minerals. Magnesium deficiency commonly results from eating a processed food diet.

Ideally, the positive and negative halves of salts separate in spatial arrangement within body fluids. This allows positive and negative charges to exist in body fluid. The difference in the concentrations across different membranes that exist between different mineral types (magnesium, calcium, sodium, potassium, hydrogen ion, chloride, bicarbonate, etc.) of charged particles allows electrical work.

Electrical work occurs when opposing minerals flow down their concentration gradient. The release of these minerals toward equilibrium releases energy that the cell can use. When minerals flow toward equilibrium they discharge the energy contained in the membrane. The membrane recharges by the continuous supply of ATP provided by the cell power plants (mitochondria). The energy released when ATP deteriorates to ADP pumps minerals back up their concentration gradient. Magnesium is one of the minerals that charge the membrane. Remember, the typical American diet proves largely deficient in magnesium content. Magnesium deficiency in the blood vessel elevates the blood pressure.

Recall, all magnesium supplemental salts are not created equal. Some preparations save their manufacturer's money, but have nasty side effects that prove mild when compared to the best prescription drugs. Choosing intelligently between the many brands on the health food store shelves requires some knowledge. For example, some brands lack sufficient magnesium content to effectuate a response in lowering blood pressure.

In addition, magnesium is only part of the salt contained in the different brands' pills. As a consequence, any weight stated on the bottle has only a fraction of this weight as true magnesium content (the salt is made up of positive and negative halves). Magnesium forms the positive half. Both halves have weight. If one looks carefully at the label, sometimes there is the exact weight per tablet of magnesium content called the elemental weight. The salt weight will be the weight of it per tablet (100mg, 200mg, etc.).

All magnesium salts are not created equally because the negative half, which is not magnesium, has properties of its own. For example, magnesium citrate is a powerful laxative. Citrate is named second denoting it to be the negative half by chemical nomenclature convention. This powerful laxative effect most owners can do without unless they are evacuating their bowels for surgery or medical procedures.

Magnesium oxide is another salt sold inappropriately over the counter. It is poorly absorbed and possesses potential as an oxidizing agent (chapter 1). The oxide component of the salt is like ingesting trash in pill form, which needs water to remove it. Most store bought magnesium salts are composed of oxide, which is a tissue oxidant and has no useful purpose. Oxide is body trash.

Examples of both absorption and the safest second half (the negative half) are magnesium amino acid chelate, magnesium aspartate and magnesium malate. Many companies offer magnesium preparations that are too weak unless one swallows the entire contents of the bottle each day. This provides an example where alternative medicine can undeservedly acquire a bad name. Weak and ineffective preparations of various herbs and supplements abound. For the best strength and quality of magnesium, the Source Naturals brand is safe.

If one chooses to begin a trial of magnesium supplementation to lower their blood pressure, the support and competence of a knowledgeable physician is necessary. The effective dosage ends up being between 300-1000mg of elemental magnesium a day. This total daily dosage should be divided between meals. Magnesium is a mineral and needs adequate stomach acid for absorption. Owners who have healthy gastrointestinal tracts will secrete maximum acid that follows a high protein meal. This becomes an important consideration when attempting to absorb this much magnesium each day (digestions chapter). Lastly, in some types of kidney disease magnesium supplementation is ill advised.

Potassium Deficiency and High Blood Pressure

When one consumes potassium at a sub-healthy rate compared to sodium, high blood pressure can be a consequence. The ability of the kidney to remove excess fluid depends on having adequate potassium compared to sodium. The healthy body maintains an optimal ratio between the two. Certain dietary choices diminish this ratio and high blood pressure results in these susceptible owners.

Before the days of processed food this problem was much less prevalent. Processed food encourages this problem due to the sodium that is routinely added and the removal of potassium and magnesium (see mineral table). This relationship is not discussed straightforwardly in the medical physiology textbooks, but has been observed clinically. It is included here to plant a 'question mark' for the possible solution to blood pressure problems being the imbalance between potassium and sodium.

An imbalance here leading to high blood pressure makes sense in light of the huge amount of sodium that food processing

adds. **This alone upsets the delicate balance between these opposing minerals. Natural food diets result in a greater than three to one ratio of potassium compared to sodium. A processed food diet reverses this ratio.**

In the case of magnesium and potassium, a deficiency of natural foods in the diet sets the stage for these minerals to unbalance. Unprocessed meats, nuts (unsalted), vegetables, whole grains, dried beans, and fruits provide examples of real foods that contain balanced amounts of minerals. In contrast, as stated many times previously, processing food causes the mineral ratios to reverse.

Sodium is critical to extend the shelf life of food. Fast food is usually loaded with added salt. The act of processing food depletes its magnesium and potassium content. Some bodies prove ill-equipped to deal with this deviation from the natural way that food grows. Excess sodium retains water trash and high blood pressure results.

Mineral imbalance can lead to elevated blood pressure and stress affects the mineral content in the body. These facts tie together, by a common interdependent thread, the four mechanisms for blood pressure elevation at the kidney level: ***The stressed owner is a trash water retention machine.***

Steroid Message Content - A Determinant of Blood Pressure

The fourth example of how the kidney can misdirect trash water removal and lead to high blood pressure is found in the overall message content of the steroid hormones that the kidney receives. A high quality steroid mixture that interacts with the kidney, directs the proper use of energy. This occurs only in the healthful state. As the quality of the steroid mixture that reaches the kidney decreases, health consequences occur.

Many women just before their period experience the effects of lower quality steroid hormones reaching their kidneys. Premenstrual bloating and fluid retention (trash water accumulation) evidence this fact. Hormonally, just before menstruation the content of natural progesterone falls off dramatically. Abnormal progesterone prescription substitutes do not count here because they do not behave like real progesterone in the promotion of fluid loss. The dramatic fall of real progesterone causes the sudden loss in informational message content which directs the kidney to dump extra body fluid (diuresis). Alternatively, pregnant women experience the

opposite situation with their frequent urinations secondary to their elevated progesterone levels.

This brings up one explanation for those few obese owners who have low normal blood pressure. The physician that takes the time to check his/her obese patient's 24-hour urine will often find one, several or all of the following hormone and their respective metabolites aberrations; elevated estrogens, diminished anabolism, sub-optimal thyroid function and/or increased cortisol metabolites (section two). Realize most of these obese patients also suffer from high blood pressure.

However, in the few obese patients who evidence and low blood pressure types their 24-hour urine results explain their protection. In many of these patients excessive progesterone metabolites are found. Remember, progesterone is a powerful diuretic. Apparently, progesterone more powerfully encourages water loss compared to the cortisol ability to retain it.

A simple concept to help understand why sodium raises the blood pressure but potassium lowers it follows. Realize that the vast majority of sodium in the body occurs outside the cells. This part of body fluids is called the extra-cellular space. The extra-cellular space contains the fluids that bath the outside of cells and includes the fluid in the blood stream. Water is attracted to dissolved minerals.

For this reason, excessive sodium expands these spaces. Conversely, the vast majority of potassium resides inside the cells. This is called the intra-cellular space. Likewise, water is attracted to potassium dissolved inside the cells. For these reasons, potassium has little effect on raising the blood pressure because it pulls water into the cells. Potassium also promotes wrinkle free cells because of this fact. However, excess sodium powerfully expands the extra-cellular space that includes the blood vessels volume. Because it powerfully attracts water to the space where it dominates, the higher its concentration the more water flows towards it to maintain the osmotic constancy requirement of the body.

Expanded extracellular space volume translates into high blood pressure unless the kidneys deal with the imbalance. Visualize the ongoing 'tug of war' of where water follows being determined by the balance between sodium and potassium. The dominant minerals, by far, between the extracellular and intracellular space respectively.

Men and woman when subjected to chronic stressors of various types develop fluid retention. Recall, baggy eyelids following late nights out and early to rise out of bed experiences. If the process becomes chronic it can lead to high blood pressure because of the increased fluid in the pipes. Stress elicits a change in the hormone message content reaching the kidney, which effectuates a change in the way the kidney handles mineral balance.

The western medical standard often ignores these basic hormonal mismatches that lead to disease. Instead of direct intervention to return optimal hormone quality, they employ symptom control medicinal approaches. These are always attended by all the consequent side effects. Sometimes prescription medication is warranted. However, many toxic and dangerous side effects are avoidable when the holism of what science has revealed are included in the workup.

These first four fixable causes for elevated blood pressure are only the beginning of what is known when the holism of what science has revealed is included in the treatment plan. There are many effective, non-toxic ways to treat high blood pressure early in the disease process. This can only occur if an owner is informed and motivated to heal. Tying together all four factors that contribute to the kidney allowing trash water accumulation and consequently high blood pressure is critical.

Stress and Dead Food Consumption Combine All Four Reasons for High Blood Pressure into an Inter-connected Web

By avoiding real food and adding in daily stress, blood pressure elevation becomes likely because these processes lead to trash water accumulation. When physicians fail to learn this fact, they dutifully prescribe medications that peripherally alter the trash water imbalance. These approaches always have side effects. Side effects lead to more prescriptions and medical procedures. Some of these scenarios can be avoided. When the goal is avoidance of symptom control approaches, these four interconnected determinants need adequate consideration - insulin level, stress hormone level (cortisol), potassium intake relative to sodium intake, and magnesium content.

Chronic stress elevates aldosterone and cortisol output from the adrenal glands. High cortisol and aldosterone accelerate potassium loss but promote sodium retention. Cortisol levels approach 200 times those of aldosterone. The kidney's receptor for retaining sodium listens to cortisol better than it does to aldosterone (the 11-beta hydroxylase receptor). Yet, physicians receive information that persuades them to think that aldosterone is all-important for salt and water balance (see informational substances chapter).

When the kidneys chronically receive high sodium relative to potassium in the diet blood pressure problems, in some, eventually manifest. Mantra: Higher sodium relative to potassium mineral intake is found in processed food.

Chronic stress hormone release compounds the problem because it leads to an exacerbation of blood vessel fluid retention. Stress hormone (cortisol) does this because it directs the kidney to accelerate the loss of potassium but retain sodium. These two effects result from the kidney being directed by stress hormone to misdirect water and minerals.

Around middle age when the potassium deficiency becomes more pronounced the kidneys begin to deteriorate (hypokalemic nephropathy). The longer the potassium deficiency causes injury, the more likely the need for permanent blood pressure medication. When the kidneys suffer damage, medication is required to normalize blood pressure.

For this reason, it is imperative that physicians begin to counsel their high blood pressure patients early on in their disease process before permanent kidney damage eventually occurs. When patients implement this advice on how to increase potassium relative to sodium in their diet they diminish their tendency toward high blood pressure in stressful situations. Blood pressure stabilizes because they now have a more proper amount of sodium compared to potassium arriving in their kidney filters. Water will be less likely to accumulate within the blood stream because with less sodium intake its retention propensity exacerbated by stress becomes less significant.

An overlooked consequence of a low potassium diet concerns a long known fact: When body potassium lowers more insulin becomes necessary to do the same job (insulin resistance). This provides a vicious hormonal cycle. High insulin necessitates higher cortisol to keep blood sugars normal (the antique weight scale) and powerfully stimulates fat cell growth. Lastly, the increased insulin needs brought on by chronic potassium deficits explains how these people often appear as one type of Syndrome X owner (metabolic Syndrome).

Recall, Syndrome X owners exist on an accelerated tract to an old body. Their fundamental defect involves elevated insulin levels in a setting of increased stress. Low potassium and low magnesium diets with elevated sodium intake makes these owners' disease process worse. A high stress hormone output explains, in part, how Syndrome X patients age so quickly and have high blood pressure (heart chapter).

Recall, health requires that anabolism balances with the catabolism. Elevated cortisol output chronically communicates the emergency message and this fact helps explain the increased catabolism associated with this syndrome. Realize, bodies that chronically perceive emergencies channel energy into survival pathways (catabolism). The survival pathway becomes the norm instead of rejuvenation. Rejuvenation depends on sufficient anabolism. Trash water removal is a rejuvenation activity.

When the body directs energy into survival pathways, wear and tear becomes more likely secondary to the lack of cellular repair. Adequate repair proves necessary to slow aging. One of the reasons that Syndrome X owners' age quickly is because they have high insulin and cortisol derived diseases.

Important point to emphasize: They also have lower IGF-1 levels. This dirty little secret greatly increases their insulin requirement (liver chapter). Increased insulin becomes desperately needed because falling IGF-1 means that fuel nozzles are scarce.

In this section, the more pertinent point to consider in the mineral balance scheme of things concerns the huge contribution to the severity of Syndrome X type owners' clinical outcome secondary to the mineral imbalanced diet. Chronic mineral imbalance intake around middle age eventually overcomes the kidney's ability to correct the altered mineral content it receives. In the case of Syndrome X owners, they add to their problem by consuming processed foods that exacerbate mineral imbalances. In turn, one mineral imbalance concerns potassium deficiency that causes excessive insulin need (insulin resistance).

The last of the interconnected four basic causes of elevated blood pressure addresses magnesium deficiency. This deficiency is common in Americans who consume processed food. In addition, excess sodium intake, in a setting of chronic stress, makes the magnesium deficiency worse. Part of the stress response consequence involves magnesium leaving in the urine in order to conserve sodium because the body thinks combat is forthcoming. This detail explains why the two mineral deficiencies usually occur together following chronic stress (life). Making matters worse, when potassium depletes often times the kidney will excrete magnesium instead. Realize although potassium is the dominant intracellular mineral, magnesium is second. Visualize the low voltage effect eventually manifesting in those that have stress and insist on eating processed foods year after year.

Assessing Hormones Contribution to Trash Water Accumulation

Often times if an accurate twenty-four hour urine test discloses imbalances in steroid hormones it may be unnecessary to manipulate the hormone mismatch directly. Using the holism of what science has revealed can often effectively counter the mismatch. In the case of elevated stress hormone secretion, supplements like magnesium and potassium, along with sodium restriction, allow for an effective counter regulatory response promoting fluid removal. In other cases it becomes prudent to facilitate a more harmonious steroid profile.

Each owner proves unique in their kidney appropriation of water and minerals in their regulation of blood pressure. This uniqueness will present itself in the diagnostic workup. Part of the workup requires including the unraveling of the hormonal mess that causes a kidney-derived problem. The twenty-four hour urine test will also provide the relative excretion rates of these important minerals.

The Inter-relationship between Cortisol, Insulin, and Blood Pressure

The message content that the kidney receives determines, in part, the resultant blood pressure. This relationship emphasizes the interrelationship between cortisol and insulin. Insulin secretes when carbohydrate absorbs from dietary sources or when mental stress inappropriately directs the liver to dismantle protein into sugar. Bottom line: Excess blood sugar requires insulin to normalize it. alternatively, between meals, as the blood sugar falls, death would shortly follow because insulin would direct the liver and fat cells to suck every sugar molecule out of the blood stream unless an effective counter response is mounted quickly. Healthy owners can do this by secreting effective amounts of Growth Hormone, glucagon, epinephrine and cortisol that raise blood sugar (the counter response).

> **Recap: Before an effective explanation of how excessive cortisol plays a role in countless middle aged blood pressure cases occurs, a few summary remarks need to be re-emphasized (see below).**

Please note that part of the unhealthy body's problem, when the blood fuel falls between meals, concerns their diminished Growth Hormone secretion abilities that lead to less IGF-1 (among other causes for falling IGF-1 explained elsewhere). Less IGF-1 means that more insulin becomes necessary to deliver fuel (insulin resistance). Less Growth Hormone means that when these bodies fast or exercise a more violent blood sugar raising mechanism saves them from death (Joiner-Bey's term). Namely, cortisol, epinephrine and glucagon differ from Growth Hormone because they promote gluconeogenesis. Gluconeogenesis denotes the process of converting body proteins into sugar. Remember, defense of body protein proves necessary if one wants to preserve their lean body mass. Recall, only Growth Hormone protects body protein content between meals and when one exercises.

Protein comprises the metabolically active component of body tissue. In other words only protein consumes calories. Enzymes, actin, myosin, mineral pumps, certain hormones and hormone receptors provide examples of proteins that consume calories. This fact
explains the central aging mechanism operating when Growth Hormone falls and these owners find themselves between meals or exercising. These owners burn their metabolically active tissues (proteins) just to stay alive because their primary hormones are off kilter. As a consequence, their metabolism slows. Diminished metabolism causes these patients to feel and look older (see liver chapter for more details).

The opposite sequence of hormone release occurs when mentally stressed. Mental stress causes cortisol release, which directs the elevation of blood sugar inappropriately. For this reason, Growth Hormone release slows dramatically in the chronically stressed owner secondary to the elevated blood sugar. Remember, falling blood sugar proves as the major stimulus for Growth Hormone's release. Its deficiency leads to less IGF-1 secretion because IGF-1 secretion depends on sufficient Growth Hormone release.

Eventually insulin needs to be secreted to return the blood sugar to normal. The extra insulin becomes necessary because with mental stress no physical challenge ever comes. Therefore, the extra fuel is not needed. When healthy, the overall effect is to keep a constant amount of sugar in the blood stream.

However, as IGF-1 levels fall insulin secretion rates must rise so as to remove the excess sugar. IGF-1 can be thought of as the major insulin of the body outside of the liver and fat cells.

Healthy people have at least one hundred times IGF-1 compared to insulin. Unhealthy people have less IGF-1. Recall, the two fuel nozzle hormones of the body are insulin and IGF-1. When IGF-1 falls the fuel nozzles beyond the liver become scarce. Consequently, they need more insulin to pick up the slack in sugar removal. See below for why simple body anatomy shows that this is unhealthy. This also explains why unhealthy people when stressed secrete more insulin: They have less IGF-1 to mop up the inappropriate elevation in blood sugars that mental stress causes.

Actually glucagon, Growth Hormone, and adrenaline are also part of the counter response to insulin. Around middle age Growth Hormone becomes less involved in the prevention of low blood sugar compared to cortisol (section two).

There is a subtle, but important clinical point often missed between the inter-relationship of cortisol and insulin after IGF-1 levels have fallen off: Excessive cortisol becomes necessary only because abnormal amounts of insulin pummel the liver in the fasting state (a falling blood sugar). Recall, insulin releases from the pancreas via the portal vein where it confronts the liver containing 200,000 pure insulin receptors per liver cell. Visualize the consequences of insulin releasing abnormally while the blood sugar falls. The insulin message within the liver always instructs it to remove sugar from the blood stream for storage. Most of this sugar is stored as fat and cholesterol. Hence, the relationship between cholesterol and insulin levels because its levels within the liver determine HMG CoA reductase activity.

Because of the abnormality of needing insulin while the blood sugar falls, its arrival within the liver worsens the falling blood sugar before any of it spills beyond the liver to help with the fuel nozzle deficiency (i.e. fallen IGF-1 level that delivers fuel beyond the liver and fat to the hungry body cells like muscle and organs). Realize the beauty of not needing insulin during the fasting or exercising state because ample IGF-1 exists. IGF-1 is also called the non-suppressible insulin like activity of the blood stream in the older literature.

Another important point; normally, insulin releases from the pancreas while the blood sugar is rising. However,

> the pathological state denotes the consequences of increased
> insulin need (popularly called insulin resistance) during a falling
> blood sugar in order to stay alive because the cells beyond the
> liver remain hungry until a fuel nozzle arrives. Unfortunately,
> very few physicians are taught about the fundamental role of
> IGF-1 delivering fuel beyond the liver and fat cells. The older
> textbooks in fact acknowledge it making up over 93% of the
> insulin activity in the body. What happened to this knowledge?

Around middle age, for the reasons listed above, cortisol becomes one of the main counter-weights to insulin. The more insulin that weighs down on one side of the scale, the larger the counter weight amount of cortisol that needs to balance the scale (normalize the blood sugar). A vicious cycle of response and counter response is created when the average middle-aged owner is eating high amounts of carbohydrate, attempting to fast, exercise and/or experiences stress. Mental stress raises blood sugar and this requires more insulin to bring it back to normal. This produces a cycle of disease that begins when either one of these opposing hormones isn't optimal. **Remember, the root cause concerns the fallen IGF-1 and hence increased insulin need. Increased insulin need in turn requires increased cortisol to counterbalance the abnormality of needing insulin while the blood sugar falls because most of the insulin secreted becomes trapped within the liver and compounds the falling blood sugar! Excessive cortisol causes sodium retention and this elevates the blood pressure of many middle-aged owners.**

Recall, only six grams of sugar, under euglycemic (normal blood sugar) conditions, circulates within the entire blood stream of a 70kg individual. The blood stream can absorb about two grams per minute following carbohydrate meals. The brain consumes about four grams per hour of carbohydrate or $1/15^{th}$ of a gram per minute. Remember, with the exception of red blood cells and nerves, all other body cells consume mostly fat as fuel. Now, add in the complexity of either stress or excess carbohydrate consumption that rapidly upsets the euglycemic state. Middle-aged owners often have lost some of their weight versus counterweight fine tuning abilities. For this reason, to ignore the obvious consequences of omitting these powerful factors in physiological upset proves as folly.

Most patients are capable of making some life changes and habit cessation if they understand that it will help in their healing. Many patients appreciate an opportunity to heal, even if it requires effort and commitment on their part. It involves helping patients understand that when the hormone message content within is chaotic, their behavior as well as health will deteriorate. Health deteriorates when the kidney receives the wrong message about what to do with trash water. Trash water will accumulate when the stress response initiates. Part of the physical manifestation of trash water accumulation is blood pressure elevation.

In the case of Syndrome X typified by high cholesterol and high blood pressure a careful analysis of the 'antique weight scale' situation between insulin, IGF-1 and cortisol will help in the motivated patient. In all three of these conditions improvement occurs if the physician and patient work together to unravel this vicious cycle.

In summary, the kidney's role in organic acid removal, mineral balance, and blood pressure control have been reviewed. The last subsection of this chapter was complex, but necessary if one desires a better understanding for the full healing abilities of the most powerful medicine of all, water. The body's ability to cleanse itself becomes hopeless when inadequate supplies of pure water occur. The mineral proportions in the diet and the quality of the hormones that direct the kidney influence taking out the trash water.

The Most Powerful Medicine of All

Water is the most powerful medicine of all. Five of the six taking out the trash organs require ample water to carry out their waste removal functions. The sixth, the immune system doesn't directly engage the services of water, but its workload increases without the adequate supply of clean water. The colon requires sufficient clean water or constipation and backwards absorption of putrefaction molecules occurs. The lungs need adequate water in their respiratory secretions or thick mucus plugs the airways. The kidney's need water to remove excess minerals and water-soluble toxins. The skin needs adequate water content to prevent wrinkling and allow adequate sweat formation. The liver needs adequate water in its bile secretions to prevent stone formation in the gallbladder.

Clean water deficiencies cause salt retention in the form of waste and mineral excesses to occur. As these accumulate, the body begins sequestering these wastes that eventually injure delicate tissues because there isn't enough water to remove these toxins.

The sequestering site depends on the toxin type. Uric acid preferentially stores in the big toe areas and in gouty tophi (hard bumps) formation. Salts of calcium build up in the kidney's drain system and form kidney stones. Imbalances between serum phosphate and calcium concentrations cause the chemical solidification reactions that precipitate calcium salts in the blood vessel walls, the joints, and create osteophytes (bone spurs). Other organic acids that fail to excrete can react with molecular structural components and lead to deformation injuries.

Some water supplies have diminished usefulness because they already contain toxins. Toxins accumulate in the water supply from industrial wastes, agricultural chemicals; urine derived pharmaceutical metabolites and automobile gaseous emissions.

Some beverages act as drying agents or diuretics. Diuretics cause more water to be eliminated when they are consumed than the water they contain. Commonly consumed diuretics are coffee, tea, and alcohol. Consequently, unless adequate supplemental clean water is taken along with these beverages the body will sequester toxins.

The chronic consumption of soda pop beverages causes unique damaging effects to the skeleton. Certain carbonated beverages contain phosphates without calcium forcing the body to use its own calcium to eliminate phosphate from the system. For this reason, chronic soda pop abusers risk developing calcium deficiency in their bones. Fortunately, the universe was constructed so that beer is free of phosphate and thus will not damage the bones like soda pop.

Some air supplies require increased clean water consumption such as in environments where each breath inhaled contains acids. Smog describes the most common source. Some of these acids absorb through the act of breathing and the kidneys eliminate them. The kidney will fail without abundant pure water.

Physicians from antiquity realized old age involved a drying out process. In many ways this still proves true. Now additional understanding of how the decrease in essential hormones leads to the drying out of body tissues comes into play. Dry body tissues become brittle and weak. Altered minerals ingestion accelerates hormonal decline and the drying effect. The proper hormones within, proper mineral intake, proper activity level, stress management, and adequate supplies of clean water all help the kidney prevent the shrinkage into old age.

Proper Garbage Removal Allows the Kidneys to Facilitate the Cellular Force Field

As has been previously stated, the body is an electrical system that maintains itself by properly proportioned and appropriate concentration of opposing minerals. Sufficient water content allows proper concentrations of minerals in the different tissues. It is the kidney's job to maintain the water content at 67% of the total atom weight content, remove waste products, and maintain the ability of the cells to generate an optimal electrical charge. The quality and proportion of the minerals (electrolytes) used by the cells to power the cell batteries depend, in part, on the kidney. The kidney responds to this after the digestive tract makes minerals available.

After the digestive tract extracts the minerals from a meal, the kidneys evaluate which minerals to retain and which to eliminate as waste. The kidney responds to the hormone messages that it receives. Healthy owners have high quality message content that directs the kidneys in the wise use of its energy.

Healthy owners also choose optimal mineral content in their diet so that the correct ratios of minerals become available to the kidney. These in turn distribute at the cellular level. Only when these processes occur can an owner make it past middle age with appropriate mineral balance. Much of that feeling of getting old comes down to the loss of the cell voltage (section five).

In summary, the kidneys oversee mineral balance. They depend on the quality of the message content (type and amounts of hormones delivered), the adequacy of nutritionally balanced mineral intake, the functional abilities of the digestive tract, and the adequate supply of clean water. Attention to these four variables can have powerful effects on regaining health from diseases like arthritis, high blood pressure, fluid retention, and osteoporosis. Unfortunately, excesses and deficiencies of the minerals constantly confront the kidney when a processed food diet becomes the norm. It is truly a miracle that they perform so diligently under the adverse circumstances of their owner choosing imbalanced minerals intake year after year.

The Interrelationship Between the Kidneys and the Liver

The kidneys are in partnership with the liver in taking out certain types of trash. The liver begins detoxification of a water insoluble trash by making it soluble. Many vitamins and cofactors prove necessary for this process such as vitamin C, glutathione, the methyl donor system of vitamins, glucuronic acid, etc. The liver then transfers many of the inactivated molecules to the kidney for elimination. The liver inactivates other toxins and then excretes them into the bile for removal by a bowel movement (liver chapter).

Significant amounts of ammonia are created everyday as a waste product from breaking down any of the 20 different amino acids and converting them into sugar (gluconeogenesis). It also occurs somewhat from the breakdown of other nitrogen containing molecules, like nucleic acids. It is the liver's job to removes ammonia from the circulation and convert it into urea. The urea manufactured in the liver excretes into the blood stream where it travels to the kidneys for excretion in the urine.

To a point, adequate urea levels allow the kidney to conserve water. Urea facilitates the ability of the kidneys to concentrate the urine. Higher specific gravity (waste concentration) becomes possible when dehydration forces prevail. Still other evidence exists that urea provides important immune stabilization effects that are not yet clearly understood. This shows that sometimes a toxin, if allowed to build up, has biochemical usefulness within normal parameters. It also elucidates how the liver-kidney trash removal partnership provides for the removal of urea.

Another class of substances depends on the kidney-liver partnership and causes the urine of healthy owners to foam: The amount of urine foam depends on the quantity of urinary steroids that have become water-soluble after the liver tags them with glucuronic acid. Glucuronic acid proves necessary to make steroids water-soluble so the kidney can excrete them in the urine. When steroids combine with glucuronic acid they make foam in water. Hence, a crude index of the steroidal adequacy can be obtained if one notes the amount of suds created in urine when it is shaken up. Who knows? Maybe steroids combined with glucuronic acid is just one of the clever ways to make soap that washes off the kidney's tubule dirt that collects over time. If this turns out to be true, it will show another example of the perils of scientist thinking inside the box.

Beyond the liver and kidney partnership is an equally important partnership, the kidney, skin and lung partnership. Like the kidneys, the lungs and skin concern themselves with waste removal. The next chapter discusses how one heals their lungs.

CHAPTER SEVENTEEN

LUNGS

The cellular factories deposit acid in body fluids. The lungs remove the majority of this acid load in the form of carbon dioxide gas. In contrast, the kidneys remove the organic acids that these factories produce. The lungs prove incapable for this task. Similarly, the kidney proves unable to remove carbon dioxide as gas. In this way, these two organs work together for the removal of toxic acids. Lactic acid provides the one exception because the liver removes it (liver section).

Diminished acid removal is the last function of the lungs to be compromised when they are diseased. Long before acid buildup occurs, the ability of the lung to deliver oxygen decreases. Initially, diminished oxygen delivery occurs only when demands increase.

The fact that automobile air filters (oxygen delivery) proves more vulnerable to malfunction (lung disease) than the exhaust system (carbon dioxide removal) offers an illustrative analogy. Diminished oxygen delivery through the air filter initially only occurs when the gas pedal is floored. Later, oxygen intake diminishes as the air filter becomes further compromised. Finally, late in the deterioration of engine performance, inadequately combusted fuel begins to belch out of the exhaust pipe and buildup in the engine.

The reason oxygen delivery falls more quickly than carbon dioxide removal, when the lungs are diseased, concerns the fact that oxygen has less affinity to enter the blood stream compared to the ability of carbon dioxide to leave it. Realize, filling the oxygen sites as a unit of blood passes through the oxygen chambers in the lungs is a critically timed event even in the healthiest of lungs.

The consequence of this, as various processes injure the lungs, then is that oxygen entry into the body falls off before carbon dioxide builds up. Oxygen entry falls off because there wasn't much 'wiggle room' to begin with. Oxygen entry into the body at high levels only occurs in the best of lungs.

The analogy holds for a car's air filter size and design. Auto manufacturers design each type of air filter with the assumption that the car owner will change the filter regularly before airway delivery diminishes. If the auto owner fails to change the filter, performance will fall dramatically. Damaged air filters diminish performance for the same reasons that lung air exchange chambers performance will fail. There is decreased oxygen delivery to both the car engine and the cell fuel combustion chamber (cell mitochondria).

Just as a dirty air filter in an auto causes decreased ability to burn gasoline, so to diseased lungs are adversely affected in their ability to deliver oxygen to the many cellular combustion chambers. Cells contain combustion chambers (mitochondria) that burn fuel vigorously only in the presence of adequate oxygen. Visualize that owners who contain diminished oxygen are those who also have weak burning power plants in their cells.

Eventually, far advanced disease in the lung causes carbon dioxide buildup. Resistance to this buildup occurs because carbon dioxide moves from the lungs more readily than oxygen enters into the body. The important exception occurs when the lung allows carbon dioxide to build up in order to compensate for another disease process that drains away body acid.

Medical physiology textbooks remain complicated in their explanation of these details. Better life decisions are necessary here if the body is going to have maximal oxygen delivery. Effective oxygen delivery into the tissues serves as a hallmark of youth. Conversely, as owners' age, oxygen delivery systems coincidently fall off. Diminished oxygen delivery leads to an increase in cellular trash because cell power plants burn in a 'soot-like' manner without it.

Consciously induced hyperventilation provides a way to understand the importance of having the right amount of acid in the body. Ten to twenty rapid deep breaths usually will produce the earliest manifestations of acid deficient caused disharmony. The breathing rate and depth are carefully regulated by the autonomic nervous system. Rapid breathing in excess of metabolic demands rapidly decreases carbon dioxide content (a major source of body acid).

Contrast this to running for a train. Here the increased demand for oxygen causes increased production of carbon dioxide gas (intake balances with need and the acid content remains the same). The body needs just the right amount. Too much acid and too little acid produce internal disharmony.

Cells need to have the right amount of acid to create the proper electrical environment. Too little carbon dioxide creates the symptoms of light-headedness, numbness around the mouth, and tingling in the fingers. Accelerated breathing (anxiety) is responsible for much of the misery caused by the loss of carbon dioxide. Anxiety stimulates the autonomic nervous system inappropriately leading to an accelerated breathing rate that exceeds demand. Eventually this can produce numbness and tingling in the digits and facial areas. Breathing into a paper bag, in these instances recycles exhaled carbon dioxide back into the body and alleviates these symptoms.

Carbon Dioxide Leaves More Readily Than Oxygen Enters

Carbon dioxide leaves the body with less effort than oxygen enters the body. Two factors contribute to this phenomenon. First, gases move from a high concentration toward a lower concentration. A dramatic difference exists in the atmospheric concentrations of oxygen compared to carbon dioxide. There are greater than 500 oxygen molecules for every 1 carbon dioxide at any elevation.

In contrast, the waste gases of expiration contain about the same concentrations between oxygen and carbon dioxide. The reason for this is that venous blood entering the lungs for expiration is depleted of oxygen after delivery to the tissues. At the same time it is rich in the waste gas, carbon dioxide.

Visualize a red blood cell as it leaves the capillaries depleted of oxygen and enriched with carbon dioxide. Consequently, the concentration of carbon dioxide when it reaches the lungs becomes many times higher than the atmospheric concentration of the gas. For these reasons, the body has more difficulty obtaining adequate oxygen inside the body compared to the ease of expelling carbon dioxide out of the body.

The rate of movement of a gas proves proportional to the difference in the concentrations between the chambers. Living cells constantly generate carbon dioxide gas. Approximately 100 times more atmospheric concentration of this gas occurs when it reaches the lung chambers. Oxygen however occurs in less than a one to four concentration difference between the amounts in the venous depleted lung chambers compared with the outside air. In the lungs, oxygen and carbon dioxide move in opposite directions. Carbon dioxide gas, because it occurs at a much higher concentration in the lungs compared to atmospheric levels, it moves more rapidly out of the body. Similarly, higher oxygen atmospheric levels (sea level) suck oxygen into the body more rapidly because the oxygen gradient between the environment and the lungs is wider.

A useful construct towards understanding the difference in the rate of carbon dioxide leaving and oxygen entering the body occurs when visualizing concentration differences as the 'steepness of the road'. The 'steeper the road', then the faster the gas moves. Carbon dioxide has a greater difference in concentration in the body compared to the atmospheric concentration of carbon dioxide. It moves more quickly down the 'steeper road', whereas the road for oxygen is less steep and hence it moves slower.

The second advantage for the ease of movement for carbon dioxide relates to the fact that different gases have different affinities to dissolve in fluids. Carbon dioxide dissolves in the blood stream much more avidly than oxygen. The more a gas can dissolve in a liquid (the blood stream) the more quickly it can enter that liquid.

Lastly, the hemoglobin protein contained within the red blood cells increases the oxygen and carbon dioxide carrying abilities of the blood stream many fold. As hemoglobin sucks oxygen out of the liquid component of the blood stream a continuous concentration difference is created while the blood flows in the lungs. Healthy owners are able to fill their hemoglobin oxygen carrying sites in the short time it takes for the blood to pass through the gas exchange chamber (the alveoli). Aging occurs when there is a decreased ability to fill the hemoglobin with oxygen in the specified time it exists in the oxygenated chamber (aveolus).

Common lung diseases manifest when dysfunction occurs between these all-important gaseous balances. Diseases that originate in the lungs lead initially to diminished oxygen transport. Diminished oxygen content leads to an increased likelihood of toxin accumulation. Toxins accumulate when there is less energy available because cells cannot burn toxins as fuel without sufficient oxygen in their combustion chambers (the mitochondria). Scientists discuss these facts in terms of aerobic (with oxygen) contrasted to anaerobic (without oxygen) fuel combustion. Without oxygen, the waste product, lactic acid begins to accumulate quickly in the cells.

Lactic acid damages tissues when it occurs at high levels. It does what other acids do to delicate cellular structures when allowed to accumulate in excess. Recall, too much acid or too little acid alters the electrical properties of the different and delicate intracellular contents. Examples of cellular contents are structural proteins, enzymatic machines, and charged ions. Lactic acid accumulation doesn't move out of the cell with the same ease as carbon dioxide gas.

Gases are wonderful. They move with ease from high concentrations to low concentrations. Lactic acid is not a gas. Consequently, cells possess a limited ability to release lactic acid once it begins to accumulate. Recall, certain nutritional deficiencies cause excessive lactic acid to form (chapter one). Insufficient oxygen around to meet metabolic demands is the mechanism that most doctors are trained to consider. It is important to emphasize that the reader recall the additional nutritional deficiencies that cause excessive lactic acid formation (chapter one)

When an owner exceeds exercise ability or suffers from specific nutritional deficiencies, his/her cells can go down the dead end road of burning sugars anaerobically. The ability to burn sugar anaerobically is limited by the amount of lactic acid the body can handle. Lactic acid forms as a consequence of anaerobic sugar metabolism. In contrast, aerobic metabolism consumes oxygen and involves a process where carbon dioxide gas forms as the waste product.

Carbon dioxide gas exits through the lungs. In contrast, lactic acid clears more slowly by processes in the liver and cannot exit through the lungs. Death or the intervention of common sense limits the amount of lactic acid production that the body will allow. Clinically, lactic acid accumulation evidences itself as sore muscles. It is the job of the liver to remove lactic acid from the blood stream (liver section).

Anatomy of Lung Vulnerability

Understanding the vulnerable areas of the lung is enhanced if some basic anatomy is reviewed. There are 300million balloons (alveoli) in each lung held in a basket of capillary vessels. Capillaries are the smallest of all vessels and so small that only one red cell can fit through them at a time by squeezing forward from the rhythmic pressure created by the heartbeat. These vessel walls are only one cell thick, which allows for the smallest of distances between the gas chamber (the balloon) and the red blood cells.

Upon entering this chamber, the red blood cells are loaded with waste gases and deficient in oxygen content. Each red blood cell has on average only .7seconds to change gases by dumping off carbon dioxide and loading up with oxygen on its billions of hemoglobin carrier sites. Each red blood cell needs to accomplish this before heading out for another transport trip.

The transport trip for each oxygen ends when it arrives at a distant, hungry cell where lower oxygen content allows it to be sucked off its carrier protein, hemoglobin through the process of deforming as it traverses through yet another tight capillary. This distant cell location is also one of increased waste gas and this high concentration difference allows hemoglobin to begin gathering waste gas for the trip back to the lungs. Around and around in the

378

circulation describes the life of the red blood cell. One way or another, lung disease interferes with the blood becoming fully oxygenated during its .7-second time allotment in the gas exchange chamber, the alveoli.

The Lung Disease Industry

Asthma illustrates the limitations and toxicities of mainstream medicine's approaches for one of the most common lung diseases. Alternatively, healing only begins to make sense after examining the other side of the scientific story. Asthma also exemplifies that lung disease decreases the ability of the body to remove trash. A diminished ability to deliver oxygen to the trash removal organ systems is the byproduct of asthma. With out adequate oxygen, all trash removal systems suffer diminished function. Consequently, learning how to heal diseases like asthma also develops the lungs ability to improve all six of the other trash removal organs.

Asthma - An Example of Symptom Control Versus Healing

Asthma provides a good place to contrast the symptom control medical approach with the holistic approach. Cause and effect treatment strategies have healing potential. Contrast these two different philosophies, with asthma care as a prototypical example. This journey illuminates how doctors in training often only receive partial information.

Omitting, key scientific facts in regard to the asthma disease process leads to unnecessary medication and side effects. A minority of asthma patients will still need some patented prescription medications to control their symptoms. However, the majority benefit by more holistic strategies.

The conventional explanation for causalities of asthma considers one or more of three interrelated processes. First, concerns the process of over reactive airways (bronchial tubes spasm). The asthmatics' airway tubes internal diameter contract (spasm) for various reasons. Spasm of the air tube (the bronchioles) leads to the musical wheezing sounds of asthma. Second involves the process of excessive mucus plugging. Many of these types of asthma sufferers are not diagnosed because they lack the characteristic wheeze of reactive airways. The mucus buildup can also diminish the diameter of the airway tubes. Often these lung exams are remarkable by there subtle decreased breath sounds.

Lastly, the process of the airway tubes themselves swelling and decreasing the internal diameter of the tube. Swollen tubes, like spasmodic or plugged tubes, are less able to move air back and forth. Like mucus, swelling of airways can fool physicians because wheezing sounds may be absent.

The wheezing symptoms of asthma are supposed to be from excessive spasm in the airways, swelling of these airways, and concurrent mucus overproduction. These three processes lead to the increased effort of moving air back and forth. These three processes lead to blood traveling into the lowered oxygen content lung chambers and as a consequence the red blood cells carry diminished oxygen.

Obviously, red blood cells that are not fully loaded with oxygen when they exit the lungs cannot deliver oxygen efficiently. These three mechanisms of developing asthma are very real. However, a deeper inquiry into the reasons why airways spasm, collects mucus, and/or swells often leads to healing.

For example, one cause of asthma concerns those owners who have adrenal dysfunction that causes wheezing, mucus plugs, and swelling in their airways. In fact, a significant number of asthma cases are caused by a dysfunction in one of the six links in the adrenal health chain (adrenal chapter). Consequently, without sufficient inquiry into the health status of suffering asthmatics' adrenal function, these patients will be condemned to symptom control. Logically it then follows that failure to recognize how healing happens causes these owners to suffer unnecessarily.

Unfortunately, patients who have asthma symptoms from additional causes lead these patients into receiving the highest doses of toxic medicines available (additional causes explained below). Understand, patients fail to respond because its cause has not been recognized.

Failure here requires that their symptoms be combated with ever-increasing use of debilitating medicines. For example, some asthma patients have bronchospasm, swelling and mucus plugging from nutritional deficiencies. Often, digestive malfunction describes their primary cause of breathing difficulties. Non-toxic restorative approaches are available for them instead of the more conventional and toxic medications.

Asthma care in America today exemplifies the consequences of treating symptoms rather than causes of a disease process. Mantra: symptom control always has side effects and toxicities. The western medical standard of care usually includes some or all of the following prescription medication types: patented derivatives of cortisol (a steroid), patented forms of adrenaline derivatives, patented forms of caffeine (the xanthine class that is usually theophylline or aminophylline as the prescribed form), the membrane stabilizers, and leukotriene inhibitors (inflammatory hormonal fat inhibitors).

All of these drugs have some utility and circumstances where they are indicated. However, there are often safer ways to heal from asthma that are largely free of side effects. In general, healing involves identifying ways to treat more centrally the imbalance that causes asthma.

A holistic approach will include nontoxic airway relaxants (salts of magnesium), herbal or hormonal mucus dissolvers (lobelia and/or correcting inadequate thyroid function and IGF-1 levels), substances that keep the balloons open because many asthmatics have an unrecognized tendency towards balloon collapse (surfactant deficiency), attention to adequate stomach acid, and the nutritionally derived airway spasm promoters (sulfites, phenols and others).

Also emerging concerns that stomach acid deficiency consequences occur in many asthmatics and need to be addressed. This deficiency causes partially digested proteins to leak across their bowel wall and activate their immune system. In some patients, the food allergies cross reacts with lung tissue leading to swelling, spasm and mucous. Consequently food allergy by this mechanism continues to evolve as a primary consideration.

In addition, the holistic medical approach considers other common causes of asthma that occur such as diminished function of the adrenal system (any of the six links in the adrenal system chain), lowered adrenaline (epinephrine) to nor-adrenaline (nor-epinephrine) ratio arising from of a methyl donor deficiency, diminished thyroid and/or vitamin A, and the imbalances between certain vertebrae, the skull, and the sacrum that impair lung function (craniosacral therapy considerations). Finally, zinc deficiency causes asthma.

Holistic Considerations - What Causes Asthma?

1. Deficiency of magnesium that leads to airway spasm
2. Inadequate stomach acid production with consequent decreased magnesium and zinc absorption
3. Increased mucus production from inadequate hormone levels
4. Inadequate surfactant production
5. Diminished adrenal system function
6. Diminished thyroid and/or vitamin A activity that

decreases the ability to respond to epinephrine's message content to relax the airway
7. Methyl donor deficiency
8. Cranial sacral therapy indications when there has been some sort of back trauma
9. Dietary determinants like, phenols, sulfites and sulfates
10. Stomach acid deficiency caused food allergies
11. Zinc deficiency caused asthma

Magnesium - An Airway Relaxant

Many asthmatics respond to aggressive magnesium supplementation because it relaxes airways for the same reasons it lowers blood pressure. Arteries and the airways are composed of a rich supply of smooth muscle. Magnesium relaxes smooth muscle. The smooth muscle layer in the arteries and airways reduces the internal diameter when they contract. In the case of contracting arteries, blood pressure rises. When the smooth muscles contract in the airways, the flow of air out of the lungs diminishes. When encountering extremely cold air the airways should contract to facilitate adequate warming of the inhaled air. However, inappropriate airway contraction causes wheezing.

Holistic physicians have observed the therapeutic effect of intravenous magnesium administered during acute asthma attacks. This has led many to make this their preferred acute intervention. Jonathan Wright MD and Alan Gaby MD have developed an acute asthma intravenous protocol that contains high doses of magnesium. They named this formulation the "Meyers Cocktail". It contains varying amounts of magnesium content, vitamin C, and high doses of many of the B vitamins, emphasizing B6 and B12. This preparation, when administered properly, can halt the most severe asthma attacks. Close follow up and monitoring are indicated because intravenous repetitions may be needed. Ideally this would be included in the protocols at the emergency rooms.

In contrast, the medical industry treats acute asthma attacks with high doses of the patented cortisol type steroids. Synthetic (patented) versions of cortisol type steroids frequently produce side effects. The side effects occur because by changing the shape of the cortisol hormone to obtain a patent, the message content changes. Recall, it is the precise shape that carries the message contained in a hormone. Altered message content changes the way that the body receives directions to spend energy at the DNA level. The altered DNA activity that results leads to altered structural and enzymatic protein production. These alterations produce their own side effects that often require additional prescription medications to curtail.

Intravenous magnesium on the other hand is relatively free of side effects. The exceptions regarding side effects are the occasional Viagra-like effects in woman and rectal fullness sensations in men (Wright 1998). The additional need to monitor blood pressure arises because magnesium proves also as a powerful anti-hypertensive. Magnesium also promotes regular bowel movements and some people experience this sensitivity. Unfortunately, traditionally trained physicians probably have not heard about magnesium usage in the treatment of asthma.

Adequate Stomach Acid in the Prevention of Asthma

Adequate stomach acid forms a prerequisite before proper mineral absorption occurs (digestion chapter). Consequently, failure within the stomach to produce sufficient acid causes deficient magnesium absorption from the diet. Realize, many asthmatics fail to manufacture adequate stomach acid and consequently develop an imbalance between calcium and magnesium. Sometimes, asthma is a consequence of this problem and results from excess calcium relative to magnesium. This situation tends to promote smooth muscle contraction.

The airways are lined with a smooth muscle layer and remain vulnerable to spasm when inadequate magnesium occurs. In these situations, the contraction properties of calcium fail to be counterbalanced by sufficient magnesium after it becomes deficient. Magnesium absorption depends more on adequate stomach acid production than does calcium.

Here lies the mechanism for imbalanced magnesium to calcium in the smooth muscles. Clinical practices that attempt to reliably measure stomach acid secretion abilities are procedurally cumbersome. For this reason, trying acid supplementation is often undertaken without insisting on the documentation of a deficient output (section three). By this mechanism, acid deficiency contributes to the development of asthma.

More recently an explanation for the increased histamine like content in the asthma patients' lung has come to light. It also involves the consequence of diminished acid secretion on two levels. The first level involves the dependency of the stomach acid-producing enzyme, carbonic anhydrase, activity to sufficient zinc. Unless sufficient zinc is present this enzyme cannot make stomach acid. The vicious cycle involves the fact that sufficient stomach acid is required before zinc and other minerals can absorb into the body.

The second level involves the fact that angiotensin converting enzyme (kinase) found in high concentrations within the normal lung requires zinc, as well, for its activity. Insufficient activity of this enzyme here causes abnormal amounts of bradykinin to accumulate. Increased bradykinin possesses histamine like activity and encourages the mast cells to release excess histamine as well. Histamine like substances causes swelling of the tissues (inflammation). When was the last time that anyone heard about a conventionally trained physician inquiring into his/her asthmatic patients' zinc status?

Excess Mucus Plugs the Airways of Asthmatic Lungs

The normal lung tubes continuously secrete a sticky film that traps dust and foreign invaders. The airway tubes are lined with motile hairs (cilia) that transport the trapped dust and invaders toward the trachea. To function properly, adequate water is the necessary mechanism for taking out the trash. The cilia need sufficient water content in the sticky film that coats them. Cilia move this film properly only when the viscosity in this film remains optimal. Thick mucus begins to develop when the water content diminishes. Certain hormones and plants help to ensure that the water content of this sticky film increases sufficiently. Only when sufficient water remains available in the respiratory mucus can the cilia continuously remove the film and debris out of the lungs.

Substances that increase the water content of mucus are called mucolytics. Examples of common mucolytics are lobelia, ginger root, and licorice root. Excess mucus commonly plagues the asthmatic lung. Lobelia inflata is a plant that benefits the dissolution of the overly producted and accumulated mucus. Ginger root is also a consideration for a natural way to decrease mucus thickness. In addition, licorice root often has a beneficial effect on the over production of thick lung mucus.

Often the thickness and production rate of lung mucus proves to be a problem stemming from abnormal hormones. Some asthmatic lung tissue does not recognize thyroid message content even though they secrete adequate thyroid hormone amounts. Thyroid message content is important for lung cells regarding their ability to keep the mucus production rate in check.

Low thyroid function causes increased mucus throughout the body. One of the places mucus collects when thyroid function is low is in the breathing tubes. This situation commonly occurs in the thyroid resistance syndromes (thyroid chapter). Unfortunately, when a physician tests for this problem in the thyroid in the conventional manner, the blood tests will often come back deceptively normal. However, peripheral thyroid resistance is one of the causes for asthma. Here the physician will need to look clinically for other clues of thyroid deficiency (thyroid discussion-section two).

The inter relationship of thyroid hormone with vitamin A requires consideration. As does the possibility that thyroid deficiency at the cell level will lead to increased mucus accumulation. The drying out effect that accompanies old age also explains some of these mucus abnormalities (section five).

Today, modern science can explain the hormone imbalances and molecular part deficiencies that allow water to escape from one's cells and mucus. However, this science routinely presents in disjointed and convoluted discussions that fail to unite key facts. The consequence often being physicians and owners are not taught to think about simple healing solutions that postpone the shrinkage into old age and thick mucous accumulation. These facts are explained in the intro of section five but a few brief introductory comments follow.

One reason sufficient thyroid hormone levels help keep mucous viscosity optimal occurs by an often overlooked hormone cascade that its presence allows: **The amount of thyroid in the pituitary determines how much Growth Hormone it manufactures**. This being sufficient allows adequate release of this hormone whenever the blood fuel begins to fall off. Growth Hormone arrives at the liver and when the liver is sufficiently healthy it releases ample amounts of fuel and IGF-1. However, many asthmatics fail to make sufficient IGF-1 in their livers because they have adrenal defects. Defective adrenal function means that DHEA will often be compromised. DHEA secretion rates form a primary determinant of how much IGF-1 the liver manufactures. Pretty boring stuff so far eh?

Well it becomes more interesting after one realizes that one of the additional old names for IGF-1 was sulfation factor. Sulfation describes the critical step in glycosaminoglycan (GAG) formation. Only when GAG forms properly can it retain optimal water. The addition of sulfate creates a powerful electrical charge that draws in water. Mucus largely consists of GAG. Some asthmatics suffer from problems in one or more of the above hormones. For the reasons listed above, they cannot form optimal mucous and instead form dry plugs.

Patients need to be informed that mainstream medicine frowns upon Growth Hormone and androgen replacement (DHEA) therapy for asthmatic owners. They purport to have ample unbiased studies that link these therapies to cancer's development and its accelerated growth. Yet, they fail to mention or consider some big inconsistent details: If all the negative fear about Growth Hormone were true, a good nights sleep, youthfulness, fasting, pregnancy and athletic training would all constitute an increased risk factor for developing cancer. Realize, all of the above are well documented to increase Growth Hormone release and hence IGF-1 as well. In addition, pregnancy, youthfulness, happiness and athletic training associate with a higher DHEA secretion rate. However, epidemiological studies have shown all of these traits to lower the risk of cancer's development.

The renaming of the nonsuppressible insulin like activity of the blood to insulin like growth factor type one (IGF-1) helps also to instill more fear still about growing cancer, as well. Note: This author has repeatedly encountered the tactic of renaming important physiological determinants like IGF-1. This effort isolates knowledge and allows for increased demand for what is for sale.

Also note that this economy-boosting tactic must ignore the fact that the highest pure insulin type receptor concentration occurs on the liver and fat cells at about 200,000 receptors per cell. Breast tissue composes itself from mostly fat. Overweight females are generally considered to be at increased risk for developing breast cancer. High insulin levels are a must before an owner can gain body fat. Yet no one counsels these breast cancer victims about insulin reduction techniques.

Instead IGF-1 receives the blame as a supposed central risk factor for tumor growth (section one). If this were so then athletic training, adolescence, a good nights sleep, fasting and pregnancy all would then be risk factors for developing cancer. In all five of these conditions, the IGF-1 levels are encouraged towards many times higher than occur in most middle-aged people. However, epidemiologic studies show that each one of these situations provides protection and does not seem to be a causative factor for cancer's development. Also as IGF-1 decreases with age, the health decreases as well (expanded discussion elsewhere).

Some asthmatic owners have severe glandular defects resulting decreases in Growth Hormone and/or androgen secretion. Either one of these defects will lead to decreased IGF-1. Some asthmatics have severe adrenal secretion defects that lead to less IGF-1 manufacture within the liver. When IGF-1 decreases then insulin must increase (see liver chapter). The more insulin increases, the more the fat maker message content within the body. A rising insulin level and a falling IGF-1 more often occur when cancer develops rather than the reverse. These facts give the average asthmatic something to consider the next time their physician orders supra physiologic doses of abnormally shaped steroids, which powerfully raise the blood sugar and inhibit Growth Hormone release. Blood sugar on the rise requires insulin to remedy. Insulin is the fat maker.

Surfactant Attention is Warranted when Balloon Collapse Causes Asthma

The alveoli in the lungs function like balloons. Collapsed balloons (alveoli) can't contain oxygen so the blood in the baskets surrounding these flattened balloons enters and leaves without exchanging gases. The more balloons that collapse, the less oxygen delivered to the cells. Only in the most extreme cases will waste gas build up in the body.

The mechanism for balloon collapse has been understood for quite some time in caring for premature infants. Unfortunately, this same mechanism that causes balloon collapse and breathing difficulties is ignored for anyone beyond infancy. Breathing difficulties result in these little patients because they fail to produce adequate surfactant. Surfactant deficiency also causes breathing difficulty in other age groups.

Surfactants have the property of forming suds (foaming agents) when in a liquid and it is shaken. The lung balloons are kept from collapsing by the presence of surfactant. Surfactant deficiency is one of the causes of asthma.

Surfactant's ability to keep the balloons open is better understood by visualizing an ordinary rubber balloon. Anyone who has attempted to blow up a balloon notices that the hardest part involves the initial expansion effort. After this initial expansion, it becomes much easier. Now expand the problem to 300 million alveoli once the gas content has completely expired. These spherical structures want to collapse purely from physical forces and inflating them, once collapsed, becomes analogous to the difficult infusion for that first bit of air into a rubber balloon times 300 million.

In healthy infants and adults the body design addresses this problem by continually producing fresh surfactant in the millions of balloons contained in each lung. When the interior of the balloons contains adequate suds (surfactant), breathing becomes easier. This property of surfactants (the ability to keep balloons open) arises because they function as surface tension reducers. This proves secondary to the law of Lapace as it refers to spherical bodies and the forces that want to collapse them.

Surfactants consist of modified fats attached to sugars that facilitate suds formation. The suds keep the chambers from collapsing. The lung chambers (alveoli) produce just the right amount of surfactant. Unfortunately, surfactant deficiency in clinical practice is mostly recognized in premature infants.

Unfortunately, the quality of surfactant production in adult and pediatric asthma patients remains often ignored. This leads this type of asthma sufferer down the road to receiving the highest doses of prescription medications. These patients have a sub-optimal response secondary to ignoring the central problem of their needing foaming agents (surfactants) before their breathing normalizes. In other words, this fact describes a group of asthma patients whose disease cause results from surfactant deficiency.

As was previously stated, the science behind the consequences of surfactant deficiency has been recognized in the care of premature infants. Typically, aggressive use of patented cortisol derivatives is administered in this surfactant deficient group of infant asthmatic patients. These medications are effective because synthetic corticosteroids are one of the hormones that increase the production of surfactant. Adequate surfactant levels lower the work of breathing.

Somehow after infancy the medical establishment ignores the consequences and causality of surfactant deficiency as it relates to the disease process of asthma. This practice occurs despite the long known association of surfactant deficiency and the eventual development of emphysema. Realize, most asthmatics develop emphysema in their later years.

This association makes mechanical sense when considering that with time if a balloon remains collapsed it will die off secondary to continued oxygen deprivation. Surfactant deficiency, along with lung cell atrophy, will result when certain hormones remain deficient. For this reason, perhaps a more thorough inquiry is warranted. Emphysema (i.e. COPD) is the medical name denoting loss in the total number of balloons that each lung contains.

The need arises to look at surfactant deficiency at a deeper level. This deficiency is often a biochemical marker of a more central deficiency. Certain growth factors are needed by the lung tissue to remain healthy (thyroid hormones, vitamin A, DHEA, and cortisol). Further insight into the deficiency of these growth factors and the presentation of asthma is substantiated by the emerging recognition that many asthma sufferers have abnormal twenty-four hour urine output of one or more of these hormones. Science has revealed the consequences of surfactant deficiency. For this reason it makes sense to include its consideration in the management strategies of this lung disease.

The majority of surfactant is composed of modified fat that confers an electrical charge on the inner surface of the balloon. The repulsive charge increases as the balloons collapses. As these chambers deflate with expiration, the charges become closer to each other. Like charges repulse each other. Each one of these modified fats has a positive charge and when these charges move closer together (expiration) an increasing electrical repulsion occurs. The electrical force created in the alveoli as it contracts generates a propensity for the alveoli to inflate with the next inspiration. Deficiency of this electrical force toward inflation of these alveoli occurs when a deficiency of these electrically charged fats (surfactants) occurs. For these reasons, it is important to evaluate whether or not an asthmatic has a surfactant deficiency.

An interesting aside consideration also occurs at this juncture of considering the properties of adequate surfactant and the different ways that this can be achieved (toxically versus non-toxically): The medical industrial dogma states that corticosteroids (cortisol like medications) are so effective in the long-term maintenance of asthma care because they alter the inflammation process that is supposed to be occurring in refractory asthmatic cases. What they often fail to mention is that science has long ago revealed that cortisol like medications directly stimulate surfactant production.

Patented versions of cortisol-like medications stimulate surfactant production, but a big price is paid. Mantra: the practice of chronically hammering owners cells with abnormally shaped cortisol-like prescriptions can lead to health consequences (altered immune function, decreased cellular rejuvenation activities, obesity, adrenal gland atrophy, etc.).

Leaving out a real possibility of why steroids (cortisol types) improve breathing in these asthma patients covers the scientific tracts that can lead to healing. The trail to healing

these patients is further concealed by medical physiology textbooks alluding to the fact that attempts to increase surfactant delivery through oral intake have proved ineffective. The truth is more accurately stated as: endogenous surfactant production cannot be increased until improvement in the hormones that direct its production occurs. Specific hormones lead to improved surfactant production. However, it is important to first touch on how certain plants help in certain cases.

All is not hopeless if one includes the consideration of certain plants that possess surfactants. Further research is warranted, but encouraging results have been achieved with high quality ginseng. Panax ginseng root, that is at least 7 years old, possesses a class of substances called the glycosides. By definition all glycosides possess the ability to form suds (foam).

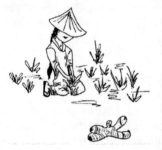

In order to avoid confusion, the active ingredient in ginseng is best thought of as a steroid contained in a package. While this steroid is still in its 'package', it possesses properties of the surfactant class. The intelligence of the body decides whether it needs ginseng as the glycoside or as the broken down (package removed) weak steroid building block for the production of other steroids.

An interesting degree of inconsistency occurs in the medical literature, if one inquires into the utility of the plant glycosides as surfactants. Medical dictionaries and textbooks go on about how all plant glycosides are not orally absorbable. They further go on to caution the reader that if given intravenously they lead to rupture of cell membranes. The inconsistency of this statement reveals itself when one understands that a very important heart medication used for over 200 years comes from this class of plant substances. If one reads the literature for the class of drugs coming from the foxglove plant that make the various digitalis derivatives, it states that they are from the class of substances called the glycosides. It is further stated that absorption of most glycosides is almost 100% orally! There is nothing about the need to worry about these drugs causing cell membrane rupture. This information saves the inquiring reader the common pitfalls that are holding back the usage of this valuable group of plant substances in the treatment of asthma.

Assessing the Adrenal System in Asthmatics

The adrenal gland is responsible for adequate secretion of DHEA and cortisol. Visualize the healthy adrenal secretion as balanced between anabolism and catabolism. However, one or both of these hormones secretion rate often proves to be abnormal in the asthmatic owner. An imbalanced antique weight scale conceptually represents the hormonal imbalance operating in asthmatics. The majority of these owners have a DHEA and/or cortisol deficiency. Many times it is their respective metabolites that prove defective. DHEA, cortisol and their respective metabolite imbalances shows up in the twenty-four hour urine test.

Here a big problem arises because Western-trained physicians do not routinely understand how to check for these important values. The few that do check for DHEA metabolite levels, often find them to be diminished. Remember, leaving out the all-important metabolites diminishes the predictive value of inquiry as to the root cause of asthma. Correlating with this finding is the tendency for other lung problems to be associated with adrenal insufficiency. Therefore by not treating the adrenal deficiency it may allow asthma patients to suffer unnecessarily (adrenal chapter).

Compounding the problem concerns the fact that conventional physicians are trained to treat only one side of the antique weight scale in an asthmatic patient, the cortisol side (catabolism). Consequently, they fail to ask what happened to their asthmatic's anabolism (DHEA) secretion. Making matters worse, conventional physicians often treat asthma owners with both supra-physiologic doses and abnormally shaped versions of cortisol. Realize that administering cortisol like message content further suppresses the anabolism component of the recipient patient's adrenal secretion. This fact explains another reason why these lopsided approaches lead to unnecessary side effects. Only when real hormones (real cortisol and DHEA) are used in amounts sufficient to correct the deficiency can healing occur without side effects.

Remember, cortisol needs to be appropriately counter balanced with adequate DHEA. When these two hormones remain in oppositional balance lung health can occur. Healthy adrenal glands secrete both DHEA and cortisol, in appropriately proportioned amounts. This happens in an optimal ratio and at the same time. In some cases, asthma becomes a disease of diminished adrenal output of DHEA and/or cortisol. This relationship provides an explanation for how medicinal plants like ginseng help in the treatment of asthma. These plants provide a source of steroid precursor that could be the reason that the weakened adrenal gland then increases its production of these hormones. The antique weight scale comes into balance again concerning these two opposing hormones.

The advice and monitoring of a competent physician proves invaluable in helping an owner return to balance in the safest way possible. Asthma disease often involves adrenal dysfunction. The evaluation for how the adrenal system can fail is important (adrenal chapter). The challenge is to discern where the basic defect lies that causes a patient to suffer from asthma.

Thyroid, Vitamin A, and Lung Health

Healing asthma requires a cognizance of thyroid and vitamin A message content in the lungs. These hormones deliver their instructions at the level of the lung cells DNA program (genes) and deficiency at this DNA level causes disease. These hormonal effects are in addition to the message content of both cortisol and DHEA directed at the lung cell DNA. All four of these level-one hormones prove necessary in order for the DNA program to activate the proper protein synthesis. Only lung cells containing the appropriate proteins can be healthy. Unhealthy lung cells sometimes manifest as asthma and the resolution of this disease needs to include an assessment of level one hormones production rates.

The importance of adequate thyroid hormone in the lung, colon, kidney, liver, immune system, and skin has been known for over one hundred years. Experiments on dogs that had their thyroids partially removed established at necropay what the cell consequences were in these organ systems. In the lungs, kidney and liver the changes were striking. These organs had a marked increase in scar tissue (fibrosis).

Thyroid is a central growth factor for these tissues and without it these organ systems cells begin to atrophy (die). When scar tissue forms where there was once viable tissue, the organ suffers from diminished function. Here emerges a recurrent body theme that cells need direction on how to spend energy. The loss of thyroid message content leads to a diminution of rejuvenation. Scar tissue replaces functional cells because cells die without adequate directions for rejuvenation.

These old time scientific observations become even more powerful today because it is known that the more thyroid hormone (within normal), the more the pituitary produces Growth Hormone.

In turn, the more Growth Hormone released the more IGF-1 released, if DHEA levels remain adequate. IGF-1 can be thought as the nutritional adequacy marker of the tissues (the fuel nozzle to the functional tissue beyond the liver and fat).

Vitamin A is similar to thyroid in that it is a necessary growth factor at the level of lung cell DNA programs (genes). Its message content provides instruction on developing the maturity of the cell (differentiation). Only when cells mature can they produce the cell product, which is inherent in that cell type. The cells that line the lung air passages need to make many secretion products, surfactants, and mucus. Unfortunately, many asthmatics that receive conventional treatment are never counseled on these scientific facts. Unfortunately, still other deficiencies occur in the education of conventionally trained physicians that prove equally problematic in other nutritionally based causes of asthma.

Nutritional Deficiencies Present as Wheezing

Nutritional deficiencies can contribute to the severity of an asthmatic tendency from an imbalance between the forces in the blood stream versus the forces in the autonomic nervous system. This tug of war occurs in blood vessel tension and breathing tube tension. These same nutritional deficiencies cause many cases of curable blood pressure problems (blood pressure chapter) as well.

Basic physiology textbooks teach that when the sympathetic nervous system activates, the airways should open up. This major message for the airways arrives from the sympathetic nerves stimulating the adrenal medulla to release epinephrine. Sometimes, part of the asthma problem centers on inadequate epinephrine release secondary to specific nutritional deficiencies. In contrast, nor-epinephrine released by the adrenal into the blood stream proves weak at relaxing the airways. For this reason, the majority of the adrenal medulla secretion should be epinephrine.

Recall, epinephrine can only be manufactured in the adrenal medulla when a nutritionally intact methyl donor system occurs. Normally, the major airway relaxation occurs from stimulation of the sympathetic nerves to the adrenal glands to release 90% epinephrine and only 10% nor-epinephrine. The optimal ratio of adrenal medulla release is important in the prevention of wheezing when stimulated by the sympathetic nerves.

Above and beyond the simple opposition of magnesium towards calcium, only epinephrine message content in the blood stream is powerful enough in its ability to relax the airways. Owners who suffer from nutritional deficiencies in vitamin B6, vitamin B12, methionine, folate, serine, tetrahydrobiopterin, SAMe, and/or vitamin C will not be able to manufacture sufficient epinephrine in their adrenal glands. Consequently, the much weaker nor-epinephrine will tend to be released and with progressive deficiencies these owners will wheeze. The above nutrients make up the methyl donor system except for tetrahydrobiopterin (partially made from folate) and vitamin C.

Unfortunately, owners who eat a processed food diet will likely develop deficiencies in one or more of these nutrients. Bodies respond to a methyl donor deficiency in different ways. Some experience wheezing as the primary manifestation of their methyl donor deficiency. Recall under the best of circumstances the body requires a methyl group at the rate of one billion times a second!

Epinephrine synthesis only remains possible when all the above nutritional cofactors remain available. For this reason, a deficiency here could be another cause for asthma. Supplementing with some of these nutritional factors in the Meyers cocktail (intravenous route of administration) leads to an improvement in breathing. For this reason, including these additional specific nutrients would probably make the Meyers cocktail even more effective.

Maintaining adequate epinephrine levels leads to an improved breathing ability. This explains why the patented inhalers like Alupent and Proventil have an epinephrine-like molecular structure. It also probably explains why Chinese herbs like Ma Hung (ephedra) receive bad press almost daily from the official view of the universe.

Epinephrine at normal dosages tends to not raise blood pressure significantly because it increases blood flow to the heart, muscles, and liver. Whenever blood flow increases in these three areas, the diastolic blood pressure decreases despite epinephrine decreasing blood flow to other areas of the body. This excludes the brain where the blood flow is held constant. Ma Hung has a similar effect on both blood flow and airway caliber as epinephrine does.

In contrast, nor-epinephrine decreases blood flow everywhere (except the brain). For this reason, nor-epinephrine dramatically raises blood pressure. Visualize a fixed amount of blood contained in the blood vessels. The pressure will go up acutely when these vessels contract and will go down when they relax. In addition, nor-epinephrine proves very weak in its message content toward relaxing the airways. These two differences between epinephrine and nor-epinephrine form important considerations when attempting to balance airway tube caliber.

The difference between the blood pressure effects of nor-epinephrine and epinephrine, explains a lot about patented bronchial-dilators. The patented bronchial dilators tend to be closely related to an epinephrine-like molecular structure. However, if a pharmaceutical company marketed a nor-epinephrine-like bronchial dilator two things would happen. First, the bronchial dilator with nor-epinephrine-like molecular shape would be very weak. Second, blood pressure would tend to rise and this is an unacceptable side effect. Pharmaceutical companies are smart enough to know the importance of avoiding this side effect. Strokes are not good for their bottom line.

The active ingredient contained within Ma Hung is ephedrine. Ephedrine proves structurally very similar to epinephrine. Taken orally, under the guidance of a knowledgeable physician, this will be more effective.

The eventual goal involves the adrenal glands producing epinephrine in adequate amounts. This is best accomplished by taking live food sources of the B vitamins. B vitamins taken this way more readily absorb. Tetrahydrobiopterin is best obtained from royal bee jelly or as its precursor, folate. Vitamin C is best in powder form. The amino acids serine and methionine can be obtained in a health food store or by eating eggs daily.

Another effective method for correcting methyl donor deficiencies involves the use of intravenous vitamin replacement therapies. Naturopathic physicians are a good source for these treatments. The Meyers cocktail intravenous preparations are one example of how naturopathic physicians can help. These physicians are very good at intravenous vitamin replacement protocols. The intravenous route will often jump start a nutritionally deficient body. This approach allows time to sort out possible absorption problems that are common in asthmatic owners.

Asthma-Influenced by Energy that Heals Versus Energy that Maims

Another consideration proves important for healing asthma that is probably the hardest one for the western owner to grasp. When energy flow problems cause asthma, cranial-sacral therapy dramatically relieves the blockages. It has to do with the emerging understanding of the energetic and rhythmical pulsation occurring from the bones in the skull down through the spine and on down into the sacrum. When this energy isn't flowing properly or has blocked areas, there becomes either a deficiency or excesses of these energies within the organs. The wrong energy pulsation will throw the recipient organs out of balance. This explains why the chiropractic technique called cranial-sacral therapy achieves some dramatic benefits.

Some cases are never forgotten. A 17 year-old asthma sufferer tried all the above approaches only to fail. Fortunately, her father took her to a competent chiropractor where this cranial-sacral technique was used and in just two office visits the patient's asthma resolved. This young patient had fallen while skiing several years before. This led to a jamming of the energy pulsation within her spine. This fixation for reasons that are not explainable in the officially sanctified view of the universe led to the symptoms of asthma.

Phenols, Sulfates, and Sulfites Sensitivities and Asthma

Sulfite sensitivity is known to be associated with asthma. A possible explanation for this common observation involves the known association of asthma and DHEA deficiencies. The connection of these two facts allows a thread of understanding between sulfite sensitivity and asthma. DHEA, when attached to sulfate or sulfite, is relatively off limits to tissues like the lung. There are numerous enzymes in the blood stream that constantly trap DHEA with available sulfite or sulfate. The higher the levels of sulfate or sulfite, the more likely it is to trap DHEA. Since some asthmatics have a diminished DHEA level already, adding sulfites in the diet will further decrease the DHEA availability. This is an explanation for why some asthmatics are sulfite and sulfate sensitive. The twenty-four hour urine test is applicable here to help discern why some owners have asthma.

Zinc deficiency caused asthma

Recall zinc is necessary for the enzyme in the lung, Angiotensin Converting Enzyme (kinase) to inactivate histamine like message content. Histamine like message content is called bradykinin. In turn bradykinin levels encourage the mast cells to release stored histamine. This chain of events explains the most common side effect of the blood pressure lowering medications called Angiotensin Converting Enzyme Inhibitors being a dry cough! Also realize that many asthmatics suffer from excessive histamine and ignoring this relationship only makes it worse! Adding insult to injury concerns the stomach's acid secreting ability depends on sufficient zinc as well but the ability to absorb zinc depends on sufficient stomach acid!

Food Allergies and Asthma

Connect the fact that most asthmatics secrete stomach acid poorly and this means they absorb zinc sub-optimally. Now consider the consequences of failing to mount a strong stomach acid secretion towards a protein containing meal: Partial protein breakdown results.

Partially digested proteins fragments can penetrate the digestive tube of some asthmatics because recall in some of these cases they have diminished GAG formation. Diminished GAG formation causes leaky gut. Partially digested protein leaks into the blood stream and activates the immune system. Certain protein sequences found in food also coincide with protein sequences found in certain body tissues like lung, nervous system, joints and kidneys.

Currently it remains a mystery why food allergy presents as Multiple sclerosis, rheumatoid arthritis, colitis, asthma, or glomerulonephritis in different individuals. For now accept that food allergy is emerging as a major cause of common disease processes. For these reasons, the mainstream should begin to wake up to the work of physicians like Jonathan Wright, MD who wrote *Why Stomach Acid is Good for You.*

It has taken this author over 20 years to unlearn some of the out there is the allergen dogma. Consider, if one is allergic to a food, the dosage here is roughly over a trillion times the dose of any environmental allergen like dander, mold or dust. For this reason, find the food allergen and the lesser allergens often become manageable.

Unfortunately conventionally trained physicians only check IgE antibodies. However, IgG antibodies are now known to contribute profoundly to diseases like asthma, multiple sclerosis, colitis, Crohn's disease, thyroiditis, adrenalitis, oophoriitis, pernicious anemia, neuropathy, rheumatoid arthritis, and other autoimmune diseases. Because of this, this type of testing in the next few years will revolutionize the ability of these patients to heal from these diseases. Lastly, always remember when dealing with the above types of disease, the physician must endevor to increase the repair rate (hormones) while eliminating the injury mechanism (food allergies).

The lungs are one of the organs that help take out the trash water. Lungs remove trash water in two ways. They exhale waste gas, carbon dioxide, from the blood stream. They also deliver oxygen to the tissues that is necessary to incinerate the constantly generated trash occurring in cells. The disease of asthma results in the diminishing ability of the lungs to exchange gases. Asthma treatment strategies were contrasted between symptom control and cause and effect modalities.

Mantra: Cause and effect is always preferable to symptom control. Paradoxically, in the treatment of asthma, too little attention is devoted to the cause of this disease. In the next chapter, the saga for the damage inflicted by symptom control medicine continues within the largest organ of the body, skin.

CHAPTER EIGHTEEN

SKIN

The skin is the largest organ system of the body. The skin not only removes certain types of trash, but also protects the body from outside trash entering it. The skin serves as a protective barrier and a trash water excretion organ. Two distinct layers of cell types compose this organ. The deepest layer, the dermis, lies over the subcutaneous fat. The dermis constitutes the last layer outward in the body that contains blood vessels. The hair shafts and sweat glands imbed in this layer. On top of the dermis lies the epidermis that has no direct blood supply. Its survival depends on the lower level dermis for the diffusion of nutrients and oxygen.

On top of the last living layer of epidermal cells are approximately twenty-eight layers of dead epidermis. The integrity of these dead layers forms a crucial determinant for the protection of the lower skin layers. Processes that alter this protective coating will increase the injury rate to the lower layers. What the skin does and how it sustains harm is the focus of this chapter. Also, once harmful skin conditions are identified, common solutions are presented.

Looking at the needs and dilemmas of the typical plant leaf on a hot summer day facilitates an understanding for the needs of healthy skin. Shriveled, crinkled plant leaves result from similar causes that lead to sagging and wrinkled skin. For this reason, processes that facilitate continued plant leaf vitality also tend to promote youthful skin.

Plant leaves, like skin, need a vapor barrier to trap moisture content within its cells. A vapor barrier prevents rapid water loss in dry environmental conditions. Maintaining optimal water content in the skin and leaf cells heavily depends on the integrity of this vapor barrier.

A plant's vapor barrier derives from it secreting a wax layer onto the surface that covers the cell. Wax is really just a slightly modified fat. However, without adequate fat to form a layer over skin cells, these cells suffer from a deficient vapor barrier. For this reason, fat provides an important deterrent to water loss. Adequate fat (oil) allows the top skin layer of dead cells to remain water filled.

The importance of having adequate fat intake in the diet proves cornerstone for minimizing the dehydrating forces. Dehydrating forces occur in two common environmental extremes. First adequate fat on the skin surface prevents water loss on a hot summer day. Second, adequate fat prevents water loss in the middle of winter when the heater has taken optimal humidity out of the air. For these reasons, excessive wind and the low humidity of some locales lead to the fast track approach for the development of the withered skin look.

These facts also explain why owners on a low fat diet prematurely wrinkle. Fat deficiency causes acceleration in the crinkling forces of the skin. Crinkling forces accelerate when the body lacks sufficient dietary fat (oils). Remember, dietary fats facilitate the development of a vapor barrier. The most pronounced wrinkles usually begin as deep creases beginning at the inferior lateral margin of the nose and extend downward toward the lateral border of the mouth.

Instead of counseling owners on ways to maintain an effective skin vapor barrier, western medicine concentrates on avoiding the ultraviolet rays of the sun. It is true that total exposure levels accumulated during a lifetime and form one determinant for how fast skin ages. However, leaving out other major factors in the formation of an effective strategy to maintain skin youthfulness promotes an incomplete view of what science has revealed. Preservation of healthy skin comes with more complete knowledge.

Healthy skin facilitates the kidney's job of toxin removal through the act of perspiration. Perspiration allows the kidney to obtain backup help for the removal of many toxins and mineral imbalances. For these reasons, daily perspiration facilitates health. One additional benefit concerns the hydration that perspiration provides to the outer skin layers. Added moisture in these outer layers adds to the youthful appearance of skin.

Ultraviolet Radiation

Knowledge is often ignored regarding the needs of the skin and its relationship to the role of ultraviolet radiation and skin damage. Depletion of the ozone layer over some locales on the planet has led to a dramatic increase in skin cancers. Unfortunately, there has been little inclination by the industrialized countries to curb the destruction of this important life-protecting layer. Refrigerators and air conditioning units slowly leak ozone-depleting molecules.

Consequently, increased radiation reaches the planet as this protective layer diminishes. Diminished atmospheric protection causes the skin to suffer from excessive exposer to the damaging effects of unnatural radiation. This damage occurs by its ability to knock electrons off of biological molecules in the upper layers of the body. As was discussed earlier this process describes how biological oxidation (rust formation) begins. For this reason, the curtailment of the increased radiation contained in the thinner atmosphere forms another determinant of skin vitality.

Mainstream Medicine's Mystery Determinant of Skin Vitality

The quality of the message content (hormones) which reaches skin forms a powerful determinant of who will age gracefully versus who will age quickly. Yet, for reasons that remain unclear, this consideration continues to be missing from clinical consideration. Skin cells, like other body cells, depend on direction from the different hormones. The messages provided from the different hormones instruct skin cells how to spend their available energy. Quality message content that arrives at the skin cell gives maximal rejuvenating stimulation to cell infrastructure investment activities. Quality message content induces skin rejuvenation and part of this message results in; the production of a highly functional vapor barrier, adequate water attracting molecules (the glucosaminoglycans), and the formation of sufficient skin protein (keratin).

Graphic evidence of the skin's dependency on the proper hormones is witnessed in adolescents that are plagued by excessive acne. Acne formation provides a clinical sign of a high androgen steroid message content in the skin that leads to excessive production of skin oil (vapor barrier). Their clinicians encourage these adolescent owners by mentioning that later in life they will have more beautiful skin than their peers. Beautiful skin comes from optimal steroid message content reaching the skin layer. The amount of skin oil produced proves directly proportional to the androgen message content. This fact is just one additional example for how the quality (hormones in types and amounts) of the message determines how a cell spends available energy.

Acne formation may occur due to excess androgen levels or an improper proportion between DHEA and cortisol. William McKenzie Jefferies MD describes in his book, *'Safe Uses of Cortisol'* how adolescents with acne have this problem. Dr. Jefferies points out that healing these patients' centers on three things. First, an accurate steroid hormone profile assessment needs to occur. Second, the treating physician also needs to be aware of the difference between supra-physiological dosing versus physiological dosing.

Finally, the downside of prescribing abnormal steroid types (patented hormones) needs to be contrasted with natural steroid replacement. Realize, the natural steroid replacement needs only to correct the documented deficiency. Adherence to this tenant avoids side effects. Simple science yet, not commonly taught in medical schools in a way that physicians understand. Individual attention to the uniqueness of each acne sufferer will allow healing for the majority.

Skin cells possess unique abilities and have unique needs when compared to other cells. Recall, the top twenty-eight layers are dead cells. These dead cells need to be been filled with three important molecular components. They are full of the protein keratin. Second, these dead skin cells contain adequate fat to protect the skin from water loss. Third, the inflationary architectural framework allows skin cells to remain filled to the brim with water content.

The framework is composed of mucopolysaccharides (GAG or also called formally, glycosaminoglycans). GAG (glycosaminoglycans or mucopolysaccharides) possess the property of attracting water inside cells. When this framework begins to crumble, another mechanism for shrinking cellular forces comes into play. The adequacy of this support framework forms another determinant for the ability of a skin cell to remain inflated with water (see below). In contrast, fat allows skin to remain inflated by decreasing water loss from above.

The skin and the digestive tube both require protective layers from the outside environment. Recall, defects in the inner protective layer of the digestive tube facilitate leaky gut syndrome. Glycosaminoglycans (GAG) compose this protective layer. As this layer continually forms in the digestive tube, it eventually degrades and it creates mucous overlying the new GAG layer.

Some scientists call the GAG layer the matrix. In fact, through out the different linings of the body such as the skin, the respiratory tract, the inner lining of the blood vessels, the GAG layer forms a protective barrier in these areas. In addition, it is this architectural support meshwork (GAG) that inflates cells, forms cartilage and connects cells together. All of these are formed by GAG. Paradoxically, mainstream medicine often fails to discuss or consider this important layer in the maintenance of health. This proves as folly because as GAG diminishes so does the owners health.

In order for doctors to appreciate all these facts about GAG, they need to know all the many alias names that describe it within the literature. Some of them are: cell coat, mucopolysaccharides, basal lamina, ground substance, cytoskeleton, extra cellular matrix and cartilage.

Additional doctor disability occurs because they have not been encouraged to remember the chemical makeup of GAG. GAG is manufactured from the molecular building blocks, glucosamine and galactosamine. These basic components are strung together and crisscrossed into chains thousands of molecules long. Furthermore, in order to attract water properly, the building blocks of each of these fundamental building blocks need additions of sulfate and acetate.

Important point: only with sufficient additions of sulfate will enough electrical charge be present to attract water. Recall, the old name for IGF-1 being sulfation factor, which describes its critical role in attracting water into the different GAG composed tissues that only then can retard the drying effect of old age.

Since GAG formation proves so important to one's overall and skin health, pertinent connecting facts for what determines its formation rate are in order. Recall, the amount of IGF-1 determines a particular body local's amount of GAG formation rate. Many physicians remain unaware of this fact because the vocabulary uniting this association has been changed. Recall, the older literature described IGF-1 as sulfation factor.

Sulfation describes the critical step in the formation of GAG utilizing the basic building blocks, galactosamine or glucosamine, where sulfate joins onto them. As long as sufficient IGF-1 instructs the locals listed above, adequate GAG forms properly. Remember, GAG cannot form properly without sufficient sulfation on each glucosamine and galactosamine.

Remember as well, the addition of sulfate powerfully sucks in water. Basic chemistry principle: the adequacy of the electrical charge within a body locale determines much about its ability to oppose gravity, which desires to squish cells flat. Therefore, the more adequate the water content, in a body area, the less shrinkage. Wrinkles on the skin are the outward expression of the shrinking process leading to old age. Why would anyone in their right mind willfully ignore the assessment of the adequacy of this process?

It is largely the GAG content of the body that opposes the forces of gravity, which desires to squish cells flat. Only when a sufficient presence of the electrically charged GAG molecules (sulfated) occurs will there be the ability to impede shrinkage imposed by gravity. Shrinkage occurs from drying out and has been recognized since antiquity to be fundamental to the aging process. Wrinkled skin provides evidence for only one component of the aging process caused by the loss of sufficient electrical charge.

Recall, IGF-1 levels depend on adequate Growth Hormone release, a healthy liver and adequate androgen (DHEA) instructing the liver to manufacture sufficient IGF-1. Preceding this is the fact that adequate Growth Hormone synthesis within the pituitary requires sufficient thyroid hormones instructing it to manufacture this hormone (50% of pituitary product). For these reasons, if any of the above four requirements fail health suffers.

Recap nerd corner: A similar vocabulary change preceded the old name of IGF-1 being called sulfation factor. This name change helps to propagate yet another disconnection in physicians' minds regarding IGF-1's important role in sugar metabolism. This older name calls IGF-1, the nonsuppressible insulin like activity of the blood. **The old name sheds light on IGF-1's important role in sugar metabolism**. The new name helps to instill fear of the same molecule being a growth factor for cancer cells. This spin on science requires ignoring the fact that all healthy people have high levels of IGF-1. Change the name and you can better manipulate how physicians think.

Another powerful disconnection results from the fact that insulin amounts, in almost all medical textbooks, are measured in micro units or micromoles. However, IGF-1 is measured in nanograms. This helps to perpetuate the concealment of the fact that ideally IGF-1 occurs at levels many times greater than insulin. If more physicians were aware of this fact they would begin asking why the body design would do this. The next step would be economic disaster for the medical industrial complex.

Some important facts about fat and a few more that mysteriously have been kept a secret

Recall the Four Important Roles for Body Fat (lipids):
1. **Cell structure and water retention (simple fats and cholesterol)**
2. **Hormone precursors**
3. **Fuel**
4. **Brain fats keep nerve cells happy**

Specialized Lipids (fats), fatty acids, triglycerides, and cholesterol make up the basic structural fats of the body. These building parts are often used as covering for trillions of cell membranes. These occur as part of the cell covering structure for the plasma membrane and organelles (cell factories). These structural fats integrate between varying combinations of interspersed proteins. Both the simple structural fats and the more complex, specialized structural fats compose membranes. The complex group contains lipids with extra molecular parts like phosphate or choline. Ultra-specialized fats have additional properties in body function by their role in specialized cells and organelles.

Beautiful skin demonstrates the importance of structural fat. It polishes the surface and prevents shriveling by retaining water. Prevention of cellular water loss describes a major function of fat. Inadequate fat content, in type or amount, causes or accelerates water loss. Shriveling and cellular inefficiency occur when water content decreases.

Second, certain lipids (fats) behave as informational substances. These can be thought of as hormonal fats and derive from the essential fatty acids. The body cannot produce essential fatty acids. They must be acquired through dietary sources and absorbed by the digestive tract.Essential fatty acids can be transformed into message carriers (hormones). Hormonal fats have their own message content contained in their precise shape. Hormonal fats promote information exchange between neighboring cells. Scientists call these essential fatty acid derived types of hormonal messengers the ecosanoids. As a consequence, the availability of essential fatty acids, which the body needs to make certain hormonal fats play a role in the prevention of heart disease, arthritis, and inappropriate immune activation.

Ecosanoids can be further divided into three groups: prostaglandins, leukotrienes, and lipoxin. All of these ecosanoids derive from arachidonic acid, linoleic acid, or linolenic acid-the only known essential fatty acids. Dietary choices and the higher level hormones circulating in the body determine what type of essential fatty acid eventually develop into hormones in cells (See ***Entering the Zone*** by Barry Sears). Consume fats that lead to a prevalence in anti-inflammatory, heart disease preventing, and immune system optimizing types of message content. Sources for these types of essential fatty acids are found in cold-water fish, borage oil, evening primrose oil, algae and vegetables.

In order to have good message content, there needs to be the right higher hormones. Only when more glucagon and less insulin hormones secrete will proper directions exist for the good precursor hormonal fats to be manufactured from the dietary derived essential fatty acids (see *Entering the Zone* by Barry Sears or the hierarchy of hormones in section two).

Some owners consume diets that lead to the promotion of skin inflammation, heart disease, inappropriate activation of the immune system, because these diets contain inflammation producing fatty acids (informational substance precursors). **In addition to promoting inflamed looking skin, these disease exacerbating hormonal fat precursors occur on all cell surfaces when insulin predominates.** The partially hydrogenated fats (Tran's fats) also contribute to this process. Some body processes will activate inappropriate message content when the disease promoting types of fatty acids make up an owner's cell membranes. They promote the above diseases because they contain inappropriate message content.

Recall that the third role of fat in the body is to serve as fuel. Per gram of weight, fat provides triple the energy content of protein, and double the energy content of carbohydrate. Only optimal hormone content (message content) permits accessibility of this excellent fuel source to the cells for caloric needs. Which hormone dominates the message content determines the fat access availability for fuel needs. If the wrong hormones dominate message content then the fat cell content becomes off limits as fuel. This condition, and all the complications to other body systems, traps the body in obesity (see section two).

The fourth role of fat concerns the electrical circuitry of the central nervous system. These electrical insulator types of fats possess unique types of components that provide for maintenance of proper nerve conduction and health. **The fact that the human brain has more fat weight than nerve cell weight illustrates this point.**

Beautiful Skin Depends on Adequate Rejuvenation Message Content

Recall that Steroid tone provides a construct that helps quantify the quality of the mixture of blood stream information carried by these important types of body hormones. The steroids are among the most powerful body hormones because they each carry specific message content, inherent in their unique shapes, directly to the DNA. Each specific type's message, inherent in its precise shape, individually directs the trillions of cell DNA programs (genes).

Consequently, too much or too little of a particular steroid causes either excess or deficiency for that message respectively.

Realize, healthy people always have the proper amounts of these most important hormones. This occurrence results in the proper amount of repair to rest ratios within the body cells. Middle age begins to occur when the quality of the information delivered to the cells by these most powerful hormones begins to deteriorate. Many of the consequences of middle age have a large component of causality in deteriorating message content (specific hormones).

Almost all the body cells possess a complete genetic program. Gene activity determines which proteins are manufactured. Recall, the sufficiency of protein (nitrogen balance) determines the metabolically active component of the body. Remember, the genes provide nothing until the right hormone arrives. The genetic program activity determines cell repair rates, rejuvenation rates, functional ability and the overall integrity of the cell. Paradoxically, mainstream medicine often overlooks the central importance, for continued youthfulness of all bodies relying on its cells receiving the correct message content.

Steroid tone is measured by a well-run twenty-four hour urine test. It provides a hormone report card for these most important body hormones. Recall, the more optimal the amount of the different steroids proportional to one another, the higher the steroid tone becomes. Adequate rejuvenation and repair activity occurring within requires a sufficient amount of steroid tone. A high steroid tone signifies that there are proper proportions of message content among the various steroids. In other words, the catabolic message content balances with the anabolic message content.

Unhealthy owners always possess poor hormone message content. Their health will continue to deteriorate until improvement in the quality of the message that directs their cells occurs.

Recall that Steroid pressure provides another useful construct that helps to visualize the behavior of steroids once released from their glands of origin. Only the most powerful hormones (steroids, vitamin A, and thyroid) can access any body tissue or chamber. Essentially no barriers exist to their penetration. The amount of their presence within the body periphery (the joints, bones and skin) is determined mostly by their initial amount of release from their gland of origin.

Like smoke in a room, which moves from a high concentration towards a lower concentration periphery, it is also similar to how steroids diffuse towards the periphery of the body kingdom. Because the skin lies at the periphery, a falling steroid pressure shows up here first. Paradoxically, mainstream medicine ignores this helpful fact for predicting who will benefit from natural hormone replacement to slow wrinkle formation.

Visualize, a poor steroid generation rate at the source (the adrenals and gonads) diminishes the pressure head. It is the periphery tissues that suffer first. A falling steroid pressure manifests as wrinkled skin, painful joints and osteoporosis. The periphery of the body kingdom is the most vulnerable because the presence of rejuvenation message content falls off here most severely because these tissues are furthest from the source of this information.

Steroid tone quantifies the quality of the steroid message content reaching the body cells. Different types of steroids have unique and precise shapes. It is the unique shape that conveys the message. Change the shape and the message content changes.

Steroid pressure quantifies the amount of a specific steroid reaching the body cells.

For example an adequate androgen message directs sufficient rejuvenation activities. In contrast, inadequate androgen message content leads the body's cells to fall into disrepair.

The signs of disrepair show up first in the periphery:

The skin

The joints

The bones

Simple science being discussed here, yet, not commonly taught in a way that physicians understand. In its place, the peripheral approaches to skin health are pandered in the forms of patented drugs and surgical procedures.

The Most Powerful Hormones and Skin Health

Remember, only one small group of hormones exist that are powerful enough to directly instruct the DNA program (genes) of a cell. The quality of their presence instructs cells on what genes to turn off or on. There are a few other hormones that can influence the cellular DNA program by indirect means. Most hormones cannot affect the DNA at all. The membership of these powerful hormones with direct DNA interacting ability includes all of the steroids, vitamin A, and thyroid hormones.

Vitamin A plays a powerful role in overall skin health. Adequate vitamin A at the skin cell level allows for the proper message content in its DNA program to activate the production of proteins necessary for a healthy skin cell. It also instructs skin cells to differentiate (grow up). Cell immaturity forms a central feature of cancer cells. How many skin cancer patients suffer needlessly simply because no one counsels them about the importance of vitamin A adequacy?

Vitamin A is found in yellow and orange vegetables. Natural dietary sources of vitamin A come in a precursor form called carotenes. The precursor variety cannot become vitamin A without sufficient Thyroid hormones instructing the liver (yet another debilitating effect of hypothyroidism).

The Epidermis is Vulnerable – It has no Blood Supply

The top twenty-eight layers of skin consists of dead cells that are filled with keratin, water sucking support framework (GAG) and all of this is covered with oil (fat). Approximately, below the twenty-ninth layer of the epidermis is alive. The skin and cartilage cells have no direct blood supply. Consequently, its nutrient delivery and waste removal processes prove to be particularly vulnerable to hostile forces. As a consequence, these two tissues types need optimal conditions to function normally. For example, without a direct blood supply, the skin becomes more vulnerable to environmental oxidative damage. This occurs from toxins in the air, bathing water, and from chemical hazards that contact the skin. The realization that these processes occur helps owners devise ways to minimize ongoing oxidative damage.

This explains why cigarette smokers often develop prematurely aged skin. Cigarette smoke contains carbon monoxide that lowers the oxygen carrying ability of the blood (chapter 1). The outer living layers of skin cells have no blood supply and are more vulnerable to a fall in the oxygen content in the blood. Less oxygen lowers the energy available for use in cellular rejuvenation. Nicotine contained in cigarette smoke compounds this effect because it constricts the blood vessel supply in the lower skin layer (dermis). Lastly, cigarette smoke contains many rust producing substances (oxidizing agents) that further compromise skin cell health.

Bald Men Have Nice Skin

Hereditary male pattern baldness is generally thought to occur from increased concentrations in the scalp of the powerful androgen, dihydrotestosterone (DHT). High levels in the genetically sensitive male direct energy out of the hair follicles causing a dormancy hair type formation. It's as if so much energy channels toward the skin that the build up choke off the surrounding hair follicle's nutrient supply. Once a hair follicle is deprived of its nutrient supply this leads to a very small dormant hair. The dormant hair takes the place of a normal hair.

Men with male pattern baldness usually have youthful skin. This provides another clue to the inner workings of androgens in the body. Androgens direct energy into the skin and a youthful quality results. There will always be examples of secondary processes robbing men of their hair. In these cases the nice skin rule may not apply. In general, the majority of men who develop male pattern baldness have extremely nice skin.

The youthful skin observation ties into the old adage regarding adolescents with excessive oily skin. The youths with excessive oily skin tend to have increased acne. The oily skin is known to lead later in life to the nice skin that becomes the envy of their peers.

These observations have a biochemical basis. Increased androgen content in the skin directs the cells to perform cellular rejuvenation. High androgens in the skin direct excessive oil production. Too much oil on the skin surface provides excess food for skin bacteria. The excess androgen of adolescence leads to increased acne, but as this level falls with age it becomes less of a problem. In contrast, deficient androgen message content, at the skin level, leads to thinning, shriveling and sagging skin.

Gray Hair

What happens when a hair turns gray? One by one the gray hairs form and eventually coalesce into the many.Understanding the building blocks of hair coloring leads to insights into the possibilities. Pigment producing cells in the skin and hair are called melanocytes. Melanin is the pigment they make. The darker the hair color or skin color, the greater the amount of pigment each cell makes. Blonds and red heads have the least total pigment so they have the least amount of melanin stores. Conversely, darkly pigmented peoples have the most reserve of this pigment.

Intense and prolonged stress has long ago been noticed to accelerate the loss of this pigment leading to gray hair and mottled skin. By understanding the building blocks that make up this pigment the first clue into the process is provided. Melanin is made up of two amino acids occurring in equal amounts and strung together in an alternating sequence that forms long chains. The two amino acids are tryptophan and tyrosine. Each of these amino acids undergoes modification before being linked together in a way that produces the light trapping properties of melanin.

One possibility is that the demands of stress activate the central nervous system in a way that tremendously increases the need for neurotransmitters. Some of the brain's main neurotransmitters are epinephrine, norepinephrine, dopamine, and serotonin. The first three neurotransmitters derive from the amino acid tyrosine. Serotonin derives from the amino acid tryptophan. This could explain the mechanism for diverting pigment producing building blocks. They could then be used to make more neurotransmitters during prolonged stress.

The second clue comes from the knowledge that cortisol production rates increase in stressful situations. Cortisol directs cellular energy out of infrastructure investment and into survival. Skin cell pigmentation production involves infrastructure investment and therefore turns off during prolonged stressful situations. In addition, the chronic elevation of cortisol tends to deplete DHEA production. For this reason, owners who suffer from a diminished pigmentation pattern should inquire into their DHEA and its metabolite levels with a twenty-four hour urine test. DHEA and its metabolite levels reflect pigmentation levels in the skin.

Proposed premise: Prolonged stress under the direction of increased cortisol production directs energy out of the melanocytes for making tyrosine and tryptophan molecular building blocks into melanin. These cell types are consequently deprived of the needed synthesis of melanin for hair and skin pigment. Instead these building blocks divert into increased production of neurotransmitters that are needed to survive stress. Deprived of their growth factors (DHEA), some of the melanocytes begin to die and will never again make pigment in that area.

Realize the master hormone (ACTH) that directs the adrenal to release cortisol and DHEA (chronic stress and aging depletes the proportion of DHEA) comes out of the brain with a companion molecule with the misleading name of melanocyte stimulating hormone. This name leads one to predict that with increased melanocyte stimulating hormone that coincides with increased cortisol more pigment will be produced. This proves true in only a limited distribution of skin.

All other observed effects of prolonged stress lead to an increasing tendency for gray hair formation and blotchy skin. However, owners do develop skin changes under the influence of increased melanocyte stimulating hormone (MSH). The increased MSH occurs only when the master hormone, ACTH increases. Increased pigmentation over the neck, extensor elbow surfaces and creases in the hands and feet describe the skin changes that result after the chronic elevated release of cortisol, ACTH, and MSH. There may also be an increase in liver spots in the facial area.

An explanation for this, at first, seeming conundrum is found at the level of the adrenal gland itself. Normally when ACTH activates the adrenal gland, it releases adequate DHEA and cortisol at the same time. Chronic stress changes this ratio with time to more cortisol and less DHEA. DHEA seems to be a necessary growth factor for healthy skin and hair pigmentation. Conversely, excess cortisol hastens the re-direction of energy out of rejuvenation and into survival.

Alternatively, recall that low thyroid function causes both accelerated graying and thinning of hair. Now recall that Growth Hormone is the major defense of body protein while one is in the between meal state. Hair color and amount arguably comprise some of the body's expendable proteins during stress. Chronic stress suppresses Growth Hormone release. Connect it all together with the dependency of Growth Hormone on the level of Thyroid hormones reaching the pituitary!

> (Side bar) The purpose of this discussion on gray hair formation concerns how some scientific thinking proves inconsistent. Inconsistent science limits the bigger picture. The bigger picture involves what may be occurring in how the different body hormones direct energy usage patterns. Changes in energy usage patterns alter the nutritional status of cells. Once the nutritional status of cells, like the pigment producing cells in the skin and hair follicle alters functional changes occur.

As was previously explained, the peripheral tissues are most vulnerable to falling quality of steroid types (decreased steroid tone) and overall amounts (a fall in steroid pressure). The fall in steroid tone and pressure has predictable consequences that occur first in the periphery of the body. The periphery for nutritional supply and waste removal is found in skin, joints, and bone tissues. Looking at the skin in the mirror evidences falling steroid tone and pressure around middle age.

Skin appearance and texture depends on the maintenance of adequate steroid tone and pressure. Skin exists on the periphery and a fall in either of these two cell youth determinants will show up here first. Healing the skin begins with an assessment of hormone levels in the body. Remember, steroids powerfully determine gene activity or silence. Gene activity determines which proteins are made. The proteins' quality of presence determines the metabolic rate and much about structural integrity. Consequently, youthfulness depends on defense of body protein. Hopefully this sequence of events makes it more apparent why a sufficient scientific assessment of hormone adequacy should be included in the routine office exam.

The skin of physically fit owners regularly encounters high quality and optimal amounts of the different steroids. Conversely, unhealthy owners will have a diminished quality of steroids as well as diminished amounts in their skin. Understanding the need to have high steroid tone and high steroid pressure summarizes one of the cornerstones of the healthy skin. There are other hormones that affect skin health by their timing and amount, but it is the steroid-type hormones (also include vitamin A and thyroid) that are the most important. For these reasons, understanding how to attain optimal steroids in the body will expedite healing.

An important skin hormone facilitates the message of the level one-hormone types. Although the steroids instruct the DNA programs to make cellular proteins, it is the responsibility of IGF-1 to allow nutrient uptake by most cells. An owner can have great steroid tone and pressure, but an insufficient regeneration response because of a nutritional deficiency in the cell (liver chapter).

Even those owners with extremes of steroid mismatch states can begin healing once the deficiencies and/or excesses have been identified from a laboratory evaluation (see 100,000 mile exam). To grasp the concept of steroid tone, think of its quality ranging from a cellular melody (highest tone states) in healthy extremes, all the way down the continuum of varying levels of cellular noise. Noise creates a chaotic message and is therefore unhealthy in regards to the steroid message directing the cell how to spend energy.

Building on this concept is the construct of steroid pressure that can alternatively be thought of as the volume. The volume of either occurs as a melody versus the loud noise possible in unhealthy states. Unhealthy states are consistent with loud noise. Excessive amounts of the steroids prove as destructive as the wrong steroids directing a cell's DNA. In some owners the melody is great, but the pressure remains low because their gonads and/or adrenals fail to make adequate steroid pressure.

The owners' adrenals and gonads create the 'pressure head' for steroids. For vitamin A, the liver usually determines this hormones release rate. Vitamin A stores and releases from the liver as needed. The processed food diet proves typically deficient in vitamin A. Thyroid pressure generates from the thyroid gland. The steroid-like hormones produced here behave like a gas defusing from a high concentration to the far periphery of the tissues.

When the skin no longer receives adequate steroid tone and/or pressure, its cells behave like other cells when sub-optimal informational direction occurs. Like other cells, skin cells need direction on how to spend cellular energy. This is largely determined by which DNA programs (genes) turn off or on in a cell.

Important point: gonad and/or adrenal insufficiency first appears in the peripheral tissues of skin, joints, and bone. This is obvious when studying the chemical behavior of molecules like steroids. Anatomically, the skin is the outward periphery of tissues and consequently is last in line with the receiving of hormones and nutrients.

Pressure gradients for oxygen and steroids are lowest when they travel to the periphery. The outer living layer of skin is also more vulnerable because it has no direct blood supply. The skin relies on the slower process of diffusion of nutrients and hormones down their concentration gradient.

Excess fat can hide the earlier stages of gonad and/ or adrenal insufficiency by stretching the dermal layer of skin in a misleading way. This shows up in subtle ways to the trained eye. These owners often have a bloated look that coincides with how the dermal layer feels. Owners often fool themselves into thinking things remain great when the bad hides amongst the fat. Missing the earliest clues of falling steroid pressure and tone necessitates a prolonged recovery.

The skin forms the outward expression of peripheral tissues. Logically, deficient steroid output or quality shows up here first. The facial skin begins to lose its firmness, fine wrinkles appear, and puffiness follows. The general process makes their face less recognizable compared to the face of their youth. Certain processes increase steroid pressure and tone and therefore slow these developments (explained above and below).

Close in onset to these facial changes are the first signs that the joints are less capable. They begin to creak and ache. Later in the process, the upper back begins to hunch over. As the steroid deficiency progresses, the internal organs begin to shrink and falter. This happens when organs no longer receive sufficient message content directing their cell types in the wise use of their cellular energy.

Each owner's body has its own subtle unique order in which different cell types respond to insufficient message content. No one will deteriorate in the same sequence as another. But as steroid imbalance progresses, this body wasting syndrome becomes more predictable. These owners have a look of someone who has been beaten down by life. At this stage, the joints become widely involved with degenerative osteoarthritic changes. This causes deformity, pain, and loss of usefulness. Other processes contribute to cellular age. For the reasons outlined above, the peripheral tissues suffer first from the ravages of diminished message content that allows these cells to age more quickly.

Skin – Taking Out the Garbage

The skin is well supplied with sweat glands that operate on the same principle as the kidneys. The sweat glands depend on aldosterone to determine the final mineral composition of sweat. When aldosterone levels remain high, the sweat contains high amounts of potassium and the body conserves sodium. However, when aldosterone levels stay low the sweat becomes high in sodium and the body conserves potassium. Many other toxins excrete through the sweat glands and in this way the skin provides aid to the kidneys.

Taking out the garbage that piles up in the peripheral tissues of the skin domain occurs in two ways. First, drink water. Skin cells exist anatomically on the periphery and will be most vulnerable to dehydrating forces. Extremes of environmental drying situations will only exacerbate an ongoing deficiency of the most powerful medicine of all. Adequate water intake promotes adequate water content in the skin. The skin dries out first when body water content decreases.

The second method of taking out the skin garbage involves perspiration. Traditional medicine men living in the northwest illustrate the power of this for taking out the skin garbage. These people have nice skin because they sweat in their lodges regularly and flush the garbage out of their peripheral tissues. It also facilitates hydration of wrinkled skin. People who exercise to the point of breaking a healthy sweat will notice their improved skin appearance following a work out. With increased pollution from all sources, it makes sense to include effort in the regular flushing of the peripheral tissues through breaking a sweat.

Skin and Nutrition

Many skin conditions directly result from nutritional deficiencies. As was previously mentioned, one group of nutritional deficiencies derives from the inappropriate hormonal fats precursors that line the dermal layer of skin cells. These fats contribute to inflammatory conditions like psoriasis, seborrhea, and dermatitis conditions. Optimizing hormonal fats (ecosanoids) will go along way toward healing skin conditions. The right hormonal fats are only possible when attending to diets that encourage the right hormones (level 2 hormones). The right essential fatty acids are also required in the diet.

Summary of the inflammatory conditions of the skin as they relate to nutritional fat

1. Avoid inappropriate hormonal fats (polyunsaturated and partially hydrogenated fats)
2. Optimize the level two hormones ratios between insulin and glucagon, by consuming a diet that encourages this.
3. Consume the best hormonal fat precursor sources (olive oil, fish oil, borage oil, and primrose oil).

The astute reader may notice that flax seed oil is missing from the above list for sources of essential fatty acids. Flax seed oil does contain large amounts of the essential fatty acids. However, flax seed also contains other oils that require it to be refrigerated, protected from air, and protected from light. Once flax seed oil gains entry inside the tissues, it is exposed to heat and oxygen. This reactive combination allows the other oils in flax seeds to oxidize.

The oxidation propensity of flax seed is well documented in the house painting industry. Oil based paints of yesteryear were formed from flax seed oil. Flax seed oil is also known as linseed oil. Linseed oil was chosen because of the speed at which its other oils oxidize when exposed to air and heat. Once oils become oxidized they harden and this process proves inconsistent with body health. What makes good house paint does not make healthy cell membranes.

Vitamin C is also important for the support layer of the outer lying epidermis. Recall, the internal layer of skin support tissue is called the dermis and contains a blood and nervous supply. The integrity of the dermal layer determines the elastic quality of the skin. Sufficient skin elasticity occurs when this layer contains optimal amounts of the connective tissue proteins of collagen and elastin. Vitamin C serves as a critical ingredient needed for the manufacture of this connective tissue layer because it serves as a cofactor in its synthesis. Without adequate vitamin C there is insufficient ability to manufacture this important layer. By this mechanism, deficiency of the dermis layer creates another way for the skin to deteriorate.

Like vitamin C, both A and B vitamin deficiencies are also possibilities in causing skin disease. Live food sources for these vitamins are emerging as superior in their ability to be utilized by the body. Processed food diets lead owners to become deficient in either or both vitamin A complex and B vitamins. Recall, vitamin A deficiency dramatically increases the likelihood of skin cancer because it instructs the skin cell DNA program on how to differentiate (mature). Skin cells stay immature without adequate vitamin A message content. Immaturity forms a central property of cancer cells. For this simple reason, physicians should be encouraged to inquire into the vitamin A status of skin cancer patients.

So far the skin, kidney and lungs role in removing body trash have been reviewed in this section. The last organ, the liver, contributes powerfully to these overall efforts. In addition, the liver determines where fuel ends up in the body. Hungry cells begin when the liver treats fuel inappropriately. Health requires that the liver do the right thing for its owner.

CHAPTER NINETEEN

LIVER

Understanding the liver's role, in where fuel channels, facilitates a deeper appreciation for how obesity is only one symptom of many other diseases. These diseases often begin in middle age. They include heart disease, adult onset diabetes, high blood pressure and muscle wasting.

Healing from middle-aged disease involves helping one's liver to do the right thing. An overview of what other things the liver performs is also included in this chapter. One of the big components of causality in the aging process concerns the liver misdirecting its available energy. This chapter explains how the liver can be encouraged to perform in the best interest of the body.

The liver serves multiple roles in the body. The tasks of the liver can be arranged into five main groups.

Disarms and removes toxins
Controls the availability of fuel in the blood stream
Facilitates the assimilation of fat into the body
Stores and releases minerals, vitamins and hormones
Manufactures and releases transport proteins into the blood
serum.

Each of these five main liver tasks proves fundamental to health. The assessment for how the liver performs in these five main areas is often superficially addressed. Longevity requires that all five of these liver tasks perform at efficient rates. **In one way or the other obesity has a component of causality in a sick liver.** Sick livers manifest from toxic injury (see subsection below), the wrong message content that instructs it to do inappropriate things with body fuel and from poor nutritional choices.

Disarm and Remove Toxins

The liver needs certain molecular parts to disarm many different types of toxins that are encountered when the owner creates or ingests them.

Toxins made by every day processes:
Natural body waste
Drugs
Ingested toxins
Cookware
Food additives
Food pollutants
Air pollutants
Water pollutants
Herbicides
Heavy metals
Toxins absorbed from an unhealthy colon

The liver has a choice on how it will disarm any toxin. There are five common mechanisms for the initial inactivation of toxins. In general, all five of these processes facilitate the next phase of liver detoxification. In the initial stage the liver machinery creates a molecular appendage, which it can use to attach the final removal compounds to. This allows the toxin to become water soluble or inactive. The final removal compounds cannot attach until one of five initial reactions occur (molecular appendage types).

The five initial liver deactivation methods are:
Oxidation
Hydrogen addition
Hydration (addition of water)
Cleavage through hydrolysis (removal of water)
Removal of chloride, fluoride, bromide or iodide
The trouble with these processes concerns the fact that they each tend to create reactive intermediates. The liver needs protection from these intermediates. The protective molecules needed by the liver are commonly called antioxidants or 'rust retardants'. The better the supply of these substances in one's liver, the more protection one has from liver injury. The greater the load of toxins, the more antioxidants needed. More antioxidants become necessary because they will be used up quickly.

The basic list of needed liver antioxidants is:
Vitamin A Vitamin E
Vitamin C Bioflavonoids (berries)
Selenium Zinc
Coenzyme Q10 Pycnogenol (grape seeds)
Lipoic acid (real foods only)

Thiol that are found in garlic, onions, and cruciferous vegetables.

These anti-oxidants are the basic protectors of the liver tissue. The liver cells need the protection of anti-oxidants because of the reactive intermediates created when the liver begins the first phase of deactivating and/or removing a body toxin. Certain vitamins and nutrients are also needed by the liver to power its molecular machinery that performs the task of disarmament.

The basic list of these vitamins is:
Vitamin B1 Vitamin B12
Vitamin B2 Lipoic acid
Co enzyme Q10
Vitamin B3 Pantothenic acid
Folic acid
Vitamin B6 Phospholipids like lecithin

Overall key point: The liver must begin the initial attachment of molecular appendages without releasing reactive molecules that can oxidize its cells. The earlier above list of antioxidants prevents the oxidants (reactive intermediaries) from causing liver rust. These initial deactivation steps require specific vitamins to power the enzymatic machinery needed for these activities. Once the liver cell has created the various appendages on a toxin, it needs to proceed on to deactivation.

The basic choices for the final reaction in toxin removal are the addition of:
Sulfate
Glucuronic acid
Glutathione or n-acetyl cysteine
Acetate
Methyl
Certain amino acids: glycine, taurine, glutamine, ornithine, and arginine

Depending on the final solubility characteristics, the deactivated toxin will either be excreted in the bile or blood stream. When excreted in the bile it will be removed in the feces. However, poor bacteria content in the colon can prevent this and, in these cases, the toxin reabsorbs back into the body. Some toxins reabsorb because the wrong bacteria rip apart the deactivation appendage that the liver attached. Consequently, bowel health forms an important consideration for continued liver detoxification ability.

When a water-soluble toxin excretes into the blood stream, it heads for the kidneys. Ideally, in this way the kidneys remove large amounts of liver-neutralized toxins. For this reason, many toxins and hormone excesses that the kidney removes must first be made water-soluble by the liver. These include ammonia, steroids, prescription medications, small chains of amino acids, and heavy metal complexes.

Fortuitously, the liver exemplifies one tissue that possesses remarkable capabilities for regenerating new cells until its underlying architecture disrupts. Scientists call disruption in the architecture state of the liver, cirrhosis. This healing compromises because cell regeneration disorganizes. Visualize, at the level of cirrhosis the energy template of where cells belong disrupts (section six). When the energy template disrupts a progressive cellular disorganization ensues.

The liver is responsible for the up take of ammonia. The majority of ammonia production generates from amino acid breakdown when protein converts to sugar (gluconeogenesis). The ammonia formed in the breakdown process converts to urea in the liver and exits in the urine. The kidney has the ability to excrete a limited amount of ammonia. However, it is the liver that neutralizes the majority of this toxin.

Overall point to comprehend: Once the liver neutralizes a toxin it uses the bile or the kidneys to remove them (many environmental toxins and prescription drugs). The liver requires numerous nutritional factors to effectively remove toxins and this ability greatly diminishes without sufficient nutrition.

A rich system of blood vessels (liver sinusoids) exists in the liver. These arrange to allow immune system scavenger cells room to grab unwanted material out of the blood stream. Blood flows directly towards them via the portal vein that is the drain for all the blood in the intestines and colon. Jeffery Bland, PhD, discusses the above concepts further in *Clinical Nutrition: A Functional Approach*.

The Liver Determines Fuel Availability

Inappropriate fuel types in the blood stream cause diseases like diabetes, heart disease, strokes, and peripheral vascular disease. These diseases can have their origins in the liver. When the liver treats fuel types inappropriately, the blood vessels begin to break down. There are two common examples of inappropriate fuel types released by the liver with consequent blood vessel injury. First concerns the high blood sugar of diabetes. The second mechanism involves the high rate of liver synthesis and release into the blood stream of LDL cholesterol found in heart disease and one type of diabetes. In both cases excesses of these fuels injure the blood vessels inside walls. In both cases the liver creates and releases these fuels inappropriately and this causes the excesses found in these diseases. The cause of inappropriate release of fuel excesses results from the liver receiving the wrong hormones messages that direct it incorrectly.

Healing involves attention to lifestyles, adequate nutrient intake, and hormone balance at the level of the liver. Instead, owners are often told the hopeless mantra about the cruel hand that genetics has dealt them. The typical approach sells drugs and procedures. However, healing still involves improving the types and amounts of hormones that instruct the liver on whether to store or release fuel.

Like other organs, the liver dutifully follows the message content it receives. Healing involves an assessment of the proportions of the hormones that deliver message content at the level of the liver cell. Only when the proper amounts of hormones instruct the liver will these diseases begin to heal.

The overall hormone message delivered to the liver determines whether the liver takes fuel out or puts fuel into the blood stream. Five main hormones determine how the liver directs fuel - insulin, glucagon, Growth Hormone, cortisol, and epinephrine. The message content arriving at the liver determines whether the liver will manufacture fuel in storage forms (glycogen and LDL cholesterol) or release them as readily combustible types for use in the cellular power plants (mitochondria). If the liver is in storage mode, it does this by removing fuel from the blood stream. Realize the liver synthesizes LDL cholesterol particles with storage in mind. Even though the liver eventually releases them, their design is such that they head for the storage destinations: including the macrophages that line the arteries and the abdominal fat cells.

The opposite situation occurs when the liver releases sugar and fatty acids into the blood stream. The sugar released readily accesses the cells when adequate IGF-1 is present in the blood stream. Once inside the cells the sugar and fatty acids either combusts inside cell power plants or serves for structural components in the cell. Realize, four out of five of the above hormones encourage this type of fuel release.

It helps to arrange the hormones interacting with the liver into the 'antique weight scale' analogy. This arrangement reveals that only insulin falls on the side of the scale tipping it in the direction of storing fuels (glycogen and LDL cholesterol). The other four hormones (at the level of the liver) counter storage and encourage the power plant accessible types of fuel release by the liver into the blood stream.

The insulin predominant hormone situation allows a tremendous increase in fat and cholesterol manufacture because insulin behaves like the liver's fuel tank nozzle connection. It preferentially desires to fill the liver cell fuel tanks because of its initial site of release, the pancreas, dumps it straight into the liver via the protal vein. This anatomical fact means that whatever the insulin secretion rate the liver will always receives the highest amount of insulin message content. Recall, the 200,000 pure insulin receptors lining each liver cell. Visualize the insulin trap within the liver. Also recall, the enzyme that manufactures cholesterol, HMG Co A reductase, depends on insulin to activate.

When the liver cell fuel tanks fill up with carbohydrate in the form of glycogen (up to 100 grams only if adequate potassium remains available), insulin instructs the liver to make the extra sugar into fat and cholesterol. This explains why one needs insulin for fat cell growth and in the storage of liver glycogen.

However, the above listed counter regulatory hormones can overpower insulin message content that directs carbohydrate and fat storage in the liver (each to varying degrees). Counter regulatory hormones direct the liver to dump stored fuel into the blood stream for usage in cell power plants. These hormones presence are appropriate to prevent a falling blood sugar.

The body perceives a falling blood sugar threat between meals and during mentally or physically stressed states and the counter regulatory hormones levels elevate. Visualize in tow out of three of these cases the blood fuel tends to deplete. For example, the fat stores are needed during intense and prolonged exercise. Exercising muscles and heart prefer fat as their fuel source. Carbohydrate storage is limited to about 400 calories in the liver and about 1600 calories in the muscles. Glycogen stores eventually deplete and in the case of prolonged exercise, the body needs other fuel sources for energy. A 150 pound athlete with 15% body fat has access to 22.5 pounds of fat times 3500 calories per pound of fat (about 80,000 calories). The proper counter regulatory hormones allow access to the tremendous fat fuel storehouses.

Nerves and red blood cells rely exclusively on sugar for all their energy needs. This fact explains the desirability of adequate counter hormones that direct the additional release of fat. Hence, processes that conserve glycogen for the nerve and red blood cells enhance endurance because nerve and red blood cell's optimal function are preserved when their sugar supply remains available. This happens when the muscles and heart have access to more fat for their energy needs. Conversely, exercising owners that insist on promoting high insulin states compromise their red blood cells and nerves due to sugar stores being consumed more quickly.

Recall, insulin levels normally fall towards zero during exercise because IGF-1 efficiently delivers the fuel. As explained through out this manual unhealthy owners develop increased insulin need (insulin resistance) to stay alive while between meals despite the fact that the blood sugar is falling. Insulin within the liver always directs the liver to uptake fuel out of the blood stream. Remember before any insulin makes it beyond the liver it must first traverse the 200,000 pure insulin receptors per liver cell. This anatomical fact means that very little insulin makes it beyond the liver trap. Remember, unhealthy owners desperately need fuel nozzles, beyond the liver and therefore accept the complication of insulin initially compounding their falling blood sugar. Visualize the insulin trap within the liver before a little insulin makes its way beyond it and out into the circulation to serve as a fuel nozzle. Recall, there only two fuel nozzles that deliver fuel to the hungry body cells, insulin and IGF-1.

Realize, the desperate situation of needing insulin in a setting of a falling blood sugar causes health consequences because insulin always arrives at the liver first. Insulin within the liver always instructs the liver to store energy (sugar and fat). This means, in these cases, insulin competes with the ability of the liver to dump sugar and fat into the blood stream and create more sugar from amino acids.

The only thing that saves these owners from death is an excessive counter regulatory hormone response that effectively competes with the insulin blood sugar lowering effects. Visualize the violence of competing message content within the unhealthy owners liver whenever they fast or attempt to exercise! How many seizure disorders arise solely because the counter response fails in certain owners and allows the blood sugar to fall below the seizure threshold?

Unfortunately most physicians are not taught that this violent situation arises only because IGF-1 has fallen off and the hungry body cells need a fuel nozzle from somewhere. Remember, it's the anatomy of the insulin secretion pathway that makes insulin the villin here because it first confronts the 200,000 pure insulin receptors per liver cell (the insulin trap).

Key point to understand: insulin release while the blood sugar falls is abnormal and only occurs in desperate situations like increased insulin need (commonly called insulin resistance as if it remains a mystery). Scientists currently diagnose these patients as having Syndrome X (metabolic syndrome or insulin resistance syndrome). They are diagnosed by finding elevated insulin levels during the fasting state.

Insulin message within the liver always directs fuel storage activities. Most fuel storage occurs as fat and cholesterol. Also realize that it is abnormal for insulin to be needed during the fasting or exercising state when the blood fuel falls.

In contrast, it is normal for insulin to release following meals while the blood sugar rises so that a certain nutritional proportion sequesters within the liver in anticipation of the next fasting state. Also, in the healthy owner who is between meals or exercising, they do not need insulin! Instead, as their liver releases stored sugar and fat it also releases adequate IGF-1 to serve as the fuel nozzle for hungry cells. Healthy owners by this mechanism avoid both the need for insulin and hence the excessive need for the counter regulatory hormones while the blood sugar falls. Recognize the difference in design for what the IGF-1 versus the insulin fuel nozzle was designed to perform.

Longevity and exercise performance critically relate to the balance of hormones that instruct the liver. When these hormones improve not only exercise ability but also heart disease, blood vessel disease and diabetes risk and its complications diminish as well.

Insulin Causes Fuel Storage as Fat or Glycogen

The counter regulatory hormones, glucagon, Growth Hormone, cortisol, and epinephrine all cause the liver to release and synthesize readily accessible fuels into the blood stream. Initially, insulin will only direct the liver to remove sugar from the blood stream for storage as glycogen (if sufficient potassium remains available). It can store about one hundred grams of sugar in this manner. Sedentary owners exist with livers that are almost always full of stored sugar. In this case, insulin directs the liver to make the excess sugar into fat and cholesterol that are packaged for the fat depots. These depots are in the fat cells and in the macrophages that line the arteries. At the level of the liver, insulin is the only hormone that promotes storage of fuel. The other four hormones oppose the message content of insulin at the level of the liver.

Recall, before the liver makes carbohydrate into fat it requires insulin message content. Visualize the excess fat and cholesterol stimulated by higher insulin levels pummeling the liver's 200,000 pure insulin receptors per liver cell via its pancreas portal vein connection. This favors higher cholesterol and fat synthesis rates occurring with increased insulin need (i.e. a fallen IGF-1).

Also, insulin directed fat manufacture results in the butter fat variety [it is packaged as hard fat (LDL cholesterol)]. This fact has been known for over forty years. Recall, as well, that when one eats butterfat and their liver contains adequate B vitamins their liver converts it into olive oil components. Certainly, a mind twists to understand and therefore has been fully taken advantage of to keep doctors in the dark.

Glucagon counters insulin by four ways in the liver. First it stimulates the liver to change available amino acids into sugar (gluconeogenesis). Second, it stimulates the release of stored sugar (glycogen) from the liver into the blood stream. Third, it stimulates the release of stored liver fat into the blood stream. Glucagon's message content makes body fuel available. Fourth, the glucagon message content decreases liver derived cholesterol and fat synthesis from carbohydrate. When cholesterol and fat are manufactured at slower rates, LDL cholesterol levels in the blood stream will go down.

Growth Hormone has some of the same effect on the liver as glucagon does. **There are two important exceptions**. It inhibits the conversion of amino acids into fuel. This is known as a protein sparing effect (it promotes positive nitrogen balance). Consequently, when Growth Hormone levels are high, it counters the ability of glucagon to convert protein into sugar.

The advantage of having high Growth Hormone levels relative to the other counter regulatory hormones concerns the fact that it conserves protein. Realize, it is important for athletes because muscles are made from protein. In addition, metabolism depends on the adequacy of energy consuming proteins. It is important to emphasize the contrast that all other counter regulatory hormones to insulin are catabolic toward protein stores.

The second different effect about the Growth Hormone message content, compared to the other counter hormones to insulin, regards its ability to direct the liver to release insulin-like growth factor (IGF-1). When this hormone is outside the liver, it acts like insulin by facilitating the muscle and organ cells to take up fuel (sugar). Remember that in healthy owners insulin-like growth factor (IGF-1) is found at levels greater than 100 times that of insulin in the blood stream. Realize this liver secreted hormone negates the need for insulin while the blood sugar is falling and does not stimulate the liver to make fat and cholesterol.

A longevity advantage occurs when IGF-1 levels are high. High IGF-1 levels depend on three things; an adequate release of Growth Hormone, a healthy liver capable of high rates of IGF-1 manufacture, and adequate DHEA levels to stimulate the liver cell DNA programs to direct the manufacture of IGF-1. Remember, also important concerns Growth Hormone synthesis rates dependency on ample thyroid hormones arriving at the pituitary (50% of pituitary gland output).

Growth Hormone's effects on the body need to be understood in a tandem-like fashion. Once the tandem of Growth Hormone release followed by IGF-1 release is recognized one can avoid the confusion discussed in the scientific literature. Medical physiology textbooks describe Growth Hormone as a diabetogenic hormone. This is a half-truth except when the liver is diseased or Growth Hormone production becomes abnormally high. Abnormal increases in Growth Hormone levels can occur with the disease acromegaly and with high dose Growth Hormone replacement therapy. However, healthy livers with adequate androgen (DHEA) message content promptly release IGF-1, sugar and fat when Growth Hormone levels rise within normal parameters. Important point: Sufficient IGF-1 release powerfully lowers towards zero the amount of insulin required to bring fuel into the cells beyond the liver and fat cells.

Cortisol is the next counter hormone to insulin's message content. Cortisol powerfully counters insulin in its ability to remove sugar molecules from the blood stream. Cortisol directs the liver to release stored liver sugar and fat into the blood stream. It also instructs the fat cells to release fatty acid fuels into the blood stream. In addition, it acts on the protein stores of the body and causes them to release amino acids into the blood stream (increases catabolism or causes negative nitrogen balance). The liver then sucks up the released amino acids for processing into sugar.

The process of gluconeogenesis denotes the conversion of liver-sequestered amino acids into sugar. Because it destroys protein for fuel generation it causes a negative nitrogen balance. Protein stores comprise the majority of nitrogen content in the body. The metabolic rate depends on sufficient calorie consuming proteins. One way scientists denote this is by discussing nitrogen balance. Negative nitrogen balance is another way of discussing catabolism. On the other hand, positive nitrogen balance is another way of describing increased anabolism.

Physician's Sidebar

Normally, Growth Hormone will counter a diabetes tendency by its message that directs the release of IGF-1. IGF-1 behaves like insulin in the circulation. This happens because of the tandem effects of Growth Hormone release followed by the liver simultaneously releasing IGF-1, sugar and fat. Medical physiology textbooks focus on the fact that Growth Hormone initially causes the release of sugar into the blood stream. However, the tandem of IGF-1 release that normally follows causes the peripheral uptake of sugar out of the blood stream (i.e. outside the liver). It is the tandem of Growth Hormone release followed by IGF-1 release that prevents the overall rise in blood sugar. The insulin-like effect of IGF-1 explains why Growth Hormone, in normal amounts, lowers insulin requirements in patients who have a normal liver and DHEA and/or testosterone level. It also explains the observation why normal DHEA levels lower insulin requirements. Insulin requirements lower because normal DHEA levels instruct the liver DNA programs to increase the amount of IGF-1 manufactured. IGF-1 releases when Growth Hormone levels elevate. The IGF-1 released, acts like insulin in the cells outside of the liver (the periphery). In the periphery, IGF-1 directs many cells to take sugar out of the blood stream. When adequate insulin-like growth factor secretes, the insulin needed to normalize the blood sugar decreases. Some physicians feel that insulin, outside of the liver in the healthful state, is unnecessary beyond very low levels.

IGF-1 has the additional benefit of facilitating the uptake of cell nutrition and minerals. IGF-1 occurs at 100 times greater the amount of insulin in the circulation when an owner is healthy. This makes sense since there is about 100 times more insulin like activity needed to direct the proper nourishment of the cells outside the liver and fat. The highest pure insulin type receptor concentration occurs on the liver and fat cells at about 200,000 receptors per cell. Whatever the insulin release rate because of the anatomy of the pancreas secreting into the portal vein straight into the liver, the liver always receives the highest message content of insulin.

High levels of IGF-1 diminish the need for insulin in the cells outside the liver and fat. Conversely, low levels of IGF-1 require an increased insulin secretion because a sugar load will require more insulin to return the blood sugar to normal following a carbohydrate meal. However, healthy owners have more than 100 times IGF-1 in their blood stream as compared to insulin. In contrast, unhealthy owners suffer pancreas and liver strain because more insulin forces the liver into sucking excessive sugar out of the blood stream (first pass effect). The extra insulin also increases the rate of LDL cholesterol synthesis. The imbalance between insulin levels and IGF-1 levels creates a situation that favors increased body fat formation. Here, the fat cells are happy but other body cells remain hungry beyond the liver until their IGF-1 fuel nozzle again rises to more optimal levels. Picture the liver as the nutritional hog of the body while other body cells are forced into hoping that some insulin makes it beyond the liver trap and out into the circulation where it can serve as an alternate fuel nozzle.

Extremely high cortisol release tends to deplete the body protein content. The metabolically active component of the body consists of protein. Diminished protein content logically extends to the need for fewer calories per day. It also causes smaller muscles, bones and organ size because this is where the protein comes from. High cortisol release occurs with stress and when Growth Hormone levels have fallen. Remember, only Growth Hormone can protect body protein content during times of stress (fasting, exercising, between meals, worry, etc.)

Physician's Sidebar

Cortisol instructs the liver cell DNA. The liver cell DNA, when instructed by cortisol, leads to the formation of certain cell receptors. These types of cell receptors are needed to recognize hormones that are not as powerful as level one-type hormones (section two). Only level one-type hormones, like cortisol, can directly instruct the DNA programs. For example, cortisol directed receptors are necessary to recognize adrenalin (epinephrine) and glucagon. These are level three and two hormones respectively (see the hierarchy of hormones). The liver will be unable to recognize the message content of epinephrine and glucagon without sufficient cortisol. Cortisol deficiency sets up a situation of the 'lesser hormones' not being able to deliver their message content (elevate the blood sugar in this case). The only other counter regulatory hormone to insulin, Growth Hormone, will cause the release of IGF-1 that exacerbates low blood sugars when the liver fails to release enough sugar between meals.

Compounding the problem concerns how cortisol further exacerbates low liver glycogen stores because it also determines the amount of glycogen synthase made within the liver. The name Glycogen synthase describes exactly what its role is in sugar metabolism within the liver. Here lies a little recognized mechanism for how low blood sugar occurs between meals: insufficient cortisol within the liver that in turn causes deficient Glycogen synthase manufacture. Without sufficient Glycogen synthase there cannot be adequate glycogen storage for the between meal state.

Low blood sugars (hypoglycemia) are the hallmark of diminished adrenal reserve (see adrenal chapter). The adrenal gland manufactures all body cortisol. Deficient cortisol in the setting of high insulin will lead to diminished blood sugar levels. Unfortunately, many of these hypoglycemic prone owners are prescribed frequent feedings. This approach leads to weight gain and a compounding of problems with the passage of time.

However, a **24-hour urine test** will document diminished adrenal cortisol and/or its metabolites production. Occasionally, the additional test of Cortrosyn challenge (beyond the level of this discussion) of the adrenal reserve function will be needed to elucidate borderline cortisol reserve.

There are several considerations for healing from diminished adrenal function. First, dietary changes for correcting carbohydrate and mineral imbalances are a strong start. Second, the results of the 24-hour urine test document the scope of the steroid imbalance that includes cortisol deficiency. In some cases replacement with real steroid hormones becomes necessary. In others, diet and life style changes suffice.

Customizing replacements to actual needs prevents side effects from cortisol replacement. In addition, changing the carbohydrate and mineral content of the diet prevents side effects. The replacement program often includes other adrenal steroids as indicated by the 24-hour urine test. When these factors are considered together, side effects are reduced or eliminated.

Epinephrine is the fourth counter regulatory hormone that opposes insulin. Epinephrine acts like cortisol in its ability to free fatty acids from the fat stores. However, its release powerfully inhibits insulin secretion. Ephedra acts in a similar manner to epinephrine. This fact explains its weight loss effect. Blood pressure elevations from either one are unusual (chapter three). In contrast, norepinephrine powerfully raises blood pressure.

The more effective a natural remedy the more it gets bashed in the media by fear tactics. Aspirin like medications kill more people in one week than have probably ever been harmed by ephedra. Yet, aspirin can be bought over the counter and ephedra has mostly been outlawed.

Recall, the other counter regulatory hormone, Growth Hormone acts mostly in the liver in its opposition to insulin. However, in one important way both insulin and Growth Hormone share a common message theme: These two hormones both have in common the conservation of body protein. Insulin conserves body protein following meals while Growth Hormone conserves body protein between meals (fasting and exercising).

The Liver Controls the Body Fat Content

Diabetes and heart disease are often diseases that are secondary to the liver receiving poor informational direction. Ninety percent of all diabetics have an excess of total body insulin. Similarly, most heart disease owners also suffer from the effects of excess message content from insulin (increased insulin release rates). When insulin is the cause, these diseases, begin with poor message content at the level of the liver.

The poor message content arises from excess insulin. The liver cell dutifully follows the message content it receives. Insulin in the liver opposes Growth Hormone, epinephrine, cortisol, and glucagon message content. The balance of message content between the hormone insulin and the other four counter regulatory hormones comprises a major determinant in the risk of an owner for developing these two diseases.

The complete cholesterol profile that is typically performed on an annual basis sometimes provides clues as to the summation of message content in one's liver. However, some owners may have a normal blood cholesterol profile, but an obese body. **Only 50**

percent of heart disease victims had abnormal cholesterol. The other fifty percent had normal cholesterol.

The fact that most heart disease owners are obese around the middle points to the fact that they secrete way too much insulin because it is always a pre-requisite for body fat (see Syndrome X). With more insulin, more message content exists to create and maintain fat and cholesterol. High insulin leads to stuffed macrophages that line the inside of arteries with LDL cholesterol. Fat laden macrophages eventually plug an artery even if the blood cholesterol is normal.

Whenever the lab results are sub-optimal or the owner is obese, several things need to be considered and investigated. With this and some life style changes, the excess insulin caused diseases are often effectively curtailed. Altering the message content that the liver receives proves critical. When these primary factors are ignored symptom control medicine becomes all that is possible.

Healing from heart disease or diabetes involves alleviating one or more of these message abnormalities at the level of the liver:

1. **Unfavorable insulin and glucagon ratio of message content in the liver**
2. **Potassium deficiency leads to insulin resistance connection**
3. **Growth Hormone connection**
4. **Excess**
5. **Deficiency**
6. **Cortisol excess**
7. **Normal pancreas**
8. **Wounded pancreas**
9. **Thyroid status**
10. **Growth Hormone when the liver is unhealthy**
11. **Excessive proinsulin levels**
12. **Excessive estrogen levels**
13. **Low androgen levels**

A key difference occurs between the disease processes of diabetes and heart disease. The difference concerns the elevated blood sugar within the diabetic. However, these two diseases share a common pathology: Remember, ninety percent of diabetics have elevated insulin secretion rates and the majority of atherosclerotic heart disease involves elevated insulin secretion rates, as well. However, in most adult onset diabetics, their body fat has finally elevated to the point (genetically determined) where their pancreas can no longer handle the increased insulin need and the blood sugar rises.

Five Basic Reasons for Elevated Insulin Need

Insulin need rises when Growth Hormone levels fall off (recall its thyroid hormone dependency), IGF-1 levels fall (recall its androgen dependency), total body potassium decreases (recall the typical American diet), chronic stress predominates and/or carbohydrate consumption increases. When a pancreas cannot meet the insulin demanded by the excessive presence of any one or more of the above conditions, the blood sugar will rise. By definition, when blood sugar rises beyond 140, diabetes is diagnosed. However, the same process of elevated insulin plugs up the blood vessels of the typical heart diseased owner. The pure heart diseased owner, who is not diabetic, can still make enough insulin to keep his blood sugar normal. **Here lies the common fundamental common link between adult onset diabetics and most atherosclerotic heart disease victims, elevated insulin secretion rates. Picture all that butterfat being turned out by these unsuspecting owners on a low fat diet!**

Many heart disease patients start out with normal blood sugars and only after many years their pancreas becomes exhausted. This commonality between these two diseases explains why mainstream medicine is finally acknowledging that at the time of diagnosis of adult onset diabetes, heart disease is presumed to already exist. **Ninety percent of diabetes and the majority of heart diseased owners have elevated blood insulin secretion rates. The high insulin levels that occur in both diseases lead to increased blood fat abnormalities.**

However, in the case of the adult onset diabetic, the amount of insulin needed exceeds the ability of their pancreas to excrete enough insulin. Adult onset diabetes results, when any one or more of the above five processes causes the pancreas to exceed its ability to excrete enough insulin. In all five situations, higher insulin output is required (commonly discussed as insulin resistance). High insulin levels direct the liver to make excess LDL cholesterol. In turn, the excess LDL cholesterol released from the liver into the blood stream causes the vessel walls to collect LDL cholesterol in the macrophages. Fat and cholesterol collecting in one's arteries describe only one of several mechanisms of injury. The elevated blood sugar of diabetics describes an additional mechanism that injures the blood vessel.

Mainstream medicine tends to focus on normalizing the blood sugar with the price paid in the form of health consequences from the increasing insulin message content. For example, conventional physicians are taught to peripherally address the increased insulin caused, cholesterol and fat making side effects, with cholesterol lowering drugs. They are also taught to prescribe blood pressure medication for the high blood pressure caused by excess insulin or mineral imbalance (Blood Pressure chapter). However, healing requires that insulin levels come down rather than pummel the liver with potentially toxic medication.

That insulin feeds fat formation in one's arteries is particularly disturbing when one realizes how mainstream medicine treats many adult onset diabetics because they sidestep the central determinant, excess insulin need. Unfortunately, the majority of diabetics are treated by methodologies that raise insulin levels even further. This may normalize blood sugars, but it will only make the fat accumulating in their arteries worse. Clinically the higher insulin levels show up as a worsening cholesterol profile. The cholesterol profile worsens with these treatment strategies because the higher the insulin release rate the more the liver receives message content to make cholesterol and fat from the sugar taken out of the blood stream.

As was previously stated, mainstream physicians are taught to remedy the worsening cholesterol profiles with various types of statin drugs. Statin drugs inhibit the cholesterol making enzyme, HMG CoA reductase. However, biochemistry textbooks discuss the fact that if the insulin message content decreases, this enzyme turns down its activity level naturally. In addition, the enzyme HMG Co A reductase turns down its activity further when glucagon levels within the liver elevate (see below). Rather than educate physicians about these buried and ignored facts the symptom control approaches still remains the standard of care. Mantra: these common symptom control approaches are always accompanied by side effects and have nothing to do with how one heals.

Physician's Sidebar

Another common symptom control approach to treating adult onset diabetes involves the metformin like drugs given to increase 'insulin sensitivity'. Their most common side effect, metabolic acidosis, provides a clue for how the increase in insulin sensitivity comes about.

Red blood cells and exercising muscles provide reliable sources for the constant creation of lactic acid. Normally, the liver removes this to keep the blood pH balanced. However, anything that poisons the liver will decrease its ability to perform this important task. In addition, a decreased conversion of lactic acid to pyruvate, a sugar intermediary, will lower the gluconeogenesis rate as well. A lowered gluconeogenesis rate, in turn, will decrease the rate at which the liver can dump sugar into the blood stream. This mechanism lowers the amount of insulin needed. However, this is probably not the primary effect for how these drugs lower insulin requirements.

Remember the more IGF-1 available the less insulin required. Also remember that the bulk of IGF-1 binds to a carrier protein called insulin like growth factor binding protein (IGFBP). Associated with this complex of IGF-1 and its binding protein is the acid labile subunit (ALS). A rise in acid content within the blood stream allows ALS to undergo a conformational change, which frees up circulating but bound IGF-1 to help insulin with fuel delivery (an increase in insulin sensitivity).

An additional insight occurs that regards the natural process of increases in insulin sensitivity when the blood turns acidic. It has long been recognized that anaerobic exercise (weight lifting) raises Growth Hormone levels many more times than does aerobic exercise. Here again it is the rise in lactic acid levels that seem to increase Growth Hormone secretion. Drugs like metformin tend to raise lactic acid levels, as they pummel the liver, and this fact recreates the rise in lactic acid seen with anaerobic exercise. As Growth Hormone levels increase the secretion rate of IGF-1 rises as well. In addition, the IGF-1 within the blood stream becomes more helpful with sugar removal because the ALS fragment has undergone a conformational change. Rather than the mainstream textbooks and eduction system helping physicians to understand the important roles that Growth Hormone and IGF-1 have in insulin sensitivity, they are given piecemeal information. Piecemeal-educated physicians enable drug sales to increase but the overall healing suffers.

Passive patients require these symptom control approaches but what about those owners who desire healing? The first step in healing an insulin-excess disease is to understand which type an owner may have. Contrary to the mainstream medicine approach to adult onset diabetes numerous additional causes for this disease process exist. Before healing can occur, the afflicted needs to know, which process causes his/her disease?

All of these previously mentioned nine factors affect the message content at the level of the liver by their unique effect on the amount of insulin message content present. **Remember that obesity has a powerful association with both heart disease and diabetes. The nine groupings below help explain why. When one understands why they have a disease, they can begin to heal. Healing is facilitated when one's physician inquires into which type of liver message abnormality promotes a given owners disease process.**

Insulin and Glucagon Message Content in the Liver

It is more accurate to say the activity of the cholesterol-manufacturing enzyme in the liver, HMG Co A reductase, is determined by the ratio, in amount, between glucagon and insulin. This fact elucidates the advantage of high protein/good fat and low carbohydrate diet because it will tend to increase glucagon levels relative to insulin. Similarly, stress management and regular exercise will tend to improve this ratio (see exercise and muscles chapter). Owners, who eat steak and eggs while simultaneously decreasing carbohydrates, will tend to see a drop in their cholesterol (see digestion of fat). There are other factors that influence blood cholesterol level, but this ratio is all-important in most owners. Without attention appropriately placed on an improved insulin and glucagon ratio healing a blood cholesterol problem becomes difficult.

Diminished Potassium Leads to an Increased Insulin Need

It was explained earlier that a fall in total body potassium leads to insulin resistance (more insulin is needed for the same sugar load). Increased insulin traveling out of the pancreas means that more fat and cholesterol-making message arrives in the liver. By this mechanism, diminished body potassium has detrimental effects to the insulin and glucagon ratio. However, this mechanism of altered blood fat creation from the liver is rarely recognized in America today.

This basic defect arises because owners who subsist on a processed food diet stuff their cells chronically with the wrong mineral ratios. The body was designed to intake at least three times as much potassium as sodium. Unfortunately, processed foods contain a reversal of this natural mineral requirement (see mineral table). Consequently, around middle age the kidney begins to falter in its ability to conserve potassium and excrete excess sodium.

The potassium deficiency of middle age means less of this mineral becomes available to bring the blood sugar down following a carbohydrate meal. A potassium ion is necessary to bring one sugar molecule inside a liver cell for sugar storage purposes. This is also true for all cells except in the brain and red blood cells.

Inadequate potassium causes the pancreas to eventually secrete extra insulin. Note that the textbooks emphasize the fact that low potassium availability causes inhibition of more insulin release out of the pancreas. However, they fail to mention that as more potassium is sacrificed from the cells that eventually insulin releases again. This fact occurs because the pancreas senses the delay in the blood sugar fall after eating.

This abnormal cycle explains why those on chronic diuretic therapy eventually develop diabetic glucose tolerance curves. These owners experience insulin resistance because the basic defect is not enough potassium to uptake the sugar into the liver and other body cells.

It is actually slightly more complicated than this because of the IGF-1 that is released between meals. Recall, potassium deficiency also impedes the storage of sugar as glycogen because a fixed amount of potassium per gram of glycogen in the liver needs to be present. Remember as well that the liver manufacture of fat and cholesterol does not depend on potassium levels.

This explains why the extra insulin that occurs in these situations will preferentially activate the fat making machinery in the liver. This happens whenever the liver receives excess insulin message content. In contrast, the healthy body has ample potassium to facilitate the rapid liver uptake of sugar out of the blood stream following a meal and to make glycogen. It also has sufficient circulating IGF-1 to facilitate sufficient organ and muscle uptake of sugar that lessens the liver proportion of sugar removed out of the blood stream during blood sugar rising events (following meals and stress). However, potassium inadequacy gives the advantage to the liver because the liver can still bring down the blood sugar by making cholesterol and fat.

Recall, ideally, blood sugar falling events (being between meals or with exercise) causes the liver stored potassium, sugar, fat and IGF-1 to secrete together. With adequate potassium, IGF-1 can promote the uptake of nutrients. Potassium and other nutrients are needed for cell energy and rejuvenation (i.e. strong, large muscles). However, with insufficient potassium, the blood sugar normalizes more by the liver than by the peripheral cells (*hungry cell syndrome*). Visualize the tug of war between insulin and IGF-1 determining where fuel flows. Also visualize that adequate potassium availability helps fuel delivery with both IGF-1 and insulin release.

The dependency of insulin on adequate body potassium exposes a defect in the high protein diet proponents. It clarifies how the fruit and vegetable proponents contribute a piece of the puzzle that pertains to diets that work. When both of these pieces correctly re-unite, a superior diet and cholesterol profile becomes possible.

The high protein diet premise improves when adding in the optimal ratio of potassium to sodium mineral content. This combo drastically lowers the insulin message content needed by the body. A lower message content of insulin will improve the ratio between it and glucagon. This will allow less cholesterol and fat synthesis in the liver. In turn, diminished cholesterol and fat synthesis leads to improved blood cholesterol. When less insulin becomes necessary the pancreas strain diminishes. In the case of diabetes, the need for extra insulin becomes less likely.

Growth Hormone Connection - What Message the Liver Receives and its Effects on Diabetes and Heart Disease
Growth Hormone Excess

Excessive Growth Hormone tends to promote diabetes when its level exceeds the ability of the liver to secrete the consequent insulin-like growth factor (IGF-1). Recall, within the liver it promotes the release of sugar and fat into the blood stream. Also important concerns the simultaneous release of insulin-like growth factor (IGF-1) that Growth Hormone causes.

IGF-1 acts like insulin out in the periphery; muscle and organ cells. IGF-1 helps insulin take sugar out of the blood stream. The diseased liver cannot release sufficient IGF-1. This defect occurs at varying degrees of severity. Elevated GH with a diminished IGF-1 release will cause the blood sugar to rise. When the blood sugar rises the pancreas attempts to normalize it by secreting insulin.

When blood sugar rises beyond the pancreases' ability to manufacture the insulin necessary to counter act the excess Growth Hormone, diabetes is born. Growth Hormone excess can occur either in acromegaly or with high dose Growth Hormone replacement protocols. Important point: It is the increased insulin, in the above scenario that leads to altered blood cholesterol profiles. When this occurs heart disease and eventually diabetes become more likely.

Within this subgroup of owners that may get diabetes are those with a wounded pancreas. Their High IGF-1 levels are their only protection from full on diabetes. Sometime in adulthood as the IGF-1 levels fall these owners develop diabetes. They can usually be recognized clinically as those atypical looking diabetics that have large muscles and diminished body fat for their age.

This is a rare type of physique for any diabetic and should alert the clinician to look into the fasting insulin, C-peptide and IGF-1 level. Also serum iron studies (screen with ferritin level) identify those owners whose pancreas was damaged by its accumulation. Again these rare types of diabetic patients have as their fundamental defect a wounded pancreas and as their salvation the particularly strong ability to make IGF-1.

This type of diabetic patient benefits from insulin treatment because insulin deficiency, and not IGF-1 deficiency drives their disease process. In contrast, the typical emaciated insulin dependent diabetic usually suffers from IGF-1 deficiency first (a wounded liver). In these cases, the IGF-1 defect eventually exhausts his/her pancreas (beta cell burnout) and diabetes develops.

For this reason, measures that raise IGF-1 early in the disease process could save some of these owner's pancreases from total burn out. However, physicians would first have to know to check a fasting IGF-1 level. Paradoxically, this is not usually part of the mainstream education content.

Growth Hormone Deficiency

For different reasons, problems with blood sugar control occur in this situation. Blood sugar will tend to rise because less liver direction occurs to release insulin like growth factor (IGF-1). Recall, normally IGF-1 levels occur at levels greater than 100 times those of insulin in the blood stream of a healthy owner. IGF-1 helps insulin with taking nutrition out of the blood stream and into the cells.

Consequently, with less IGF-1, more insulin must be secreted for the same sugar load. The increased demand for insulin exhausts the pancreas of some owners and diabetes develops. Sedentary lifestyles promote declining Growth Hormone secretion rates. Conversely, hormonally intact owners that exercise, have higher Growth Hormone levels. That means less insulin will be required because of the increased liver stimulation to secrete IGF-1. Less insulin creates less message content in the liver to make fat and cholesterol. Athletic training will decrease cholesterol levels for these reasons.

Clinically, Growth Hormone deficient owners express as one type of syndrome X (metabolic syndrome) patient. Their

fundamental health defect results from a fall off in their IGF-1 levels. Healthy people have over 100 times the IGF-1 compared to insulin within their blood streams. The liver is large and the pancreas is small. The smaller pancreas, when forced to increase its insulin production rate many fold eventually exhausts itself. Realize, a small fall in IGF-1 levels requires a marked increase in insulin production to offset the deficiency in the total amount of fuel nozzle hormones for the body cells outside the liver and fat. Recall, as well, the insulin trap of 200,000 pure insulin receptors per liver cell that allows very little secreted insulin to make it beyond the liver. Again, increased insulin need for survival more accurately describes the 'why' better than the hopeless dogma about increased insulin resistance as remaining an unsolved mystery.

IGF-1 levels fall from three basic mechanisms; liver injury, decreased Growth Hormone secretion rates and diminished DHEA (testosterone) levels, which direct the liver DNA to make IGF-1. Recall, Growth Hormone instructs the liver to secrete IGF-1. Also recall, sufficient Growth Hormone manufacture within the pituitary depends on adequate thyroid hormone levels.

Excess Cortisol Levels - The Message the Liver Receives Depends on the Health of the Pancreas

Excess cortisol creates obesity and/or borderline diabetes. In either case the blood vessels sustain damage. The phenotype distinguishes which process occurs. The 24-hour urine test confirms the physical exam and blood findings. With increased cortisol, owners with a normal pancreas, tend to become obese. With the passage of time, they will tend to appear cushingoid (moon face, buffalo hump, stria on the abdomen, panus formation on the abdomen, muscle loss). If the cortisol level elevates high enough, they can reach the upper limit of their pancreas for insulin production and diabetes results. Important point: It is the insulin that makes them fat. It is the cortisol that elevates their blood sugar and sucks down their body protein content (catabolic effect).

Mainstream physicians are generally groomed into thinking that cortisol directly makes these owners fat. This is not true. First, the elevated cortisol inappropriately directs the liver to begin creating and dumping sugar into the blood stream. This results from the fact that when cortisol levels increase, the body thinks there is an emergency. However, mental stress still causes increased cortisol, but here, no physical challenge ever comes and the body eventually recognizes the increased blood sugar as inappropriate. When the body recognizes the increase in blood sugar as inappropriate, insulin levels begin to rise. When increased insulin secretes into the portal vein, because of body anatomy, the liver receives a higher message content to make fat. Visualize the insulin trap within the liver. Increased fat synthesis leads to weight gain.

Unfortunately, the second group of increased cortisol producers is often missed clinically because they lack body fat and this fools physicians. Any owner who has heart disease and appears on the emaciated side of physical body habitués deserves a deeper inquiry. Although they have increased cortisol output, they could have a 'wounded' pancreas.

Wounded pancreases cannot increase insulin production to match the increased sugar output of high cortisol. Instead these owners rely on their IGF-1 to eventually bring their sugars back down to normal. Increased blood sugar proves only transient but the return to normal levels delays. The prolonged increase in blood sugar has oxidizing effects on the blood vessels (increased glycation rate, otherwise known as an increased rate of blood vessel rust formation).

In these cases, the normal fasting sugars are almost always normal, but the glucose challenge and hemoglobin A1C tests are not. These owners acquire blood vessel injury from the episodic elevations of blood sugar levels following the cortisol surges or carbohydrate binges. Increased blood vessel injury occurs from the rust processes that high sugar causes to the vessel walls. **These types of patients provide another situation for which insulin shots will prolong life because their insulin deficiency is at the root of their disease process.**

Further complicating these owner's health problems concerns the fact that they also crave sugar. They crave sugar because they lack sufficient insulin. Sufficient insulin is required so that the blood fuel can stay constant between meals because it encourages the liver to store sugar.

Normally, between meals the release of Growth Hormone occurs when blood fuel first begins to fall. The arrival of Growth Hormone at the liver that is stuffed full of glycogen, which insulin directed following the last meal, causes sugar, fat and IGF-1 to release. The IGF-1 delivers the fuel to the hungry cells in the between meal state.

However, in these types of afflicted owners their insulin release was inadequate, following their last meal, so their glycogen stores prove insufficient. **Here lies the mechanism for another type of hypoglycemic prone owner.** These types present clinically as emaciated in their muscle mass and have very low body fat. They get hypoglycemic because they lack sufficient insulin to instruct the adequate storage of sugar within their livers to get them through the between meal state.

Thyroid Hormone Levels

Thyroid hormone levels form a determinate of how fast the cell power plants can utilize blood fat. Consequently, owners with low thyroid levels suffer from a diminished ability to utilize fuel in their power plants (mitochondria). Also visualize their feeble livers secondary to the diminished thyroid message content arriving at its DNA programs (genes). Scientific experiments performed on dogs that had their thyroids partially or totally destroyed clearly showed the consequent pathological changes at the level of the liver. Without adequate thyroid, the liver becomes pathologic because it lacks appropriate instruction at the level of its DNA programs.

The thyroid hormone also determines how many mineral pumps are present within the 70 trillion cell membranes. At rest, the largest amount of calories burn from recharging these 70 trillion cell batteries (charging up the cell voltage by concentrating mineral differences about a membrane). Logically it follows then that as the numbers of the mineral pumps increase so does caloric expenditure. Remember the thyroid message partially concerns itself with instructing the body cells DNA program (genes) to manufacture more mineral pumps.

The more mineral pumps that exist, the more calories burned while an owner rests. Scientists call this the basic metabolic rate. In general, the metabolic rate depends on four things: the amount of mineral pumps, the sufficiency of other energy consuming proteins, adequacy of potassium and magnesium and the strength of the furnace flame within the mitochondria. Thyroid hormone plays a role in all four or these important processes.

For these reasons, weight gain propagates until someone helps the thyroid hormone level to increase towards normal. Nuclear fallout, spent rocket fuel and other contaminants around the world have poisoned millions of owner's thyroid glands. Rather than educate physicians properly about the need to check the thyroid more completely, countless owners are falsely reassured that their thyroid hormone level is fine (see thyroid section).

Recall, thyroid hormone levels within the pituitary determine how much Growth Hormone is manufactured. Growth Hormone adequacy defends body protein content while the owner fasts, exercises or is between meals. Cognizance here allows one to realize that higher normal thyroid function to be desirable rather than the standard of care today, which falsely reassures those that are above the bottom 2.5% of a thyroid poisoned population (outside two standard deviations). Coincidentally, maybe, by setting the normal range to absurdly low values more statin and antidepressant drugs become necessary (Barnes).

Growth Hormone and the Unhealthy Liver

Unhealthy livers are unable to release adequate insulin-like growth factor (IGF-1) when Growth Hormone instructs them to do so. **As a consequence, the Growth Hormone released can be diabetogenic in these situations.** Injured liver cells still make fuel available when directed to do so long after their ability to make proteins curtails.

The liver manufactures the blood stream amount of insulin-like growth factor (IGF-1, sulfation factor, or also called the nonsuppressible insulin like activity of the blood stream). Many different reasons arise that cause the liver to become metabolically defective. Some of them include poor nutrition, excessive liver toxin exposure (alcohol, prescription drugs, putrefaction of the colon contents with liver reabsorption), poor trophic hormone levels (cortisol, thyroid, androgens, etc.) fatty liver and excess iron storage.

It is interesting that many medical textbooks emphasize that Growth Hormone is diabetogenic (promotes diabetes). Sensationalizing this rare possibility leads to yet another example of how physicians' thinking gets groomed into the more profitable ways to treat disease. Instead of saying that Growth Hormone is diabetogenic when the liver is sick or the amount of Growth Hormone exceeds the ability of the liver to produce IGF-1 they propagate a half-truth. To tell the whole truth would facilitate a curiosity for the importance of IGF-1 for blood sugar control.

Insulin - Pro-Hormone Levels

Insulin is first made within a 'package', the pro-hormone, that converts to insulin before its release into the blood stream. Certain situations create an increased release of the pro-hormone form of insulin (in its package). This occurs when the pancreas is forced to increase insulin production in response to some other body condition (obesity, high carbohydrate diets, insulin resistance). When this occurs the effectiveness to remove sugar from the blood stream diminishes per amount of pancreas secretion. The pro-hormone seems to retain some of its message content in the ability to make the liver create fat from sugar. This also happens in the growth of fat cells.

High Estrogen Levels Will Increase Insulin Need

There has been a flurry of media attention toward supposed new evidence about increased estrogen levels and the increased risk for heart disease. All along the evidence for this predictable association has been buried in the medical textbooks.

This chain of events is high estrogen leads to increased Growth Hormone release but it also simultaneously curtails the liver's release of insulin like-growth factor type 1 (IGF-1). The decrease of IGF-1 and the increased Growth Hormone message causes the sugar release to be uncompensated because there is a diminished release of IGF-1. In this situation, the blood sugar will rise higher than it does when excess estrogen is not present (a diabeticgenic effect of excess estrogen).

The body eventually senses that the blood sugar is elevated and insulin secretes out of the pancreas. The increased insulin secretion rate required to shore up falling IGF-1 causes the liver to receive increased message content to change sugar into fat and cholesterol. Recall, insulin levels within the liver primarily determine energy storage ability and most energy stores as fat.

Cholesterol and triglycerides are the two types of pH neutral fat that the body manufactures. Carbohydrate sequestered by the liver converts into fat and cholesterol under insulin's direction and eventuallysecrete into the blood stream as LDL cholesterol. In these situations, the blood has more LDL cholesterol and the triglyceride levels will be higher when measured. Triglyceride levels are only the summation of all the fatty acid derived fat in the blood stream (the fatty acid derived content of HDL, LDL, and VLDL cholesterol). While cholesterol is the body's other type of pH neutral fat it not derived from fatty acids. LDL, VLDL, and HDL all contain various amounts of triglyceride, phospholipids, specific proteins and cholesterol by definition. Both high blood stream exposure rates to liver released triglycerides and LDL cholesterol are associated with an increased risk of heart disease.

For completions sake, a side detail needs to be discussed briefly as to why women tend to have higher HDL cholesterol levels. The clue as to why involves the observation that most women tend to gain weight evenly spread out between their trunk and limbs. In contrast, men collect fat mostly on their trunk (android distribution). This clue leads to a solution when one realizes that the enzyme, lipoprotein lipase evenly distributes throughout women's bodies but remains mostly present in the truncal areas in men. Lipoprotein lipase is the enzyme that chews on the triglycerides of LDL transforming them into HDL. Estrogen levels control the enzymes distribution.

Low Androgen Levels

Many diabetic's disease traces back to a fall in their androgen levels for one reason or another. Early on in their disease if their physician recognizes this deficiency, when it occurs, total pancreas burn out can be avoided. In addition, many of the complications of diabetes such as: blood vessel pathology, colitis, and digestive tract dysfunction are made worse when androgen levels stay low.

Prediction: in the near future more attention as to whether insulin dependent diabetes resulted from liver injury first or pancreas injury first will come into the mainstream spotlight. The liver injury first variety has a component of causality in low androgens. Pancreas strain occurs whenever androgens fall because IGF-1 levels consequently fall off as well.

Physician's Sidebar

The important role of IGF-1 and the amount of GAG formation on the lining of the blood vessels, colon and stomach was previously mentioned. Briefly, IGF-1's presence in these tissues controls the important step of sulfation for these molecules creation. In fact the older literature called IGF-1, sulfation factor. Recall, a fall of the androgen message content in the body directly causes IGF-1 to fall off throughout the body. In turn, less IGF-1 instructing the adequate sulfation of the blood vessel lining causes defective GAG to form.

A deficiency in this layer paves the way for an increased injury rate in these tissues. Add in the unmanaged high blood sugars of the uncontrolled diabetic and the injury rate accelerates. For this reason, restoring the androgen level to normal makes sense as an additional step beyond blood sugar control alone.

Liver Facilitates the Assimilation of Fat from the Digestive Tube

There is a system in the liver for breaking down spent hemoglobin molecules by utilizing certain parts of these aged hemoglobin molecules, bilirubin, for the manufacture of bile. Bile facilitates the ability of the digestive tracts to absorb dietary fat and in the excretion of certain body wastes that the liver processes. The bile system is anatomically like a 'tree' in the liver. The smaller branches of bile containing the fluid coalesce into larger bile containing branches until they all converge in the common hepatic duct. The bile system tree has its root in the gall bladder that lies outside the liver. Salts of cholesterol are also used in the chemical concoction called bile (digestion chapter). All the constituents that make up bile facilitate the assimilation of dietary fat. When the liver becomes sick, the bile can back up into the blood stream. Jaundice results because of these components backing up in the blood stream. The hemoglobin breakdown product, bilirubin, being too high causes the yellowish skin color changes of jaundice.

The message content that the liver receives can help or hinder the fat content in the blood vessels and body. Equally important to overall body health concerns the molecular parts needed by the liver to deactivate numerous toxins.

The Liver Stores and Manufactures Vitamins, Minerals, and Hormones

The liver stores many vitamins such as vitamin D, A, and B12. In the case of vitamin A, the liver also manufactures its transport protein, retinol-binding protein. When carotene (dietary vitamin A) absorbs from the diet, it requires a capable liver to split carotene in half. Every carotene split in half creates two vitamins A's. Some owners begin to turn yellow when their liver becomes unable to split this apart.

Vitamin A is best thought of as a hormone. The vitamin A 'hormone' belongs to the most powerful class, the level one-type hormones (see hierarchy of hormones). All level one hormones share the unique ability to regulate the DNA programs (genes). Healthy owners have ample vitamin A stored in their liver.

Part of the ability to intake nutrition at the cellular level depends on the liver storing adequate potassium. A high potassium diet facilitates this ability. One potassium ion moves one sugar molecule out of the blood stream. Cells need adequate potassium to stabilize the proteins in the body cells. The size of muscle cells serves as an example of the importance of adequate potassium.

IGF-1 is a level two hormone made in the liver and its blood levels determine the ability of muscle and organ cells to uptake nutrients out of the blood stream. Once nutrients are inside a cell, they can be incorporated into power plant generation activities or regeneration projects. IGF-1 activity also depends on adequate potassium release from the liver. Normally potassium and IGF-1 release from the liver at the same time. Owners who possess high potassium and IGF-1 stores in their liver have a health advantage. Recall, the rate of IGF-1 manufacture in the liver is determined by the amount of DHEA and testosterone that reaches the liver DNA programs. In turn, the amount of IGF-1 released by the liver is determined by the amount of Growth Hormone released from the pituitary. **Common factors that encourage the release of Growth Hormone from the pituitary are exercise, fasting between meals, high pituitary dopamine levels, low pituitary serotonin levels and low blood sugar. Conversely, high estrogen depresses the ability of Growth Hormone to cause IGF-1 release from the liver.**

Physician's Sidebar

Here lies the mechanism for how high estrogen levels cause insulin resistance (higher insulin need). Insulin resistance occurs because more insulin is needed when IGF-1 secretion rates diminish. This happens when estrogen, at high levels, inhibits IGF-1's release from the liver. The IGF-1 released diminishes despite the concurrent estrogen enhanced GH increase that directs the liver to dump sugar into the blood stream. This leads to the need for more insulin to return the blood sugar to normal. A diabetogenic effect of high estrogen operates in these cases. Instead, the textbooks propagate the half-truth of Growth Hormone being diabetogenic. While in fact, Growth Hormone only becomes diabetogenic when the liver is ill, high estrogen levels occur, or it secretes at abnormally high rates like in acromegaly.

IGF-1 essentially proves ineffective in the liver and fat cells for directing these types of cells in the taking of nutrition out of the blood stream. In contrast, insulin is less effective for directing the uptake of sugar in cells like muscle, but many times more effective in directing the liver and fat cells to remove sugar for storage because of its lower blood stream concentrations and receptor concentration differences.

Anatomically the liver always receives the highest amount of insulin message content whatever its secretion rate. A fat making consequence of increased insulin regards the fact that it is most effective in the liver and fat cells for taking nutrition out of the blood stream. This fact results from the liver and fat cells having the highest pure insulin receptor concentration of all cells in the body, around 200,000 per cell.

In contrast, IGF-1 proves more effective for facilitating

cells like organs and muscles in their up taking of nutrition. Increased estrogen then promotes the need for increased insulin to make up the deficit of IGF-1 in the peripheral cells. However, because increased insulin always hits the liver first the cholesterol and fat making machinery abnormally activate in these situations. This fact explains the increased LDL cholesterol and triglycerides seen in women on high estrogen prescriptions.

Also note that pregnancy is a high estrogen state but possesses a growing placenta. Here the placenta secretes human placental lactogen that stimulates it in turn to make more IGF-1. Unfortunately, oral contraceptive usage and excessive menopausal estrogen replacement dosages both provide situations where a placenta is absent. These common conditions need to be carefully thought out for these reasons.

The Liver Manufactures Most Transport Proteins in the Serum of the Blood Stream

The liver makes most of the many proteins circulating in the blood other than the immune proteins. Many liver manufactured proteins are needed for diverse reasons. The liver manufactured proteins include transport proteins for the different steroids and minerals (iron and calcium). The liver also makes the clotting protein that prevents bleeding when a blood vessel tears. Lastly, the liver makes stress survival type proteins.

Common examples of liver manufactured proteins by type

1. **Transport proteins**	**molecules transported**
Sex hormone binding globulin	estrogen and testosterone
Albumin	Some calcium and some progesterone
Thyroid binding globulin	thyroid hormones
Retinol binding protein	vitamin A
Cortisol binding protein	cortisol
Insulin-like growth factor **binding proteins**	insulin like growth factor
Transferrin	iron
Ceruloplasmin	copper

2. **Blood clotting proteins**
        Factors 1-12
3. **Acute   phase   reactant**

proteins that secrete during stress

  Complement proteins
  Fibrinogen
  C reactive protein
  Interferon
  Ferritin
  Ceruloplasmin

This concludes the taking out the trash discussion involving the liver, skin, lungs and kidneys. The colon's role for trash removal was discussed in section three. In the next section, the immune system will be discussed in its taking out the body trash role. In addition, the sixth principle of longevity will be developed by looking at the organ systems that best exemplify this important principle.

SECTION FIVE

SECTION FIVE *450*

PRINCILE SIX: MAINTAIN CELLULAR CHARGE 451

CHAPTER TWENTY 463

    CARTILAGE WITHIN THE JOINTS 463

CHAPTERTWENTY-ONE 478

    IMMUNE SYSTEM 478

CHAPTER TWENTY-TWO 501

    IMMUNE SYSTEM AND THE JOINTS 501

CHAPTER TWENTY-THREE 508

    BONES 508

PRINCILE SIX: MAINTAIN CELLULAR CHARGE

Avoid Low Cell Voltage Syndrome

While alive, the cells must generate and maintain an electrical charge. This all-important electrical charge is contained in various membranes.   A few of these membranes are the cell membrane, mitochondrion membrane, nucleus membrane, lysosomal membrane, and endoplasmic reticulum membrane. Membranes selectively control which molecules move in, out or around a cell (the force field).

In addition, the strength of electrical cell charge (voltage) generated provides the energy that a cell draws upon to accomplish cellular work.   In general, all membranes in the cells and around the cells possess electrical charges.   Bottom line: The quality of these electrically charged barriers determines how much work is possible and the ability to defend the cell from harmful ions.

As was previously mentioned, brand new car batteries are similar to healthy cells.   When the battery or cell remains charged and it activates, it can perform work by discharging electrical energy.   In the case of batteries, the post begins to oxidize inside and out in a few years.   Consequently, as time passes the electrical gradient between the positive and negative posts possess less energy.   As batteries age the metal posts oxidize and form corroded terminals that are consequently less capable of performing energetic work.

Similarly, the oxidation (rust) process that occurs in a cell jeopardizes its maximal charging abilities.   The consequence being, oxidations of cellular components decrease its productive capacity. This in turn eventually leads to worn out cell factories.

It is more accurate to say that in the battery and the cell less productive capacity is secondary to both the process of oxidation and decreased electrolytes (minerals) in the fluids. These two effects result in a decreased electrical charge with the consequence of there being less energy output from a battery or a cell.   When the battery is unable to deliver adequate charge it is replaced.   Likewise, corroded and depleted cells are best repaired or diminished function manifests.

During the life of the battery the clues to its decreased energetic capacity are subtle, until one day it fails. The analogy between car batteries and the cells is similar for why cells lose electrical vitality.   Cells are different in regards to the ease of their repair and replacement once oxidation or altered electrolytes (minerals) damages them.   Healing here involves repair of the damage to the cell charge systems.   One of the ways to comprehend how to heal is to appreciate the similarities between cells and car batteries. Later, their differences will be explained.

As has been introduced before, the various cells are like different sized car batteries, but now the next level of understanding needs to occur. The size of the charge varies with the different cell types. Each cell type has an optimal charge that is necessary for efficiency in the life of the cell. Efficient living cells have achieved the right proportions of opposing electrolytes (minerals) around their membranes. All healthy cells maintain an optimal charge by maintaining high intracellular concentrations of potassium and magnesium. These two electrolytes (minerals) are electrically opposed by high concentrations outside the cell of sodium and calcium.

Batteries, including cells, charge by moving minerals against their concentration gradient around the membrane. It is the membrane difference (outside versus inside) between the various mineral concentrations that determines the strength of any battery. As this important difference decreases, the energy in the membrane decreases.

Cells charge their membranes by moving opposing minerals against their concentration gradient. This is an energy requiring process. It is the mitochondria (power plants) that constantly supply the ATP energy packets that are used to re-concentrate the minerals against their concentration gradient. However, minerals moving down their concentration gradient, through specific channels, release energy as the cell performs the work of living. Realize, the more extreme the concentration differences about the membrane between these few minerals the more energy it contains. This dynamic process creates a living little battery.

The living cell battery serves two basic purposes. First, it is the electrical charge of the cell membrane that blocks out unwanted molecules. By this mechanism, when a cell membrane fully charges maximal protection exists for the contents inside the cell from outside hostile ions. In contrast, when the membrane charge depletes below a critical threshold, these, always lurking ions harm weakened cells. Summarize, the life of the cell depends on the membrane charge to protect it from external, harmful molecules.

Second, the cells, in order to perform certain biochemical reactions, must discharge some of the energy contained in their membranes. Recall, this process is much like a car battery that performs electrical work by discharging the energy contained by the difference of mineral concentrations between the two different battery posts.

Certain processes diminish cellular batteries. When they occur, each type causes two immediate consequences to any cell. First, as was previously stated, if cellular charge is too low, the cell becomes vulnerable to a massive influx of damaging charged ions. Among these ions are high concentrations outside the cell of calcium and sodium. When a cell becomes vulnerable, due to low cellular charge, ions like calcium rush in and irreversibly harm numerous structures. Visualize that the cellular charge acts like a force field that requires adequate electrical energy for its maintenance.

Examples of these harmful processes occur with decreased oxygen delivery, decreased fuel availability, or an increased stimulus to membrane excitability (discharge) beyond the cells energetic ability to recharge itself. All three of these processes can be permanently destructive to cellular contents within minutes to the more metabolically active tissues (brain) through the mechanism of hostile invading ions introduced above.

The second consequence resulting from membrane energy depletion is that there will be less energy available within the cell to perform the job of living. As has been previously introduced, this job requires sufficient electrical energy to occur within the cell membrane. When the electrical energy contained in the cell membrane diminishes, life-sustaining work becomes less possible. This mechanism also describes one of the reasons owners' cells age.

This section concerns how the principle of cellular charge must be optimized in order for health to continue. Like the other principles of health, a failure to satisfy this requirement will subdue the body's performance despite the other six being in full operation. The satisfaction of the principle of cellular charge is interdependent on the other principles to come to its fruition. The combination of interdependent principles can be thought of as: Avoid *low cell voltage syndrome.*

This section will explain the different organ systems that best exemplify the principle of cellular charge. Basic explanations will be given as to how these organs function in regard to this principle. In addition, the other six principles will be touched upon where they are pertinent.

Next level discussion of Cellular Batteries are like Car Batteries

The entry of charged metal ions, like calcium and sodium, into cells is carefully regulated (gated). This process occurs simultaneously with potassium and magnesium flowing outside the cell. Cellular function is possible only when calcium and sodium flow into the cells and potassium and magnesium flow outside the cell. There is a price for this function: The ions that are flowing down their concentration gradient deplete the electronic energy contained in the cell membrane. Consequently, the cell power plant (mitochondria) must continuously provide energy packets for recharging the cell membranes. Visualize the force field.

Adequate cellular charge energy determines the ability of the cell to obtain the proper proportions of molecular supplies and these supplies need to be constantly available. This consists of raw fuels (carbohydrate, fat, and the twenty different amino acids), correctly proportioned minerals, specific vitamins to process the different raw fuels into refined fuel, and oxygen to power the furnace.

Recall, all cells need proper informational direction on how to spend available cellular energy contained in these molecular supplies. The energy availability in the mitochondria depends, in part, on which hormones direct the operation of this facility. Remember, mitochondria function depends on ample thyroid hormone. Adequate thyroid message content instructs a cell's mitochondria to burn fuel more efficiently (section two).

Cells age when either or both of these processes begin to occur. All cells need adequate molecular replacement parts and proper informational direction on what to do with these parts. This section combines these two processes and explains cell charge and the consequences to cells when the cell charge system fails.

When cell charge systems fail they become like old car batteries with oxidized posts. In living cells, occasionally ions (fluoride, lead, calcium etc.) slip inside and react with intracellular structures (an oxidation process). Their mechanisms of destruction are the same, as when unsupervised, these charged ions irreversibly bind delicate intracellular support structures and machinery (enzymes). This binding often times causes deformation because shape and size matter in the molecular world.

Incapacitation of enzymatic machines and structural support systems follow. This process in turn blocks breakdown and removal of the molecular junk that results. Junk contributes to the intracellular landfill of useless protein structures and oxidized fat. Dysfunctional proteins and oxidized fat fail to participate in the chemical reactions of life.

The body's systems of chemical reactions that sustain the life process depend on a proper gradient occurring between certain opposing minerals. These differences create an electrical force field that can also be partially discharged in the performance of cellular work. The high concentration of magnesium and potassium inside the cell are opposed by the high concentrations of sodium and calcium outside the cell. This difference allows an electrical gradient that the cell can harness. Electrical energy contained in the membrane is constantly used and therefore requires recharging. Remember, the electrical energy of the cell battery is maintained by the gradient between calcium and magnesium and sodium and potassium, as well.

Recall, this is similar to a car battery that continuously needs to be recharged while the car burns fuel. In the body the combustion of the raw fuels; protein, fat, and sugar can only occur after all three are processed into a common combustible derivative called acetate. Acetate is the simplest fatty acid. Acetate is only combusted when exposed to oxygen in the cell's power plants (mitochondria). Combustion of acetate here creates carbon dioxide and water.

The acetate requirement for the power plants is analogous to the fact that different power plants, in the physical world, require specific fuels inherent in their design. For example, some require gasoline and others require natural gas. Similarly, the body's power plants are designed to only combust the fuel called acetate. Processing protein, carbohydrate, or fat creates acetate. Recall, numerous and specific vitamins prove necessary to convert these three different fuel groups to acetate. For these reasons, owners who become deficient in one or more vitamins suffer a diminished ability to burn fuel in their power plants (section one).

Important longevity points: The power plants allow the recharging of cellular batteries and healthy cells avoid unnecessary oxidation. Adequate cell charge (the force field) prevents oxidation by preventing the inappropriate penetration of un-channeled ions inside the cell. The prevention of inappropriate calcium entry into the cell requires an adequate force field (cell charge) at all times.

Appropriate and inappropriate ways exist for calcium to enter a cell. When calcium enters through appropriate cell channels the energy liberated allows for useful cell function. The cell has many reasons to keep calcium within these appropriate channels. Calcium within the appropriate channels allows it to be pumped back outside. In order for this to happen energy packets (ATP), created in the mitochondria, are used up and the membrane receives a slight recharge from having less calcium inside the cell. This process describes the basis for how the cell charges its membrane energy content (cell voltage).

However, living cells must constantly power up energetically against the influx of calcium through inappropriate channels. Unfortunately, when calcium slips inside a cell inappropriately it is analogous to an intracellular missile. Calcium outside of appropriate channels will damage inside the cell structures. It is the strength of the electrical charge contained in the membrane that protects the cell from harmful penetration of ions.

Examples of cellular energetic depletion occur when the blood or oxygen supply compromises (drowning or cardiac arrest) or if vulnerable tissue activates membrane discharge beyond its energetic capacity to maintain adequate cellular energy (seizure). All of these mechanisms injure cells because they all allow depletion of the cellular membrane electrical charge (the force field) with a resultant massive influx of inappropriate calcium. These inappropriate ions flood inward when the membrane energy becomes depleted. Once inside the depleted membrane energy cell these ions readily react detrimentally with intracellular contents (Salpolsky).

Cell batteries must maintain a full charge to maintain health. Fully charged cell membranes maintain mineral balance. Mineral imbalance results from a diet of processed food. America is a land of diseases caused by nutritional deficiencies. Many owners remain unaware of the sickening consequences when they arrive at middle age after eating a processed food diet. These unfortunate owners stuff their body cells, year after year, with the wrong ratio of minerals contained in processed food.

Middle-aged owners are also often not aware of the need for optimal hormonal direction that determines how their cells are directed to spend energy. Realize, only good hormonal directions allow appropriate use of available energy. Conversely, poor hormonal directions lead to the inappropriate use of energy. One example of poorly functioning energy directions within a cell concerns the consequence of diminished cellular charge.

The typical middle-aged American can be typified as an owner who contains diminished cellular charge. These cells cannot maintain their charge without adequate molecular parts and proper hormone direction. The depletion of cellular charge shows up clinically as fatigue, high blood pressure, more fat, less muscle, bone weakening, memory loss, depression, and irregular heart rate. From this menu of ailments a common denominator arises that explains the perfect American way to become weak and fatigued: The loss of cellular charge describes this determinant for how youth is lost.

The American Method of Becoming Weak and Fatigued

As has been mentioned many times, the mineral content of processed food has been significantly altered from its natural state. Important recap: Real food is high in magnesium and potassium. The body was designed to eat food in the natural state for cell charge to remain strong. Now it is time to put these facts into a workable construct for how maintaining mineral balance allows for avoiding *low cell voltage syndrome.*

Processed food, among other depletions, is low in these nutrients. The other mineral aberration contained in processed food concerns its unnaturally high sodium content. The food industry adds sodium to prolong the shelf life of these processed products. Sometimes processed food is only relatively low in regard to the magnesium and potassium content because of all the sodium that has been added. Either way, the mineral content of processed food has been significantly diminished from the natural state (see mineral table).

When an owner eats these processed foods and experiences chronic stress his/her health becomes further compromised. Recall, stress hormones alter the ability to remove extra sodium from the body and this causes fluid retention. Stress hormones also increase the loss of magnesium and potassium from the tissues creating further health consequences.

Important points to recall: As a general rule, 4,000 mg of potassium day, 1000 mg sodium, 300 mg of magnesium, and 500 mg of calcium are needed every day. Most Americans consume the reverse ratio between sodium and potassium (see mineral table). The ideal mineral ratio occurs when there are normal kidneys and adrenals. Extremes of environmental heat or exercise habits increase sodium requirements. For these reasons, individual variation exists on the optimal amounts of minerals needed. However, this general reference will put most owners back on the path to adequate cellular charge.

When owners consume cellular food that confers these mineral ratios, their body's can effectively charge its cell batteries. This remains true even when an owner experiences stress. If the kidneys have not been damaged from the processed food diet, their blood pressure should drop off, as well. This becomes especially true when a concomitant effort to diminish insulin production and obtain optimal vitamin status occurs (chapter three).

Seven Reasons the Potassium Deficient Diet Leads to Old Cells

The importance of ample potassium in the diet has been over looked as a determinant of health. The half-truth about the desirability for a low sodium diet has been substituted for an appropriate emphasis on potassium. Also, the preoccupation about the importance of calcium for the bones obscures the need for magnesium. The truth would include a balanced discussion of all four important minerals. A real food diet provides the only way that these four minerals correctly proportion in consumption relative to need. The focus here will be on potassium only to allow clarity on how mineral balance proves fundamental to health. Potassium provides an excellent example of the importance of achieving appropriate ratios of mineral intake.

Optimal potassium facilitates:
1. **Stability and conservation of protein**
2. **Protection of the kidney**
3. **Insulin efficiency and function**
4. **Red blood cell flexibility and health**
5. **Choice of normal testosterone with normal blood pressure versus normal blood pressure from medication with a consequent decreased testosterone production**
6. **Electrical charge of the cellular force field**
7. **Optimal cellular function**

Potassium and Protein

Potassium availability forms a crucial determinant of the cellular ability to hold onto protein. Adequate potassium content within a cell is necessary to stabilize its protein content. For every gram of protein, 2.6 milliequivalents of potassium are needed. Consequently, those who consistently eat low potassium diets begin to notice an increase in body fat and a decrease in muscle mass around middle age.

One method for the loss of muscle derives from inadequate potassium and/or excess sodium intake. In addition, chronic stress accelerates potassium loss, which contributes to muscle loss. Recall, the additional powerful role that Growth Hormone plays in defending body protein content while an owner fasts, exercises or is between meals. Here, the focus concerns mineral content, like potassium, for preserving protein levels within the body.

This mechanism explains how muscle wasting can result from the body experiencing a potassium deficiency. The body will raid the cells (98% of potassium stores) for potassium if it is not provided in the diet in order to maintain its serum levels (2% of potassium stores). The price of raiding the inside the cell storehouse of potassium concerns the obligatory loss of cellular protein. When cells give up protein they lose structural and functional integrity. Notice the routine serum potassium depended upon by mainstream physicians is not very reassuring when these ratios are realized.

Potassium and the Kidney

It has been known for many years that low potassium diets carry the risk of kidney damage. For this reason, a processed food diet and stress increase the risk of hypokalemic nephropathy. The kidney damage will increase when the potassium deficiency persists. This type of kidney damage can lead to high blood pressure (hypokalemic nephropathy).

There is a correlation between kidney damage and high blood pressure caused by potassium deficiency. Many owners in America remain uninformed about this simple consideration. The longer the time that the owner spends with symptom control, the longer the potassium deficiency will exist to do further damage.

Recall from section one that the common laboratory test method for potassium only measures the serum (blood stream component) of potassium. Two percent of body potassium is found here and it is the last to deplete even when a substantial deficiency occurs in the other 98% outside the blood stream. The other 98% of body potassium resides inside the cells. In order to survive the stress of processed carbohydrate intake, which is largely devoid of potassium, the cells must sacrifice their potassium to the serum (explained in next subsection). This makes the serum look good long after health has suffered from this deleterious process. This means the common lab test mentioned above can give false reassurance about the true status of body potassium content.

The Function and Efficiency of Insulin

The effect of insulin lowering blood sugar requires potassium. One potassium ion associates with each glucose molecule that enters a cell, under insulin's direction. As a consequence, the more carbohydrate in the diet, the more the need arises to increase potassium consumption. For this simple reason, owners who fail to consume potassium in their diet, often suffer form increased insulin exposure caused health consequences.

They will become insulin resistant, meaning for a certain sugar intake more insulin is required to bring the blood sugar back to normal. The increased insulin level required will tend to stimulate the liver to uptake excessive sugar compared to other body organs. In these cases, excessive insulin pummeling the liver increases the manufacture of sticky fat and cholesterol particles, called LDL (section one). In other words, the prolonged higher blood sugar preferentially stimulates the secondary liver sugar removal pathway that does not require potassium. Only the brain, red blood cells, and liver can remove blood sugar without potassium. All other cells require adequate potassium to feed on the sugar in the blood stream.

In these situations, potassium in the cells is eventually sacrificed to the blood stream. Cells donate potassium when more carbohydrates are consumed than there is potassium available (processed carbohydrate). Over time the body begins to become depleted in cellular potassium (98% of body potassium resides here). With a greater potassium deficiency the ability of the cells to donate potassium for sugar uptake slows.

Less potassium in the cells means they eventually become less able to part with it. In contrast, healthy owners' cells promptly donate potassium quickly. This allows the blood sugar to return to normal because sufficient potassium remains available. Remember, potassium depletion accelerates when an owner experiences stress because it accelerates potassium loss because it causes increased cortisol release.

It is important to take note for how the textbooks discuss these above facts in confusing ways. They emphasize that low potassium inhibits insulin secretion. If this were the actual end result, all potassium deficient individuals would develop diabetes. Some possibly do but most suffer from delayed ability to lower the blood sugar following meals (diabetogenic glucose tolerance curves).

However, slowly but surely the cells of the body, to varying degrees, sacrifice their potassium and suffer functional consequences, but eventually the blood sugar returns to normal (insulin again releases from the pancreas as the additional potassium flows into the blood stream). These facts provide something for the average owner to think about the next time they indulge in processed food.

All seven principles must be applied in life. An owner could be practicing all other six principles of health and fail only because they have not been counseled to turn off the desire of the liver to make more sticky fat (butter fat). They need to know this important mechanism for how a potassium deficiency will increase insulin's fat maker role in the body.

Red Blood Cell Flexibility

The red cells possess the feeblest electrical charges of any cells. These cells are often the first to sacrifice potassium content to keep the serum potassium level normal. For this reason, a mild potassium deficiency can be missed when the doctor only checks a serum potassium level.

When red cells lose potassium content their ability to charge their force field diminishes and they weaken. Weak red cells are less effective at squeezing out their contents of nutrients, oxygen, and hormones at the capillary level. In addition, red blood cells with diminished flexibility raise blood pressure (chapter two).

Testosterone and Blood Pressure

Normal testosterone synthesis with a normal blood pressure becomes impossible in certain owners that eat a processed food diet. The combination of high salt with low potassium and magnesium commonly lead to high blood pressure. These situations are often treated in the mainstream medical paradigm with ACE (angiotensin converting enzyme) inhibitors that lower aldosterone production. Unfortunately, the aldosterone level is the rate limiting step for testosterone production as well as other steroids. Conventionally trained physicians are trained to reduce aldosterone levels. Unfortunately, the fundamental role that aldosterone plays in all the steroids biosynthesis is largely down played or ignored (section two).

A real food diet allows for normal aldosterone levels and normal blood pressure. It contains high potassium and magnesium but low sodium. In some owners, only by placing careful attention to these electrolytes (minerals) being properly proportioned in their intake can they avoid blood pressure problems. The body was designed to consume the mineral proportions that are provided by the real food diet. Conversely, the processed food diet violates a basic body design theme in that the mineral proportions are drastically altered. Individual variation occurs for how long a body can tolerate an aberrant mineral intake.

The analogy to understand how a processed food diet will eventually harm owners' cells is similar to purposely violating the composition of battery fluid. Just like batteries, human batteries were designed for specific mineral intake. Although remarkable resilience to chronically reversed mineral consumption occurs, a tolerance limit exists. Cells that reach their tolerance limit behave in electrically aberrant ways. Electrical aberrancy is the culprit, but aldosterone is blamed.

Western trained physicians are taught to decrease aldosterone levels when blood pressure elevates. Aldosterone will only elevate blood pressure when the minerals within become imbalanced. The elevated aldosterone effect further exacerbates when stress also occurs because this further promotes potassium and magnesium losses while retaining sodium (a cortisol effect). Sodium retention causes fluid retention. The fluid retained causes the rise in blood pressure.

Simple truth: the dominant mineral in a given body compartment determines the attractive force for water to follow. The higher the water content within, the greater the pressure becomes. For this simple reason, excessive blood pressure often results from excessive water within the blood vessels.

Important point: Sodium is the major mineral inside the blood stream and this explains why its excess so avidly raises blood pressure (it pulls water into the blood vessel and this raises the tension). In contrast, potassium is the major mineral inside the cells and this causes its abundance to pull water inside cells (wrinkle free cells). Also remember, stressful situations push the advantage into fluid going into the blood stream and out of the cells (sodium conservation and potassium loss occurs during stress).

> Next important point: Aldosterone compared to cortisol on a per weight basis is many times more powerful in its sodium-retaining role. However, two salient points make cortisol more powerful for fluid retention in the body reality. First, cortisol occurs at levels approaching two hundred times those of aldosterone. Second, the receptor that both aldosterone and cortisol bind to within the kidney, which causes sodium retention, binds cortisol many times more avidly. These two facts taken together allow the largely fictional story about aldosterone as the villain to at least surface as a possibility (see more evidence in chapter three).

For these reasons, owners who experience stress, but consume the proper mineral ratio become less vulnerable to fluid retention induced high blood pressure. This occurs because they possess the proper mineral balance and this means they will tend to tolerate a higher aldosterone and cortisol level. Visualize ample potassium in the cells as a sufficient 'tug of war' event that counterbalances sodium in the blood stream, which pulls water into the pipes. Recall, sufficient aldosterone allows a proper stimulus for the production of other steroids. Proper mineral consumption, for this reason, forms a determinant of the rate of steroid synthesis.

Most physicians are schooled in the vague principle of a low sodium diet only. Very few doctors are aware of food types that are low in sodium such as real food. Even fewer physicians understand the importance of increasing the potassium and magnesium containing foods in the diet. Real food is high in magnesium and potassium. Only, real food provides ample potassium and magnesium, which counters the ability of sodium to pull water into the blood vessels. Processed food has less magnesium and potassium content, but increased sodium content. Only when physicians understand the facts about the different natural mineral proportions can they begin to counsel on diets that will heal. Owners heal from correcting cellular charge related health problems.

The Cellular Force Field

The amount of potassium forms a central determinant of the cellular ability to keep out unwanted molecules. The potassium level permits the membrane to maintain a protective electrical charge (a higher cell voltage or force field). Consequently, when a potassium deficiency exists there is less protection. Eventually, this leads to the destruction of the cell. Sodium is over abundant in America and potassium deficiency is prevalent. However, to maintain cellular health, there must be proper proportions between sodium and potassium within the body.

Potassium Availability and Cell Charge

Cell charge is directly proportional to the amount of potassium available inside the cell. Adequate potassium levels are necessary for optimal cellular function. Owners with diminished potassium content have weak cells that cannot accomplish the same function as properly nourished cells. The availability and proportions of potassium, sodium, calcium, and magnesium determine how much work a cell can perform.

Owners that understand the importance of this mineral ratio take the time to create a diet that reflects this. A real food diet will naturally provide these ratios and amounts (see mineral table). When this consideration becomes habit another principle is better satisfied of the seven.

These first four minerals help introduce the idea of cellular charge (cell membrane voltage). In addition, certain organ systems also exemplify this process when they charge themselves. For example, there are other molecules that the body uses to charge different anatomical areas that occur outside of cells (cartilage matrix). Some of these additional molecules will be explained in the chapters that follow. Although these organ systems may use different molecules that occur outside of the cells (the matrix) the principle of optimal function requiring an electrical charge proves similar. The joint tissue of the body provides the first illustrative example.

The Concept of the Electrical Extraction Architecture That Keeps Cells Inflated

Consistently present among the cells, but beyond the view of the electron microscope, exists an important anti-aging architectural framework. This sub-microscopic architecture solves the problem of internal cell pressure. Inside the cell and neighboring cells stack on top of and around every cell: This creates pressure. Gravitational pressure desires to squish the cells flat. Healthy owners have a high integrity framework operating inside and around each cell that opposes the force of gravity. Gravity is opposed because sufficient architectural framework in the body possesses an adequate electrical charge. It is the electrical charge that opposes the gravitational forces from expressing cellular fluid.

One of the reasons owners age involves the fact that this sub-microscopic framework becomes compromised under certain conditions. When the electrically charged framework of a cell crumbles, cellular collapse appears clinically as the shrinkage of old age. As water squeezes out, the framework of the cell begins to collapse and everything becomes smaller.

Physicians dating back to antiquity noted that aging involves a drying out process within the body. Today, this consistent observation has a molecular explanation. Yet, mainstream medical practitioners often fail to appreciate this simple fact.

The architectural framework attracts sufficient water by the amount of its electrical charge. When a sufficient electrical charge exists, in the framework, water sucks inward to further inflate this framework creating wrinkle free matrix, cartilage. Healthy cartilage contains sufficient electrical charge, which opposes the gravitational force and this allows water to attract sufficiently. However, unhealthy cartilage lacks sufficient electrical charges and consequently dries out.

Overly ripe fruit wrinkles for the same reasons those body cells or its supportive matrix shrink and wrinkle. In both cases it involves the loss of the electrically charged, and hence, water-sucking framework within. The difference concerns that the healthy body continually recreates new electrically charged framework. Adequate framework, which possesses sufficient electrical charges, powerfully sucks water into a body area. In contrast, its deficiency allows the gravitational forces to squeeze water from the cells.

For this simple reason, processes that accelerate this sub-microscopic framework's deterioration also accelerate the shrinkage into old age. Conversely, processes that re-enforce this framework's continued rejuvenation maintain a prolonged youthful vitality. The cartilage cells serve as an excellent example for how this electrically charged architecture (matrix) keeps itself in repair. Their ongoing repair process exemplifies the importance of adequate electrically charged architectural framework.

CHAPTER TWENTY

CARTILAGE WITHIN THE JOINTS

Many things can go wrong when the integrity of the sub-microscopic framework becomes compromised and cellular collapse begins. Once the framework begins to give way, re-inflating the cell becomes difficult. For this reason, understanding ways to slow down deflationary cellular forces is most effective early in the aging process.

The same electrically charged architecture that is responsible for keeping the majority of the cells inflated also applies to the joint cells. The difference concerns the amount of reinforcement-architecture needed because of the environmental variations that the different cell types experience.

Healthy joints need a few basic molecular building parts supplied on a regular basis. Joint cells also need adequately equipped cellular factories. Cellular factories must be able to manufacture new framework structures during the entire life of the cell. In turn, cell factories need informational direction that can only be delivered by contact with high quality hormones. Joints are on a path to deterioration unless these three requirements are present.

In one way or the other inflammation follows from the repair rate not keeping up with the injury rate. It seems rather counter intuitive at first that prevailing shrinking forces lead into swelling and pain. It helps to think about the disruption to a cell's function when its anatomy alters. Part of the altered anatomy change concerns the loss of a formidable barrier to the penetration of harmful molecules always lurking outside the cell. Not only do the electrically charged architectural framework molecules attract water but they also form a selective barrier to harmful molecules. Also, if water escapes from inside the cell it collects outside of it leading to swelling. Swelling is one component of inflammation. Swelling tissues cause pain.

Mainstream physicians receive very little educational emphasis about how one continues to possess an optimal electrical water-sucking grid (matrix) throughout their body. This fact becomes quite disturbing when one realizes that this electrically charged architectural framework associates in many important body locations. Some examples are: inflates the inside of all body cells, forms the major component of cartilage and spinal disc material, connects and supports the outside of all body cells, lines the inside surfaces of all blood vessels, lines the respiratory tract, it lines the entire length of the digestive tube and is the substance that inflates skin cells so that they remain wrinkle free. Awareness of these facts explains why many diseases have a component of causality in the disruption of this electrical water-sucking grid. Some common electrical water sucking grid associated diseases are: colitis, heart disease, asthma, arthritis, and the complications of diabetes. This fact becomes more believable when one realizes that each of the above diseases operates with a component of inflammation.

Part of the mainstream medical confusion about the extensive involvement of this grid in so many diseases concerns the additional disturbing fact about the many disjointed alias names that are used to describe it. In order to appreciate that the above listed body locals all contain and rely on this electrically charged-architectural and water-sucking meshwork, a physician would need to know that the following alias descriptors mean basically the same thing: glycosaminoglycans, cytoskeleton, ground substance, basal lamina, mucopolysaccharides, extra cellular matrix, cell coat, cell wall, cartilage, and mucous layer to name a few.

Ignorance further propagates because the molecular makeup of these many ways to name the same substance largely remains ignored. The most accurate chemical descriptor for the above alias names is glycosaminoglycans (GAG). GAG derives from the molecular building blocks, glucosamine and galactosamine. These basic building blocks string together and form chains that crisscross with other chains thousands of molecules long. In addition, it is the addition of various amounts of sulfate and acetate to each glucosamine and galactosamine that powerfully attracts and retains water. This property results from the fact that these two molecular additions are electrically charged and therefore attract water. Important point: only when galactosamines and glucosamines contain the proper electrical charge additions will water content remain adequate.

For these reasons, many practitioners observe patient benefits by supplementing with glucosamine and galactosamine. However, there are additional determiners for how much of this electrical water sucking grid a body manufactures. The central more important determiners involve increasing the repair rate while slowing the injury rate. The injury rate concerns harmful toxins within one's blood stream that penetrate a cell's protective barrier. Part of the injury rate can be slowed with methods that digest or neutralize toxins within the digestive tract (see below). The repair rate concerns three factors: 1) the nutritional completeness to provide molecular replacement parts, 2) the amount of antioxidants and anti-inflammatory molecules within a cell that serve to neutralize harmful invaders, 3) the quality of one's repair hormones within.

Before discussing these three determinants of properly inflated and un-inflamed cells the contrast of mainstream medicine's treatments needs mention. More people die from complications of aspirin like medication every day than have ever died of ephedra. Yet, millions of dollars continually channel into various media outlets expounding on the wonders of these related drugs. In contrast, media campaigns continually warn about the severe dangers of ephedra consumption.

Similarly, simple and effective strategies for promoting joint health remain largely ignored and in their place the more toxic, but profitable, symptom control methods receive favorable comment. Even though some of these over the counter medications kill owners, little consumer protection exists. A healthier level of skepticism for these tactics evolves with each passing day. For these reasons, owners increasingly employ healing strategies instead of the mainstream symptom control solution pandered by the complex.

Nutritional molecules and elements necessary for the formation of new electrically charged architectural framework:

> **Magnesium**
> **Zinc**
> **Potassium**
> **Selenium**
> **Glucosamine and galactosamine**
> **Sulfur containing compounds like MSM**

Antioxidants that prevent cell damage
> **Quercitin**
> **Milk thistle**
> **Oregon grape root**
> **Stinging nettle extract**
> **Tocotrienols extract**
> **Resveratrol**

Nature's anti-inflammatories
> **Tumeric**
> **Ginger**
> **Ashwagandha**
> **Quercitin**
> **Chinese skullcap root**
> **Feverfew**
> **White willow bark**
> **Rosemary**

Substances that help digest and neutralize toxins
> **Super oxide dismutase**
> **Bromelain**

Hormones that increase the repair rate of body tissues
> **Testosterone**
> **DHEA**
> **IGF-1**
> **Growth Hormone**
> **Aldosterone**
> **Thyroid hormones**

> **(Note: these hormones are all interrelated)**

Around middle age many owners begin to suffer the consequences of diminished hormone secretion quality. Hormones deliver messages to cells that instruct them what to do. The many different types of body cells are faithful servants that only do as the messages delivered by the hormones direct. Here lies the middle-aged problem: deficiency of hormone rejuvenation message content allows cells to fall into disrepair. One of the consequences of disrepair concerns the diminished amount of new electrical water-sucking grid molecules manufactured. Visualize that a similar process occurs within an overripe piece of fruit. In both processes water escapes and the object in question shrivels.

The quality of the GAG layer, like other body tissue components, depends on specific hormones that direct its manufacture rate. Again the major reason that many physicians do not understand this concept concerns the way these facts are organized within the textbooks. Additional confusion arises because of the many alias names given to a single important hormone for forming fully charged GAG throughout the body.

As was previously mentioned, the current medical literature calls this important GAG manufacture rate-determining hormone, insulin like growth factor type one (IGF-1). Older literature describes this same hormone as: sulfation factor, somatomedin C, and the non-suppressible insulin like activity of the blood stream. Some holistic physicians feel that by disconnecting important hormones, like IGF-1, by renaming and separating it from the other literature perpetuates physicians practicing in the dumbed down state. The dumbed down state of practice results when doctors are not taught simple holistic facts about how the body heals. Everyone suffers from the dumbed down state except the medical industrial complex.

The sulfation factor name for IGF-1 describes its critical rate-determining role in the formation of fully electrically charged GAG. GAG that fails to contain fully charged additions possess a diminished ability to retain water. Simple science being discussed here, yet, not taught to physicians in a way that they can understand its importance in avoiding the shrinkage into old age manifestation.

Diminished water content leads to wrinkled cells and the shrinkage of old age. In fact, beyond the hysteria to avoid the sun and sell sun blockers this major determiner for youthful skin remains ignored. Remember, skin wrinkles result from the same process that causes over ripe fruit to wrinkle. This truism extends to other body cells as well. The amount of fully charged GAG in an apple or a body cell type largely determines its ability to hold onto water. Human cells require adequate IGF-1 to re-synthesize GAG as it deteriorates. Because ripened fruit lacks hormones they rot and wrinkle as their GAG content diminishes.

It now becomes important not to confuse the IGF-1 released by the liver into the blood stream with its amount inside the body cells. Recall, healthy people possess 100 times IGF-1 levels compared to insulin within their blood streams. IGF-1 helps the cells outside the liver and fat cells in their procurement of body fuel (sugar, fat and amino acids). IGF-1 and insulin are best thought of as the body's "fuel nozzle hormones". Just as filling a car fuel tank with fuel requires a nozzle, similarly the body cells require a fuel nozzle, which these two hormones provide. The alias name for IGF-1 that best describes its fuel nozzle role is the nonsuppressible insulin like activity of the blood stream.

In contrast, IGF-1 within cells delivers a message of cell rejuvenation and repair. Think of its role inside cells as a continuation of its nourishment and revitalizing message that begins with its help outside the cells. Part of rejuvenation and repair concerns the manufacture of fully charged GAG. Only fully charged GAG (sufficient sulfate concentration additions) prevents the shrinkage into old age. For this reason, one of the major reasons that young people have fewer wrinkles involves their greatly increased IGF-1 levels.

Around middle age IGF-1 (sulfation factor) begins to fall off and this results in less fully charged GAG formation. The lower the GAG charge level the more water leaks out of the body tissues (the drying out process of old age). Skin wrinkles exemplify one example of this process. Other diseases for the same reason have a component of causality from diminished GAG content in their area of pathology. For example: the thick mucous of the asthmatic, the copious mucous in the colitis patient occurring when GAG fails to form properly it breaks down at an accelerated rate into mucous, the decreased GAG content that causes much of the disease process of osteoarthritis, the decreased GAG in the blood vessels of some diabetics, and the decreased GAG in the blood vessels of some heart disease patients.

While the above diseases' severity cannot be entirely explained by GAG deficiency, in each case, a profound contribution to the course of these diseases arises from their association with diminished GAG. Since the above diseases cause so much suffering and are part of the shrinkage into old age, the determinants of IGF-1 (sulfation factor) presence deserve mention within the clinical setting (section two). This sadly is not yet the case.

Remember, inflammation within the body arises from the repair rate not keeping up with the injury rate. Anti-oxidant levels, nutritional status and the amount and quality of the repair hormones determine the repair rate. The injury rate subdues by limiting environmental toxin exposure, avoiding inflammatory fat consumption, and supplementing with digestive enzymes. One can observe the glaring reality that the medical industrial complex fails to advise owners in all of the above considerations. In its place, it sells the symptom control measures.

FACILITATING THE HEALTH OF JOINTS

Joint Cells Need Molecular Building Materials to Make Cartilage

Joint cartilage has three basic components; collagen (a structural protein); modified simple sugars that contain varying added amounts of nitrogen, acetate and sulfate groups (GAG); and ample water to inflate the structure into a hard rubber consistency. These raw material components are capable electrical charge generators in the body. Recall, the strength of electrically charged molecules, within an anatomical area, determines the ability to attract water despite the opposing gravitational forces that want to squeeze water from a cell or body support structure. Before owners can have enough of these electrically charged molecules, their cartilage cells require an adequate supply of the necessary building blocks.

Cell Factories are Vulnerable

In general, cartilage cells are affixed to the end of the bones. They are usually on the ends of two bones to form a joint. Cartilage serves to cushion the trauma of gravitational forces. Each cartilage cell contains many factories that produce and secrete structural framework. These cells are spaced far apart between the electrically charged frame works they weave. It is important to emphasize that in between the cartilage producing cells lay the elaborate framework that is in need of constant repair and maintenance. Healthy cartilage cells are capable of producing adequate new framework structure. Realize, healthy framework contains a sufficient electrical charge.

The cartilage cell factories produce the electrically charged framework. The wide spacing between the cartilage cells, with the intervening support framework, makes sense functionally because cartilage cells are given more gravitational stress than other types of cells. This occurs because of the added structural support role that they play.

As a consequence, each cartilage cell needs to be re-enforced by more surrounding support framework due to added gravitational pressure created by its weight-bearing role. The other extreme is provided by the red blood cell that needs almost no outside supporting framework. Less support framework is necessary because they are floating inside the blood stream where the imploding force is less. In general, different body cells need unique amounts of electrically charged support framework to defend from being crushed. Cartilage cell factories produce an extreme amount of this protective framework because of the role they play.

Joint Cell Factories and Message Content

The third element required for healthy joints is high quality message content contained in the hormones. Many different organs and

468

glands provide these messages to the joint cells. Like other cells, cartilage cells depend on receiving quality message content to direct the use of cellular energy appropriately.

Three Omissions Perpetuating Joint Destruction

The biochemistry of joint health is not discussed in a straightforward way. This leads to erroneous thinking that comes from three main areas. First, there is a failure to remember that the human body cannot digest wood. Second, there is confusion regarding which hormones are centrally responsible for directing the joint cartilage cell. Third, owners are not counseled regarding the importance of facilitating the removal of joint trash water. Avoiding these pitfalls allows healing.

Chondroitin is a Wood-like Molecule

When clinicians prescribe chondroitin to be taken orally, they are asking their patients to digest a wood-like molecule. If human bodies' digestive tracts were equipped to digest wood, these endorsements would be valid. However, human bodies cannot digest wood.

Wood (cellulose) is made of glucose molecules strung together in a beta linkage. Beta denotes the angle of the repeating sugar molecules linkage that humans cannot split. Human's digestive systems can split (digest) alpha linkages. However, the human digestive tract machinery is ill equipped to dismantle beta linkage into its glucose building blocks.

Dietary fiber is cellulose or plant wood. Cellulose has water-conserving properties in the colon because the indigestible beta linked sugar molecules remains osmotically active. This linkage is the reason lettuce and grass provides so few calories to the digestive tracts of humans. In contrast, life forms like rabbits, horses, cows, and termites have the ability to digest this beta linkage. Hence, they derive caloric benefit from the liberated simple glucose contained in the fiber.

It is important to emphasize, human digestive tracts can only break down the alpha linked glucose molecules contained in complex carbohydrates. Members of this group include potatoes, grains, pasta, breads, and corn. Human bodies also store sugar fuel (glycogen) in the alpha linked arrangement.

A problem arises when clinicians endorse the consumption of chondroitin by mouth in the hopes of helping joint tissue regenerate. The building blocks making up chondroitin are in fact useful for part of the renewal reactions in cartilage synthesis. However, consuming chondroitin by mouth is futile because the building blocks making up its structure are linked together in a beta like arrangement. Oral chondroitin supplementation is nothing more than an expensive form of dietary fiber. Human bodies' digestive tracts machinery cannot access and split the building blocks making up the chondroitin molecule. Hence, it is not absorbed out of the digestive tract as molecular building blocks (section three).

The other part of the endorsement usually involves glucosamine sulfate. This is a simple molecule and is readily absorbed when taken orally. Glucosamine sulfate is a necessary building block molecular component, but it is only part of the crucial molecules that are needed for new cartilage synthesis. Galactosamine in conbination with glucosamine is much more powerful in contributing to healing because the other critical building block molecular component is galactosamine. For this reason, ideally supplementation protocols for healthier joints would include both glucosamine and galactosamine because healthy joint cartilage is composed of these building blocks.

Until a reliable source of galactosamine occurs, supplementation with commercially available gelatin will help because it is composed of partially digested cartilage. These partially digested products contain both glucosamine and galactosamine. Complete digestion of gelatin would enhance the effect, but it is currently unavailable.

Building Blocks and the Hormones that Oversee Construction

A mental picture of these structural building blocks after processing in the joint (cartilage) cell is helpful. Galactosamine and glucosamine are derived from galactose and glucose by the addition of varying amounts of sulfate, short carbon chains, and nitrogen containing groups (amino groups). Synthesis of these compounds under youthful circumstances is routine and not complicated. Realize, the manufacture of these fully charged and modified sugar building blocks can only occur when there is adequate message content from a hormone, insulin-like growth factor type 1 (IGF-1 or also called sulfation factor). When owners are young, there are ample amounts of this hormone being produced and delivered to the chondrocytes (cartilage producing cells).

Unfortunately, as owners' age, total body production of this hormone decreases. Supplementing with glucosamine and galactosamine makes sense as age progresses because providing these building blocks somewhat sidesteps the obstacle of the falling IGF-1 message content. However, when message content falls, there is less direction for the manufacture of more of these fully electrically charged components. For this reason, synergism is achieved when methods that increase insulin-like growth factor (IGF-1) production are included in the treatment protocol. Ideally, lifestyle choices that promote high hormone tone will raise the hormones necessary for joint rejuvenation (section two).

Key point: The material that makes up the supporting framework occurring inside and outside of all the body cells is similar. At the molecular level, the same molecular material produced in excess outside of cartilage cells is also around most other body cells. The supporting framework occurring outside the cell is called the extra-cellular matrix. The supporting framework that expands the cell from inside is called the cyto-skeleton. Throughout the body the adequacy of the cellular support framework prevents the flattened look of old age and depends on these same three criteria as are necessary for cartilage health.

Visualize the different cells as different types of fruit. The different cells and different cell membranes become analogous to the different skins of different fruits. The cytoskeleton becomes analogous to the different fruits internally. When fruit is ripe they have a firm consistency and resist pressure forces. However, as fruit ripens they begin to lose water and become mushy. Eventually they begin to wrinkle. Mushy fruit occurs for the same reasons as mushy and wrinkled cells. They have in common the loss of the electrically charged supporting framework (GAG-sulfate) that expands them and holds in the water content.

All these galactosamine or glucosamine derived products are composed with an alternating sequence of one of the simple sugars (either glucose or galactose). These molecular associations extend into chains that are made from thousands of simpler molecules. These long chains are precisely crisscrossed and reinforced generously with the protein collagen. The resulting molecular structure is like the steel support structures contained in the skyscrapers. These molecular 'sky scrapers' have the additional property of being electrically charged. Consequently, the adequacy of IGF-1 (sulfation factor) determines the message content that directs the critical step of adding sufficient sulfate to the backbone of this repeating sequence. Realize, sulfation adequacy largely determines the strength of the electrical charge in these anatomical areas. In turn, the strength of this electrical charge powerfully determines how much water remains in a cell, despite gravity.

Building Block Properties and Joint Health

The presence of galactosamine and glucosamine type molecules is critical to joint health. Pivotal point to achieving prolonged joint health involves realizing that these building blocks need to possess the right electrical charge properties (adequate sulfate additions). Only then are they able to powerfully suck water into the framework. This framework is created by their formation into long chains of electrically activated building blocks. These molecules are elaborately crisscrossed to make up the overall structure. The electrically charged chains result in a mesh net configuration. The higher the electrical charge, the more powerfully water is drawn into the meshwork.

Joints are a sophisticated combination of shock absorbers and a hinge. The shock absorber feature works best when adequate water is lubricating into and out of the cartilage. Old age begins to occur when the flow of water into and out of the shock absorber diminishes. Cartilage (shock absorber) needs to possess enough crisscrossed (electrically charged) chains made up of modified and hence electrically charged building blocks, glucosamine and galactosamine, to be healthy. Healthy joints are only possible when these repeating units occur in optimal amounts, contain sufficient electrical charges and are associated with adequate water. The molecular meshwork allows water to be electrically sucked into the joint space whenever joint pressure is released. The water is then squeezed out when pressure is re-applied. The ebb and flow of water moving back and forth serves two important functions. It creates a cushion (shock absorber) for the traumas inflicted by resisting gravity. Secondly, it is the way joint cells eliminate waste and take in the nutrition they need.

Cartilage cells (chondrocytes) have no direct blood supply making them critically dependent on adequate water flowing back and forth. This flushes waste and brings in nutrients.

Processes that contribute to the degeneration of the cartilage architecture are ones that create the presence of less elaborately crisscrossed chains derived from galactosamine, glucosamine, and collagen. In addition, the degree of diminution of the electrically active meshwork that results parallels the decreased function in the joint tissue.

Joint Deterioration – Part of the Solution

Whenever there is a process that decreases the performance of the electrical meshwork abilities, a vicious cycle of continued joint deterioration is normal. With decreasing electrical power to suck in water, there becomes also an ever-increasing defect in the ability to achieve adequate waste removal and nutrient delivery.

Part of the solution involves providing adequate, preformed building blocks necessary to jump-start the synthesis of new framework material. If the other joint cell needs are satisfied there will be an optimal response toward regenerative healing.

Joint Deterioration - the Rest of the Solution

Cartilage cells depend on reliable message content delivered to them via the informational substances (hormones). These messages direct them on how to spend energy. Cartilage cells are no different from other cells throughout the body in regards to their need for informational direction. Differences exist in that they are more vulnerable because they have no direct blood supply. These isolated cells critically depend on the functional power of the electrical sucking grid (healthy cartilage) for waste removal and nutrients intake. In addition, as the electrical power of the meshwork begins to fail a corresponding decreased ability to attract informational substances also occurs. Making matters worse, with less power to suck in water, a corresponding drop in the amount of informational substance arriving at the cartilage-producing cell manifest simultaneously. Less message content directing cartilage production leads to less work performed.

Owners on an accelerated path to old age have poor hormone tone (section two). Poor message content results from sub-optimal hormone types and amounts being the norm in these owners. Some nutritional supplementation programs fail, for this reason, to deliver the desired benefit in these owners. Nutritional supplements for joint health can only benefit those owners that have some message content from the informational substances hormones) direction the joint cells to utilize it. This fact describes the second failure occurring in clinical medicine: Clinicians have good intent when they instruct their patients in the need to take nutritional supplements, but fail in assessing whether their patient has adequate hormone tone to derive the intended benefit.

Important recap: Hormones direct the cells in energy expenditure. Healthy owners have optimal message content (optimal anabolism versus catabolism) from the right amount of each hormone occurring at the proper times and for the proper duration. Conversely, unhealthy owners suffer from diminished quality in their message content leading to the inefficient usage of energy (insufficient anabolism and perhaps exaggerated catabolism). Over time, inefficient use of energy results in breakdown of tissue. This result predictably occurs from the cells not receiving the message to invest appropriately in cellular rejuvenation. Simple science being discussed here, yet, once again not taught in a way that physicians understand.

When clinicians fail to inquire sufficiently into the status of their patient's hormone tone, they often observe diminished clinical results if hormone tone is the problem. The science exists to measure many of the body's hormone levels. Healing becomes facilitated when an assessment is made where an owner's message content lies. It can be between the extremes of healthy joints and the deteriorating processes that result from poor hormone tone.

Ensuring that adequate Growth Hormone, androgens, and thyroid hormones reach the joint cell constitute fundamental considerations in the management of improving joint health. Opposing these hormones effects by inhibition are the counter-regulatory hormones estrogen and cortisol. These hormones provide inhibitory effects on the regeneration abilities of joint cells. However, patentable estrogens and cortisol derivatives are big business and therefore, a disincentive exists to advertise the well-documented downside resulting from their excessive usage

Cortisol Injections - The Other Side of the Story

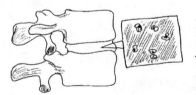 Many owners by age forty have received at least one cortisol injection delivered into a painful joint. Most often it involves a finger, shoulder, or knee. Most people remember the dramatic improvement that followed these injections. Some are lucky and no further problems arise. The upside of these injections involves the power of the cortisol message to diminish inflammatory activity within an injured joint. Unfortunately, this rosy outcome is unusual because of the often-unmentioned side effect: This type of injection inhibits the message of rejuvenation in the joint. As a consequence, the lack of rejuvenation increases the likelihood of further degeneration. In other words, the cortisol message amplifies from the injection and the rejuvenation message dwarfs.

The majority of these cortisol injectable formulations are designed to remain localized and active for about six weeks meaning the injected joint will receive decreased message content for rejuvenation and repair during this time. The usual consequence, by the time the medication wears off is that further joint deterioration occurs. Joints deteriorate when there is a lack of message content directing rejuvenation (insufficient anabolism).

One example of suppressing joint rejuvenation is the spinal disc injection. This procedure involves using patentable cortisol derivatives and is a favorite practice of many specialists. Too often the injured disc, after initially seeming less painful (appearing better clinically), succumbs to the biochemical forces that result when cellular energy is directed away from rejuvenation. The consequence of ignoring this detail is often the need for a surgical procedure. This does not mean that there is never an indication for cortisol injections, but rather patients should be included in the risk versus benefits analysis.

Excessive Estrogen Inhibits the Joints Rejuvenation

The second major counter-regulatory hormone that directs energy away from ongoing joint rejuvenation arises from excesses of the estrogen group of hormones. Over twenty different estrogens occur in nature. Basic medical textbooks counsel on this fact. The discrepancy regards what science has revealed contrasted to what is being practiced in the clinical setting. Too much estrogen message content directly inhibits rejuvenation in joint cells. This consequence occurs with the environmentally acquired estrogen mimics (section two) in both men and women. In addition, it results from taking inappropriate amounts of estrogen replacement therapy.

Whenever estrogen's message content rises too high, at the cartilage cell level, there needs to be an increase in the counter weights (increased IGF-1, androgens, and thyroid hormones). Without an effective counter hormone response these cells do not direct energy into cellular rejuvenation (see estrogen effects in the liver chapter). Basically, like other tissues, cartilage cells need sufficient IGF-1 or these cells deteriorate. IGF-1 levels in cartilage cells depend on sufficient Growth Hormone levels. Recall, high estrogen levels promote Growth Hormone secretion but inhibit its ability to promote IGF-1 levels. If this situation becomes chronic joint deterioration begins.

Androgens – Messengers of Cartilage Rejuvenation

On the opposite extreme of informational content are the androgen hormones that are manufactured mostly in the gonads (ovaries and testes) and the adrenal glands that rest on top of the kidneys. There is a small amount of these steroids manufactured in the brain itself. Men tend to make more androgen and therefore initially have a joint longevity advantage. Women's tendency for joint deterioration is exacerbated by the medical custom of ovary removal and then failing to supplement them with adequate androgen replacement therapy. Some women without their ovaries have strong enough adrenals to manufacture adequate androgen. Adequate androgen allows enough message content to direct the joints to both repair and rejuvenate. However, the adrenals of many women are not up to the task of increased androgen manufacture. As a consequence they suffer from an increased likelihood of joint problems. In addition, the joints of many males have the disadvantage of joint insults acquired early in life that exceed the ability of the body to repair the damage.

The Cartilage Cell's Dilemma

Cartilage cells exist with an ongoing dilemma. While awake, constant compression and decompression occurs as an owner goes about the activities of living. Rest provides opportunity for rejuvenation when the right informational content reaches the cartilage cells. Recall the analogy of the antique weight scale. Often disease states originate from this loss of balance between the opposing hormonal forces. When energy moves too far in any one direction in the body, imbalance occurs and this proves detrimental to continued health.

Cortisol message content is involved in joint health as a counter-regulatory hormone. Any hormone will convey different message content that depends on the tissue with which it interacts. This subtle point is often missed when trying to understand the effects that a simple molecule like cortisol can have on different tissues.

Cortisol is a powerful and important hormone that counter-regulates many other hormones. For example, there is the tug of war of cortisol opposing the actions of insulin. However, cortisol has another counter-regulatory role in a different body tissue, cartilage cells. Here it is anti-inflamitory. Visualize joint cells are caught between the 'weight' and the 'counterweight' of opposing hormones (anabolism vs. catabolism).

Understanding balance between these opposing messages facilitates comprehending the terms existence of a cartilage-producing cell. On the deficiency extreme there occurs the tendency to swell as physical traumas are inflicted on these cells. If one were to take any other tissue outside the musculoskeletal system and compress and decompress it for any length of time, it would become inflamed (swollen). The process of swelling when tissue is overused is mediated by the release of informational substances that give the cells permission to begin swelling. Swelling of tissue is perceived consciously as pain.

However, within the musculoskeletal system the body eludes this problem by secreting small amounts of anti-inflammatory cortisol into these tissues just before the owner wakes up each morning. Cortisol powerfully inhibits inflammation. The risk of this process comes in the form that sometimes an operating deficit of the counter hormones to cortisol develops. Too much cortisol message content leads a cell into disrepair. The anti-inflammatory message content has the side affect of inhibiting ongoing cellular rejuvenation (anabolism).

Ideally, when healthy owners rest their counter response to cortisol remains optimal in the form of released androgens and

Growth Hormone. The net effect that occurs appropriately allows cycles of cellular rejuvenation that balance with cellular rest. The counterweights to cortisol message content are the androgens and Growth Hormone. These hormones stimulate joint cells to invest in cellular infrastructure investment activities and encourage factory synthesis of new meshwork (cartilage, the extra-cellular matrix). Without adequate cortisol secretion into the musculoskeletal tissues each morning, an owner would soon become stiff and swollen.

Conversely, inadequate counter response from both the androgen class of hormones and Growth Hormone will lead to painful and stiff musculoskeletal tissues as well. This common disability results from the disrepair following secondary to a chronic inadequate message to these cells to invest in rejuvenation. Battle cry: the practical operational principle concerns awareness. Awareness allows attention to the necessary balance between opposing hormones that allows health to continue.

Joint Health - Taking Out the Trash Water

Adequate elimination of toxins and waste is the third requirement for the facilitation of joint healing. Overlooking the need for the most powerful medicine of all, water, is behind many joint ailments. The joint cell cells produce waste on a regular basis. Adequate free water intake removes the waste generated in the cells.

Recall, the cartilage cells, within the joints, are more vulnerable to toxins and waste buildup because they have no direct blood supply. Sufficient water squishing back and forth is necessary to remove the waste and toxins. When the joint cells do not receive adequate water between the joint spaces, the tissues begin the process of sequestering (see taking out the garbage chapter).

The effect of an inadequate water supply is exacerbated by diminished thyroid function. Recall from section four that this defect affects all six garbage removal organ systems. Further obstructing this discovery concerns the lack of appropriate clinical attention into the physical signs of low thyroid function at the tissue level (seven links of the thyroid health chain).

Instead mainstream doctors often dutifully check their patients' thyroid function superficially by obtaining often only a TSH (Thyroid Stimulating Hormone) level. This occurs despite the medical physiological textbook fact that events like stress will depress TSH (the fear or pain of the blood draw). Undertreatment also occurs because doctors are not taught to think about the advantages of higher normal thyroid function, like increased Growth Hormone instructing the joints to make IGF-1 and hence they remain vigorously intact. Accumulating evidence suggests that at the very least patients should be instructed to take an armpit temperature before getting out of bed. If the temperature is more than one degree below 98.6 degrees then thyroid hormone replacement should be considered (Barnes).

Recall, Thyroid function determines how much Growth Hormone the pituitary manufactures. A healthy lifestyle allows for sufficient Growth

Hormone release. In turn, Growth Hormone arriving at the liver, instructs it to conserve body protein (longevity advantage), release stored sugar and fat, and to release IGF-1. Sufficient IGF-1 avoids *hungry cell syndrome* and also avoids the need for excessive insulin (insulin resistance).

Inadequate thyroid message leads to, at the level of the joint, trash water accumulation and this causes the afflicted owner's joints to hurt. Sometimes healing the hurt is only an accurate thyroid test away. Sometimes the afflicted owner only needs to realize the potential contained in the most powerful medicine of all, water.

This concludes the discussion of joint health and how it depends on electrical charging abilities. Like cartilage cells that produce matrix material that possesses a electrical charge, the immune systems' cells must also generate a electrical charge to power its weapons of destruction. Hence the voltage of the immune system cells determines whether or not the body prevents invasion of hostile forces from tumor cells, bacteria, fungus and virus's. The next chapter is all about how this happens and what these cells need.

CHAPTER TWENTY-ONE

IMMUNE SYSTEM

Most owners have been supplied with a standard equipped immune system. The different powers contained in this standard equipment contain far-reaching longevity potential. Scientist like big words and often make matters worse by the numerous examples of non-communicating duplicity among the many different competing ways to say the same thing. The end result is usually disempowered owners. This means that owners enjoy less ability to choose intelligently between 'hype' and 'helpful'.

Less obvious is the confusion that disjointed scientific writings has on a physician's ability to offer their patients the best advice. Duplicity of scientific vocabulary and information overload provide effective methods for the suppression of how healing takes place. One way around this involves going back to basic medical textbooks and reviewing what is known about a subject.

A presentation of the big picture has the power to facilitate healing many immune imbalances through insight. Insight allows for seeing cause and effect relationships. At this level, symptom control medicine begins to look less attractive.

The sixth principle is that of cellular charge adequacy. This principle is exemplified in the immune system because these cells require a highly functional 'power grid' to supply the energy needs that arise when their weapons of destruction (immune system) activate.

The Standard Equipment of the Immune System

The different elements (soldiers) in the standard equipment immune system can be conceptually divided into the army, navy, air force, and Special Forces. This will serve as the analogy for this system. Each service has a weapon of destruction. The effectiveness of these forces is constrained by the military budget of the body. The budget is composed of the energy available to power these various defenses. The types and amounts of hormones available to the cells control the use and distribution of this budget. The level one (section two) hormone quality is the congress. They are either wise or foolish in their appropriations.

The types and amounts of more powerful hormones (level one type hormones) determine the immune cell energy budget. Once the energy budget is decided, the communication system carries out the directives. One of these systems can be thought of as the E-mail system of the immune cells. The E-mail system communicates among the different types of soldiers and weapons. The quality of the message content (immune system

E-mail) in this lesser communication system orchestrates where and when different immune system soldiers deploy towards. It gives them their individual orders. Technically, this communication system is still a hormone system because it contains message content carried in the blood stream. Many basic types of soldiers need to be available to defend the homeland.

All immune cells (soldiers) arise from one of three main areas: the thymus, the lymph, or the bone marrow. The basic immune cell types are leukocytes, lymphocytes, macrophages, eosinophils, basophils, and mast cells. General requirements exist before these different immune cell types (soldiers) become well populated in proportion to the other forces. In addition, they must be well equipped with their unique weapons, have properly constructed components that make up the different immune cells, and operate with the different communication systems that can either help or harm the defense systems.

The Immune System Communication

Communication systems (hormones) differ with the different soldiers while they are out in the field. The 'E-mail system' is known as cytokines among the various soldier types. The E-mail system is capable of sending many types of messages that can become complicated by the use of big words and duplicity of expression. Some scientific descriptors are words like interleukin, tumor necrosis factor, and interferon. These names are unnecessary if thought of as different E-mail message types. The E-mail is a type of hormone that the immune system cells use for communication. The different types of immune system cells secrete different types of E-mails that contain unique message content intended for other immune cell types. The immune cells receive these E-mails via the blood stream or lymphatics. Occasionally they can be delivered out into the tissues.

The E-mail choices that each immune cell type is capable of secreting into the blood stream are limited to short cryptic communiqués. These communiqués are the way that the different soldiers and weapons in the immune system communicate to one another. The type of E-mail secreted into the blood stream forms one of the determinants of immune system readiness for defending the homeland. As a general rule, the more all seven principles of health are actualized, the higher the quality of E-mail message that will predominate.

The immune system is composed of various types of armed forces and each is equipped with weapons of destruction. When this system is well numbered and equipped there is a formidable obstacle against potential enemies that want to invade the homeland. Also, potential enemies are created form the rebel cells within.

The military budget directors determine the strength and size of each of these forces and the weapons they use. The budget directors are made up of powerful hormones that determine the amount of body energy available for defense purposes. The qualities that the collective budget directors impart determine the overall maintenance schedule, number of new recruits, and repair activities that are allowed from total body resources.

There are four basic determinants of the overall readiness of the immune system:
1. **The size of each type of soldier population (army, navy, air force, and special forces)**
2. **The amount of weapons that each soldier type is allotted (each type of immune system cell has a special way to destroy the enemy)**
3. **The nutritional integrity available for the construction of the various components that create the operating system of the immune cell**
4. **The overall tone of the message content that the immune cells receive**

E-mail is only one type of message content within the larger system. The other message content delivers via the blood stream, as well, and originates from a large number of different body locations. It will be explained shortly how these different types of messages interrelate. Healing the immune system is best understood by explaining the overall design.

Processes that organize optimal message content in E-mail confer a performance advantage for the owner. Conversely, processes that impair the quality of the message content in the E-mail system weaken the body's performance. Remember, E-mail is just a construct to help lump together one class of hormones, which are secreted by the immune system cells.

Immune system cells secrete other types of hormones. All hormones contain message content, destined for delivery to other cell types. In the case of immune system cells, these hormone messages are designed to communicate almost exclusively with other immune cells. One of the immune system cells' hormone types is best conceptualized into a general group by the construct of E-mail.

Sometimes the quality of E-mail communiqués can be rebellious in nature and contradict the desires of the budget directors (powerful hormones that act like a congress). In these situations increasing the forceful presence of the budget directors (level one hormone amount) is required to subjugate the rebellious E-mails sent by the various soldiers. When different soldier types send out rebellious message content disease can eventually result such as allergies, autoimmune disease, asthma, and various skin afflictions. Adding to some of these disease processes concerns an additional type of soldier message system.

Each immune cell 'soldier type' comes equipped with another communication system. This standard equipment is most analogous to each soldier having voice of its own. This type of message content can communicate with other soldiers in the vicinity of the cell that sends the message. The length of time that the message lasts is only one to two seconds. This is similar to the voice being only heard as it is articulated and only as far as the voice will carry. This 'voice' equipment feature of the standard immune system is called the ecosanoids.

Molecular reality of this concept is more complicated: This 'voice' feature is really yet another hormone class known as the ecosanoids. Recall, all the different hormone classes (levels 1-4) all contain message content that delivers via the blood stream. Realize, all hormones deliver their message content in the blood stream initially. However, the ecosanoids are unique because they are only locally heard and short lived messages that are analogous to the voice message in many ways.

The ecosanoid class of substances contains the prostaglandins, leukotrienes, and lipoxin and these are all made from essential fatty acids. The final amounts among the three choices above largely depend on the types of ecosanoid precursors produced and are also determined by diet. In turn, this quality determines the adequacy of the various voice communication possibilities in an owner.

For example, if an owner indulges in processed food consistently for their essential fatty acids source, he/she will be more inclined to make the pro-inflammatory types of voice messages. The problem with loading the immune system cells with the pro-inflammatory essential fatty acids involves the fact that certain diseases arise when these messages predominate. A few examples are certain types of asthma, some allergies, some autoimmune disease, and some skin problems.

In contrast, owners who obtain regular high quality essential fatty acids from cold-water fish, fresh vegetables, borage oil, evening primrose oil, and olive oil make more anti-inflammatory hormonal fat precursors. These foods supply the non-inflammatory essential fatty acids to the immune system cells. For this simple reason, many inflammatory aches and pains that begin in middle age can be resolved by a simple change in these 'voice messages' that are communicated by the different soldiers.

Choosing real foods in place of the processed foods will increase these hormone precursors on the wiser owners' immune cells. When the hormone precursors contained on immune system cells are of the non-inflammatory variety, a diminished ability to propagate diseases exists. Notice, taking this step before committing to a symptom control approach, with its attendant side effects, improves the immune system naturally.

Healing doesn't require controlled double blind studies although it would be a nice validation. These studies are rare when profit is at stake. Healing has no side effects and some argue this should always be tried first.

The 'voice' system that delivers inflammatory message content describes a cause for owner suffering. The complex largely ignores this fact. A bigger mental picture develops the ways to heal. Healing from the inflammatory diseases that result from poor message content in the immune system is possible. For these reasons, understanding the interplay between the different message systems within the immune system plays a significant roll.

In the world of humans, the lifespan of spoken language occurs only during the moment of articulation. It also only operates over the distance that it can be heard. In addition, the louder the voice the farther it will carry. Contrast the 'voice' system (ecosanoids) of communication with the more powerful and far reaching E-mail system (cytokines). E-mail communiqués capably travel throughout the homeland via the blood stream whereas vocal (ecosanoids) communicate locally (brief existence of 1-2 seconds). The short lifetime of these 'vocal' messages necessitates adequate nutritional supplies and appropriate dietary choices.

Consequently, nutritional fat choices determine the type of 'speaking manners' that these local vocal messages communicate. They also depend on other factors: Some of these general factors are whether a soldier is properly equipped, properly fed with quality rations, and the quality of the energy in the soldier's environment. Unfortunately again, traditional medicine fails to place appropriate attention on the environment in which these 'soldiers' operate.

One aspect of the environment involves the emotional state of the owner. Environmental energies are in part determined by the qualities of the emotions that an owner experiences. These energies range from those that heal to those that maim cells (section six). The quality of emotional energy circulating denotes a concept quite foreign to many western owners.

Opening to the possibility that the Western view of the universe contains inconsistencies allows one to access even more possibilities for healing. Science has revealed the importance of the emotional environment and the energy it contains. For this reason, emotions are another determinant of how well the immune cells function (section six).

Immune Performance and Longevity

The different performance parameters of the immune system depend on certain nutritional building blocks. Nutritional imbalances lead immune cells towards disease risk possibilities. The quality of the essential fatty acids in the diet is only one determinant of maximizing immune cell performance. For example, the immune cell power plants also require specific vitamins to generate maximal energy to power its weapons of destruction. Weapon performance ties directly into the energy that powers them.

The ability to deliver oxygen and fuel to the immune cell furnaces forms two determinants of the energy available for living. The trapping of energy from this combustion process, which occurs in the cellular mitochondria, fills part of a cell's energy requirement. When immune cells cannot sufficiently power up their force fields they lack energy to defend their homeland. Requirements exist beyond fuel and oxygen that crucially impact power plant performance.

For example, immune cells succeed at trapping the energy created only if sufficient molecular building blocks remain available. Only when the heat energy of combustion is trapped can it be converted to useable energy packets. However, the trapping of the heat energy of combustion requires numerous vitamins and cofactors. The energy packets are required for cellular work and in the case of immune system cells for the work of defending the homeland.

Think of the ability of the cell to perform its specific function as being analogous to the ability of a car engine to move the vehicle down the highway. Superior automobile engines deliver more energy (gas combustion) transfer to the drive train. In other words, less gas wasted translates into more (efficient combustion of energy) efficient movement in the vehicle. In contrast, inferior automobiles waste energy (gas) and this causes less efficient combustion that equals fewer miles per gallon.

This situation can exist in body cells. These cells lack one or more of the nutritionally derived molecular parts that prove necessary to trap cell furnace heat energy to power cellular electronics (force fields). Immune system cells functional prowess critically depends on the ability to generate a large voltage that can fire upon the enemy (respiratory burst).

For this reason, immune system cell performance depends on the general process of electronic charge that the cell membrane contains. Recall, the membranes' charge directly affects the energy available for work in a cell. The immune system cells need more energy because they activate the weapons that defend the body. It takes adequate membrane energy for these weapon systems to function properly.

The immune system cells need adequate supply lines of certain key molecular parts or immune cell energy becomes compromised. As a consequence, the deficiency of critically needed molecular components (vitamins and cofactors) causes the power plant to generate heat instead of supplying defensive energy. This means that over time the furnace flame diminishes despite the presence of adequate hormone direction. Recall these appropriate molecular parts are required to process fuel (sugar, protein, fats) into acceptable shapes before they can combust inside the furnace flame (mitochondrial respiratory transport chain) in the presence of oxygen.

Think of a gasoline engine that requires gas instead of unrefined oil. Similarly, cell furnaces are 'engines' that require a precise fuel, acetate, that they can combust. Like oil that must be refined into gasoline before a car engine can utilize it, the cells need to refine raw fuels (protein, carbohydrate, and fat) into refined fuel, acetate. Many owners suffer from infections, feel overwhelming fatigue, or even succumb to cancer because certain types of their cells are nutritionally deficient. Here, their immune cells cannot protect them.

> (side bar) The science that discusses these basic principles has existed for years. It often lies buried in confusing descriptors. Owner empowerment is bolstered when some of these basic (but less profitable) understandings are brought back into the discussion that concerns this complex subject.

For these reasons, the immune system exists with a ravenous need for specific nutritional components. Immune system defects can be one of the first places that malfunction when vitamin supply lines become compromised. Deficient molecular replacement parts often leads to diminished cellular force fields (*low cell voltage syndrome*). In the immune system this can manifest as frequent infections, chronic fatigue, and eventually as cancer.

For these reasons, the ways the cells charge themselves becomes relevant to longevity. Immune dysfunction often has at its roots the deficiency of overlooked nutritional molecular components that prove necessary to power its weapons of destruction. Vitamins and proportioned minerals allow for superior cell performance (adequate cell voltage). They often accomplish this feat by virtue of the cellular charge that becomes possible when the right supply of these ions (minerals) and building blocks occurs.

Overseeing all this activity are specific hormones that direct the use of energy in the immune system. For this reason, the relationship between hormone tone and the nutritional adequacy available to power cellular charge is critical. Vitamins and other nutrients allow the hormonal directions to be followed. Outstanding hormones provide very little if the owner is deficient in certain vitamin-like substances. An owner with a vitamin deficiency, in a setting of high hormone tone, is analogous to a fine tuned engine that has had its transmission and drive train progressively degraded by improper lubrication.

For this reason, appropriate nutritional components must occur in the presence of effective hormonal direction. When the body contains nutritional components, but doesn't have good hormone tone, use of available energy flows in improper directions (section two). It is important to emphasize that the relationship between the directors (the hormones) and the adequacy of available molecular building parts and minerals proves critical to avoiding *low cell voltage syndrome*. It makes possible the sixth principle of optimal cellular charge. Realize the quality of the hormones within forms a determinant of the sixth principle. Only when the immune cells have both of these determinants in operation can the owner defend himself with optimal cellular charge.

The Immune System and the Hierarchy of Hormones

Level 1 - Hormones

The powerful Level 1 hormones are the generals and the only hormones that directly instruct the immune cell DNA programs (genes) to turn off and on. This group of hormones contains the steroids, thyroid hormones, and vitamin A. The quality of this mixture forms a central determinant of the competency of an immune cell. This group of hormones can access almost all tissues and move freely into the nucleus of the cell to instruct the DNA. The consequence being, which hormones arrive here, determines what genes become active or silenced. Remember the genes provide nothing until the right hormone arrives.

For example, the cortisol message content directs the white blood cells known as lymphocytes into cellular rest and decreased new cell production. Consequently, with insufficient cortisol message content inappropriate activity of these types of immune system cells occurs. These are the immune cells that manufacture antibodies appropriately and inappropriately. For example, overstimulation and excessive cell numbers of these types of cells causes allergies, some asthma, some autoimmune disease and various other diseases. Also recall, when thyroid hormones directions diminish the immune cellular furnace (mitochondria) decreases in its burning capabilities (section 2). Finally, vitamin A deficiency leads to a lack of DNA direction for immune system cells to grow up (differentiate).

For these basic reasons, this class of hormones powerfully sets the stage for what the other 'lesser' hormones must confront before their influence can be felt within the different immune cell types population. Recall, all other hormones are limited by the body tissues they can penetrate and by not being allowed to directly influence DNA programs (genes).

Level 2 Hormones

In the hierarchy of hormones, level 2 includes insulin, glucagon, Growth Hormone, cytokines, and prolactin. These are made from various sequences of amino acids that confer precise messages to different and specific cell receptors throughout the body. The effectiveness of theses hormones depends on the presence of their unique cell receptors sufficient presence. Recall, the level 1 hormones need to 'set a stage' that directs the manufacture for the level 2 hormone receptor that fit on a specific immune cell. Only when this occurs can a level two hormone have an effect in directing how that cell spends its energy content (storing energy versus its combustion).

Once these amino acid chain type hormones (level 2 hormones) deliver their message, the cellular digestion machinery disassembles them. However, before disassembling, they leave a 'directive' that instructs the cell in its available energy options. These options are only available for few seconds once activated because they are precursors to the level 4 hormones. In the case of immune cells, this directive affects how reactive they become to immune stimulants (appropriate and inappropriate). This is accomplished by affecting which hormone fat precursors are allowed to form on the immune cell surface, which are precursors to the level 4 hormones (explained below).

This directive is accomplished through level 2 hormones providing an influence on which level 4 hormone precursors will be possible. By this mechanism, level 2 hormones play an extensive roll in the domination of level 4 hormones. For this reason, (recall from section two) the ratio of insulin versus glucagon levels will powerfully affect, which level four hormone precursors are possible.

In the case of immune cells this directive affects how reactive they become to immune stimulants (appropriate and inappropriate). The type of predominant level two hormones instructing the immune cell largely determines this reactivity. The level 2 hormones accomplish this by affecting which level four hormone precursors are allowed to form on the immune cell surface.

The level two hormones, glucagon and insulin, are largely determined by an owner's diet preferences. The relative levels between these opposing hormones determine what level four hormones are possible. For this reason, wise choices in food consumption allow advantageous level 4-hormone precursors to form. However, poor nutritional choices adversely affect the types of level 2 hormones released.

For example, too much insulin prevents the 'good' level four hormone precursors from forming. By this mechanism, dietary indiscretion produces immune dysfunction. The immune problems that occur from hormonal mismatch include allergies, painful joints, painful tissues, immune compromise, etc. Extreme cases can lead to the inability to destroy cancer cells that are made daily (Sears).

Level 3 Hormones

Level 3 hormones direct blood flow. The ability to perform this function is established by level 1 and 2 hormones. Level 3 hormones include epinephrine, serotonin, histamine, dopamine, nor-epinephrine, and acetylcholine. In addition, this level of hormones critically depends on adequate intake and absorption of amino acid precursors in the diet. For this reason, nutritional deficiencies lead to impaired blood flow in afflicted owners (because the manufacture of these types of hormones requires many different vitamins). In general, the manufacture of level 3 hormones requires some or all of the following nutritional cofactors and vitamins; B1, B2, B3, B5, B6, B12, SAMe, folate, magnesium, vitamin C, and tetrahydrobiopterin. Realize these have proven biochemical validity (expanded discussion in chapter three and section six).

(side bar – Hopefully by now the reader sees advantages in their physician inquiring into the nutritional status of patients that suffer from blood flow problems, like high blood pressure. Unfortunately, many physicians receive inappropriate education for how nutrition affects blood pressure and blood flow. The power of the pharmaceutically influenced education is truly amazing. This fact is not meant to criticize the many devoted but conventionally trained physicians. However, it is emphasized here rather to point out the missing educational guidance that their training involves. Matters are made worse by the ways text books are worded and organized that steers many curious physicians down erroneous thinking paths that perpetuate the complex's interest.)

By this mechanism, the immune system is often only as good as what absorbs nutritionally. Many owners suffer from disease processes caused by unrecognized mal-absorption of critical nutrients. This is particularly relevant within level 3 because these hormones need many nutritional factors that must be present before their manufacture occurs. For these reasons, immune system diseases worsen from deficiencies in level 3-hormone production. Failure to recognize this factor increases the need for the symptom control approaches.

Both nor-epinephrine and serotonin tend to raise blood pressure and histamine tends to lower it. Histamine also increases blood vessel wall permeability, which allows certain immune system cells to penetrate the tissues and reach their destination more quickly. In contrast, although epinephrine raises blood pressure slightly, it confers an immune advantage by keeping allergy and asthma tendencies inactive. For this reason appropriate attention to one's methyl donor system makes sense with these two diseases because epinephrine synthesis requires methyl. Recall,   under the best of circumstances, the body requires a methyl about one billion times a second! How many allergy and asthma problems arise simply because the physician fails to address a methyl donor deficiency (lung and blood pressure chapters)? In addition, epinephrine's presence avoids the leaky capillary side effect which histamine causes. Again, this detail sheds light on why epinephrine-like ephedra was most likely banned because it cost pennies a day and proves in many ways superior to the popular anti-histamines marketed by pharmaceutical companies (section six).

Level 4 Hormones

Level 4 hormones include the weapons of destruction employed by a functional immune system and the 'voice'system operated by excreting the hormonal fats. This level of hormones has only a local effect and last only for a few seconds. Similarly, in the world of humans, limitations of the voice exist because it can only be heard while speaking and only over the distance it can travel. Likewise, in the analogy of level 4 'voices', these are short-lived hormones that can only be heard by neighboring cells for an instant. Two examples of level four type hormones occur that pertain to the immune system.

First, the ecosanoids are made from the essential fatty acids and depend on absorption from the diet. As was mentioned above, the types of level 2 hormones, which predominate, determine the hormonal fat precursors formed from the essential fatty acids ingested. Recognize that though all hormones contain message content, the level 4 hormones existence time is extremely short-lived and as a consequence they cannot travel very far from their point of origin.

Recall, even if an owner manages to consume adequate essential fatty acids, they can still develop immune system diseases from the wrong level 2 hormones' domination. The main level 2-hormone opposition for the immune system occurs between insulin and glucagon.   Insulin promoting diets increase production of the wrong hormonal fat precursors on the cells and alter immune function with time. In contrast, diets that promote more glucagon promote the creation of desirable hormonal fat precursors that line immune type cells. Overall point: when the good hormonal fat precursors dominate, immune cell's can respond appropriately.

A Level 4 Hormone - An Immune Cell Weapon

The second type of level 4 hormones is made from oxidizing nitrogen to nitric oxide. The cells that line the arteries, the endothelium, manufacture the hormone nitric oxide that produces local vasodilatation. In these cells, nitric oxide is released in much lower concentrations and contains hormonal properties. Nitric oxide that occurs at low levels is one of the ways local blood vessels are directed to relax, a hormonal effect.

In contrast, within the immune system it is generated in concentrations many times greater than needed for hormonal effects and becomes a weapon of destruction when it releases. For example, high production levels occurring in the macrophage cells allow nitric oxide to exert toxic effects on targeted recipient cells. Macrophages roam the body in search of an enemy. However, these sufficient nitric oxide production capabilities depend on key nutritional components. These nutritional components are thiol, tetrahydrobiopterin, niacin, riboflavin, and adequate arginine.

Macrophages need sufficient amounts of these nutritional factors to generate sufficient 'killing gas' (nitric oxide). As mentioned above, these are adequate thiol (found in garlic and onions), tetrahydrobiopterin (made from folate), niacin (vitamin B3), and riboflavin (vitamin B2). In addition, arginine is required because it is needed to donate the nitrogen group that starts the conversion into nitric oxide. All of these nutrients must be present to produce nitric oxide. If any one of these becomes deficient, nitric oxide production becomes impossible. As a consequence, any deficiency among these cofactors tips the advantage to foreign bacteria, virus, yeast, and cancer cells. Making nutritional compromise worse concerns the fact that this gas lasts only a few seconds before it is deactivated.

Nitric oxide poisons foreign organisms and cancer cells only when high enough concentrations arise by a functional macrophage. This is analogous to automobile exhaust fumes (carbon monoxide gas) that only kill when a high concentration is generated. Similarly, when the immune system remains healthy, it can generate sufficient nitric oxide to become a toxic gas when released upon the enemy.

A methodical approach assesses where an owner is in the different levels of energy directors (hormones). Focus on the hormone 'generals'(level 1 type hormones). Then consider successive steps down through the level 4 type hormones. Concurrently, an assessment of the nutritional needs of the immune system should occur. These two insights lead to healing.

The Immune Cellular Charge Adequacy and Nutrition

The nutritional needs of the immune system are no different than that of other energized cells in the body. However, the magnitude of body dysfunction brought about by poorly nourished immune system cells makes their needs paramount. Nutritional deficiencies often show up in immune cell performance long before a serious disease manifests. To avoid symptom control paradigms, the owner needs to be empowered to 'think outside the official box' when thinking in terms of nutritional vitamin needs.

Sound science exists to expose the weakness and inconsistencies brought on by detrimental practices of the profit driven approaches pandered towards immune dysfunction. One of the most extreme and tragic outcomes of ignoring the central role of the immune system that regards health versus disease is found in the way main stream medicine treats cancer. Despite this avoidance dogma, the role that specific vitamin-like nutrients play in the immune cell ability to power weapons and their cellular force fields is still critical to a healing response.

For example, the different immune cell types need to have adequate supplies of 'energy packets' in order to power these systems. All the proper hormones instructing the immune cells to defend does little good if the energy force to power the weapon system is missing molecular components. The opposite is also true. Poor hormone instruction can be equally destructive to defense systems directed against disease. It usually is a mixture of these two interrelated processes that leads to disease. Healing involves a cognizance of interrelating health principles.

Specific nutrients are needed to burn fat and carbohydrate in the immune cell furnaces. The ability of an immune cell type to destroy unwanted cells is directly proportional to the amount of energy contained in the cell membrane force field (cellular charge used in the respiratory burst). The ability of the cell to function directly relates to the amount of cellular energy available. Fully charged immune cellular batteries capably power their weapons of destruction.

(side bar - A startling reality arises out of Americans' preference for dead food (processed food) in place of live food (nutrients are intact). There is healing power contained in live foods and because of this changing the diet can change the owner's health for the better. Unfortunately, the downplayed role that optimal nutrients play in healing from diseases like cancer arises from the way the complex grooms (neuro-linguistic programming) the thinking patterns of doctors and patients.

However, adding back the holism of what nutritional science has revealed, includes the nutritional needs of the immune system that powerfully affect its performance capabilities. This approach allows an underutilized way to heal to surface. This can be accomplished in some instances without the cut, burn, and poison approaches pandered by the complex. At the very least, even if cut, burn and poison approaches were utilized, it makes good scientific sense to inform owners about maximizing their immune system performance. Realize, the more holistic approach is routinely done in countries like Germany that do not operate within a profit driven health care system.)

A major impairment operates in the immune system of many owners because of their chronic decision to eat dead foods in place of live food. This fact is further effectively down played by arbitrarily low official daily values of key vitamins. Exacerbating even this ignorance, involves the practice of minimizing the importance of certain nutrients chemical instability.

Nutrient instability secrets are the result of not educating the public. The public is not educated about the loss of vitamin content once food has been processed, fortified, or cooked. Even official publications that the public rarely reads (USDA 1996) acknowledge that most Americans are deficient in multiple vitamins and minerals. Many of these deficiencies are caused by processed foods that contain little nutritional value. Realize this fact receives little press coverage.

A properly functioning immune system powered to its full potential contains great protective strength. Cancer cells form every day within the body. However, initially new cancer cells are not the determining event, but rather it is the deficiencies and accumulated toxicities that impair one's ability to address the routine daily event of cancer cell destruction.

Early on, cancer cells are feeble in their ability to create energy. Initially they can only use sugar for a fuel source. Cancer metastasis cells usually burn this fuel anaerobically, which further limits their energy attainment. It is the energetic discrepancy between normal immune system cells and cancer cells, which gives the body a major advantage. Nutritional deficiencies decrease this advantage.

The importance of increasing the energetic advantage in the immune system cells is critical to realize. Enemies want to harm the body. Countering this ongoing process are the immune cell weapons that need ample energy to power them with. Nutritional deficiencies lower the amount of energy packets created in an immune cell. Ample energy packet formation is necessary to allow body defenses to function properly.

Critical nutrients prove necessary for trapping energy from fat combustion. Similarly, specific things are necessary before carbohydrates can be maximally utilized in the formation of these energy packets. Most of these nutrients allow the immune system cells to trap fat and carbohydrate combustion energy after processing them into acetate. In turn, the usable packets created can be used to power the defensive weapons. However, when any of these critical nutrients become deficient, the immune cellular power plants (mitochondria) lose more energy to heat. More heat equals less ability to trap energy for cellular function.

Carnitine, pantothenic acid, vitamins B1, B2, B3, B6, and coenzyme Q10 are the molecular components needed to trap energy packets before fat derived acetate combustion occurs. If a deficiency exists in any of these nutrients the immune cell finds itself compromised in its ability to create energy packets (ATP) from fat. Insufficient ATP causes the dependent cellular power systems to diminish.

When this happens two different detrimental processes occur that depend on which nutrient becomes deficient. First, the severity of certain deficiencies directly limits how much of the fat converts into acetate. Without acetate formation, combustion cannot occur within the immune cell power plant. The second detriment concerns the fact that some of these deficiencies make the combustion process more wasteful. When this happens less energy packets form, but an increase in heat (waste energy) production occurs.

Several factors influence why Americans today are deficient in one or more nutrients. First, most of these vital nutrients are extremely heat and light sensitive. Consequently, owners who subsist on processed foods are likely to become deficient. Second, a highly functional digestive tract is critical to proper nutrient absorption. For example, around middle age owners develop mineral imbalances because of poor absorption capacity arising in their digestive tract cells. In many ways, owners are only as good as what they absorb.

It is important to emphasize that specific nutrients prove crucial for immune cells to form energy packets (ATP) from fat. For example, carnitine moves fatty acids into the outer furnace compartment. This is the first layer of 'armor' in the mitochondria. Carnitine is the shuttle carrier of the body for common sized fatty acids destined for combustion. Unfortunately, it is not often realized that deficiencies in carnitine manifest clinically as rising blood fat and as one type of heart failure.

SAMe, vitamin B6, vitamin B12, lysine, and vitamin C are required in tremendous amounts for the manufacture of carnitine. Recall, the SAMe dependency connection to a highly functioning methyl donor system that under the best of circumstances requires a methyl at the rate of one billion times a second! The carnitine nutrient is also available by consuming meat that has not been over cooked. Realize though that some people fail to absorb it properly even with a normal ingestion rate. Interestingly, professional athletes consume carnitine because they have know that its cellular levels form a determinant of how fast the cell can suck fat into their cellular power plants.

In addition, immune cells need ample pantothenic acid in order to manufacture coenzyme A. Co Enzyme A is the carrier of acetate into the ignition chamber (the electron transport chain in the mitochondrial cristae). Realize the role of Pantothenic acid concerns the strict fuel requirements of the cell power plant in that it can only combust one size of 'briquet' (acetate). This requirement is similar to power plants in the physical world that can only burn a specific fuel. Remember, the raw materials of fats, proteins, and carbohydrate must first be processed into acetate 'briquettes' before they can be combusted in the cellular power plant.

Fatty acids always contain even numbers of carbon in their chains. Coenzyme A is necessary to accept the two carbon fragments (acetate) that are broken off of fatty acids sequentially in the mitochondria. Once acceptance occurs, Coenzyme A derived from pantothenic acid, acts as a carrier of these 'briquettes'. For this reason, a deficiency of pantothenic acid reduces the amount of Coenzyme A. Less Coenzyme A means less available briquettes to stoke the cellular power plant flame. Pantothenic acid is contained in diminished amounts within most B complex vitamin formulations. Consequently, owners are advised that this could be a weak link in their nutrient supplementation strategies.

In addition to carnitine and pantothenic acid sufficiency, the availability of vitamins B1, B2, B3, B6, and coenzyme Q10 in the immune cell determines how much of the power plant flame energy can be trapped into energy packets. Without these, cellular function becomes progressively impossible. A failure to trap the power plant flame energy creates only heat.

This situation is analogous to power plants in the physical world. They only create heat if they cannot trap some of the combustion energy and convert into to the energy packets of electricity. Power plants in the physical world require specific functional components that facilitate the conversion of raw energy into electricity. Likewise, in the cell power plants, a deficiency of any nutrient diminishes the ability of the mitochondria machinery to trap combustion energy packets (ATP). In deficiency situations, the more heat energy formed the less energy packet formation possible. Now realize, each of these additional vitamins listed above becomes a facilitator for trapping some of the combustion energy in the cell power plant.

Unfortunately, a coenzyme Q10 deficiency is likely in owners who consume the class of cholesterol lowering drugs known as the statins because the same enzyme, HMG Co A reductase, that begins the manufacture of cholesterol also begins the manufacture of coenzyme Q10. The statin drugs lower cholesterol by poisoning this common enzyme in the liver. Heart cells and immune system cells require tremendous amounts of Co enzyme Q10 to power their functional components. For this simple reason, body health depends on the liver manufacturing adequate amounts of Co enzyme Q10.

This fact will probably eventually explain both the suspected increased cancer rate and increased incidence of heart failure in some of those owners who chronically consume these types of medication. In the case of cancer, it probably has to do with the decreased energy that the immune cell has available to power the weapons of destruction against the daily occurrence of cancer within the body. Fortunately, most owners on these prescriptions could avoid them entirely if they became committed to a low carbohydrate diet, optimized their hormones (section 2), ate mineral balanced foods, and absorbed sufficient nutrients (section 3). Even for those that have a rare form of dyslipidemia or lack motivation to change, they could at the very least ingest high quality coenzyme Q10 supplements.

One other major side effect comes from inhibiting HMG Co A reductase activity. The drug companies currently twist around this side effect in a clever promotional way (inflammation and heart disease in the heart chapter). For now, anticipate more insights on the statin drugs revealed in section six.

Carbohydrate as a raw fuel source in the immune system cell requires additional vitamins before it converts into acetate. Remember, only acetate burns in the immune cell power plants (like all other body cells). So the immune cell confronts a similar dilemma, as it does with the other raw fuels when it suffers from specific nutrient deficiencies (processing fat and amino acids into acetate). It is important to realize that specific nutrients need to be present before manufacturing carbohydrate-derived acetate occurs.

Be aware that a deficiency in any one of these cofactors forces the immune cell to burn sugar anaerobically (like cancer cells). Without sufficient amounts of any one of these five nutritional cofactors sugar cannot be processed inside the mitochondria and the anaerobic metabolism limitation occurs. Bottom line: Without all of these five factors, no way exists, to cut the head off of the three-carbon intermediate (pyruvate) of sugar breakdown into two-carbon (acetate). Consequently, deficiencies here, force the immune cell into anaerobic metabolism.

Recall, metastatic cancer cells initially lack the ability to burn fuel aerobically. This occurs even with all the nutritional factors because they usually possess deficient cellular machinery and initially suffer from a poor blood supply. For this reason, an owner who wants to survive cancer would insure the availability of these nutrients within their body.

Burning sugar is inefficient and wasteful when anaerobic metabolism is involved due to the obligatory creation of lactic acid. Lactic acid builds up and manifest clinically as sore and painful tissues. It is the liver's job to slowly accept the lactic acid, generated within cells and released into the blood stream, for converting it into pyruvate (a three carbon sugar intermediary).

There are many sufferers of fibromyalgia whose main problem arises from their decreased ability to handle sugar (high carbohydrate intake is bad). Their condition magnifies by the below listed nutritional deficiencies. Remember, suboptimal thyroid and adrenal gland deficiency also operates in fibromyalgia syndrome. For these reasons, if these suffering owners receive appropriate treatment for improving their thyroid hormone levels and adrenal function, they improve (adrenal and thyroid chapters). In addition, many of these patients also have stiff red blood cells that need to be addressed (chapter two).

Diseases like chronic fatigue, a cousin of fibromyalgia, often has an immune dysfunction component. Part of this dysfunction results from nutritional deficiencies regarding the combustion of carbohydrate. Recall that in order to convert the three-carbon intermediate of sugar breakdown to a two-carbon briquet (acetate) adequate amounts of **all** five nutritional molecules need to be present: Lipoic acid, vitamin B1, pantothenic acid, vitamin B2, and B3 all must be available or this important process will not occur.

In contrast, fat combustion deficiencies tend to decrease cell energy as the severity of the deficiency intensifies. Realize fat only burns up aerobically. In other words there is no such thing as anaerobic metabolism for fat.

However, sugar burns aerobically or anaerobically. Which process occurs depends on the adequacy of certain cellular reaction facilitators derived from the diet. In the case of sugar combustion preparation, all five of these factors need to be present in the cellular machine complex called pyruvate dehydrogenase complex. This complex enzyme machine cleaves the three-carbon fragment, pyruvate, to form the two-carbon molecule, acetate. Remember, only acetate forms the perfect briquet for the cellular power plant.

When any of these five vitamins becomes deficient, the breakdown of carbohydrate leads to lactic acid formation. Clinically this buildup evidences itself as sore muscles. Remember, this enzyme, pyruvate dehydrogenase, needs all five vitamins or it will not function. Think of this enzyme's nutritional needs as an all or none requirement.

Owners that have this type of deficiency when carbohydrate, excess becomes their fuel source, contain diminished energy in their afflicted immune cells. Recall, lower energy occurs in cancer cells early on, because anaerobic combustion of carbohydrate provides their only fuel source. Here, the immune cell and cancer cells are forced into a feeble low energy state (*low cell voltage syndrome* surfaces again but from a different reason).

The immune system advantage over cancer cells concerns the increased energy contained within the immune cell when all nutritional factors remain present. Unfortunately, this advantage disappears when deficiencies occur. Recall that the liver provides the only route for lactic acid processing. For this reason, high levels of lactic acid that form daily hurt the ability of the liver to detoxify other problem molecules (prescription drug metabolites) and this in turn causes additional injury and inflammation in the body.

For these reasons, owners who are ill can consider intra-muscular or intra-venous vitamin replacement therapy to revitalize their cellular situation. However, thiamine injections need to be done cautiously because of the risk for occasional anaphylactic reactions. Here, intra-muscular reactions tend to be less severe.

An important additional consideration involves the fact that lipoic acid is a common vitamin missing from most multivitamins. This fact describes another mechanism for disease development. Taking supplements doesn't necessarily prevent nutritional deficiencies. Only sufficient lipoic acid along with the other B vitamins prevents this above mechanism from manifesting as lactic acid excess.

Realize lipoic acid is not commonly present in multivitamins. Consequently, B complex vitamins do little good for preventing this process until it becomes available. Summary point: Cells need sufficient amounts of all of the above five nutritional molecules or lactic acid builds up. Excessive reliance on the anaerobic pathway weakens the immune system by the above-mentioned mechanism.

Oral therapy with a combined effort of both more live foods in one's diet and high quality supplements makes sense in the absence of overt disease. The owner needs to be cautioned to remain mindful of the fact that he/she will only derive benefit from that which he/she absorbs.

The above nutritional discussion has proven biochemical validity within the mainstream biochemistry and medical physiology textbooks.

When the above nutritionally dependent processes occur smoothly an owner's immune system cells can charge themselves up fully. Conversely, when the above nutritionally dependent processes become enfeebled the immune cell charge weakens (*low cell voltage syndrome*). Paradoxically these biochemical requirements of cellular charge have yet to become incorporated within most clinical settings. When owners fight for their lives it seems rather cruel to withhold this knowledge in favor of more lucrative ways of treating these common illnesses.

Nutrients that DNA Needs to Behave Itself

The methyl donor system denotes a process in the context of the immune system that gains particular importance when trying to understand another way to lower the risk of cancer. Removal of the abstractions contained in scientific literature becomes the challenge. Often the ill owner fails to identify the power of the methyl donor system to heal their physical form because of the abstract way this information conveys.

A central problem for cells arises when the methyl donor system depletes: A depleted methyl donor system allows an increase in the number of cells that want to misbehave. Some of these cells become cancer cells. Cancer cells display properties that disregard total body protocol. One way the body stabilizes cellular DNA programs (genes) involves the methyl donor system. Cancer cells uniformly contain inappropriately activated DNA programs (genes).

The methyl donor system serves many functions such as epinephrine biosynthesis, estrogen metabolism, hormone deactivation, and specialized brain fats manufacture. Pertinent here, regards its additional role for stabilizing the DNA in the 70 trillion or so body cells by the addition of methyl groups.

The addition of a methyl group to many biologically active molecules confers either activity or silence depending on which biological molecule receives this molecular addition. In regards to the immune system, adequate methylation rates on the DNA do much to stabilize cellular rebellion. In other words, effective methylation rates occurring on the DNA lower the police force needs of the immune system.

Think of it as a reduction in anarchy among the cells. The cells behave when they contain adequate methyl groups on specific DNA programs. This allows the job of the immune to become easier in regards to its surveillance of rogue cells.

Methyl is a very simple, small molecule in comparison to most biologically active molecular components in the body. It contains one carbon and three hydrogen atoms. Often times it becomes proportional to a biological molecule wearing a 'crown'.

The crown analogy proportions the methyl group for how it changes the size and shape of an average body molecule. Despite its simplicity, it confers powerful abilities to activate and silence some of the most important molecular players such as DNA programs (genes), steroid hormone types, level three hormone types, quality of brain fats, and blood vessel health.

The quality of the cellular DNA methylation rate is determined by which and how much steroids, thyroid hormone and vitamin A reach the DNA program of the cell. Recall, interdependency exists in the relationship between hormone tone and nutritional adequacy. Cellular activation or deactivation of DNA programs (genes) conveys directly by the amount and type of level one-type hormones present. Only level one-type hormones instruct the DNA directly (section two).

Recognize that some of the above mentioned steroid-like hormones accomplish silencing of the DNA programs (genes) by methylation. Still other level one-type hormones can activate these same programs by the process of de-methylation of a cellular DNA segment. Recall, each level one-type hormone contains message content inherent in its precise shape and this determines the message delivered to the DNA. By this beautiful design feature, different level one type messages (hormones) effects the DNA program in opposing ways. Consequently, one of the main on and off switches involves whether DNA programs are methylated or un-methylated

In order to minimize the risk of cancer both optimal amounts of level one type hormone instruction and a nutritionally supplied methyl donor system must be available. These interdependent facts provide powerful measures that can be acted upon toward controlling rebellious DNA total body load.

Craig Cooney PhD in Biochemistry wrote an insightful book *Methyl Magic*, 1999. His career long research into many body processes that rely on an operational methyl donor system has lead him to estimate that methyl groups are changing places at one billion times per second. This estimate describes the rate at which an owner runs the risk of their genetic program rebelling. Genetic program rebellion is a centrally observed feature of cancer cells' behavior.

One billion times a second the body needs to supply methyl groups somewhere in the body. Dr. Cooney and other medical texts provide a short list of documented roles for methylation; synthesis of melatonin, epinephrine, acetylcholine, carnitine, creatine, and lecithin; deactivates histamine and dopamine; estrogen metabolism; DNA methylation; myelin sheath integrity; in repair of damaged proteins; and homocysteine conversion back into methionine.

All of the above processes are central to lasting or regaining health. The methyl donor system critically needs to be nutritionally supplemented. A healthy methyl donor system occurs when SAMe (S-Adenosyl methionine) levels stay high and homocysteine levels remain low. However, the cell must possess the nutritional components to continuously recharge SAMe.

Simplistically, one billion times a second the body uses SAMe when it donates a methyl group and becomes homocysteine. The ability to recharge SAMe determines the yardstick for how well the methyl donor system performs. For this reason, owners who are methyl donor deficient tend to have elevated blood homocysteine levels.

One billion times a second the body needs to have adequate supplies of SAMe. Deficient ability to recharge to SAMe leads to rationing among methyl donor related vital processes. In some owners the DNA begins to become unstable causing rebellious cells. In others the adrenals supply of methyl becomes deficient causing epinephrine synthesis to suffer. This leads to elevated blood pressure (heart chapter) and/or asthma (lung chapter).

In still others the methyl donor deficiency manifests as a delay in the elimination of histamine. This decreased ability to eliminate histamine leads to a worsening of allergy symptoms. Unfortunately, conventionally trained physicians usually prescribe symptom control methods (antihistamines) before suggesting correction of underlying nutritional deficiency possibilities, if ever. This is not meant as a criticism, but as a red flag that something is missing from the educational emphasis of conventionally trained physicians.

Basic medical biochemistry textbooks contain methyl donor reactions. However, these facts are rarely applied in the clinical setting. All the molecules in the methyl donor system are concerned with keeping SAMe levels sufficient. In order for SAMe to recharge, there has to be adequate serine, vitamin B6, Vitamin B12, and folate in the tissues. Some authorities feel that the official government recognized minimum daily requirements for these nutrients are too low. These nutrients are necessary for the prevention of methyl donor deficiency.

Concern exists within the mainstream regarding the addition of methionine in the methyl donor supplementation programs. Methionine is an essential amino acid (the body cannot manufacture it). SAMe contains methionine that degrades to homocysteine each time it donates a methyl group to another biological molecule. Understand, the absence of a completely functioning methyl donor system causes blood levels of homocysteine to raise as available SAMe is consumed.

Elevated homocysteine levels are a well-recognized risk factor for blood vessel disease. In most owners, the homocysteine level will only rise when one or more of the other members of the methyl donor system become deficient. In this light, all the hype about limiting the intake of methionine in the diet seems ludicrous because the real problem results from some other component of the methyl donor system being deficient. For this reason, the curtailment of the essential amino acid methionine proves unwise in most cases. Instead,, correction of the methyl donor supply team deficiency remains the recommended course of action.

Some clinicians endorse the consumption of SAMe. This has been shown to be of great benefit in treating some forms of depression and insomnia. This results because it is used to manufacture epinephrine (a mood elevator in the central nervous system) and for melatonin (necessary for a good nights sleep) both of which require SAMe.

SAMe contains methionine meaning without an adequately recharging methyl donor system, the supplementation of either one of these will lead to a rise in the blood homocysteine levels. In extremely deficient cases this will occur at the rate of one billion new homocysteine molecules a second. Without attending to maximizing the methyl donor system nutrients, the supplementation with either one of these will lead to elevated blood homocysteine levels.

This causes many owners to suffer the consequences of elevated blood homocysteine levels, such as heart disease. In most cases elevated homocysteine result solely from inattention to vitamin status. Recall, increased homocysteine levels serve as an indicator that one or more vitamins within the methyl donor system has depleted.

Rarely, genetic defects occur in one or more enzyme machines that facilitate the transfer of methyl groups in the methyl system. The most famous of these genetic diseases is known as homocystinuria that results from the enzymatic absence of cystathionine synthase. Normal owners use this enzyme to transfer the methyl group from serine to reform methionine from homocysteine.   Folate, vitamins B6, and B12 are also required to complete this series of reactions.   Even in cases of this rare genetic condition, the consumption of methyl donor nutrients proves beneficial.

In addition, some researchers like Cooney, Bolan and Sears feel that DNA gone awry leads to some of the autoimmune diseases including systemic lupus, multiple sclerosis, and fibromyalgia. Other research would emphasize placing equal attention to restoring adrenal health in these autoimmune diseases (section two). Still other research clearly shows the additional role that undiagnosed food allergy plays in these disease processes (section three).

The importance of methylation in the prevention of autoimmune diseases is underscored by the fact that drugs that tend to cause lupus (hydralazine, quinidine, and procainamide) all have the ability to decrease certain immune cells' DNA methylation rates. Methylation is important in the prevention of diseases concerning the central nervous system. For example, the cerebral spinal fluid of multiple sclerosis and fibromyalgia patients contain elevated homocysteine levels. Both of these diseases seem to have an immune system malfunction component. Recall, deficient adrenal steroids occurring in some of these patients could also explain their methylation problem.

(side bar - Sufferers of these diseases should be advised in healing their methyl donor system and inquiring into both their adrenal and thyroid gland derived steroid tone (section two). Steroid-like content should involve adequate attention on evaluating the adrenal status of these owners. This inquiry becomes particularly important for multiple sclerosis sufferers because of the remission that occurs while these patients are pregnant. Pregnancy produces high progesterone and cortisol levels.

Multiple sclerosis patients have a disease process where progressive injury occurs to the nerve sheath (myelin sheath) surrounding the nerve. Most clinicians feel that this disease involves an autoimmune component. These facts argue that cortisol and possibly progesterone regulate the immune system in ways, as yet, that are not appreciated.

Less commonly known, however, concerns the fact that progesterone contributes significantly to the continued health of this nerve cell over layer, the Schwann cell. Unfortunately, most patients with multiple sclerosis, under the care of conventionally trained physicians, do not have their progesterone status evaluated. As a consequence they do not receive the benefit of a state of the art twenty-four hour urine test for analysis of their steroid metabolites.

In addition, many multiple sclerosis patients have toxic levels of heavy metals in their bodies. A hair screening analysis and heavy metal provocation test can evaluate the heavy metal factor.

Finally, multiple sclerosis sufferers often suffer from severe food allergies. Jonathan Wright, MD has led the way on developing the best screening tests for where these allergies come from. In addition, Catherine Willner, MD, who is a Mayo clinic-rained neurologists, understands quite clearly the association of MS and food allergy provocation.)

Additional ways to acquire a methyl donor for the recharging of SAMe occur within the body. When pressed, the body can rip methyl groups off of other molecules. Unfortunately, this desperate approach comes with the price of a deficiency in the type of molecule from which the methyl group was taken. For example, the conversion of testosterone into estrogen by the enzyme aromatase frees up one methyl with each occurance. When this occurs one methyl group frees up for use somewhere else in the body. This desperate method for obtaining methyl groups has the powerful side effect of decreasing testosterone and increasing the estrogen message content.

The body sacrifices many active biological molecules that contain methyl groups when the supply of methyl donors becomes deficient. This variability between how individual owners prioritize the rationing of methyl groups helps explain individual clinical variation. For example, individual variation occurs in the possible diseases that can result when abnormal adrenal steroids occur (adrenal chapter).

In still others, the DNA programs become unstable. These types are at increased risk for cancer. In others the DNA molecules that require methylation preferentially receive the little methyl that remains available. In others, hormone manufacture like epinephrine in the adrenals dramatically falls off and this leads to asthma and/or high blood pressure (lung, blood pressure and heart chapters). Recall, epinephrine biosynthesis requires methyl. In still others, the breakdown of allergy producing histamine is curtailed. Histamine deactivation requires methylation. How many allergies arise from a simple methyl donor deficiency?

Finally, in some, the protective specialized fat coating (the myelin sheath) around nerves can become deficient in its molecular supply. A major component of this coating comes from lecithin. When adequate lecithin fails to be obtained in the diet (low fat diets) it can only be made from an adequate functioning methyl donor system. Unfortunately, each molecule of lecithin requires three SAMe molecules to properly form. For this reason, owners that insist on low fat diets and become methyl donor deficient and increase their risk for brain fat deficiencies. Recall, the brain contains more fat weight than nerve weight.

This reveals an additional role that diets play in helping or exacerbating the methyl deficiency. Certain fats are needed in such large amounts in the nervous system that diets lacking these fats put a tremendous strain on the methyl donor system. This depleting process occurs in addition to having all the right vitamins because diets deficient in certain fats require that these be obtained from using up large amounts of methyl. For this simple reason, the need for methyl increases tremendously because some diets prove deficient in preformed nutrients like choline, lecithin, and carnitine. Conversely, owners who consume adequate amounts of these nutrients help their bodies because they save their methyl donors for the other reactions critical to life

One billion times a second a methyl group is needed. In some owners with deficient methyl donor states, it forces their immune system to police the increased numbers of rebellious cells. Methyl donor deficient owners have increased rebellious cell numbers because the DNA behaves inappropriately. Inappropriate DNA program activity creates extra strain on the need for policing cells. Cancer cells are the most extreme example of this process.

Also, it was mentioned earlier, the fact that inappropriate immune cell activation can also be secondary to other problems. The autoimmune problem can also occur when the level one-type hormones are of poor quality and amount. In addition, autoimmune problems can fester when the poor integrity of the digestive tract occurs and this allows foreign shaped molecules into the body. Foreign molecules activate the immune system. Trouble begins when body tissues cross react. For example, when joint tissue is mistaken for foreign material, the owner's immune system attacks inappropriately and injury occurs.

CHAPTER TWENTY-TWO

IMMUNE SYSTEM AND THE JOINTS

Sometimes the immune system and joint disease are inter-related. This relationship stems from the fact that bacteria, fungi, and virus' have a cell wall that is supposedly absent from human cells' outer coating. Actually, it is more accurate to say human cells have an under developed outer coating that is derived from various combinations of glucosamine and galactosamine. These same building blocks are used in the outer cell coating of these other organisms, as well. The difference lies in how much of this support framework surrounds a certain type of body cell. Cartilage cells have more of this molecular material around them than any body cell type.

This architectural framework lies outside the cartilage cells. Scientists long ago declared that by definition mammalian cells lack sufficient framework to call it a cell wall. This confuses and limits the way people think because there are structural similarities between human cells outer coating and those of the bacteria, virus, and fungi. For all practical purposes, the human cell wall is just under developed. Consequently, if the immune system fails to function within normal parameters, it can inappropriately cross react with joint tissue because it confuses it with a foreign invader (bacteria, fungus, or virus). This misguided activation is analogous to microscopic missiles launching into joint tissue.

There is some technical truth in the delineation between the difference in the cell wall material in bacteria, fungus and virus' versus the human cells outer coating. The difference centers on the ability of this framework to protect these single cell life forms from environmental extremes of temperature, humidity, and saline fluids. Human cells could never survive these environmental conditions.

However, similar molecular building materials surround both human cells and pathogens. In all cases these materials are organized into supportive architecture that keeps the outside of the cell from collapsing. Human cells differ in the tightness of the weave that results from their containing sparser interlocking chains of these molecules crisscrossed and woven together. The end result being that the human cell is unprotected from these environmental extremes because of its loose molecular weave.

These similarities explain how the immune artillery can make mistakes between human cells and pathogenic organisms. These mistakes become more likely under altered circumstances. Joint tissues are potentially one of the most vulnerable to these mistaken attacks by the immune system because they have the most abundant amount of these

501

substances surrounding each cell. These building blocks when altered and arranged in unique sequence under normal circumstances alert the immune system that an invader cell is present. Under normal conditions the immune system can tell the difference in the outside architecture of human cells by sequence and type of the building block components.

The immune system is poised to recognize the material making up the cell walls of invading organisms. The molecular material (glucosamine and galactosamine-like building blocks) is also found in surrounding body cells (but most prominently in cartilage cells). Remember; because of this similarity the potential always exist for an inappropriate immune system attack on the joint tissues.

Under normal circumstances the immune system cells capably differentiate the sequencing of the invading organism cell wall and human cell coatings. However, these sequence differences are so slight that cross reactivity occur against some owners own cartilage cells under certain conditions. This explains one of the causes of rheumatoid arthritis. Once the immune system has been activated against a specific sequence, massive joint destruction ensues.

More physicians have come to understand when the digestive tract leaks, dysfunction occurs in the immune system and sometimes affects the joints. Leakage, here, allows seepage of partially digested proteins to obtain access into the blood stream. Partially digested proteins are immunologically reactive. The immune system design causes it to activate against any sequence of amino acids longer than three. When this occurs the possibility arises that this sequence exists in the joint tissue.

A healthy digestive tract poses an impenetrable barrier to large molecules like specific protein sequences unique to each food. However, if the unique amino acid sequence of say, milk, were to slip inside the blood stream even partially intact, it would activate the immune system. When the immune system activates against foreign sequences, a chance arises that these same sequences exist in the joint tissue. This starts the process of joint destruction and explains one possible mechanism for rheumatoid arthritis.

The amino acid sequences that make up the protein componet of cartilage are unique in each owner. Joint cartilage is also made up of varying amounts of glucosamine, galactosamine, glucose, and galactose. Understand, these building blocks interlace with different types of protein, like collagen. The overall scheme is that building block molecules are arranged in chains of thousands, crisscrossed with other chains, and then wrapped together on a bed of the protein, collagen. These individual building blocks are further customized by the addition of varying amounts of sulfate, amide, and acetate groups.

When these molecular building blocks occur individually in the blood stream, they are too small to activate the immune system. Recall, this reoccurring body theme: The body places new molecular building parts inside the blood stream and transports them to their building sites. These individual molecules are too small to activate the immune system. A similar process occurs when the digestive track first breaks down a protein into its individual amino acids and these are assimilated and transported in the blood stream to building sites (digestion chapter). Like undigested protein containing invaders (bacteria, viruses and fungi), partially digested food proteins, acquired from the diet in those lacking sufficient stomach acid and suffering from leaky gut, allows these partially digested protein fragments to activate an immune response.

The danger of leaky gut syndrome stems from that it allows larger than normal (partially digested molecules) to absorb into the blood stream. In these situations, a grave danger of immune activation against these larger molecules arises. Some researchers feel this explains one of the reasons that infants fed solids too early in life develop food allergies. Other research suggests an association with leaky gut and other more harmful autoimmune system diseases such as; rheumatoid arthritis, systemic lupus, colitis, multiple sclerosis, Crohn's disease and scleroderma.

Furthermore, leaky gut situations are encouraged wherever the bacteria in the digestive tract are sub-optimal. This can occur with candida over growth, chronic chlorine poisoning, excessive iron intake, excessive fluoride intake, recurrent antibiotic usage, poor nutrition, and inflammatory bowel. For this reason, many holistic physicians take an active role in counseling their patients to prevent these situations.

Imbibing in clean water and taking steps to optimize the bacteria growing in the colon are good first steps in preventing a leaky gut situation. Immune cell function is sometimes tied to the health of the digestive tract. When leaky gut causes the immune destruction of the joints, improvement will not be possible until the leaky gut resolves (digestion chapter).

Still other forms of arthritis activate when certain bacteria or virus' penetrate inside a particular joint space. When pathogens begin to multiply in the joint space, the resulting attack from the immune system cells leads to joint damage. Streptococcus, staphylococcus, Lyme disease bacteria, and chlamydia are common microscopic organisms known to invade the joint spaces and activate joint destruction. Attack by these organisms is one of the times that early and aggressive antibiotic treatment is warranted over alternative treatment strategies.

A smaller group of owners suffer a seemingly unprovoked attack on their joint tissues. These owners defy explanation even after a diligent search. Research suggests that these patients suffer from damaged adrenal glands. These defects cause an inappropriate balance of message content directed at the immune system cells. The adrenals are a prime site of immune regulation by proportioning and timing cortisol and DHEA (counterweight) release. Others steroids like androstenedione and progesterone secrete from the adrenal glands as well.

The common approach to immune dysfunction involves routine prescriptions of synthetic versions of cortisol derivatives. However, the detrimental consequences can be understood by loading one side of an antique weight scale. Loading one side of the scale without considering the counter weight side causes health consequences. Understanding this fact allows one to comprehend why this approach always causes side effects. In other words, with cortisol-like prescriptions not only the inappropriate immune response subdues but the repair ability (anabolism) as well.

Commonly, cortisol-like derivatives are prescribed to suppress either inflammation or immune response in diseases like rheumatoid arthritis and systemic lupus. Recall, patented cortisol derivatives contain altered message content: The altered shape and amount deliver abnormal message content to the genes. However, the additional price from this approach involves its causing a substantial decrease in cellular rejuvenation.

Remember, cortisol like steroids (prednisone) are from the catabolic class. Excessive catabolism makes protein fair game for fuel generation. In contrast, healthy adrenal glands secrete optimal ratios of both anabolic and catabolic message content simultaneously. Mainstream medicine adherents ignore this simple fact and only treat one side of the deficiency, the catabolic side. This practice in turn exaggerates the anabolic deficiency.

Cellular rejuvenation diminishes by two mechanisms when an owner consumes cortisol substitutes (prednisone like prescriptions). First, cortisol substitutes do not contain real cortisol and therefore do not contain true message content (section two). Altered message content causes side effects.

However, additional damage occurs by increasing the cortisol substitute's blood levels because this inhibits the release of the counter weight hormones (normally adrenally released hormones, like DHEA). This second consequence occurs because the cortisol substitute's presence fools the recipient body's adrenals into to thinking that the other adrenal steroids are also available. Adding insult to this injurious practice concerns the fact that these types of afflicted owner's often suffer from diminished repair ability (DHEA) that in part caused their disease in the first place! Furthering their loss of anabolism by this mechanism accelerates the aging process by the above mechanism.

One promising new understanding in promoting a balanced approach in the treatment of systemic lupus comes out of Japanese research. Here they correctly posited that in some autoimmune diseases the problem arises from the counter hormone DHEA being too low. Dramatic improvement was noted when DHEA was given (Whitiker).

The effectiveness of DHEA makes sense in the holism of autoimmune diseases consideration, like lupus, because these types of diseases root cause often arise from adrenal glandular defects. Treating only one side of the weight scale (cortisol) exacerbates the deficiency in other adrenal counter regulatory hormones like DHEA (i.e. DHEA and sometimes cortisol are operationally deficient in this disease process). For this very important reason, cortisol needs to be counter balanced by DHEA or health consequences occur. Supplementing with only one side of the hormone balance equation leads to unnecessary complications that can be avoided if the holism of what science has revealed comes into practice.

Healing becomes possible when one realizes that healthy adrenal glands secrete DHEA and cortisol (also progesterone and androstenedione) at the same time. The optimally proportioned adrenal secretion (high *steroid tone*) consisting of these types of hormones occurs when the pituitary directs it by releasing ACTH. Unfortunately, medical textbooks fail to unite the simultaneous steroid hormone release that occurs in predetermined ratios whenever the adrenal gland activates. This relationship has been ignored for a long time. Fortunately, the re-inclusion of this scientific fact profoundly contributes to healing from diseases like systemic lupus, rheumatoid arthritis, asthma, allergies, fibromyalgia and chronic fatigue.

Take home point: Replacing only one component of a multi component system compromises the all important balance/counter balance relationship operating between different steroids. An example of this faulty practice occurs when diseases are treated with cortisol substitutes only. Making matters worse concerns the additional health consequences that occur because the pharmaceutical dosing (contrast this to physiological dosing) of cortisol-like patented drugs suppress the adrenals even further in their DHEA, and other adrenal steroid, production. Here lies a major cause of cortisol replacement associated toxicity. Here, the antique weight scale becomes totally out of balance. Knowledge of this process allows a better way to re-approximate the optimal adrenal glands secretions. This method includes both DHEA and cortisol replacement (possibly progesterone and androstenedione as well).

The final dose between these powerful hormones is individually determined. Unbalanced amounts of these hormones are usually the true culprits of these types of disease. The specific nature of the unbalanced ratio is uncovered by analyzing the results of a afflicted patient's twenty-four hour urine test. Sometimes an adrenal challenge test is required as well. Realize that the common practice of measuring steroids levels in the serum or saliva often fails to document the defect. Part of the explanation concerns that these methodologies fail to accurately assess the metabolites of steroid metabolism. Here exists the great deception occurring in imbalanced steroids caused diseases. Unfortunately, until physicians learn how to interpret 24-hour urine steroid tests accurately and replace accordingly their patients' health will suffer.

Failure to consider the status of other adrenal steroids causes many fears about cortisol. If mainstream physicians were trained in the need to assess adrenal status before they began symptom control medical treatments for disease, many owners would be saved from countless complications. The side effects from cortisone-like drugs are often traced back to a lack of this initial consideration. A twenty-four hour urine test, which evaluates for steroid output during this time period, facilitates assessment for what doses are needed for DHEA, cortisol and other adrenal steroids. Performing an adrenal challenge test provides added information in marginal cases. When these approaches are utilized there will be fewer side effects because much of the guesswork has been eliminated.

Autoimmune diseases like lupus are related to androgen deficiency (never forget to evaluate food allergies here as well). This is shown in the rate of occurrence of lupus based on gender differences.

Recall, DHEA is a precursor androgen steroid that stimulates investment in cellular rejuvenation once it converts into more powerful androgens within the recipient cell. Lupus occurs in females nine times more often than it does in males. Females depend on DHEA for 99% of their androgens. Also realize the advantage of acquiring the vast majority of androgen through a sex neutral route (DHEA) that does little to masculinize them (see intracrinology discussion in the next chapter). These facts alone warrant a detailed, and scientifically valid hormone assessment for any patient suffering from these diseases. Realize that the conversion of DHEA into powerful steroids and then into specific metabolites is beyond the darlings of the medical establishments steroid measurement protocols using saliva or serum.

Because accuracy matters in most cases, this will require a 24-hour urine sample to accurately measure a patient's steroid hormone profile. Again, blood and saliva analysis methodologies fail to measure the all-important metabolites and ignore the pulsatile release of glandular secretions. In addition, the technology (RIA) that they rely on is only a ballpark estimate at best. In fact, several scientific journals (see bibliography) have recently called these popular testing methods validity into question, especially in women, for even achieving the modest plus or minus 20% that the test touts!

All six links in the adrenal system need to be diligently investigated (adrenal glands chapter). Contrast the 24-hour glandular output to the instant of the blood draw where this value could be high or low depending on a multitude of variables. Realize that different life situations require that these most important level one-type hormones change accordingly. For example, romance, exercise, happiness, fatigue, hunger, postprandial states, and stress all profoundly influence these important glandular secretions.

When was the last time that anyone heard about a salivary or serum test aficionado pondering these variables while interpreting their patients' results? In contrast, over a typical 24-hour day, the patient usually experiences an average amount of stress, romance, nutrition, exercise and rest. In addition, the 24-hour urine test relies on superior technology called Gas chromatography mass spectometry (GC mass spec). GC mass spec allows for the accurate measurement for the 24-hour output of the all-important steroid metabolites. The types and amounts of these different metabolites guide the knowledgeable physician in recreating balance between anabolism and catabolism.

The other links in the adrenal health chain can fool the physician who only checks one link, the blood stream. For the above reasons, salivary samples and blood draws, although most doctors use these methods, sometimes do not make scientific sense. However, the truth is painful when it involves learning something new and this is what holds back the advance of this important testing method.

Another consideration occurs for why females are more susceptible to autoimmune disease: The association of estrogen usage and blood clot formation can cause an overlooked risk for adrenal injury occurring in females. The risks increase with higher dosages, prolonged sitting, cigarette smoking and obesity. The adrenal gland proves particularly vulnerable to clot formation because of its unique venous drainage anatomy. The adrenal gland has four arteries leading into it, but only one vein heading out making it susceptible to venous clot induced damage. Females who suffer clot formation here would notice a subtle decrease in their ability to participate in a quality life experience.

Unfortunately, these changes are often confused with other imbalances. Misdiagnosis causes needless suffering. Autoimmune disease, thyroid disease, hypoglycemia, depression, and, in some, hypochondria are sometimes attributable to diminished adrenal function. Again, these errors in primary diagnosis are best avoided by employing the best scientific methods available to assess the true hormone status. Steroid breakdown chemistry is complex and often confuses physicians who want to help.

Several laboratories now offer twenty-four hour urine assessment steroid profiles. Now that there are several good laboratories performing these steroid assessments, there needs to be an increase in the understanding among physicians regarding the interpretation of the results. The importance of patients' steroid status has been chronically ignored by all but the most superficial inquiries.

This fact is disturbing. The steroid class of hormones is the only hormones other than vitamin A and thyroid hormones that directly activate or suppress the DNA program (genes) in cells. Consequently, the quality of the types and amounts of steroids circulating determines the quality of DNA programs that express or repress. Gene activation determines which proteins exist in a cell. Proteins comprise the metabolically active components of the body. Youthful cells require sufficient protein. One component of the aging rate results from diminished protein content (lost anabolism or negative nitrogen balance). In turn, with fewer life-sustaining reactions occurring, metabolism slows and the shrinkage of old age begins.

All other hormones act on the periphery in their ability to influence DNA programs. Only the steroid-like class of hormones plays the central role in youth versus' old age. The time has come that this basic central consideration in health versus' disease comes to the forefront. Adrenal evaluation needs to be clinically considered for those whose immune system begins to malfunction in the middle of their earthling experience.

The upright position is another important part of the earthling experience. Since the upright position defies the laws of gravity the skeletal integrity becomes impossible without bone cell health. Like other body cells, bone cell health requires a few basic ongoing things occurring in an interdependent manner.

William B. Ferril, M. D.

CHAPTER TWENTY-THREE

BONES

Like other cell types, the bones that make up the skeleton depend on the seven principles of longevity. Above all other principles two of these centrally affect the bones: cell charge and the fact that the hormones giveth and the hormones taketh away. Unfortunately, the knowledge of these principles remains only partially acknowledged in their relationship to the bones. In the first part of this chapter, the hormones and bone health will be reviewed. Next, the cellular charge principle as it involves bone health will be discussed along with the other principles where appropriate.

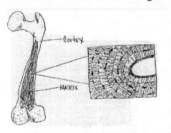

Message quality is the 'bull's eye' for optimal cellular performance. Almost weekly media sound bytes or newspaper articles discuss the 'latest information' on the prevention of the disease osteoporosis. Press coverage has been occupied with peripheral considerations while central scientific facts are disregarded about preventing skeletal deterioration.

Recently, the growing body of evidence linking the mainstream cornerstone of osteoporosis prevention, estrogen replacement therapy, to accelerated heart disease risk, breast cancer, and uterine cancer makes matters worse. Most authorities go on about the difficult decisions women face in the light of this 'new data'.

Looking into what is known about the role of estrogen in tissues it is no surprise about its role in cancer. Excessive estrogen can increase the overall tendency to develop cancer. It comes down to a failure to understand balance. Estrogen when unopposed by its counter regulatory hormone is a potent stimulus for cancer growth in estrogen responsive tissues in the breast, ovaries, uterus, and prostates in men. The central message content property of estrogen in these tissues promotes cell division. One of the central features of cancer cells is in the ability to divide (multiply).

When an owner is in hormone balance and free of environmental estrogens (section two), estrogen is unopposed in the first half of the female menstrual cycle. In optimum health (hormone balance), in the second half of the cycle estrogen is counter regulated by adequate progesterone. Progesterone serves as the counter response (counter weight in the antique weight scale analogy) putting the biological breaks on estrogens message to stimulate cell division.

Progesterone in many tissues behaves in an androgen-like fashion by directing cells to invest energy in cellular rejuvenation. This property of progesterone in the bones is one of the central prerequisites for continued bone health. Situations develop that lead to a deficient progesterone output, which allows the estrogen message to be amplified to dangerous levels. Clinically these states show up as fibrocystic breast growths, uterine fibroids, cyclical migraine headaches, thyroid dysfunction, and weight gain in the hips and thighs, and in extreme cases as cancer. Some holistic authorities believe that the more severe the progesterone deficiency, the greater the tendency to develop osteoporosis. However, this author adds that this is especially a risk if other androgens are deficient (testosterone, DHEA, androstenedione, etc.).

Bone rejuvenation should optimally occur in the monthly cycle when progesterone is the highest. Rejuvenation is only possible when the bones receive proper message content at the DNA level. Around middle age the slow decrease of progesterone message content in the monthly cycles affects the bones by decreasing instruction to rejuvenate.

The other problem in the bones of some women as they approach middle age regards their decreased adrenal performance. The adrenal abnormalities can be quite variable (section two), but the main effect results from a decreased output of androgens (DHEA and androstenedione). They can also suffer from an increase in the relative amount of cortisol compared to DHEA. Cortisol message content at the level of the bone channels energy into survival and away from rejuvenation.

Many times both their adrenal glands and ovaries become less capable in the manufacture of sufficient androgen message content. The severity of this deficit effects how fast women lose bone mass. Androgen deficiency increases bone mass loss because it contains message content that directs bone restoration.

Bones Need Sufficient Anabolism

Bone health depends more on androgens (testosterone, DHEA, etc.) than the numerous peripheral solutions pandered by the medical industrial complex. Realize the reoccurring body design theme of the androgen hormone class telling the different cells that it is important to invest energy in cellular rejuvenation reactions. Body tissues only differ in which type of androgen steroid they prefer to be stimulated by. The bone cells are no different than other cell types in regards to the need for high quality message content that directs wise use of cellular energy.

Some feeble truth persists in the consideration of estrogen for the prevention of bone loss. Bone occurs as a living dynamic tissue that constantly replaces its old electrically charged matrix with new matrix (minerals). In broad general terms, at any time approximately eight percent of the bone mass is in the remodeling stage. As a consequence, the average skeleton completely replaces itself every twelve years. This remodeling creates a tug of war between the cells that must eat bone matrix (osteoclasts) and the cells that make bone matrix (osteoblasts). Bone matrix describes the mineral and protein part of bone that occurs outside the widely spaced bone cells.

This process provides the only thread of scientific evidence for the role estrogen plays in bone health. The peripheral bone support that estrogen imparts concerns its message content. The estrogen message will impede the bone eating cells for up to five whole years after the menopause. What fails being said regards the additional hormones responsible for new bone formation. The hormones that direct bone formation are all in the androgen class (progesterone, testosterone, DHEA, etc.). When androgens are included in the healing program the bones begin to strengthen. This approach lessens the estrogen related side effects.

Many good scientist has suffered over the last few years by pointing out which hormone class is truly responsible for maintaining bone health in men and women. Osteoporosis prevention medications and the technology to detect and follow its course make big money for the complex. Though there is some doubt about a true conspiracy, there is the suspicion that this process occurs one upwardly mobile decision at a time protecting the profitable ways of treating a disease process. Therefore profitable decisions receive the advertising dollar. Little incentive exists and in some cases even a disincentive occurs for advertising the holism of what science has revealed. Owners should be aware of the reasons they have not heard of this more contrary approach).

Other hormones direct the manufacture and maintenance of healthy bones. This is found in the different rates of occurrence for developing osteoporosis between men and women. Men with healthy gonads do not develop osteoporosis even though their total body estrogen content is less than women. If estrogen were the central hormone directing new bone formation, osteoporosis would be higher in men. Consistency among reoccurring hormone themes bears out that androgen message content as being central to healthy bone formation.

Two caveats need mention for women when they deal with the androgen class of steroids. Androgens-like testosterone and dihydro-testosterone (DHT) cause marked physical masculine message content in female bodies. For this reason, exceeding the natural optimum will produce unwanted side effects. Second, healthy female owners have a remarkable process at work that protects them from developing physically masculine traits and still deliver androgen steroid message content to their target cells (bone, muscle, organ and nerve cells etc.). This process involves the action of peripheral conversion whereby weaker androgens (precursor steroids) are initially formed and released into the blood stream. Once inside the target cell they are converted into more powerful androgens. This conversion takes place

when the much weaker androgens (namely DHEA) changes to the more potent androgens once inside the target cells.

This process describes a way to deliver powerful rejuvenation message content inside female bodies, but it avoids unwanted male characteristics (hair growth, clitoral enlargement, increased aggressiveness, and acne). This fact exposes erroneous thinking when clinicians counsel patients about androgens like DHEA, androstenedione, and progesterone being relatively weak and unimportant. They forget the powerful concept of peripheral conversion (intracrinology) operating in the healthy female body. This conversion allows female cells to convert the weaker androgens into the more powerful androgens. This process occurs after the blood stream phase and thus the male characteristic side effects subdue. This process lessens the tendency for increased testosterone to areas that cause facial hair, clitoris enlargement, and/or chest hair.

Intracrinology is the term coined by Fernand Labrie, the scientist who discovered this important steroid process. In fact, once one understands the reason that DHEA is highest during the peak health years is because it provides a reservoir of both sex neutral estrogens and androgens that arise peripherally inside the target cell. Also pertinent is the fact that pound for pound of lean body mass women need just as much androgen (Labrie) as men, but they obtain ninety nine percent of it in the above described sex neutral way. Conversely, men obtain only sixty six percent of their androgen by the sex neutral DHEA route. Consequently, women are more dependent on adrenal health than are men.

Sex neutral refers to the fact that DHEA is a precursor steroid and therefore inactive (neutral) within the blood stream. However, when a body cell needs repair, if it contains the ability to activate DHEA into more powerful steroids once inside, this ability denotes the process of peripheral conversion. Importantly, after the powerful newly created steroid instructs the pertinent genes it becomes inactivated into specific metabolites before entering the blood stream again where it heads for the kidney for removal in the urine. Note that the true body androgen exposure level is not discernible without measuring these specific metabolites. Currently only the 24 hour urine test reliably achieves this measurement.

Sex neutral steroids allow the body's wisdom to create them once they penetrate inside the target cell. Even more importantly, this safety step allows the target cell to turn the active hormone (like testosterone or estrogen) into a inactive metabolite before it releases it back into the blood stream where it eventually exits in the urine. Different body areas produce unique metabolites, which spill into the urine and this allows the steroid savvy clinician to pursue clues as to what the nature of the steroid imbalance is all about.

Contrast the benefit of precursor steroid dosing, like DHEA, with the more common practice of pummeling women with steroids with a sexual attitude, like testosterone and estrogen. These

diametrically opposed messages enter the blood stream activated. Here the body's wisdom has been by passed. Prediction: in the not to distant future the wisdom of first attempting to prescribe precursor steroids as the hormonal foundation will become the new standard of care.

The power of having adequate precursor steroids, like DHEA, in men and women is due to its serving as the building block molecule for making many other steroids. For this reason, processes that harm the ability to manufacture precursor steroids have far reaching health consequences. Steroid hormone synthesis begins with the steroid building block, cholesterol. As gonads and adrenals age, these tissues begin to fail in their ability to obtain cholesterol. This initial step is necessary to start the process of making the precursor steroids leading eventually to progesterone and DHEA (the chassis for multiple other models of steroids). Bone cells are no different from other cells. They need continuous, quality cellular direction provided by hormones. The most powerful hormones are level one-type hormones because they instruct the DNA program directly.

Simple scientific truth: The sufficiency of bone cell protein depends on which DNA programs activate. As a consequence, to advise patients to comsume more calcium without increasing collegen synthesis is folly. Calcium has nothing to adhere to in the bone until gene activation directs collegen syntheses. Before synthese can occur the right hormone has to arrive to activate gene's coding for collegen synthese. This is an anabolic process. DHEA controls anabolism activity at the bone cell level.

The above paragraph provides an example of how the DNA program activity primarily depends on certain level one-type hormones that are made in the adrenals and gonads. Recall the first few steps in the conversion process towards making precursor steroids from cholesterol occur in the mitochondria.

Recall, as well, the importance of aldosterone. As aldosterone output diminishes with age, gonads and adrenals suffer a decreased ability to send cholesterol into the mitochondria (explained in the informational substances chapter). Functionally these structures can be thought of as the armored power plant of a cell. For this reason, supplementing with DHEA or progesterone to a body in possession of aging gonads and adrenals facilitates it to convert these precursor steroids to other biologically active steroids. These reactions of biosynthesis occur in the cytoplasm of the cell and are not as susceptible to the ravages of old age. Remember, as the initial conversion of cholesterol depends on adequate aldosterone message content.

Remember the important theme emphasized throughout this manual in regards to a cell's need for specific instruction from level one-type hormones on how to expend its energy. However, a little knowledge can be dangerous without a full appreciation for the importance of the power contained in the level one-type hormones. These hormones turn off and on the DNA. DNA activity determines how much and which proteins manifest in a cell. It is the proteins in the body that consume energy. One of the reasons old bodies perform less avidly and burn fewer calories occurs because of these relationships (lost anabolism).

Pregnenolone supplementation provides a prototypical example for how partial knowledge applied to lagging hormone production can have deleterious consequences. Pregnenolone is a steroid precursor that occurs on the path to DHEA and progesterone biosynthesis. It is the intermediary between cholesterol and the biosynthetic pathway to making all steroids including progesterone, testosterone, and DHEA. Think of it as the grandfather of all steroids because not one is possible unless sufficient pregnenolone occurs first.

Unfortunately, some clinicians routinely prescribe this steroid precursor with the belief that it simply jumps starts the aging gonads and adrenals in their ability to manufacture the anti-aging steroids. However, better and safer ways exist to bring about these desired results. Here, the side effects are not worth the benefits. The side effects occur because pregnenolone contains a message content that is very similar to that of the cortisol message content. Recall, if the cortisol message becomes higher than necessary, the cells move energy away from cellular rejuvenation and into survival pathways (section two).

> (side bar - The official stand is to demand double blind studies. When pursuing official policies, it is very apparent that there is significant control in what is studied and what the public receives about the results of these studies through mainstream media. It is a cozy arrangement).

This fact serves to caution owners to consult a physician who has competency and a complete understanding of steroids. Increased cortisol-like message content in the bone cell will behave as cortisol does. This becomes an unacceptable side effect in the case where bone rejuvenation is the goal. For these reasons, pregnenolone creates opposite effects to the desired effect that is to strengthen weak bones.

Often, supplementation with DHEA and/or progesterone under the guidance of a competent and hormone knowledgeable physician is the safest approach back to health. This allows for a trial in usage for several months to document objective benefits. Proving the ability of these precursors to reverse osteoporosis involves obtaining an bone density scan as a baseline before treatment. At the end of a six-twelve month trial period the bone density scan can be repeated and compared to the before treatment scan.

Progesterone cream leads to wonderful facial skin. For this reason some progesterone should be given as a cream. The cream can also be applied to the breast to help protect them from estrogen dominance. Use only pharmaceutical grade true progesterone. Without adequate potency the desired benefits fail to materialize.

Other methods of progesterone replacement exist that may be relevant for certain owners. Reputable sources for these progesterone products are obtained through a prescription to the compounding pharmacist. A physician can best advise a patient for which time of the month will be best for cream or sublingual application and when to abstain. Hormone holidays allow for the recognition of the natural ebb and flow of the cycle between estrogen and progesterone. Also realize that it is best to dose progesterone at bedtime only because while awake when there is stress it often converts into cortisol causing weight gain among other things. However, sleep is a time when cortisol production is very low (a low stress state).

An excellent summary of natural hormone replacement for women was written by Uzzi Reis's MD. His book is, **Natural Hormone Balance for Women** (Pocket Books, 2001). He explains the benefits of real hormone replacement instead of patentable hormone replacement. Overall this book is well written and informative for women past thirty-five years of age.

When viewing the disease osteoporosis holistically, the accumulated scientific evidence more accurately describes this process as originating from gonad and/or adrenal insufficiency. Lagging gonad or adrenal function leads bones down the path of deterioration secondary to the lack of hormone message content. Recall the androgen steroid message content directs the bone cells in ongoing rejuvenation. In addition, more peripheral considerations exist that potentially contribute to reversing the overall severity of the disease process. Unfortunately, all to often, it is the more peripheral considerations that receive the advertising dollar. Amazingly, these peripheral approaches dominate, without the benefit of implementing the central role that the anabolic steroids play. Could it be that this cozy arrangement maintains consumer demand for the services of the complex?

The need to supplement with powerful steroids does occur. Females who have had their ovaries surgically removed may be at increased risk for developing osteoporosis. Owners suffering from autoimmune disease and owners who have diminished adrenal reserve benefit from stronger forms of therapy. Remember, a complete twenty-four hour steroid metabolite urine test forms the basic starting point to assess for message content abnormalities. This tests an important part of the overall 'hormone report card' that helps guide the physician toward healing. (section seven)

Another caution is in order when considering steroid supplementation for a patient that has a history of a hormone responsive malignancy. These cases often occur in breast, uterine, ovarian, and prostate cancers. Counsel from a knowledgeable physician is essential. Progesterone that arrives at capable gonads and adrenals is easily converted to other steroids. Remember this important, but subtle clinical point that is often overlooked. This approach relies on the body possessing an intelligence to do the wise thing when given the chance.

The Chinese have recognized this fact for millennia in their routine supplementation with high quality ginseng to combat the lagging hormones. As a general rule, at the age of forty it is a common practice to begin supplementing with ginseng. When inquiring into why this practice is reverently adhered, interesting biochemical support emerges. Meanwhile, the complex creates smoke and mirrors tactics to discount this strategy that has been proved successful down through the ages. The public has the unenviable task of deciding whom to believe.

Ginseng contains steroid like precursors in a package. Before the package comes off, the intact ginseng molecules serve as a type of surfactant (lung chapter). This revered quality facilitates an optimal breathing function resulting from regular use. If the intelligence of the body sees need in the lungs, that is where the intact ginseng molecule will go. If more need exists in the aging gonads and adrenals that's where it goes. This property will also make the androgen message content available for increased bone structure.

When the steroid precursor package comes off, natural steroid precursors can jumpstart the aging hormone glands into renewed production of lagging steroids. Life style choices in exercise and nutritional adequacy will also influence this ability.

The use of ginseng to strengthen bones includes the need to realize that quality ginseng is the most difficult medicinal herb to find in this country. There are over 2 billion Asians and a good proportion of them are over forty years old. Good medicinal ginseng takes a minimum of seven years to grow before there is sufficient bioactive ingredient present.

Two cautions arise in the use of ginseng. Regular ginseng usage may raise blood pressure. Monitoring this should be a safety measure. Raising the androgen content can result in hair thinning in genetically predisposed males after forty. Around this age, testosterone production decreases enough in males to slow down their hair loss and increase the tendency to develop a beer gut. Here insulin levels become less opposed to the fat burning effects that testosterone creates. The tough decision becomes which facet of youth the owner wishes to maintain. A knowledgeable physician should monitor these decisions.

Some owners supplement with steroid precursors and high quality ginseng for increasing bone mass. A *hormone report card* can be obtained through a twenty-four hour urine test for steroid content before beginning any supplement program. Follow this up in ninety 90 days with a repeat test.

Ginseng builds stronger bones by stimulating steroid synthesis in the adrenals and gonads. Men usually notice a discernable increase in the size of their testicles in about seven days. Some owners do not absorb ginseng like the normal population. In these cases, it is worth experimenting with taking it on an empty stomach versus a meal containing eggs or cheese. Unfortunately, without certain vitamins, ginseng can be taken for a long time with no benefit because these vitamins are needed by the body to process it into more active forms.

Halatorrhea floribunda, suma (Brazilian ginseng), macca, pomegranates, European mistletoe berries, ashwaghanda and possibly Mexican wild yams are a few of the additional plants that contain progesterone or a similar precursor. However none of these have the thousands of years of safety and efficiency that ginseng possesses. People will continue to gather information and compare notes and eventually more will be known about these other medicinal plants. Until then, it is wise to proceed cautiously and stay in the areas where common safety guidelines are established.

There are cases where stronger anabolic steroid creams and potions are warranted. The ability of testosterone creams applied over the fracture site to speed bone healing is one of them. Another effect is in the ability of testosterone injections to facilitate ligament and joint injury healing. These are all predictable when considering the stimulatory message content that anabolic steroids play in healing these tissues. There are other hormones to consider (Growth Hormone and insulin), but they have obstacles because of potential side effects.

A case in point involved a naturopathic physician who broke his knee (fractured his proximal tibia into three pieces and tore up the overlying meniscus). He also had a 18 year history of insulin dependent diabetes. This was a concern to his orthopedic surgeon who reconstructed the joint and tibia fracture fragments with pins and plates. The concern was founded on the general knowledge that long-time, severe diabetic patients heal poorly and very slowly.

Unbeknownst to this talented surgeon was the fact that his patient had two things in his base of knowledge that powerfully enhanced his ability to heal. First, he was a faithful adherent to the pioneering work of Richard Bernstein M.D. in the solutions to diabetes mastery (*Diabetes Solution*, Richard Bernstein M.D.1998, Little Brown Co.) and this program allowed him to be entirely free of the usual diabetic complications. Corroborating this was that through strict adherence to this program his hemoglobin A1C values average around 5-5.5! Second, he applied a mixture of testosterone and progesterone cream over the fracture site daily, at this author's suggestion. This resulted in an acceleration of fracture healing time. At the time of his 4½-week exam x ray there was 9 weeks of healing when compared to healing in the normal population!

The quality of the hormones and their direct relationship to anabolic steroids greatly influences the healing processes of the bones and how cellular energy is expended. Throughout the cell types, health requires optimum message content or aging results. Clinical assessment is critical to rejuvenation and should be applied skillfully and holistically. Today's knowledge about different hormones' ability to preserve youthful properties should be fully applied in the office setting.

Other hormones (discussed below) play a less central role in the health or deterioration of bone mass but these are often the ones that physicians hear about. These along with different lifestyle choices, nutritional adequacy, and emotional energy impact bone health and the youthful state of cells.

Bones and Exercise

Exercise is a powerful stimulant for strong bone formation when an owner possesses capable gonads and adrenals. Unhealthy gonads and adrenals when faced with the physiological demands of exercise are analogous to attempting a cash withdrawal when the safe is empty. Without previous deposits, no withdrawals can be made. The inability of some owners to maintain an adequate fitness program stems from this simple truth.

Exercise proficiency is limited by the quality of the steroids being secreted in the months before starting to exercise and by current ability. Exercise encourages the gonads and adrenals to function efficiently. If they are capable, far reaching performance and longevity advantages occur. For this simple reason, some exercise can be harmful if gonad and adrenals ability to produce adequate anabolic steroids chronically fails. Exercise increases the need for message content that directs appropriate investment into muscular-skeletal strengthening.

Simply, exceeding gonad and adrenal ability to generate sufficient message content (anabolic steroids) causes soreness and potential injury. Normal training can also produce some soreness. Injury verses exercise training can be differentiated. Exceeding the level of current gonad and adrenal ability creates sore joints or ligaments after exercising. Regular exercise with cautious increases in intensity will stimulate the adrenals and gonads to increase output of anabolic steroids.

Increased demand of anabolic steroid production often goes unrecognized in owners who lack adequate response of gonad and adrenal ability. Signs of aging elicit unnecessary counseling to slow down. However, with an appropriate inquiry and effort into re-balancing lagging hormones, slowing down may not be the answer.

Once the sufficiency of level one-type hormones becomes realized an exercise program will cause remarkable restorative affects. The interrelationship between exercise and hormone quality and the bones is obvious. Weak bones can come from either a sedentary lifestyle or poor hormone production ability in the adrenals and gonads. Fortunately, healing becomes possible when awareness occurs for both possibilities. The muscles and ligaments chapter will explore this further.

The Bones and Calcium

Calcium plays a significant role in bone health. The press on a regular basis covers adequate calcium intake. The average adult contains about 2½ pounds of calcium in their body. 99% of this amount resides in the bones. Realize, dietary calcium has little effect on increasing overall absorption. Rather, absorption is determined by which hormones are present. The hormone quality also further determines where calcium ends up in the body. In addition, eating meals rich in phosphates and oxalates causes calcium to bind and exit in the formation of microscopic gravel in the stool.

One percent of calcium (free calcium) that is not in the bones needs to be carefully channeled and regulated. Organism havoc ensues when this pool of calcium changes minutely. This concept is often lost in trying to make sense of the complex medical phraseology that is in print.

Making informed choices regarding adequate calcium content requires cognizance for the need in the body to keep one percent of the calcium constant. This calcium influences whether the owner lives from one moment to the next. For example, if free calcium falls ten percent below normal, tetany promptly ensues and the next step is fatal laryngospasm. For this reason, the body possesses an elaborate system of hormones that regulate and counter regulate the one percent of body calcium content that is free on multiple levels. These hormones ensure that an adequate and constant supply of calcium is maintained.

There are two classes of hormones operating that concern calcium. The first group includes vitamin D, parathyroid hormone, and calcitonin. These hormones ensure that calcium in the free form (the one percent quotient) is kept constant to maintain life. This must occur in a wide variety of metabolic circumstances.

Parathyroid hormone is secreted from six little glands behind the thyroid. These glands promptly respond to the calcium content falling in the blood stream by secreting sufficient parathyroid hormone. This in turn increases active vitamin D formation in the kidneys and also instructs bone tissue to release calcium. Following this the increase in active vitamin D content increases absorption of dietary calcium, puts it into the accessible bone pool of calcium, and increases the ability of the kidney to retard calcium excretion in the urine.

In contrast, the role of thyroid-derived calcitonin hormone seems to speed the uptake of calcium increase in the blood stream that may occur following a meal. In other words, calcitonin hormone increases dietary tolerance for calcium because it subdues blood level spikes by by directing its efficient removal. This calcium is initially destined to the readily accessible bone calcium that is separated from true mineralized bone structure. Also realize that deficient calcium encourages the release of parathyroid hormone, which in turn promotes the absorption sequence described in the preceding paragraph.

The second group of hormones determines how adequately bone quality is being addressed at any given time. It is these and not the first group that needs sufficient quality and amount occurring with proper timing to maintain bone health. Conceptually, think of this second group of hormones as those that inhibit or promote adequate bone rejuvenation. The type and amount of steroids determines the message content for expenditure of available energy of a bone cell (anabolism versus catabolism or the quality of nitrogen balance). Realize, sufficient protein (positive nitrogen balance) needs to occur before bone mineralization can occur. In addition, these cells need adequate molecular building parts constantly supplied by a highly

functioning digestive tract. Wise nutritional choices are critical. These last two concepts have been discussed in sections two and three respectively.

Similarly, the joint spaces, like the bones and cartilage, have specific requirements before healing transpires. Hopefully, by now the reader is beginning to see the body pattern involving the interplay between the seven principles within each organ system. Joint spaces are no different but like other specific cells they have unique vulnerabilities and priorities.

Joint Space

Hinged joints have an added layer of joint lining cells surrounding the joint cavity such as fingers, toes, knees, ankles, hips, elbow, and wrists. In contrast, there are the less moveable joints occurring in the intervertebral disc, sternum with rib articulations, hand and foot joints. Both types of joints have cartilage anchored over the bone ends and anchored around the sides by tough fibrous attachments that secure the two ends in close proximity.

Additional joint cells line the hinged joints and are like hollow sponges stuffed into a joint space. The secretion of these cells is a gel-like substance. The adequacy of manufacture of this gel is one of the determinants of how well joints function. This gel is made from modified galactosamine that forms hyaluronic acid. Gelatin is made from ground up and partially digested cartilage. One of the components of cartilage is galactosamine.

When the joint cells secrete this gel substance appropriately, the hinged joints receive enhanced ability to glide with minimal friction during performance of their hinging action. In addition, water performs magic when it remains in adequate supply. Only if adequate supply of water bathes the joint compartment during the ebb and flow of daily living can the cleansing forces rinse off the gel that looks and feels dirty. Clean water deficiency describes one of the mechanisms for painful joints. When joints hurt drink abundant, clean water.

The cartilage overlying the bone ends adjacent to the joint space and looks like shinny linoleum in the youthful state. As it ages, it becomes cracked and worn. Visualize the additional joint lining cells occurring in the hinged joints as grease forming carpet layers. This mental picture facilitates defending against some of these hostilities.

This layer has its own blood and nerve supply that allows for a superior nutrition source. It also serves as a toxic waste site in the body for trash that must be removed. When this situation begins to occur, it becomes critically important that the garbage is removed. The owner usually perceives this as pain.

Instead of consuming large quantities of clean water, many are trained from an early age to consume toxins like aspirin or acetaminophen (liver chapter). This contributes to more trash water. In addition, concepts that are good for the cartilage are also good for the joint lining cells. The pain perceiving nerve fibers are not present in the cartilage, but in the surrounding fibrous anchoring ligaments that encases the joint and the joint lining cells that overly the cartilage. It is the responsibility of these pain fibers to scream out if dysfunction occurs in the joint. Unfortunately, processes that injure these nerves, like diabetes, diminish the ability to alert the owner to these types of problems.

Problems occur in the joints for the above reasons but there is an additionally important body tissue that causes owners to suffer when it becomes unhappy: The bone marrow lies within the hollow spaces of a few bones. From here, the precursors of red blood cells, the various white blood cells and platelets reside and develop into mature cells as there fellow comrades wear out and die within the blood stream.

Bone Marrow

In some of the larger bones, bone marrow exists. The potential for continued or the possibility of renewed vigor resides here. This space describes the location of pure potential for the ability to rejuvenate the blood with new cells of all types. For this reason, processes that injure the potential energy contained in the bone marrow inhibit healing until they resolve.

Some of the immune system cells have a life span of 6 hours. Without adequate maintenance of the bone marrow, there is depletion of vital cell lines. If this process continues deficiency of the afflicted cell line ensues and diseases follow.

Processes that are good for the bones are good for the bone marrow. Like in other body cells the bone marrow needs informational content that directs the wise use of its available energy. From this simple truth the lack of quality information content leads to programmed cell death (apoptosis) for many of its potential containing cell populations.

Falling quality message content occurs when disease processes injure enough kidney cells that there becomes a diminished ability of the kidney to manufacture the hormone erythropoietin. Thousands of years ago Chinese physicians determined that sufficient kidney energy is necessary for the continued optimal function of the bone marrow. They also discovered that the kidney area (the adrenals that are attached to the kidney) and their dominance over the strength of the gonads all interact to generate sufficient message content directing energy expenditure within the bone marrow.

Regretfully, in western medicine a tendency occurs to forget the holism of what the Chinese have known for thousands of years. In its place, profitable approaches to treating failing bone marrow abound. This is found in the common practice of relying on recombinant DNA technology to manufacture the complex erythropoietin hormone. This doesn't mean that this expensive technology is never helpful, but rather that many diseased owners lack the ability to pay the astronomical fees for this treatment. Fortunately, understanding the holism of what science has revealed often times allows for less costly alternatives.

It has been known for many years that adequate androgen content stimulates optimal performance of the bone marrow. The androgen class of steroid hormones is important to stimulate the different cell lines of the body to maximize potential performance.

Androgen type steroids stimulate the bone marrow to make new cells and increase the ability of the kidney to manufacture erythropoietin. For this reason, applying this knowledge in the clinical setting allows a way to sometimes avoid the more costly approach to healing. There are some cases where this costly approach is warranted, but why not include the holism of more affordable options?

Holism discussions are incomplete until the energies that heal contrasted to the energies that maim, the seventh principle of longevity, become part of the healing plan strategy. The next section explains the seventh principle and how its healing properties can be realized. In addition, the health and needs of one's nervous system, heart, ligaments and muscles are reviewed.

SECTION SIX

SECTION SIX.. *522*

    PRINCIPLE SEVEN: ENERGIES THAT HEAL CONTRASTED
TO THE ENERGIES THAT MAIM....................................523

CHAPTER TWENTY-FOUR 531

    BRAIN AND NERVES 531

CHAPTER TWENTY-FIVE 574

    HEART 574

    THE SEVENTH PRINCIPLE: THE ENERGIES THAT HEAL
CONTRASTED TO THE ENERGIES THAT MAIM THE HEART 574

    PRINCIPLES 1 AND 2 586

    PRINCIPLE 3: THE HORMONES GIVETH AND TAKETH AWAY ONE'S
HEART..587

    PRINCIPLE 4: YOU ARE WHAT YOU ABSORB 598

    THE SIXTH PRINCIPLE AND THE HEART: AVOID *LOW CELL VOLTAGE
SYNDROME* 599

CHAPTER TWENTY-SIX 604

    MUSCLES AND LIGAMENTS   604

PRINCIPLE SEVEN: ENERGIES THAT HEAL CONTRASTED TO THE ENERGIES THAT MAIM

HEALTH is a QUESTION of BALANCE

The reoccurring body theme of balance forms a prerequisite for true health. Balance reverberates all the way down to the opposing molecules that interact within a cell. Unfortunately, Western medicine often ignores this because of the reductionism logic on which it is founded.

The seven principles of healthful longevity largely involve the balance between the opposing life forces: The creative forces versus the destructive forces. Where balance exists between the two, the healthful state continues.

In each of the five sections before this one, the emphasis has been on one or two of the first six principles for healthful longevity. The next chapter concerns itself with how the central nervous system functions. The central nervous system, more than the other organ systems, lends itself to explaining how the seven principles of longevity interrelate with the each other.

Evidence exists to unite these seven principles into a comprehensive assessment of what science has revealed. Although the popular scientific method that employs reductionism at its very foundation in an attempt to explain the biochemical reactions of life has merit it lacks the seventh principle. As a consequence, at some point its investigation into health misses the interwoven theme of balance. In contrast, when science becomes more unified it brings people to the realization that a healthy life requires balance between these opposing forces (the creative forces versus the chaotic forces). Wherever imbalance occurs, deterioration and disease eventually result.

The reader is warned that this section prepares him/her for the hardest principle for the Western mind to understand, the seventh principle. The seventh principle encompasses the energies that heal contrasted to the energies that maim. With this in mind, the central nervous system will initially be explored within the consideration of the seventh principle.

A few introductory remarks about the seventh principle

Other medical scientific theories embrace the energetic understandings of balance. For example, traditional Chinese medical theory considers the life energies quality at its foundation. The foundation of their energy science uses the concepts of Yin energy that directly opposes Yang energy in a harmonious way. The harmony between these two energetic entities forms a prerequisite for health. The Chinese science of health embraces this reoccurring body theme; balance.

Conversely, the western system ignores the dynamic forces between Yin energy and Yang energy. Despite this stance, thousands of years of accumulated evidence show that enduring health requires balance between these two opposing energies. Yin energy can be thought of as quiet, calm, contemplative, reflective, cool, deep, patient, and content. Whereas, Yang energy, in contrast, is; loud, rushed, hurried, hot, shallow, and explosive, on-the-move, action and inpatient in its expression.

Evidence accumulating for more than 60 years suggests that the life force forms an *intelligent energy* grid (an energetic template) that permeates every cell. Every cell in the body is organized energetically by this living entity until death. The evidence seems to indicate that when this life force evenly distributes and remains at the right vibration frequency health continues within the body (evidence discussed below).

In contrast, the western medical approach can best be described as the '*slab of meat approach*'. The slab of meat describes all that remains when the mysterious energies that organize the human form are ignored. Unfortunately, the western scientific paradigm ignores the qualities of the life force.

Never the less, when life energy imbalances cause disease, owners in these situations will continue to suffer until this principle of longevity is applied. Sometimes they continue to suffer solely because the western medical complex fails to consider energy aberrations that can cause a disease process. Even more surprisingly, the Chinese are not the only medical theory that includes the life force energy.

Eastern Indian scientific theory has long understood the flow of optimal life sustaining energy through several Chakras in healthy individuals. Recently there have been some interesting applications of these imbalanced energy states, and how they correlate with disease. This evidence involves the other side of the story for what science has revealed but still ignores.

In this section, the ignored evidence will be reintroduced. The trouble with re-including it into the discussion of health versus disease is that many of the mainstream approaches and explanations of the inner-workings of the universe begin to look inconsistent and incomplete. Conversely, this information complements many of the alternative treatment modalities and allows them to make more mechanistic sense.

Down through the age's many wise men have contemplated the human condition. For example, Dr. Paul Brand, MD, author of the book 'Fearfully and Wonderfully Made', points out that knowledge is lost. He maintains that the Egyptian physicians of thousands of years ago could perform surgeries that cannot even be contemplated today. High technology solutions can only go so far before one confronts the ignored energy of life. For these reasons, some holistic physicians argue that the life force needs to be considered and appreciated in order to carry healing over the 'bridge'. This process unites the mainstream with the alternative modalities.

The Intelligence behind the Intelligence

The body contains approximately 70 trillion cells. The 46 chromosomes that contain the DNA (genes) within most cells are in some ways analogous to a computer encryption code. However, without an intelligent operator the encryption code hides useful information. Something is missing at the encryption (DNA) level.

Something else is needed to explain the precise and ordered unraveling and repair of DNA. Some, as yet, unseen guiding principle, superbly directs the replication of DNA and RNA. Also, the RNA directed protein synthesis, which results in elaborate and unique protein architecture, also needs direction. In addition, the direction of the construction of cell architecture involves many types of fat and specialized sugar groups. What directs how all of these fits precisely together fail to be explained by the genetic code contained within specific DNA sequences (genes).

Realize DNA segments (genes) only contain the sequencing information for the amino acid sequence contained in a specific protein. In turn, the activity of a gene depends on the arrival of specific hormones. Recall, the genes provide nothing until the right hormone arrives.

Consequently, gene activity determines the amount of a specific protein. However, genes do not contain information, which regards the synthesis of the many different and specific types of fat and modified sugars added onto certain proteins. In addition, recall, they need to be precisely arranged in three-dimensional space for life to continue. A plausible explanation for what directs these complex processes is currently beyond Western scientific comprehension.

Interesting research results exist, which provides insights into what the nature of the force is that intelligently directs the DNA. One of the early scientific pioneers, in this field, was Dr Harold Saxon Burr, a long time researcher at Yale University. In the early 1920's his research began documenting the electromagnetic field properties, found to occur in all living things. Dr Burr later named this electromagnetic field, which is present in all living things, the life field. He pointed out that if one hadn't seen their friend in over six months, new molecules during the intervening time period, would have replaced every molecule in their friend's face.

The fact that the body replaces all soft tissue molecules frequently is secondary to the body's ongoing cellular rejuvenation program. The cellular rejuvenation program occurs throughout life at varying degrees of efficiency. His research led him to conclude that it was the life field that served as an organizing template. He theorized that the electromagnetic field, which he measured, was the organizer of the structure contained within living things. He concluded that the electromagnetic 'template' preserves the pattern in the friend's face. The underlying energetic template reproduces a consistent appearance, even though the molecules themselves are different. He extended this concept to explain the mystery of embryological cells, knowing how to organize, divide and differentiate into fetal form.

Conversely, mainstream science remains unable to explain these two fundamental life processes, because they ignore theories like Dr Burr's. Specifically, no believable mainstream theory occurs to explain why one's face stays recognizable after the molecules are replaced. In addition, mainstream science is still baffled about the process of embryogenesis. Embryogenesis denotes the organized process of cell differentiation, spatial arrangement and orientation of the embryo's development.

Robert Becker, MD in his book, '*The Body Electric*', elaborated on this research. Dr. Becker comments, "Embryo genesis is as if a pile of bricks were to spontaneously rearrange itself into a building, becoming not only walls but windows, light sockets, steel beams and furniture in the process." Later on he summarized this mystery that led to his life research," As I contemplated their findings and all of biology's unsolved problems, I grew convinced that life was more complex than we suspected. I felt that those who reduced life to a mechanical interaction of molecules were living a cold, gray, dead world, which despite its drabness, was a fantasy. I didn't think electricity would turn out to be any élan vital in the old sense, but I had a hunch it would be closer to the secret than the smells of the biochemistry lab or the dissecting rooms preserved organs."

Dr's Burr and Becker are in good company: Another scientist agrees with their line of thinking in regards to solving the mystery of an organizing energy field. Albert Szent Gyorgyi won the Nobel Prize for his work on tissue oxidation and the elucidation of the molecular structure of vitamin C. According to Dr. Becker, while addressing the Budapest Academy of Science on March 21, 1941, Dr. Gyorgyi pointed out that when these scientists broke living things down into constituent parts, life slipped through their fingers and they found themselves working with dead matter. Albert emphasized, "It looks as if some basic fact about life is still missing, without which any real understanding is impossible." For the missing basic fact Albert proposed putting electricity back into science's investigation of living things. Unfortunately, more than sixty years later mainstream science is still trying to explain life within the limitation of molecular matter while ignoring the evidence for organizing energy.

The continued omission of the life force has altered medical treatment decisions. Some of the consequent treatment decisions have associated toxicities. Some of these toxicities are avoidable. In contrast, the alternative treatment modalities tend to address the importance of an owner's life force quality. This fact has resulted in alternative healing disciplines. This fact also forms a powerful common denominator between many of the alternative methods of healing. Some holistic physicians feel that the common denominator regards their common practice of improving, maintaining, and cleansing this life field. The alternative therapies believe that the life force functions more efficiently during health than in disease.

Some call the life force energy, measured years ago by Dr. Burr, *intelligent energy. Intelligent energy* denotes the property of the life force to organize molecules into complex arrangements which life requires. This fundamental requirement of living things violates the science of physics' third law of thermodynamics. The third law of thermodynamics states that molecular arrangements will tend to move in a random fashion towards more disorder. Again, mainstream medicine remains unable to explain how living things violate this basic physical law of the nonliving universe.

Some newer mathematical theories predict that the life force swirls around at speeds faster than the speed of light. The faster-than-the-speed-of-light requirement has merit because when energy moves this fast the math predicts it to behave with an organizational intelligence. Richard Gerber, MD in his book called, '*Vibrational Medicine*' explains quite well the math pioneered by Carl Muses.

Carl Muses proposed in his work on hyper numbers that when energy moves faster than the speed of light, organizational consequences occur. Dr. William Tiller of Stanford University expounded on these mathematical consequences and described this type of energy as difficult to measure within the dimension of the physical world, except that it would create a weak magnetic field. Interestingly, all living things studied, to date, create a magnetic field until death occurs.

The faster than speed of light property would help explain the above mentioned long-standing physic's enigma. Specifically, the third law of thermodynamics in physics states that energy naturally moves in a direction of more and more randomness (increased entropy). Realize life's complexly created molecules, which are precisely arranged so that life may continue, violate this basic tenant of physics. However, if one limits the third law of thermodynamics to a description of energy's behavior when energy travels at speeds equal to, or less than the speed of light, it remains consistent. Until very recently no mathematician or scientist had really thought about the consequences of energy moving at speeds greater than the speed of light.

Understanding the enigma regarding life energy violating physics' thermodynamic law is best grasped by considering the chicken egg. If one dropped a million eggs on the floor, breaking each of the eggs, there would be a mess. There would be no chick formed. The physicist would say that the third law of thermodynamics was consistent in this case. However, it is only consistent because the act of breaking open the shell kills the life contained inside of it.

Contrast this to successfully incubating any one of the eggs through its gestation time. The live chick would be formed. The baby chick provides an example of increasing complexity, which arise from uncomplicated molecules inside the chicken egg. What was just a gooey mess inside the egg somehow energetically organized into the complex multi-organ and multi-cellular baby chick.

What is the nature of this *intelligent energy* that violates the laws of physics? The theory of energy moving faster than the speed of light and behaving with an organizational intelligence provides a viable explanation for how the life force may organize matter like the gooey chicken egg into a baby chick.

Drs Muses and Tiller were some of the first mathematicians to look into how energy behaves moving faster than the speed of light. They theorized that when energy travels faster than the speed of light it would behave with an organizational intelligence with only a weakly measurable magnetic field. They thought of the physical world, for which owners have sensory apparatus to experience, as the speeds equal to or less than light dimension.

They further predicted that at speeds greater than light the measurement of the electrical properties of this type of energy would exceed today's technological capabilities. The one exception that their mathematical calculations predicted was the ability to detect a weakly measurable magnetic field. This theory is consistent with the measurability of a weak bodily magnetic field, which changes in strength and polarization during different levels of activity and consciousness level. These facts provide evidence, which would help explain life's mysterious energetic properties more completely yet it routinely remains ignored in the mainstream world of medicine.

The life energy can best be thought of as moving within another dimension than the physical world. Current technologies cannot detect energy moving faster than the speed of light. In fact this becomes the basis for claiming that it does not exist. Consequently, the mathematical theory of matter moving faster than the speed of light, which predicts that it would create a weak but measurable magnetic field, tends to be ignored.

Interestingly, research looking into the organization of the body's magnetic field, has found an unvarying energy grid, corresponding to the ancient Chinese system of acupuncture meridian lines. Science has come a long way in eloquently explaining cellular biochemical reactions. Scientific understanding is advancing about the understanding of the contents of the DNA programs (genes). Yet, the organizational principle that allows life to continue defies Western scientific explanation. Perhaps other theories are worthy, if one seeks guidance about a healing response.

Scientific theory, going back thousands of years in India and China, recognized the importance of living things containing optimal energy flow. The Indians call the life energy prana and the Chinese call it chi. Both of these scientific systems place attention to the overall quality and integrity contained within the life energy field and believe it to be fundamental to health.

In addition, the Chinese realized the quality of energy penetrating the body's trunk organs could be palpated in the peripheral pulse. This method measures the amount of chi contained within the various organs and is called pulse diagnosis. Pulse diagnosis was developed over the last several thousand years. Pulse diagnosis allows an elaborate understanding of the consequences of energetic excess or deficiency within each organ.

The electromagnetic lines, known as the acupuncture meridian lines, were painstakingly developed with their corresponding organ effects noted. Out of this several thousand years of observation, an understanding developed for ways to increase or decrease the energetic meridian tone depending on what was needed. The energetic energy tone is composed of the opposing energies, Yin and Yang. Yin and Yang imbalances lead to organ system dysfunction.

The Chinese scientific theory regards Chi as organizing life energy. This energy concept is worthy of some consideration. This theory predicts that Chi needs to be balanced by the forces of Yin and Yang within any organ system in the body or disease occurs. Investigations into Chi energy could solve the mystery about the created perpetual complexity of living things.

For these reasons, the complementary Western idea for the existence of *intelligent energy* serving as the ultimate director of the cellular biochemical reactions of life allows healing possibilities. Healing possibilities could be realized when the Chi energy (intelligent energy) improves. For example, improvement in the Chi energy improves the quality of the hormones secreted in a rhythmic and harmonious way. These alternative theories predict that the areas of body breakdown result from either Chi energetic deficiency or excess. Chi is the Chinese description of *intelligent energy*, the life force, or prana.

The merging of energy theory and what is known about the biochemical reactions of life incorporates the intermediary step of the hormones and neurotransmitters. The hormones deliver the message, which was stimulated by the *intelligent energy*. Think of these important level one-type hormones as the interface between the two dimensions.

Hence, the quality of the *intelligent energy*, within the body, becomes a determinant of how an organ directs energy expenditure. If the *intelligent energy* distribution and quality remains favorable, this communicates to the body's cells by the informational substances (hormones). Like wise, the level one-type hormones need to be of sufficient quality (adequate *steroid tone and pressure*) or the informational interface between the two dimensions breaks down.

The informational substances include the hormones and neurotransmitters. The Chinese theory regarding Chi predicts that practices, which facilitate the life-energy rhythms, will promote health by way of the informational substances. Conversely, any practice that injures the quality of the *intelligent energy* rhythms will promote aging and eventually cause disease. Western science can measure the diminished quality of informational substances. However, western science does not specifically appreciate or acknowledge the possibility of the life force energy being a determinant of these informational substances.

Conversely, the Chinese and East Indians have developed theories that explain the life force energy. Unfortunately, Western medical thought begins its treatment decisions at the level of the informational substances. Even more alarming concerns the fact that often times even this level of inquiry becomes less than adequate (section two).

The theory of *intelligent energy* can best be thought of as the organizational template which directs the overall living body processes. The quality and completeness of this life energy determines which informational substances secrete. Quality informational substances depend on a highly functioning *intelligent energy field*. This belief has long ago been appreciated and incorporated into Chinese and East Indian scientific medical thought. The belief that these energies move faster than the speed of light provides an explanation for why they prove difficult to detect by conventional technological means.

Similarly, before the understanding of television and radio waves, the presence of these wave energies in the natural environment largely went unnoticed until technology developed that measured their existence. The key to understanding this possibility regards an appreciation of the fact that television and radio waves existed down through the ages. Their properties of existence were not affected because humans were unaware of their presence.

Also similarly, today the upper limits of scientific study concerns energies which move slower than or equal to the speed of light. However, the evolution of mathematics considers the consequences of what energy would behave like when it moves faster than the speed of light. Part of these consequences includes the possibility that would explain how life organizes matter into complex arrangements. If an owner can be open to this possibility, then a mechanism for why alternative therapies improve owner vitality becomes available.

Alternative therapies are only part of the healing strategy. Often they exert their healing effect by honoring the seventh principle. However, the other six principles of longevity apply in the pursuit of the physical health of the brain and nerves.

Cutting edge scientific thought: Neurodegeneative diseases like MS, myasthenia gravis, neuropathy, Parkinson's disease, and Lou Garrig's disease are sometimes secondary to IgG food allergies (the injury mechanism). Therefore, identifying and removing these from the diet allows healing to begin. Further, replacing decovered deficiencies of neurosteroids (progesterone and DHEA) and thyroid enhances recovery.

CHAPTER TWENTY-FOUR

BRAIN AND NERVES

The brain has a unique protection system that is commonly known as the blood brain barrier. This barrier is created by the blood vessel lining cells (the 'tiles' discussed in the blood vessel chapter) within the brain forming a tight interconnected barrier. Here, the barrier is very selective on what it allows to pass in or out of the brain blood vessel. This barrier is complete except in a few areas deep within the central underside of the brain. These four small areas where the blood brain barrier fails to exist are called the circum-ventricular organs. These small areas provide a 'window' for the brain to more directly interact with the body environment. However, it also allows an area of vulnerability for unwanted substances as well.

Physicians treating for possible brain infections have to constantly keep in mind that only a few antibiotics can penetrate beyond the blood brain barrier. This anatomical fact also creates a problem when attempting to medicate brain function. For example, illnesses like Parkinson's disease subside if more dopamine makes its way into the injured neurons responsible for its manufacture. However, the trouble is dopamine cannot cross the blood brain barrier. Scientists circumvent this by providing a synthetic dopamine precursor, L-dopa that penetrates the blood brain barrier. Once it moves across the blood brain barrier, L-dopa converts into dopamine.

The blood brain barrier also creates challenges for the brain cells. One challenge for brain cells involves their continued procurement of all the needed molecular building blocks. The brain needs more molecular building parts because it is an area of high metabolic activity. High metabolic activity means that molecular parts wear out and need replacement more quickly. All this active replacement requires the use of lots of fuel and oxygen. The consequent increased combustion of fuels and oxygen necessitates an increased need for efficient waste removal and rust prevention. In addition, only some of the most powerful body hormones can gain access to the entire brain. This fact has powerful repercussions when one wants to know how to keep their brain functional.

Keeping in mind the physical blood brain barrier will facilitate the understanding of nine determinants of physical brain health. These are: 1) availability and completeness of neurotransmitters within the brain 2) availability and direction for the use of molecular building parts 3) adequate fuel delivery 4) blood vessel health within the brain 5) informational directions regarding cell architecture and rejuvenation activities 6) anti-oxidant versus oxidant activity 7) the quality of the force field that the individual nerve cells are able to generate 8) toxin accumulation 9) status of the energies that heal contrasted to the energies that maim. Overall, informed choices in the day-to-day little decisions promote brain health when one considers its nine determinants of health.

It helps to organize the seven principles of health and how they relate to the nine determinates for the brain. The brain is somewhat unique and expanding from seven to nine will facilitate a healing response.

1. Principles 1&2: blood vessel health (4 and 6 above)
2. Principle 3: hormone message content (5 above and some of 1 above)
3. Principle 4: molecular replacement parts (2 and 3 above and some of some of 1 above)
4. Principle 5: taking out the brain trash (8 above)
5. Principle 6: cellular charge of brain cells (7 above)
6. Principle 7: the energies that heal contrasted to the energies that maim brain cells (9 above)

The Nine Determinants of Brain Health

1) Neurotransmitters

The many different neurotransmitters within the mind convey specific information to the neighboring nerves. A discussion of the numerous different neurotransmitters can become really complicated. However, some of the most basic considerations will help to avoid gullibility about the medical business complex. With this goal in mind, it becomes important to obtain an overall feel for the different types of neurotransmitters. Neurotransmitter's availability depends on certain nutritional and biochemical factors. These nutritional and biochemical factors need to be present in order for a happier and more efficient brain function.

The first group of neurotransmitters is called the biogenic amines. These same neurotransmitter molecules (epinephrine, nor-epinephrine, dopamine, histamine and serotonin), when they occur within the blood stream, are known as hormones. A large proportion of this group of informational substances exerts blood vessel effects on tone when acting as hormones. Thus the terms neurotransmitter and hormone are thought of as a distinction of where in the body their action occurs and not as different molecules.

Remember, the bioactive amines are found in the nervous system and blood stream. These same molecules are called hormones when they are within the blood stream and neurotransmitters when they are within the nervous system. Someday some contrary guy will successfully propose the simplified and unifying term, informational substance. This term will take the place of this confusing arbitrary semantics drama between hormone and neurotransmitter. Until that far off day it is probably wise to maintain a grasp for this duplicity of ways to say the same thing in as complicated a way as possible.

Examples of the precursors, which form the biogenic amine types of the neurotransmitters, are the amino acids: tyrosine, tryptophan, and histidine. Tyrosine can be converted into epinephrine (adrenaline), nor-epinephrine and dopamine. Tryptophan can be converted into serotonin and melatonin. Finally, histidine can be converted into histamine. A few others exist and these will be discussed later in the chapter in order to keep the initial discussion less burdensome.

The biosynthesis of these neurotransmitters depends, to varying degrees, on a number of nutritional cofactors (synthesis facilitators). Without sufficient cofactors these neurotransmitters' manufacture becomes impossible. When was the last time that anyone heard of a mainstream physician inquiring about the nutritional adequacy of a given owners ability to manufacture these essential neurotransmitters? This failure provides yet another example for how medical schools educational content proves deficient when compared to the holism of what science reveals.

For example, the conversion of tyrosine into the above neurotransmitters occurs in an orderly fashion. Each step of the progression requires specific reaction facilitators, called cofactors. Remember, the assembly line order of progression depends on adequate molecular replacement parts for each step of the manufacture process. Logically, health consequences follow when any one of these parts becomes deficient.

Tyrosine first converts to dopa, then into dopamine, then on into nor-epinephrine and finally into epinephrine. This may sound really boring and dull but underneath a superficial veneer of these qualities await an exciting youth preserving mechanism. This occurs because when one understands the simple cofactors that are needed in order to make proper amounts of each one of these neurotransmitters one can jump on the brain functioning advantage track that leads to vitality.

In order of need in the above listed assembly line progressions of neurotransmitter manufacture are: tetrahydrobiopterin (made from folate), vitamin C, vitamin B6, and finally S-adenosyl methionine (SAMe). These are the basic cofactors that are needed in their active form or synthesis along the assembly line from tyrosine to epinephrine comes to a halt. It should be emphasized that for each neurotransmitter molecule made: one to two vitamin C molecules are used, one tetrahydrobiopterin unloads, and one SAMe degrades.

For these reasons, unless a highly functional molecular re-supply system operates, these cofactors rapidly deplete. In addition, SAMe can only recharge if adequate folate, vitamin B6, vitaminB12, and the amino acid serine remain available. Recognize, each SAMe unloaded needs one molecule of folate, vitamin B12, and two serine's available or recharging it becomes impossible. Realize the need for a real food diet rather than memorize all these picky facts.

The demands for newly manufactured bioactive amines are much greater within the blood stream. The blood stream needs more bioactive amines because here these informational substances only exist for about 2 minutes. This means that within the blood stream, these informational substances have two minutes to convey their message, once released into the circulation, before their deactivation occurs. In contrast, they exist within nerves for much longer periods of time because once released they recycle many times.

When owners become mentally, not what they used to be, the cause could be from one or more of the above nutritional deficiencies. Recall, SAMe and the molecules which recharge it each time it donates a methyl group is called collectively, the methyl donor system. Also recall, the methyl donor system is used at the rate of one billion times per second. For this reason, owners become only as good as the least present nutrient within their methyl donor system.

Serotonin

One of the most likely bioactive amines to deplete comes from the amino acid tryptophan. The unique reason for this will be explained shortly. This amino acid occurs in high concentrations in eggs, dairy products, and turkey. This obviously shows why vegans develop far ranging mental impairments. This really isn't always true. It was included just to add joy to all those that are not vegans.

Serotonin deficiency becomes more likely, compared to the other bioactive amines, because some of it changes into melatonin each day. In contrast, the other neurotransmitters recycle more efficiently each time they discharge into the synapse because they do not change into other neurotransmitters. Serotonin within the brain is felt to be involved in arousal. Deficiency in the arousal state leads to one of the types of clinical depression.

This simple fact provides a business opportunity that has been well realized with the skyrocketing sales of drugs like Zoloft, Paxil, and Prozac. These drugs work by keeping the serotonin released between nerves around longer in the active little space between nerves called the synapse. These prescriptions poison the enzymatic machine, which pulls serotonin out of the active little space occurring between nerves, the synapse.

Without these enzyme machines being poisoned every day the serotonin would only affect arousal for a normal time per excretion of it into this little space. However with the advent of these drugs, which are able to penetrate the blood brain barrier, this enzymatic machine becomes incapacitated for a while. Consequently, the increased amounts of serotonin in this little space between the arousal nerves send the arousal message for a longer time.

It should be mentioned that two of the three of the above listed popular drugs in this class, contain the most powerful oxidizing element on the planet (stronger than the oxygen radical). This cannot be good when it penetrates the blood brain barrier by being attached to the carrier molecule (see below). How much of this breaks down within one's mind setting off a frenzy of rust production? The most powerful oxidizing element of all is fluorine and will be discussed latter in this chapter. It is mentioned here to help facilitate learning in regards to the other side of the story that science has revealed about the potential down side of what is for sale by the complex.

Here come the protest and rationalizations about how these types of antidepressant drugs saved Aunt Sally, a vegan, who no one could help before. However, stop for a moment and ponder what often fails being said, concerns the rate limiting step for serotonin manufacture depending on the amount of tryptophan delivered into the blood stream. Science, long ago revealed that serotonin levels within the brain directly relate to three factors. First, the amount of tryptophan consumed in the diet. Second, the ability of the digestive tract to absorb the tryptophan presented to it. Third, concerns the necessary presence of vitamin B6, which converts tryptophan into serotonin. This means that supplementing with tryptophan, vitamin B6, in the diet, and making sure that the digestive process remains operative will do what these expensive prescriptions will do.

The reason tryptophan as a supplement remains not readily available in America today results from suspect policies occurring within the FDA. How convenient, right when these new serotonin uptake poisons were to become the anti depressant drugs of the nineties, a single source of a contaminated batch of tryptophan was discovered. Later it was found that the only reason that this batch caused severe muscle toxicity was that a single Japanese company tried to save money by changing the standard protocol by which it was traditionally made (Wright 98). Since the FDA answers to almost no one they have used this excuse into the present time and thus limit effective strength tryptophan to prescription only. The prescription only designation makes this natural treatment much more expensive

Serotonin depletion occurs because of two general processes. First, within the pineal gland there is the daily need to manufacture melatonin from available serotonin. Second, depletion occurs if there are not enough cofactors or dietary derived tryptophan present within the brain and the pineal gland. Recall, the body requires only one cofactor to convert tryptophan to serotonin, vitamin B6. Recall as well, sufficient serotonin is required daily so that enough melatonin can be manufactured from it. In addition, the essential cofactor for melatonin synthesis from serotonin is SAMe. Remember, SAMe is an important methyl donor for biological molecules within the methyl donor system, mentioned above, which depletes within the body at the rate of one billion molecules a second.

The previous discussion mentioned the need for vitamin B12, folate and serine to keep SAMe recharged (possessing a methyl to donate). SAMe needs to be recharged each time it makes a new melatonin molecule. When healthy owners go to bed serotonin release slows within their brain. Conversely, melatonin made during the day and stored within the pineal gland flows into the blood stream with the onset of sleep. In young children the amount released is much higher and this gradually decreases until melatonin release becomes quite diminished in old age.

Adequate melatonin proves cornerstone to a good nights sleep. The high levels occurring with sleeping children may explain the soundness of their sleep. The above daily draining off of serotonin within the brain in order to make new melatonin each day explains the first reason why serotonin deficiency is more likely than other neurotransmitter deficiencies.

The second mechanism for brain serotonin depletion occurs when inadequate tryptophan becomes available to satisfy the body's serotonin and melatonin needs. Serotonin deficiency can occur from either poor dietary choices or a decreased ability of the digestive tract to properly dismantle proteins. In addition, the dietary deficiency of niacin (vitamin B3) will accelerate the body's usage of tryptophan. Tryptophan usage accelerates because it can be changed to niacin. Niacin deficiency causes the disease pellagra.

Realize, melatonin release into the blood stream, from the pineal gland during sleep depletes brain stores of this substance. Melatonin escapes each night when it rhythmically discharges into the blood stream, from the pineal gland, and performs its mysterious sleep enhancing activity. The melatonin released eventually degrades and then the kidneys remove it. Logically it follows that the continual drain off of melatonin from the brain causes the continual need for new sources of tryptophan. Actually 95% of body tryptophan depletes by processes occurring in the GI tract and blood platelets (explained below). For these cumulative reasons, tryptophan continuously degrades and therefore needs to be replaced by the diet.

In contrast, the other biogenic amine neurotransmitters operate under a theme of a highly effective recycling system. The other biogenic amines recycle more efficiently because they lack drain off processes for other uses within the blood stream. The other neurotransmitters release and recycle out of the little spaces between nerves, the synapse.

Here they deliver a message that each of their unique shapes imparts. Shortly after message delivery has been completed they recycle back to where they came, the nerve ending. Because of this recycling system the same rate of depletion does not occur with the other biogenic neurotransmitters.

Recognize the majority of serotonin, in the body, occurs outside the brain. The platelets and digestive tract contain the majority of serotonin within the body. Within the digestive tract it serves as a hormone that instructs this tube on how it should behave. Alternatively, the serotonin message contained within the blood platelets involves the orchestration of clotting parameters. In addition, it encourages blood vessel spasm (vasoconstriction).

The three above additional serotonin purposes utilize greater than 90% of total body serotonin content. Therefore, when owners take drugs that keep serotonin around longer (popular antidepressant medications SSRI types), then a percentage of the effect occurs within these areas! For example, this fact explains the common experience of increased gastrointestinal distress while taking these drugs.

It should be acknowledged that there are 7 different types of serotonin receptors. The drug companies research findings, which sell SSRI like drugs, documents that the highest affinity for these drugs occurs within the limbic system in the brain. The limbic system contains only type 6 and 7 receptors.

Serotonin levels also affect the amount of the hormone prolactin released from the pituitary. Prolactin may sound like another boring hormone at first. However, a higher prolactin level leads to inhibition of gonad function. Re-including this little detail helps explain the high rate of sexual dysfunction that commonly occurs when owners take these prescriptions.

This does not mean that serotonin reuptake inhibitors are never warranted. In fact once someone is prescribed them it is a pretty tricky business to safely navigate their discontinuation. However, the risk of decreased gonad function underscores the need to consider nutritional deficiencies early in the depression presentation. No side effects arise when one heals.

For this reason, while an owner takes these types of medications they should monitor their prolactin levels. Alternatively, if sexual dysfunction occurs, obtain a well-run twenty-four hour urine test for steroids. After a competent physician analyzes it, treatment strategies that lead to correcting the steroid defects can be instituted. For example, if the gonad steroids are found to be low and continued serotonin reuptake inhibitors are still warranted then natural sex hormone (bio-identical) replacement therapy could be considered.

Histamine

The next neurotransmitter, in the bioactive amines class, to be discussed is histamine. Histamine is manufactured from the amino acid histidine. This is an important neurotransmitter and hormone. Unfortunately, the role of this important informational substance is largely ignored. Histamine likely is ignored because there is a lot of money at stake, which revolves around the popular drugs known as the anti-histamines. This has far reaching implications on how physicians and owners are groomed in their thinking patterns.

Histamine secreting nerve cells (neurons) have their center (cell body's) within the tuberomamillary nucleus of the posterior hypothalamus. From here these neuron cell bodies send projections (axons) into all parts of the brain and spinal cord. These axons carry the nervous impulse to the next nerve synapse when histamine releases. Consequently, some of these axons are several feet long! For this reason, this small group of histamine secreting neurons, which connects to all parts of the nervous system, exerts a broad scope of influence. Some examples of histamine secreting nerves influence are: consciousness, blood pressure, pituitary hormone secretion, thirst and sexual behavior.

Mast cells are one type of immune system cell that tend to concentrate within the pituitary gland. Mast cells contain histamine. This is important because the pituitary gland is commonly known as the master hormone gland. This title is well deserved because under the direction of the higher brain structures the pituitary secretes powerful hormones that control the activity of the gonads, adrenals, thyroid, pancreas, placenta, and thymus.

Important point: Histamine levels, within the pituitary, modify the release of many of these master hormones (ACTH, FSH, LH, prolactin, TSH and GH). In addition to histamine, dopamine and serotonin within the pituitary, as well, all exert a modifying effect on how the pituitary responds to commands from the higher brain centers. The textbooks imply that it is the interplay between these three neurotransmitters, which influence the response of the master hormone gland to higher brain commands.

It is important to emphasize the bigger picture of histamine's role within the brain. These include its influence on consciousness level, sexual behavior, regulation of body secretions, regulation of the release of the pituitary hormones, blood pressure regulation, drinking fluids behavior, and in pain thresholds. Histamine is especially important in activating the sleep center within the brain, the diencepahlic sleep zone.

This doesn't mean that the popular anti-histamines are of low value in some medical conditions. Rather the implication is that the public deserves a better understanding for the consequences of chronically consuming a substance that affects powerful nervous system activities. Fortunately, anti-histamines often become unnecessary when one corrects the cause of their problem.

For example, the use of DGL licorice root for gastritis or heartburn was discussed in section three. In addition, the ways to evaluate the adrenal deficiency, which causes allergies, were discussed in the adrenal chapter. Food allergies, as well, cause much untold suffering, by their ability to inflict far reaching immunological reactions (allergic symptoms are one possibility). Finally, it is coming to be known the important role that high normal thyroid function plays in immune regulation (Barnes).

Epinephrine

The neurotransmitter, epinephrine conveys a sense of alertness within one's mind. Epinephrine is the crowning glory of what can only be manufactured when all the above listed biochemical cofactors are present (the methyl donor system plus vitamin C and tetrahydrobiopterin). Epinephrine's unique message properties have gone largely unrecognized and in its place there is a tendency to lump epinephrine's actions into those of nor-epinephrine and dopamine as well.

Add to this, the biochemical sloppiness that regards the common practice of trying to explain these three above listed bioactive amines in a complicated and arbitrary system of different types of receptors. Commonly these are referred to as: alpha 1, Beta 1, and Beta 2 receptors. Unfortunately, this method of limiting the discussion regarding each of the above three's actions by this arbitrary nomenclature perpetuates many a well-meaning physician's confusion.

Sometimes it helps to ignore the discussion of these arbitrary methods of 'pigeon holing' these informational substances receptors. In its place one can begin to glean an overall picture for why the body would prefer one of these neurotransmitters to the other. For example, one complication of ignoring the interplay between the different neurotransmitters is the over prescribing of anti-histamines when the real problem is diminished epinephrine production.

Most allergies occur by a peripheral action of histamine acting as a hormone and not as a neurotransmitter. However, when owners take many of the anti-histamines they are potentially affecting the neurotransmitter availability and the peripheral acting histamine that produce allergies (among other things). This approach always has side effects because of the central role that histamine plays within the brain (discussed above).

Recall, in the immune chapter it was discussed how often times it is safer to take epinephrine like medicines for allergy control than the anti-histamines so commonly utilized. The mantra about blood pressure elevation resulting from herbs like ephedra becomes largely the hype of clever little sound bytes of disinformation when the other side of what science has revealed is included (see immune and blood pressure chapters).

Never the less, when taking powerful medicinal herbs like ephedra it is wise to be followed closely by a physician just in case there is even the slightest chance that one's blood pressure could become elevated. In addition to epinephrine like medication for the short-term control of allergies it is always a good idea to check these owners' adrenal and thyroid glands function (see thyroid and adrenal chapters).

Perspective is added when one realizes that more people die from the complications of aspirin like medication in one week than have ever died of ephedrine or epinephrine treatments. Another possible role for epinephrine like medication involves the treatment of depressive illness. Epinephrine is safer than nor-epinephrine because it does not raise the blood pressure as avidly. However, before this possibility can be realized there needs to be adequate studies performed.

Nor-epinephrine and epinephrine

In regards to the neurotransmitter role of epinephrine and nor-epinephrine, these substances can only be manufactured, when the previously mentioned cofactors are available. Briefly these are: tetrahydrobiopterin, vitamin C, vitamin B6 and SAMe. Recall, SAMe degrades at the rate of one billion times a second within the body. It needs folate, vitamin B12 and serine to recharge it each time it donates a methyl to make epinephrine. Because nor-epinephrine and epinephrine are some of the major neurotransmitters, this is an important consideration.

Realizing the extent for the continual need of sufficient supplies of the above nutritional cofactors helps one to be open to yet another cause of some cases of clinical depression. Depression is often the result of a nutritional deficiency. These deficiencies affect the ability for these parts of the brain to manufacture these important molecules (see nutrition deficiency caused depression below).

Dopamine

Dopamine is the last, for now, of the bioactive amines needing to be discussed. Dopamine can be generalized to be involved with pleasure and fine motor coordination. When the part of the brain stem concerned with fine motor coordination fails in its production and release of dopamine, Parkinson's disease begins.

Cocaine usage is generally felt to result in the increased presence of dopamine within the pleasure centers of the brain. This is generally felt to happen because cocaine poisons this brain areas ability to reuptake dopamine within these little spaces between the pleasure nerves (synapses). Therefore more dopamine remains in these spaces. The higher the dopamine level within the synapse then the more messages conveyed for the pleasure message.

There is an additional important role of dopamine as a neurotransmitter within the brain that was briefly alluded to above. This regards its effects on pituitary hormones when its level increases. Like serotonin and histamine, mentioned above, dopamine as well affects the pituitary responsiveness from higher brain centers. Dopamine levels increase within the pituitary gland when the nerve endings within the hypothalamus release it.

The hypothalamus is the area of the brain immediately above the pituitary, which controls the pituitary secretions. In turn, higher brain centers control the hypothalamus. As dopamine increases, within the pituitary, Growth Hormone release is encouraged and prolactin release is discouraged. Conversely, as serotonin increases within the pituitary prolactin release is encouraged and Growth Hormone release is discouraged.

A pivotal point in the understanding for how one retains his/her youth far longer than his numerous peers now occurs. To better understand why, one needs to recall two things. First, increased prolactin levels directly correlates with decreased gonad function. Decreased gonad function means a lowered *steroid tone and pressure* will occur. Recall, *steroid pressure and tone* adequacy determine the ability to repair and regenerate. Consequently, when steroid tone and pressure diminish the wear and tear changes inflicted by life fail to repair properly.

Failed repair accelerates the aging process. The second point was more completely explained in the liver chapter. However, briefly stated Growth Hormone provides many youth conserving properties. As owners age, Growth Hormone levels gradually decline to low levels and become really low just before death. Logically, processes that increase Growth Hormone levels will tend to increase cellular rejuvenation activities described in the liver chapter. Higher pituitary dopamine levels encourage adequate Growth Hormone levels.

An additional concept deserves brief emphasis: Pituitary levels of dopamine inhibit TSH release. Recall also that thyroid hormone levels reaching the pituitary cells' DNA programs (genes) determine how much

Growth Hormone is made within this master hormone gland. In this powerful way well meaning physicians that prescribe dopamine raising medications (Wellbutrin) can inadvertently accelerate their patients aging rate. For this reason, patients on these types of medications need to have their thyroid hormone status followed closely. Of particular note concerns the fact that in these cases the TSH level will mislead treatment decisions because these types of medications inhibit its release. Here, the more accurate free T3 and free T4 better guide dosage decisions of thyroid replacement.

Applying Biochemistry to Longevity

Millions of Americans' depression symptoms are treated with serotonin reuptake inhibitors (SSRI) medication. SSRI like medications raise the level of serotonin within the brain. Recall, increased serotonin within the brain has the potential to raise prolactin and decrease Growth Hormone. It's instructive now to return to the consequences of an increased prolactin secretion and decreased Growth Hormone secretion coming out of the pituitary gland. This situation results when serotonin levels become increased in the brain. Realize, aberrations in Growth Hormone and prolactin levels can injure certain body tissues. One example of potentially vulnerable body tissue secondary to these types of hormone imbalances is heart valve tissue.

Cardiac (heart) valves are made from specialized cartilage tissue. As was discussed earlier in the joint chapter, a big part of the continued health of cartilage relies on the quality of the message content it receives. When high quality message content occurs these types of cells are instructed to invest appropriate energy in rejuvenation activities. The big players in this regard were said to be adequate androgen and Growth Hormone. When these two hormone groups reach these cell type's rejuvenation activity becomes possible.

A few years ago certain pharmaceutical companies expressed great surprise and remorse when it became obvious that some owners who took the popular diet drug, fenfluramine (commonly known as the fen-phen diet of which fenfluramine was one of the components), developed heart valve damage. A common denominator for how these owners' heart valves were injured emerges if one applies the previous discussion in regards to increased serotonin levels within the pituitary gland. This is because drugs like fenfluramine raise pituitary levels of serotonin.

It becomes even more alarming when one realizes that the popular antidepressants Prozac, Paxil and Zoloft are all structurally related, to varying degrees at the molecular level, to that of fenfluramine. These types of drugs also tend to raise pituitary serotonin levels. It is important to recall that higher serotonin levels, within the pituitary, have been noted to raise prolactin levels and decrease Growth Hormone levels.

Now it is important to apply the above previous discussion, which regards the role of increased prolactin and decreased Growth Hormone on the tissues like heart valves. First, the increased pituitary serotonin causes increased prolactin release and this increase inhibits gonad function. The inhibition includes androgen release and production from the gonads. Second, when there is decreased Growth Hormone and androgen message content reaching cardiac valve tissue, there is a diminished message to instruct these cells to rejuvenate.

The heart valve cells need instruction to invest appropriate energy into repair and rejuvenation activities. For these reasons, with low Growth Hormone and high prolactin in operation some owners' heart valves will succumb to disrepair. This scenario provides a likely mechanism of injury for these patients' heart valves, after they ingested these types of medications.

Realize, the PDR does not group fenfluramine as a serotonin reuptake inhibitor (SSRI)! Even though its molecular configuration is like these other antidepressants. However, if one examines their molecular structures and active sites it becomes probable that the PDR division is arbitrary.

The PDR and pharmaceutical text discuss the possibility of Growth Hormone secretion depression for all of these substances including fenfluramine. In addition, the basic medical physiology text link increased pituitary serotonin levels to an increase in prolactin secretion and to a decrease in Growth Hormone secretion. It is important to point out that because fenfluramine has been known to damage heart valves, this drug probably raises pituitary serotonin levels more than the others do.

Unfortunately, very few doctors or patients are made aware of these potential dangers. Some of the confusion occurs because of the likely arbitrary divisions in classification between fenfluramine and the other SSRI drugs. Continued risk is really unnecessary if the public still had affordable access to tryptophan.

Alternatively, owners who need these medications should be followed for elevated prolactin and decreased Growth Hormone levels. These same owners should also have their heart valve function checked until the actual risks are quantitated. When either of these tests results become abnormal then supplementation could be considered to correct the deficiencies of either androgen or Growth Hormone.

A comment on perhaps a safer way to treat depression with medication

It was previously mentioned that some anti-depression medication works by raising brain dopamine levels. Increasing dopamine levels within the brain will decrease prolactin and raise Growth Hormone levels. The downside to this medication is the slight risk for seizure while taking this drug. In addition, the thyroid status needs to be monitored while on this medication (explained above and below) because dopamine depresses TSH release.

Recall, low thyroid states accelerate the aging rate mainly because T3's sufficient presence within the pituitary is required for the proper stimulation of the pituitary to manufacture Growth Hormone (50% of pituitary cells devoted to this purpose). In fact, the highest T3 receptor concentration within the body occurs here at 8,000-10,000 per pituitary cell.

This fact allows one to see perhaps another advantage for ensuring high normal thyroid function.

Beyond treating depression, the advantage of this approach arises from raising Growth Hormone levels and suppressing prolactin levels (as long as thyroid function remains adequate). Recall, the SSRI like drugs create the reverse situation in that they favor prolactin but inhibit Growth Hormone release. Most if the time middle aged and depressed owners need all the Growth Hormone they can muster and usually suffer already from a climbing prolactin level.

All drugs cause side effects. Sometimes physicians prescribe antidepressants to stabilize a bad situation. Here the emphasis regards the lesser of two evils. Choose the least toxic path to stabilize the downward spiral of depression and then work on holistic strategies towards healing the root cause of the depression.

The scientific name for this medication is burprion (Wellbutrin). Stopping short of abusing cocaine, with all its predictable sad consequences, this is one of the most reliable methods for raising brain dopamine content. Dopamine is the neurotransmitter responsible for pleasure.

Remember, if one chooses the Wellbutrin route of treatment, they need to have their thyroid function monitored. Thyroid monitoring becomes necessary because whenever dopamine levels rise within the pituitary, thyroid function depresses because TSH (stands for thyroid stimulating hormone) falls off. For this reason, when this medication causes a depressed thyroid function, the popular conventional test for TSH will be unreliable as a measure of thyroid function.

Better yet, upon awakening, obtain armpit temperatures. This provides a supportive first step but twenty-four hour urine, for thyroid function, will also be helpful. The important point here concerns the fact that Wellbutrin has potential advantages, in the treatment of depression, when its side effect profile is understood. The downside involves monitoring patients for possible thyroid dysfunction. For the reasons listed above, this will avoid missing thyroid dysfunction caused by this medication. Realize, thyroid dysfunction is more easily treated than attempting to rectify compromised gonads and Growth Hormones status.

Until dietary tryptophan or ephedra again becomes available the Wellbutrin method of treating depression is less risky to one's health than SSRI type medication. In addition, there is a group of owners who will dramatically respond to nutritional supplementation for the manufacture of the needed neurotransmitters discussed above. These healing steps can be worked into the treatment plan.

2) The Brain's molecular building parts replacement program

Brain molecular building parts include unique components. Some of the need for unique brain molecular components arises because the brain is composed of more fat than nerve in its makeup. In turn, the fats, which make up one's mind, are constructed with unique components. Unique components are needed within the brain because fat serves as insulation to prevent electrical cross firing between the different nerve cells. Adequate molecular supplies are also necessary to rebuild the brain structures that wear out. In addition, the continuous need exist to replace the nerve cell enzymatic machines that begin to breakdown.

Realize, the high metabolic rate of the brain increases the rate at which molecular parts become defective. Because the brain burns about 25% of the oxygen within the body, at normal basal conditions, it is more vulnerable to 'rusting' (oxidation damage) than are many other body tissues. As stated above, the brain is composed of more fat than nerve by weight and this fact increases the rust vulnerability many times. The increase in vulnerability results from the rusting processes creating rancid fats within the mind.

It is accurate to describe the brain as a fatty bag containing nerves, hormones and neurotransmitters. In health, the fatty bag releases in a rhythmical manner the appropriate amount of informational substances between the various nerves (the neurotransmitters). Concurrently, there is a rhythmical release, from the brain, of other informational substances into the blood stream (the hormones). The rhythm of the brain's release of information breaks down when ongoing replacement parts fail to be replaced as they wear out. This subsection concerns what the brain needs to regenerate. Since fat is the number one component which makes up one's mind its procurement is emphasized next.

Fat is the major building block that makes up one's mind

The brain is really just a bag of fat. Brain fat has well connected nerve cells within it. In addition, within the brain fat are some specialized areas that secrete powerful informational substances into the blood stream. Therefore the quality of this fat proves as a pivotal point for continued intelligence.

Some owners make the procurement of molecular replacement parts for their fat bag a difficult process. No one counsels these owners about how all their brain fat is kept in the right place. In addition, they usually have not a clue about how to take out the fat trash that begins to stink. Anyone knows that when fat becomes bad it begins to smell rancid. Also, certain fats serve as a support and cushion for the brain's delicate connections. In addition, fat keeps the electrical activity confined by its effective insulating abilities. Because the fat in the brain has so much to accomplish, it makes sense that these fats are special. Because brain fats are special and they have unique needs in order to keep them from rotting.

Myelin coated nerves provide examples of how fat's integrity within one's mind rests on the continued replacement of certain fats, which have rotted. Scientific writings frequently mention myelin coated nerves and their importance for optimal brain and nerve functioning. In fact the disease, multiple sclerosis, results from injury and breakdown of the myelin coating around these nerves. Myelin serves an example of one of the specialized fats occurring within the nervous system. Unfortunately, by naming it, myelin, a disconnection occurs for the obvious need for certain fats and perpetuates physicians recommending more peripheral treatment decisions.

Important nutritional factors need to occur in order for myelin fat to remain healthy. Additionally, certain informational substances need to be around in adequate amounts in order for optimal myelin synthesis to be maintained. Progesterone proves central for example, in the directing of adequate myelin sheath formation (see below).

Another example of the unique needs of the brain for its ongoing molecular replacement program is the neurotransmitter, acetylcholine. The choline half is a specialized fat component needed in large quantities within the mind for neurotransmitter formation and specialized fat formation, including myelin sheath formation. The need for choline is underscored by its role in the synthesis of the neurotransmitter acetylcholine. This use of choline is in addition to the important, already mentioned, synthesis of the myelin sheath.

Now that the discussion centers on fat, which builds one's mind, it is important to include the neurotransmitter, acetylcholine. Acetylcholine is derived from joining choline and acetate. The choline half, in addition, provides a component of the specialized fat (myelin sheath) needed for the structural and insulating properties within the brain. Acetylcholine is the major neurotransmitter of the brain and nerves of the body. Ample supplies of choline are easily obtained with a high fat diet.

Conversely, owners who subsist on a low fat diet make their nervous systems acquirement of choline difficult and draining to other body systems. In order to make one choline molecule from scratch, three SAMe molecules degrade unless all the recharging cofactors (see below) remain present. Alternatively,, owners who regularly ingest quality sources of choline negate the need for depleting SAMe stores. Eggs and fish prove as exceptional sources.

In addition to these first few structural components, another important molecular building block for structural brain fats is called phosphatidylcholine. Laypersons commonly call phosphatidylcholine, lecithin. The important point here is that all brains and nerves in the body need a continuous and adequate supply of these essential building blocks or neurological efficiency compromises.

For example, remember, the nervous system continually needs new sources of choline for its building block role. The nervous system uses choline for so many of its ongoing construction processes. Because these processes are so numerous within the brain, failure to include this in one's diet could eventually deplete the methyl donor system (SAMe, vitamin B12, folate, serine, and methionine). Recall, the methyl donor system already depletes at the rate of one billion times a second under normal circumstances.

When was the last time anyone heard about a Western trained physician counseling their middle aged patient, who was concerned about brain function, about this basic scientific fact? Again it is not a mean spirited conspiracy but rather a result of yet another evisceration from the mainstream medical education in regards to the importance of basic preventative and nutritional advice.

How one makes more intelligent choices on how to supply their brains with the highest quality fats is the topic of this subsection. In general terms, regular consumption of fish, eggs and olive oil are a start. Realize free range chicken eggs and wild fish make the difference because of the essential fatty acids found in them are adequate. Whereas caged and farmed fish lack these important essentials. Greens provide the wild animals with a source of essential fatty acids. Wild fish eat greens like plankton and free-range chickens eat greens as well. In addition, the lecithin found in eggs is important. Finally, the vitamins that make up the methyl donor system are fundamental, as well, in order to preserve or regain mental function.

The point is that brain structure as well as maintenance requires particular and unique molecular building parts needs. Owners who make it easier on their brains to acquire these basic essentials enjoy an advantage for brain longevity. Unfortunately, this information within basic medical textbooks presents in a scattered and confusing way. The time has come for a re-inclusion of these basic scientific facts, in a way that physicians and patients can understand. The uniqueness of the fuel delivery requirements for brain function further explains how the brain becomes vulnerable when molecular parts replacement becomes compromised.

3) Fuel delivery to brain cells is crucial

Many owners are walking around on this planet that are mentally not as clear as they once were. Complaints of brain 'fog' early on in these patients typify the presentation. Later, they go on to develop hypoglycemic events. In the extreme cases, fainting and seizure disorders can result. Many of these patients have in common fuel delivery problems within their brain.

Brain cells are more vulnerable to fuel delivery interruptions than other body cells. Two central reasons explain the brain's increased vulnerability to fuel interruption. First the brain can only burn sugar for fuel. Therefore the brain becomes vulnerable to injury when the blood sugar falls. Second, the brain has a high rate of fuel usage (high metabolic rate). If fuel supplies interrupt, brain cells' function quickly impairs.

The brain is different than most other body tissues in that its ability to uptake sugar is independent of insulin or IGF-1 levels. Thus unlike most other body cells the brain can suck up sugar without insulin like message content.

Many owners suffer form various vague forms of mental dysfunction. Sometimes these conditions occur only because their physician fails to consider issues of fuel delivery to the brain. Fuel delivery problems to the brain largely result from imbalanced hormones.

The problem for most owners that suffer from low blood sugars involves a failure in their body's ability to mount an effective counter hormone response to insulin. Excessive counter response hormones become necessary to counter insulin's desire to direct the liver to suck every last sugar molecule out of their blood stream. Often, middle-aged owners suffer from excessive insulin need (popularly called insulin resistance as if it remains a mystery). Diminished IGF-1 explains excessive insulin need.

As discussed earlier, hormones operate on a system of balance. Balanced blood sugars only occur when the proper balance between insulin and the four counter response hormones exist. The counter balance hormones to insulin are glucagon, Growth Hormone, epinephrine and cortisol.

By far, after middle age, the most important counter regulatory hormone to insulin is cortisol (see liver and digestion chapters). In contrast, youthful and healthy owners regulate their blood sugar between meals more with Growth Hormone than other counter regulatory hormones. This fact provides a pivotal health advantage occurring only in the healthiest owners. Middle-aged failure of Growth Hormone and/or its consequence, a falling IGF-1 level becomes the norm and consequently cortisol needs increase. As explained earlier this compensation causes health consequences (section two and the liver chapter).

For these reasons, healing these owners usually requires restoring hormonal balance. When was the last time a Western trained physician was seen counseling about hormonal balance being central to healing these symptoms? Again this is not meant as a criticism of the many fine physicians desiring to help their patients but rather as an observation of yet another evisceration of what the holism of science has revealed. Instead, in the place of healing, Western trained physicians are trained to prescribe frequent feedings of carbohydrate, which predictably results in a fatter patient.

Important point: A return to hormone balance allows healing brain fuel delivery problems. Contrast this approach with constantly loading the 'antique weight scale' with insulin and then constantly re-supplying the body with more sugar before insulin sucks the blood sugar down again. Alarmingly, additional methods are often employed that involve correcting the brain fuel delivery problem by encouraging excessive inferior counter weight message content. Adding to the misery concerns the fact that additional owners, for one reason or another, become enfeebled in their ability to secrete the ever increasing 'counter weight' of cortisol to the 'weight' of increasing insulin required by high carbohydrate diets, and suffer from low blood sugar episodes.

Physicians who recognize the fundamental body theme of hormonal balance in the healthful state can counsel their patients to restrict carbohydrate. A restriction of carbohydrate lowers the need for insulin. Lowered insulin leads to a lessened need for the counter hormones, like cortisol. Exercise also has a profound stabilizing effect on one's blood sugars (muscle chapter).

The above two lifestyle changes make mechanistic sense if one obtains a cognizance for the importance of balance. In other words, less counter weight (diminished adrenal function) means one needs to decrease the need for making the weight (insulin) secreting into the blood stream. Attention to this basic understanding allows the 'antique weight scale of hormonal balance' to return to optimum. When this occurs then the symptoms of 'brain fog', anxiety secondary to roller coasting blood sugars, seizure disorders from low blood sugar, and weight gain from the commonly prescribed hypoglycemic promoting diet begin to resolve (liver chapter).

4) The blood vessels within the brain

The next physical determinant of brain health involves the blood vessels. Much of what was discussed in the blood vessel chapter remains applicable to the cranial blood vessels. However, here the discussion requires additional material that emphasizes the particular vulnerabilities of the brain's vessels.

The first vulnerability of the brain vessels results from the volume of blood flowing within the brain. The brain contains 25% of the total volume of blood in the basal state. This high volume means that the brain blood vessel lining cells have a higher rate of exposure to rust producers (oxidizing agents) than in other parts of the body. For this reason, owners who have elevated levels of oxidizing agents (rust producers) and/or low levels of anti-oxidants suffer vulnerability to cranial blood vessel injury.

The second vulnerability of the brain's blood vessels arises from these vessels coursing through a closed box (the skull). Blood that leaks from a brain vessel has nowhere to go without squishing delicate nerves and ripping them from their precise connections. For this reason, processes that weaken the blood vessels do more damage to the brain than similar insults inflict elsewhere in the body.

Last, nerve cells are the most vulnerable of all body cell types to an interruption in oxygen and nutrient supply. In fact, one minute after an interruption in blood flow occurs, because of their high metabolic rate, neurons start to die. Even the high energy consuming heart cell can be oxygen and nutrient starved for up to 4 hours before it dies (myocardial infarction). This fact is partially explained by the high-energy requirements that neurons demand to power up their force fields (cell charge). Adequate cell voltage allows these cell types to maintain their action potentials and keep out injurious ions like calcium (see below).

Realize, the brain creates a higher electrical charge (cell voltage) than other parts of the body. The high electrical charge of the brain is used to power the nerves transmissions between one another (the action potential). Consequently, a loss of voltage causes the neurons to become vulnerable. All cells but especially nerves deteriorate when the energy for current generation becomes compromised (see 8 below for mechanism).

5) The hormones giveth and the hormones taketh away one's mind

Specific informational substances (hormones) direct the process for how one preserves their nerve cells physical integrity. Recall, the genes provide nothing until the right hormone arrives. Consequently, only when the proper mixtures of informational substances courses through the brain blood vessels will the nerve cells direct available energy to rejuvenate and repair themselves.

Similar to other body cells, adequate repair and rejuvenation activities depend on the nerve cells receiving the proper directions to spend energy wisely. Some of these necessary hormone mixtures direct appropriate absorption of minerals, vitamins, molecular building parts and fuel. Still other necessary brain hormones promote adequate cellular infrastructure investment and rejuvenation activities. Cellular infrastructure investment activities include: new cell machines (enzymes); new cell factories (organelles); toxin and waste removal, etc. Realize nerve cell rejuvenation activities concern repair activities. Examples of repair activities are: new outside the nerve cell support framework where it is damaged, new enzymes and mineral pumps, rotten fats replacement, DNA repair and stabilization, etc.

Mantra: The steroids like hormones (level 1) are the only hormones within the body that penetrates through all body tissues. Once these most powerful hormones penetrate one's mind they then instruct the nerve cell DNA programs (genes). Which DNA programs activate or repress centrally determines how that nerve cell spends its energy (repair vs. survival continuum). All other hormone types (levels 2 through 4) encounter limits as to where in the body they can penetrate.

For example, many other body hormones cannot penetrate the blood brain barrier. However, all the steroids, thyroid hormones, and vitamin A can penetrate into the central nervous system. Once inside the quality of their type and amount determines the appropriateness of the many different nerve cells DNA programs (genes) activity level.

The DNA contains the genes. Which genes turns on at any given time determine the quality of proteins present in nerve cells. Remember, like other body cells, the adequacy of protein content and types forms a central determinant of cell vitality. Metabolically active proteins constitute the part of the body that consumes calories in the reactions of life. Structural proteins, as well, optimize nerve cell function.

For this reason, lousy steroid amounts or types arriving in the brain result in poor gene activation. Recall the genes provide nothing until the right hormone arrives. For these reasons, in general, processes that increase the *steroid pressure and tone* will impart to owners a longevity advantage. In contrast, processes that decrease the *steroid pressure and tone* within the brain allow deterioration to occur more quickly.

Owners who enjoy optimally functioning gonads and adrenals possess the ability to direct the wise use of nerve cell energy within their mind. Optimally functioning gonads and adrenals serve this role because they capably create optimal *steroid pressure and tone* (section two). In addition, the brain can make some of its own steroids but this ability varies among different owners. This means that even when the gonads and adrenals begin to fail in some owners their brain provides an effective back up system of its own for the manufacture of its steroids. Some brains therefore enjoy a degree of protection not afforded to other body systems when the adrenals and gonads fail.

However, all three areas of steroid production (the adrenals, gonads and brain) become potentially compromised when the body perceives stress. Stress redirects the nervous system energy into survival activities and away from repair and rejuvenation activities within one's mind. Conceptualize the continuum of possible message content a nerve cell receives as efficient on down to lousy.

Modern life's complexities are stressful: time deadlines; financial worries; job security worries; relationship worries; keeping up with the Jones etc. Stress damages certain brain tissues involved in learning and memory. Stressful living increases the lifetime exposure of these brain tissues to cortisol (one of the body's main stress hormones). Recall, cortisol is a major player as an informational substance involved in redirecting cell energy into survival pathways and away from cellular maintenance activities. The body's cells can't discern if the stress is real or imagined.

Either real or imagined stress causes cortisol levels to increase. Cortisol is just one of the important informational substances that make up message content delivered to cells during stress. Excessive exposure of these brain structures to cortisol has been implicated as a major mechanism of cell death in the brain. The cortisol message channels energy into survival pathways.

Whenever energy chronically channels into survival pathways profound postponement in rejuvenation activities occurs. If stressful events occur only occasionally or are otherwise mitigated by adequate periods of behavioral and environmental restorative activities, then some delayed effects are noted in the degenerative process (section two). However, if stress becomes chronic, the daily cortisol message continuously defers the rejuvenation activities, which the brain needs for its peak performance.

Important point: Chronic high cortisol production rates direct nerve cell energy away from rejuvenation activities and towards survival pathways. The lack of rejuvenation activities leads to an increase in brain wear and tear changes. This results from the chronic message of survival being delivered to one's nerve cells. During the stress response the learning and memory centers in the brain are not a teleological part of the *emergency cell team*.

The *emergency cell team* denotes the cells in the body, which preferentially obtain ample energy during the survival response. Examples of these areas within the brain are found in the cerebellum and vision centers. Some additional examples of other body cells, which are part of the *emergency cell team*, are found in the muscle, heart, and lungs. The emergency response cell team cells, during stress, receive metabolic energy to mount the bodies perceived survival challenge. However, they are asked by cortisol message content to put on hold critical cellular maintenance activities. The difference between the two groups of body cells concerns that the emergency response cells of the body receive ample fuel delivered during the perceived emergency. Thus cortisol excess causes deferred maintenance throughout the body. In addition, chronic shunting of fuel away from the memory and learning centers contribute to brain aging.

The effects of chronic stress on the brain are exacerbated when the stressors are of an unpredictable nature in timing and intensity. The additional promoters of chronic stress changes are a feeling of hopelessness, and if the personality of the owner is emotionally reactive. Finally, the brain will age more quickly when less than optimal social support exists, as well. In the end, all three of the above exacerbations of the stress response accelerate the brain-aging rate by increasing cortisol levels.

Thankfully, the destructive effects to one's brain arising from the chronic elevation of cortisol can be somewhat mitigated when adequate counter balance occurs from the androgens. Balance between the catabolic effects (body wasting effects) of cortisol (and the other stress hormones) and regular secretions of the counterbalancing anabolic hormones (the rejuvenating and strength giving hormones) deliver restorative potential (positive nitrogen balance). Remember, cortisol delivers catabolic (uses up body structures for fuel generation) message content. In addition, recall, all steroids have the powerful ability to instruct the cells DNA programs (genes). Consequently, the relative proportions of each type determine which genes turn off and on. Therefore, the quality, timing and amount of each steroid type interacting with a given brain cell centrally determines whether it simply hangs on in survival or it efficiently repairs the wear and tear that life inflicts.

Recall, all steroids derive from cholesterol stores in the adrenal, gonads, and to a limited extent the brain. However, each steroid possesses unique message content, contained in its precise shape, for how it directs body energy usage. **Some of the steroids increase molecular part buildup activities (positive nitrogen balance) within a given cell type and these are called anabolic. Alternatively, some of them encourage burning different body structures for fuel (negative nitrogen balance) to maximize survival during emergencies and these are called catabolic.** Finally there are the steroid-like hormones concerned with maintaining the minerals within the body at an optimum level for structure and maintaining the cellular force field (aldosterone, thyroid hormones and vitamin D). The brain, like other body tissues, needs a balance between all three types of steroid message content.

Within the brain, the anabolic steroids are DHEA, progesterone, androstenedione, testosterone, and dihydrotestosterone. Different body tissues respond preferentially to the different anabolic steroids. For example, blood vessel health seems particularly responsive to DHEA and possibly progesterone. Also, brain myelin producing Schwann cells need a steady message from progesterone to optimize its nerve cell protective effects. GABA producing neurons in the spinal cord need adequate progesterone as well, or anxiety and irritability occurs. In addition, DHEA concentrates within the brain at five to six times the blood level when the brain remains healthy. Take home point; each body tissue has a specific anabolic steroid, which it optimally responds.

Examples of anabolism can be summarized in a broad way beyond the strict sense of sufficient protein that it designates. For example sufficient protein optimizes toxin removal (taking out the cellular garbage), enzyme replacement (new cellular machines), rejuvenation of the cell membrane, and the manufacture of new organelles (cellular factories unique to each cell type). For longevity considerations the trick is to have enough anabolic tone influence (optimal amounts of DHEA, testosterone, progesterone, etc.) to counterbalance the possible deleterious effects of chronic stress elicited cortisol release. As mentioned earlier certain brain structures because of their increased metabolic rate, are particularly vulnerable to increased cortisol message without adequate counterbalancing of the anabolic steroids.

Adequate anabolic steroid levels within one's mind remain possible only if several things occur regularly within the owner's body. First, there needs to be adequate functional capabilities in the gonads and/or adrenal glands. One or both of these paired glands needs to be sufficiently capable of producing the factory order of increased anabolic steroid production. If the bank vault is empty (ill or near dead adrenals and/or gonads) a response to stimulants towards increasing anabolic steroid production fails to manifest.

Unfortunately, many owners exist that suffer from toxin exposure, surgical procedures, lifestyle, and/or poor glandular constitution. For different reasons, each of these owners' glands exist with some degree of gonad or adrenal failure, which needs to be addressed before improved anabolic steroid output becomes possible. Second, there needs to be an adequate regular stimulus, to produce optimal anabolic steroids. Healthy sports competitions, regular aerobic exercise, warm nutritive relationships, as well as positive emotions (happiness, joy, forgiveness, singing, and love) all directly stimulate more optimal anabolic steroid amounts. Of course amorous romantic and sexual attractions cause bank withdrawals in the capable gonad.

Finally, it should be stressed that the steroid hormones all derive from cholesterol or more rarely from plant derived sources containing high progesterone content (natural progesterone can serve as a precursor for some of the other steroids' biosynthesis). Progesterone easily converts, once inside the adrenal or gonad tissues, to some of the other types of steroids, if the body's intelligence sees fit.

This turns out to be a practical consideration because as bodies age, a decreased ability to manufacture steroids from the cholesterol precursor route occurs. The failing rate-limiting step seems to be in the freeing up of cholesterol within the cell so it can be delivered to the mitochondria (the site of the first chemical reactions in the synthesis of the steroid hormones). Deficiencies of pantothenic acid and vitamin A seem to greatly diminish the ability of these tissues to manufacture steroids. Within the immune and adrenal chapters the reason why these nutrients prove so important was explained.

Beyond the repair and maintenance of the neurons (nerves) are the always-lurking destructive forces, which gain access to one's mind. One example of such a destructive process involves those molecular substances, which tend to promote rust within one's mind. Thankfully the properly nourished owner contains adequate molecules to counter the rust promoters.

6) The rust promoters versus the rust retardants

The next determinant of brain function regards the level of rust promoters versus rust retardants. Rust promoters are called oxidants. Rust retardants are called anti-oxidants. Alternatively, the duplicity of saying the same thing occurs by discussing a given element's electro-negativity. Electro-negativity denotes, in chemical jargon, the ability of a specific element to grab electrons (oxidize or rust) other elements or molecules. It becomes very important not to lose sight of these interchangeable terms if one wishes to avoid becoming the victim of what fails being said.

The top four rust producing atomic elements on the planet (out of more than one hundred are; fluorine, oxygen, chorine and sulfur. The ability of an element to produce rust regards their power of electro-negativity. What a certain element's electro-negativity is determines the ability of that element to rust or oxidize other molecules. Fluorine has the highest electronegativity among all the 100 plus atomic elements. This electro negativity scale gradates the rust promoting abilities relative to an interaction with all the other elements and molecular combinations possible within the world. In other words, the most powerful electron hog (rust promoter) on the planet is fluorine followed by oxygen then chlorine and finally sulfur.

Consequently, when any of these oxidizing elements arrive within the brain they had better be happy (stable) or the cellular consequence of rust formation results. Because human bodies contain greater than 60% water, some protection always exists. Protection occurs when elements like chlorine are bathed in sufficient water and then become largely free of a tendency to bind to body structures. Sufficient water creates a way for chlorine to associate loosely (dissolve) with oppositely charged elements within body fluids (sodium, potassium, and calcium).

However, this quality remains largely absent for oxygen and fluorine in the ionic form. Much attention regarding less potent oxidizing agents occurs within the media sound bites. It helps to be less gullible when one stays mindful of the big four electron hogs on the planet. Remember, these are the radicals of: fluorine, oxygen, chlorine, and sulfur. Also remember that even after the free radicals of these elements hog an electron and become ions (fluoride, oxide, chloride, and sulfide) they still powerfully desire binding to an oppositely charged body structure or cellular machine.

Most of the time the oxygen (oxide) and fluorine (fluoride) ion are the main rust promoters to be concerned with in one's mind. A prime example of the reactivity of fluoride occurs with its propensity to react with tooth and bone tissue. Sure it makes these tissues harder but what is often left out is the fact that fluorine also makes these same

tissues more brittle. Brittleness provides one measure of oxidation occurring within body tissue. Here lies the concern of elements like fluorine and oxygen in the unpaired state within one's mind.

Oxidizing agents can damage one's mind by two different mechanisms. First, and more common with oxygen but less common with fluorine, is the unstable radical. The oxygen radical denotes the state of unpaired oxygen before it steals an electron (s) from a weaker atom. This occurs with oxygen because of the process described in chapter one. Briefly, chapter one describes oxygen cleavage explosions within the mitochondria of numerous body cells. Because tremendous amounts of oxygen (oxygen gas contains two oxygen atoms bound together) get cleaved each day in an owner's life, consequent small amounts of oxygen radical are generated.

Oxygen radical occurs whenever the split of the two atoms, O2, gets outside of the 'armor' of the mitochondria chemical reaction chamber. For this reason, owners who lack sufficient ability to deal with oxygen radical leakage suffer from diseases that result from oxygen radicals injuring body cells. One proto-typical disease associated with this defect, in the unpaired oxygen mop up team, is Lou Gahrig's disease (amyotrophic lateral sclerosis). Amyotrophic lateral sclerosis involves a process that kills the motor nerves within the spinal cord. These cells die because either an increased production rate or decreased ability to neutralize oxygen radical formation occurs.

The second way that oxidizing agents (rust promoters) injure nerve cells occurs after the radical has hogged an electron. For example, the second mechanism occurs after the electron hog like oxygen and fluorine radicals have already stolen an electron from somewhere else (now they are called ions). Scientists denote this state by acknowledging a negative charge to these elements. Oxygen in this state is called oxide. Fluorine in this state is called fluoride.

Importantly, even after their radical form has hogged an additional electron and become an ion (negatively charged one), they still tend to bind to positively charged body structures. Unfortunately, when these hogs bind in this manner they alter the recipient molecules' properties and shape. Realize, the fluoride and oxide forms can do this. One needs oxygen for life and therefore curtailment here is only possible by limiting intake of the salts of oxygen (see blood vessel chapter) and in attempting to breath air that has less oxidizing properties (commonly called clean air).

Fluorine gas has two fluorine atoms bound together but if they split apart the radical is formed. In turn, fluorine radical is the same as fluoride except this name modification designates that it has already hogged an electron of its own. Important point: Negatively charged fluoride still powerfully desires to bind to positively charged structures or enzymes.

Already mentioned was the popular example of fluoride binding the tooth enamel and bone readily. Again, what often fails being said involves that it not only becomes harder but often these tissues become more brittle as well. Brittleness provides another example of the rusting process (aging process) occurring within. For these reasons, fluoride and oxide within one's mind remain a concern.

The example of fenfluramine needs to be recalled (see earlier discussion) because it contains fluoride. The fluoride contained within fenfluramine has the potential to release fluoride within one's mind. Recall, the brain's number one protection from outside toxicities involves its highly functioning blood brain barrier. Consequently, pharmaceutical agents that contain designs capable of penetrating beyond this barrier potentially cause great harm if they contain injurious atoms. The fluoride content of fenfluramine provides such an example.

For example, a journal of the American Medical Association article disclosed direct evidence that fenfluramine (one of the components of the popular fen-phen diet) damages neurons cultured in Petri dishes. About the same time of that disclosure it was discovered that fenfluramine was injuring heart valves (see earlier discussion). Three fluorine atoms occur on each fenfluramine molecule!

Even more alarming, other widely used SSRI type prescription drugs, which deliver fluoride to the brain, also occur. For example, Prozac has the same amount of fluorine as fenfluramine! The other popular and related antidepressant, Paxil, contains one fluorine. In addition, if one inquires into the chemical structure of these previously mentioned SSRI drugs, commonly prescribed to treat depression they all possess an aromatic ring. Causing even more concern involves the fact that fenfluramine has this same aromatic ring structure where the fluorides attach in the same position as Prozac. These facts point to the possibility that the popular SSRI type drugs are more related to the recalled, fenfluramine than the medical literature reveals. Awareness of this possibility makes it worthwhile to consider more completely about how one heals nutritionally from depression (discussed later).

The politics of scientific information

The take home point here is not to vilify the profit driven scientific community that operates in America today. Rather, the point is to alert the reader to yet another consequence of the fact that popular medical literature discloses only a small fraction of what science has revealed. Continued gullibility in this regard causes health consequences that the above serves as only several examples of the many that exist. This will begin to change for the better as more people begin to realize that they have been the recipients of clever advertising campaigns.

The PDR (physicians' desk reference) is actually less complete than it should be in regards to what science has revealed (authors personal opinion). Its wording accentuates the upside of what is for sale and simultaneously minimizes the risks involved. Anyone who doubts this trend can read for himself or herself about any new drug that still has a patent advantage. The reason that it is important to read the patentable drugs entries that regard this trend is that one method for increasing new drugs sales is to slam on the patent expired varieties.

In addition these advertising campaigns have been designed to steer thinking in a beneficial way. The benefits are larger profits for their most lucrative products. When one understands the down side then there will begin to be a demand, at the consumer level, for a more complete discussion regarding the options for a given ailment.

One further point about the PDR is in the realization that it has largely become an effective marketing strategy towards patients and physicians. These descriptions of the different drugs are sometimes without a picture of a drug's chemical structures. The lack of a chemical structure becomes very disabling, when one wants to understand the basics on the safety within.

One needs to stay mindful about the way drugs are classified. Drug classification can lead physicians thinking into erroneous avenues of understanding. The fenfluramine example being grouped outside the serotonin reuptake inhibitors (Prozac, Paxil, and Zoloft) when they share many suspicious overlapping structural and activity related characteristics again illustrate this point.

The long held suspicion persists about under reported side effect profiles. This suspicion becomes more justified when one becomes cognizant of the often-harried physicians workday. How much time do most doctors really have to read the fine print of these subtle PDR pieces of work? Only when the under reporting becomes outlandish, will physicians eventually observe enough suspicious clinical inconsistencies and this leads eventually to printed warnings. The more common situation involves the chronic under representation of the potential to harm a given group of owners who take different medications. If owners were again taught some of the basics about what the body processes are about, devoid of the complex abstractions, they would better be able to alert their physicians at the first signs of trouble.

Mercury as a rust promoter needs to be discussed while on the subject of scientific incompleteness and inconsistency. It is a long known fact that mercury is a nerve toxin. Less well appreciated even within the medical community concerns the duplicity of ways that pharmaceutical companies include mercury within vaccines by identifying mercury as a side name that few physicians and patients can recognize.

This nasty little fact has finally come to light thanks to many doggedly stubborn owners who kept up the campaign against the mercury contained within these vaccines but hidden under the ingredient name, thimerosal. This revelation has forced the manufactures of many childhood vaccines, to agree to reduce the mercury content within these injections to 5% of the previous amount. They now say that much less mercury is needed in them to stabilize the vaccine ingredients. Thankfully, preliminary data suggest that the rate of Autism is now decreasing.

Unfortunately, this means that for years countless children have been injected with a known neurotoxin that was unnecessary. In addition, the common flu vaccine injection also contains mercury. Adding insult to injury, some types of testosterone injections contain mercury as well.

For these reasons, it seems advantageous that physicians receive their primary scientific information from unbiased sources of scientific inquiry. This probably will only become possible when enough patients stand behind their doctors and begin to demand a little house cleaning from the grips of the FDA and rampant corrupt funding of university research by silent pharmaceutical interests. Socialized medicine has many of the same problems inherent in the current system because of the lobbying protectionism of any 'complex' interest before passage would be possible. In other words a new socialized system would tax the citizens to ensure continued 'complex' profits.

Healing paths are probably most likely to originate outside of the current system. Movements like 'keep it simple' are such beginnings. Here doctors agree to charge less but accept no insurance or government programs of any kind for out patient care. Patients pay in cash but at reduced charges because their doctor no longer has to generate huge sums of money to pay for all the paper work and time spent arguing with insurance programs. In systems like this the doctor patient relationship is again a private exchange and it has a focus regarding the number one priority of getting the patient on a healing path.

Contrast this to the frenzied demands on a general practitioner's time today. Very little of this time centers on who the patient is, where has he/she come from, what are their fears and hopes, where are they going (someplace good versus someplace bad). In the end when change comes to the way health care is practiced it will come from the patient's demands.

Politicians are scared to death of angry voters. This is why, despite the complex's best effort otherwise; there has been a gradual acceptance of alternative modalities. Slowly but surely, patients have legitimized chiropractic care, acupuncture, naturopathy, and massage therapy to their insurance companies. All the while, the various complex entities have been trying every dirty trick that attempts to marginalize the alternative therapies (see appendices at the end of the text).

The late John Lee, MD, summarized the situation very well in the introduction of his book, '**Some things your doctor may not tell you about the menopause**'. He commented on how over the last several years there had been repeated attempts to marginalize the importance of his progesterone findings. However he communicated that the complex underestimated the power of the international women's network that regards what works. In the end accurate scientific information will become available only when consumers vote out those politicians that continue to receive 'honorariums' from the complex.

7) Taking out the brain trash

The unique power supply to the brain presents unique challenges to keep the brain free of toxins. The main vulnerability within the brain lies in the obligatory requirement of nerves to only burn sugar as their fuel source. Sugar is consumed within the nervous system at a high rate in oxygen's presence. Unlike most other body organs the brain can only burn sugar in its power plants.

For example, failure of the nerve cells' power plant energy supply consequent to when blood sugar supplies fall off has toxic consequences. In addition, injury to delicate nerve cell contents occurs, from the oxygen radical. Oxygen radicals create brain trash whenever a failure in certain backup systems occurs.

One back up system involves the oxygen radical 'mop up' enzyme machines. Oxygen radicals require enzyme mop up machines that clean up the occasional unpaired oxygen (oxygen radical) that leaks outside the 'armored'mitochondria. The nerve cell prevents the creation of oxidized cell components in two ways. Both ways are discussed below.

First, it needs an effective set of enzyme machines hanging around to process the oxygen radical (reactive oxygen species) situation when it occurs. The enzymes within the nerves, which neutralize reactive oxygen species, are called super oxide dismutase and catalase. Oxygen radical formation occurs because of the shear volume of oxygen being processed for life giving combustion reactions within nerve cell mitochondria.

As stated previously, when this set of enzymatic machines proves deficient, diseases like Lou Gahrig's (ALS) result. These types of diseases kill nerve cells when oxygen radical is allowed to escape outside of the protection of the mitochondria. When reactive oxygen species are outside of the mitochondria they damage the first structure that they contact. In these cases, the damage from rust production processes eventually exceeds the best repair abilities of the nerve cells.

A similar process occurs in the retinas of premature infants that require high oxygen content to remain alive. The high oxygen content that saves them also, in many cases, overwhelms the oxygen detoxifying systems and visual impairment results from death of the nerves behind the retina. Scientists call this injurious side effect retrolental fibroplasia.

The second form of brain defense with regard to oxidizing agents is more generalized. This system of anti-oxidants is able to neutralize many different 'rust' promoters within the brain. Glutathione, vitamin C, vitamin E, garlic, and onions are all common examples of substances that perform this important task. They each work by stabilizing many different rust promoters when they react with them. Some of these anti-oxidants are rechargeable and others are only able to work one time. Consequently, nutritional deficiency of these important protective molecules causes the nerves to rust more rapidly. The brain becomes one of the most potentially toxic areas in the body because the brain has 25% of the body's blood at rest. For example, consider the blood vessel lining cells exposure to toxic oxidant insults as the blood flows by as it courses through one's mind.

One additional consideration becomes important in regards to 'rust' promoters. This consideration concerns what are the nerve cell options once a cell's molecular component has been damaged. When nerve cell molecular components become injured a repair process needs to occur.

Fat constitutes the largest molecular component within the brain and hence remains the most likely to sustain damaged. Therefore, this necessitates that adequate cellular direction exist to invest in fat rebuilding activities. In addition, to appropriate informational substances (hormones), which direct the repair of damaged intracellular contents, it needs a highly functioning landfill site (lipofuscin deposits) or incinerator (peroxisomes). The incinerator burns the damaged fats.

Lipofuscin deposits within the nerve cells as storage sites for damaged fat molecules. Also remember the requirement that there are adequate molecular replacement parts available to remanufacture the damaged structures. In the case of damaged fat replacement the owner needs to have appropriate dietary fat supplies or have a highly functioning methyl donor system to make these specialized nerve fats from scratch. Recall, by this mechanism, owners on low fat diets strain their methyl donor system.

Finally, before leaving the toxin discussion the reader is asked to remain mindful of ingested substances that have the ability to cross the blood brain barrier and move on into one's mind. Once they are inside they breakdown into elements like fluorine (fluoride usually within the body). Too many elements like fluorine place a particular strain on keeping adequate anti-oxidants around. Realize the trade off balance between less antioxidant around necessitating increases in the rate of repair and replacement of brain molecular parts.

8) The nerve cell's cellular force field

The concept of the cellular force field was discussed in section five. Because nerve cells require this property to function more reliably, than in any other body cell, a brief summary is in order. The reader is asked to recall, yet once again, the analogy of the car battery.

Car batteries operate on a similar principle, as do nerve cells. The difference between certain minerals (electrolytes) concentration need to be maximized about a membrane before both of these types of batteries charge up. The differences in mineral concentration are maximized about a membrane (or between the two posts in the case of the car battery). The greater the difference between the mineral types (across a membrane) then the battery will have more energy to perform electrical work. The nerve cell is similar in that the membrane lining it maintains a concentration gradient between different electrolytes (minerals), which allow it to perform the work of living.

Cognizance here allows one to desire the avoidance of *low cell voltage syndrome* within his/her mind. Important point: Beyond adequate minerals in the diet the nerve cell DNA (genes) needs appropriate directions to avoid *low cell voltage syndrome*. Recall, the genes provide nothing until the right hormone arrives.

Powerful hormones are needed, in adequate amounts and in appropriate timing, before the cell's DNA (genes) activate. Recall, proper DNA direction (gene activation) allows the nerve cell to make the enzyme machines, direct repair to its structures and direct the manufacture of force field generators (membrane mineral pumps) within the membrane.

For example, the force field generators (Na/K ATPase membrane pumps) are necessary for an effectively performing force field. The adequacy of pumps like these powerfully determines the ability to concentrate potassium within the nerve cell. In the end, the strength of a nerve cell's force field (cell voltage) directly relates to the amount of force field generators (mineral pumps), the minerals respective availabilities and the energy supply delegated to them. Think of these as the three basic determinants of cell voltage adequacy.

One example of the importance of the nerve cell force field (cell voltage adequacy) occurs with regards to its ability to prevent inappropriate calcium ion penetration. The nerve cell membrane can only prevent the inappropriate penetration of calcium ion when it possesses sufficient strength of charge (adequate cell voltage). Sufficient charge becomes possible only when adequate sugar makes its way into the nerve power plants. These power plants need sugar as fuel and adequate oxygen to combust it and eventually trap some of this liberated energy.

Recall, specific vitamins prove necessary before sugar processes to acetate. Only acetate burns up in the presence of oxygen within the cellular combustion chambers (mitochondria). Recall, raw fuels (carbohydrate, protein and fat) all need refining into acetate before combustion in the power plants becomes possible. Specific vitamins and cofactors are required for each (section one). However, the brain only processes carbohydrate into acetate.

The energy trapped in the form of ATP by combusting acetate in the presence of oxygen and converting it into carbon dioxide charges up the membrane by pumping certain ions against their concentration gradient. Consequently, insufficient or excessive mineral supplies interfere with efficient charging. Basically, any thing, which disrupts this process, allows the energy contained in the nerve membrane to run down. When the energy in the nerve membrane runs down harmful ions (minerals) inappropriately penetrate inside the nerve cell.

Inappropriate calcium entry into nerve cells should not be confused with appropriately channeled entrance of calcium in order to perform cellular work. The difference with the later occurs because when calcium enters appropriately it is tightly regulated and quickly pumped outside again. This movement of the calcium mineral about a membrane is similar to how a battery discharges and recharges.

In contrast, inappropriate calcium entry into nerve cells is similar to when battery post become oxidized. Battery oxidation results when the minerals inappropriately leak outside the battery and react with the post. The reader is asked to visualize the gunk that accumulates on these aging battery posts. So it is with the inside of owner's nerve cells that for one reason or another are unable to keep calcium channeled within the appropriate pathways. When calcium penetrates outside of carefully gated channels then cellular gunk begins to occur. The cellular gunk occurs when calcium reacts with delicate inside the cell structures. This inappropriate calcium reaction damages nerve cell structures.

This process describes the main mechanism for nerve cell death when either oxygen or sugar delivery become compromised. In each of these cases the energy content of the nerve membrane falls (section five) and calcium rushes inside the nerve cell. Nerve cell death begins to occur in as little as one minute (usually four minutes but in cold water drowning it can be a lot longer). In other words, calcium always lurks outside the cell wanting to penetrate inside. The electrical charge (cell voltage) prevents inappropriate calcium penetration as long as the cellular force field remains strong.

Nerve cell energy compromises from decreased oxygen, specific vitamin deficiencies and/or decreased blood sugar. Failure occurring in anyone of these processes causes the force fields strength (cell voltage) to fall off dramatically. The energy contained within the nerve cell membrane rapidly depletes when interruption of its ability to recharge occurs. A fall in membrane charge only takes a few minutes and when these situations arise massive amounts of calcium influxes into the cell. Calcium can only flood into a nerve cell, by the inappropriate channels, when the force field energy compromises. Remember, as the force field depletes calcium rushes inward and chemically reacts in harmful ways with intracellular contents.

Consequently, processes that increase a cells ability to generate a maximal force field provide a longevity and performance advantage to the nerve cell. Conversely, processes that compromise the ability of nerve cells to generate an optimal force field, lead to their injury (old age). Remember, nerve cells are particularly vulnerable if their force field diminishes for a short time.

The two main hormones within the body that determine how powerful a given nerve cells force field becomes are aldosterone and thyroid hormone. Thus a continued maximal nerve function only becomes possible when these hormones arrive in sufficient amounts (section two). Over looking the central directive role, which these two hormones play often allows owners' nervous systems to slip into the diminished energetic state mentioned above. The diminished energy state of one's nerve cells is best understood through the example of the common mineral imbalance of middle age. One important mineral particularly important to nerve health is potassium.

Potassium deficiency will diminish the cellular force field and hurt nerves at eight different levels

Potassium is the main mineral contained inside nerve cells. Nerve cells, which possess adequate potassium, are afforded energy and protection. Unfortunately the importance of ample potassium within one's nervous system is often overlooked in the clinical setting. The failure to counsel owners on strategies, which will improve their nervous systems content of potassium, has many nerve health consequences (see below). Fortunately once potassium deficiency is remedied the owner begins to heal.

The potassium-depleted nerve cells are irritable and weak. Many owners are misled by their annual lab test results, which clearly states that they have a normal blood potassium level. Remember, this blood stream measurement measures the 2% tank of total body potassium. This fact occurs because only 2% of total body potassium resides within the blood serum. The other 98% of potassium sequesters inside body cells. Confusion occurs because patients and their doctors fail to appreciate that the 98% tank will greatly diminish before one ever sees a decrease in the 2% tank within the blood stream. The unfortunate consequence of this misunderstanding is that there are a lot of owners with nerve cell potassium depletion (*low cell voltage syndrome*) but normal blood potassium test results.

The ability of a nerve cell to charge its force field (increase its voltage) is directly proportional to the amount of potassium it contains. Potassium deficiency often results from poorly informed diet choices. The consequences of poorly informed diet choices usually delays manifestation of the chronic disease expression until the onset of middle age.

Recall, the most common reason for potassium deficiency with the onset of middle age results from the American diet. Very little medical emphasis occurs in regards to the importance of the proper consumption of balanced mineral intake. Balanced mineral intake will promote the maximal nerve cell charges. Conversely, the chronic imbalance of mineral intake leads to around middle age to the tendency for mineral imbalanced related diseases. The reasons for this have been discussed in other sections but a brief review as they pertain to nerve health follows.

In contrast, real food diets (natural food that has not been processed) tend to be high in magnesium and potassium. These foods are almost always low in sodium, as well. They tend to be intermediate in their calcium content. When owners consume real food the proper mineral proportions are rather easy to obtain. In general, 4000mg of potassium, 1000mg of sodium, 500mg of calcium, and 300mg of magnesium a day will suffice. Owners that live in hot climates will need more sodium. Owners that live in colder climates may need less sodium. In addition, owners that sweat while either working or exercising may need more sodium. These mineral intakes only apply for those with normal kidney and adrenal function.

Unfortunately, owners, who have been chronically fed the reversed mineral ratios, contained in the processed food diet, eventually possess nerves that become fatigued and irritable around middle age. Nerve problems occur around middle age in America because processed food has had much of its potassium and magnesium removed (see mineral table in chapter three). A compounding of the problem occurs through the addition of large amounts of sodium to preserve the shelf life of the processed food. When owners eat these altered mineral contents for years, nerves become less able to hang on to or procure the necessary potassium.

Making matters worse, the nerve cell potassium deficiency process greatly accelerates in those owners who are under chronic stress. This occurs because stress hormone, cortisol, increases potassium loss and conserves sodium. This fact describes the second tier of a complex problem. Realize, it would be very difficult for this to occur if a given owner ate a real food diet because there would be sufficient potassium around to accommodate its increased loss.

The third tier of the nerve cell potassium deficiency problem occurs when the kidneys sustain damaged from chronic potassium deficiency. It has long been known for many years that low potassium intake constitutes as a risk factor for kidney damage (hypokalemic nephropathy). Paradoxically, very little is said about this association to patients in the clinical setting. Unfortunately, the blood pressure begins to rise when the kidneys sustain damage in this way.

High blood pressure is hard on the brain cells. If the doctor understands nutrition at this early stage he will begin to counsel his patients regarding the importance of a more balanced mineral intake contained within real foods only. However when the physician misses this healing opportunity the patient will go on to develop more kidney damage. Once the kidney sustains damage his/her blood pressure will be less responsive to a better diet. At this stage high blood pressure medication may be necessary on a permanent basis. One of the reasons high blood pressure medication becomes necessary involves protecting the brain.

The fourth tier of the nerve injury caused by the potassium deficiency problem concerns the associated insulin resistance. Insulin resistance predictably occurs in the processed food diet situation around middle age. Insulin cannot facilitate sugar uptake in most body cells without a one for one association between sugar and potassium. This means that for every sugar taken into a cell their needs to be corresponding potassium taken up as well.

However, at the onset of deficient potassium availability following meals causes the secondary system within the liver to activate. The problem here becomes exaggerated as well because the pancreas senses the delay in the blood sugar falling that potassium deficiency causes. So in these situations the pancreas eventually secretes even more insulin for a given sugar load as more potassium becomes available from within the cells (one cause of insulin resistance). This process describes one of the reasons for still becoming fat even though a given owner eats less carbohydrate. A given owner will always secrete more insulin for a given amount of sugar when their total body potassium diminishes. The delay of blood sugar normalization damages nerves because its excess forms advanced glycation end products (AGES).

Note: the medical textbooks focus on the initial inhibition of insulin secretion that acute potassium deficiencies cause, but fail to acknowledge that as more potassium drains out of the cells the pancreas again secretes insulin. However, between times while more potassium leaks out of the cells, the liver pathway for turning sugar into cholesterol and fat abnormally activates because this pathway does not require potassium. Remember, both protein and glycogen formation requires a fixed amount of potassium for their creation. However, fat and cholesterol formation from sugar does not need

potassium in order to form and this fact partially explains the abnormal cholesterol parameters seen in these patients. These relationships also describe one mechanism for how chronic diuretic therapy causes diabetic glucose tolerance curves alongside the worsening cholesterol profiles.

The liver that receives increased insulin message exposure, which arises from the potassium deficient state, contributes to the fifth tier of potassium related illness that damages nerves. The liver only needs insulin's message for it to begin sucking sugar out of the blood stream. Visualize the 200,000 pure insulin receptors per liver cell. Conceptualize the liver as an insulin trap. Insulin within the liver always instructs energy storage. The more potassium available the more sugar that converts into glycogen for storage. But its deficiency promotes cholesterol and triglyceride synthesis because these pathways do not require potassium.

In contrast, other body tissues require potassium as well to suck up sugar out of the blood stream. The increased insulin levels needed, as in the case of potassium deficiency, means that the enzyme HMG CoA reductase (that creates cholesterol within the liver) will be abnormally activated. Insulin also up regulates triglyceride synthesis as well. These enzyme machines begin the process of turning sugar into cholesterol and triglyceride (both are pH neutral fats). Important point: HMG Co A reductase is the same enzyme that the popular cholesterol lowering drugs inhibit.

Here lies yet another simple explanation for how cholesterol tends to increase around middle age. In addition, high levels of liver manufactured fat and cholesterol (LDL) tend to damage the blood supply that feeds the nerves of the body. The blood vessels in these areas plug up when the macrophages lining the arteries stuff themselves chronically on LDL cholesterol. **Recall, the older medical physiology textbooks still acknowledged that insulin directed fat and cholesterol manufacture results in butterfat but dietary butter ingestion results in the fat component turning into olive oil!**

As stated above, it is important to realize that the liver does not require potassium to convert sugar into fat and cholesterol. However, in order for it to store sugar as glycogen, a fixed amount of potassium needs to associate. Here lies yet another reason for abnormal cholesterol synthesis: Deficient potassium prevents adequate glycogen formation and promotes excessive cholesterol and fat formation (the butterfat kind).

The sixth tier of damage, which low potassium states cause to nerve cells, arises from the lessened tolerance for aldosterone within the body. Aldosterone is a fundamental player for two important nerve processes. One, it tells the nerve DNA that it is important to invest in updated cell charge components within the cell membrane. Second, it is the steroid, which determines the rate at which cholesterol converts to pregnenolone (the mother of all steroids). For this reason, aldosterone levels control the rate-limiting step for steroid biosynthesis within the gonads and adrenals (probably in the brain as well).

Nerve cell health depends on adequate steroid tone and pressure. Adequate steroid tone and pressure cannot occur without sufficient aldosterone levels. Recall from section two that its message instructs the steroid producing tissues of the body to begin the conversion process. The steroid producing tissues are found in the gonads, the adrenals and the brain. However, unless adequate aldosterone message content reaches these areas, the rate of steroid synthesis declines. A fall in steroid synthesis means that the steroid pressure and tone will fall as well (section two). Consequently, the nerve cells receive a diminished message content to rejuvenate.

Remember, the nerves of the body rely on adequate aldosterone levels to help keep the *steroid pressure and tone* at youthful levels and the nerve cell charge (voltage) sufficient. Unfortunately, the processed food diet, common in America today, only compounds the difficulty of the body's steroid producing cells receiving adequate aldosterone message content. Aldosterone deficiency will occur for two reasons. First, involves the treatment of high blood pressure states with ACE inhibitors (section one). Most of the time, these drugs become necessary, if one fails to catch the low potassium diet injury inflicted on the kidneys early on. It also occurs when an owner continues to eat a processed food diet. Recall, chronic subsistence on a low potassium diet will injure the kidneys (hypokalemic nephropathy). When the kidneys sustain injury blood pressure will rise. Not until over fifty percent of the kidney dies will the common kidney function blood test (creatinine) begin to creep into the abnormal range.

ACE inhibitors work, in part (see chapter three), by decreasing aldosterone and therefore conserving potassium. Potassium has long been known to lower blood pressure. The other mechanisms of ACE inhibitor type drugs hypotensive action were reviewed in earlier chapters. The important point, in this subsection, concerns the many owners that remain unaware of how their processed food diet proves central to their nerve disease process at multiple levels. For these reasons, if these people change their diets early on their nerves will benefit in multiple ways.

The second way that potassium affects aldosterone and therefore the nervous system steroid levels regards the fact that in some owner's atrial natruretic peptide (ANP) activates early on. This powerful hormone releases from the hearts of some owners and over rides the stimulus to release aldosterone when a high sodium diet prevails. This hormone, in these situations, keeps these owners blood pressure low at a price to their health. The first price to these owners health arises in that they will make less aldosterone and this deficiency causes a consequent reduction of the other steroids' production rates. Second, they will still tend to suffer with the consequences other than high blood pressure from diminished total nervous system potassium.

The seventh tier of potassium deficiency and the resultant nerve dysfunction arises from the diminished force field (cell voltage) that becomes possible. When nerve cells function with diminished force field generating abilities they become irritable. Certain owners are more susceptible to this side effect. It comes down to the fact that different bodies handle total body potassium deficiency in their own prioritized way. Some do a better job at conserving potassium within the nervous system until late in the deficiency process. The important point to recognize is that some cases of anxiety or irritability have their origins in potassium deficiency states.

The eighth tier of potassium deficiency produced nerve disease present as weakness and fatigue. This situation occurs because total body potassium content serves as a determinant for the amount of cell protein possible within body cells. Nerve cells need protein for their function and health even more than other body cells. Sufficient potassium within the cells of the body has been known for many years to stabilize proteins by its association. Consequently, without adequate potassium, body protein content diminishes. Nerve cell health relies on sufficient potassium content to stabilize nerve cell proteins.

The eight ways which potassium deficiency injures one's nerves serve as an introductory example for how dietary deficiencies or excesses can alter nerve function. In addition, multiple other nutritional deficiencies cause clinical depression. Clinical depression therefore can often be healed when the nutritional problem resolves.

Nutritional Deficiency Caused Depression

Imbalanced amounts of the different neurotransmitters often result in clinical depression. Mainstream medicine adherents tend to lump all these cases into the vernacular of a biochemical imbalance. While the biochemical imbalance, accurately describes the cause of their clinical problem, the solution often proves nutritional. Unfortunately, instead of applying even a little effort as to how a poor diet might contribute to depressive illness, most owners receive antidepressant prescriptions.

Many patented prescriptions have been created to address nutritional deficiencies in peripheral ways. These medications circuitously improve depressive symptoms by keeping the deficient neurotransmitter around for a longer time within the active little spaces between nerves, the synapse. However, proper nutrition also increases the amount of neurotransmitter available within the different nerve cells of the body, as well. In addition, proper nutrition replacement therapy avoids side effects.

The science behind the necessary nutritional molecular components for optimal neurotransmitter production has been understood for years. Unfortunately, instead of advising owners on ways to increase their own neurotransmitter production rates, prescription medications remain the treatment of choice.

Certain nutritional factors need to exist before sufficient neurotransmitters can be manufactured. Optimal neurotransmitters amounts prevent depression. When a certain neurotransmitter's manufacture rate fails, predictable mental symptomatology follows. Paradoxically, rather than augment the deficiency through nutritional intervention, these owners receive counsel that they have a biochemical imbalance.

By labeling depression in ways that imply genetic determinism, the owner's ability to heal him/her self appears unlikely. The truth of this intellectual roadblock proves suspect but never the less perpetuates. A disincentive exists to share with doctors and patients the ability of directed nutritional refortification to overcome many inherited weaknesses within one's DNA. In addition, the appalling nutrition contained in the typical American diet accelerates the inherited weakness. In turn, these inherited genetic weaknesses respond to symptom-control methods by peripheral pathways in the brain.

The symptom-control approach involves prescribing the various drugs that increase the length of time that the neurotransmitters occur within the little spaces between the nerves. These prescriptions do nothing to increase production of the deficient neurotransmitter. They only prolong how long the neurotransmitter signals its message within the active little spaces, the synapse.

In marginally depleted owners, this approach has potential to help, but with a price. The price depends on the class of antidepressant agent prescribed (see earlier discussion). Unfortunately, very few owners receive counseling concerning what needs to happen nutritionally, for normal neurotransmitter production rates to occur. Instead, they are told that they have a biochemical imbalance and this follows to imply that it is genetic in its causality.

However, some owners prefer a trial of nutritional supplementation before they embark on the precarious path of symptom-control medicine. Nutritional supplementation covers the other side of the story of what science has long ago revealed about the cause of some depressive illnesses. These largely untold facts include the central nutritional molecular building parts and chemical reaction facilitators (vitamins). These molecular building parts and chemical reaction facilitators prove necessary within the brain for neurotransmitter biosynthesis to occur. Thankfully, if these factors arrive in reliable and constant supplies to the central nervous system the need for prescription medicine often disappears.

Sadly, many conventionally trained physicians receive scant education about the important nutritional pathways that bring about optimal neurotransmitter levels. How convenient to leave some basic nutritional science out of the educations of the certified experts. Earlier in this chapter, the most common neurotransmitters were reviewed and some of their manufacture requirements were discussed. The previous discussion contained the potential downside of several antidepressant classes. Here a brief summary follows on what nutritionally needs to pass into the brain in order for different neurotransmitters' biosynthesis to occur.

Serotonin (arousal states): Adequate tryptophan in the diet serves as its basic building block precursor. Sufficient stomach acid and digestive juices need to secrete once tryptophan occurs in a meal. Failure to separate tryptophan from a protein containing meal results in its deficiency.

Vitamins needed for its manufacture: tetrahydrobiopterin (made from folate) and pyridoxal phosphate (vitamin B6).

567

Dopamine (pleasure and fine motor coordination): The amino acids tyrosine and phenylalanine can serve as its basic precursor building blocks. Again sufficient stomach acid and digestive juices need to secrete or deficiency occurs.

Vitamins needed for its biosynthesis: tetrahydrobiopterin (made from folate), pyridoxal phosphate (vitaminB6)

Norepinephrine (mental alertness): Dopamine is needed as its building block precursor. Sufficient stomach acid and digestive juices need to secrete or deficiency occurs.

Vitamin C is needed for its biosynthesis

Epinephrine (mental alertness): Norepinephrine serves as its building block. Stomach acid and/or digestive enzyme deficiencies lead to scarcity of this important neurotransmitter and hormone.

Sufficient SAMe allows its biosynthesis to occur. Because one SAMe donates its methyl for each epinephrine made, it becomes rapidly depleted without the methyl donor system adequately recharging it back into its active form. Methyl Donors recharge system includes: Vitamin B12, Vitamin B6, folate, serine, and methionine. SAMe deficiency shows up as an elevated homocysteine level with laboratory testing of a blood sample. How many clinically depressed owners arise solely from a simple methyl donor deficiency nutrient?

Understand that tyrosine and phenylalanine lead to the sequential manufacture of dopamine, followed by norepinephrine, and lastly, epinephrine. Epinephrine deficiency is most likely because specific nutritional deficiencies anywhere along the assembly line will prevent its manufacture. Where the nutritional deficiency occurs becomes the point that a neurotransmitter's manufacture stops. In other words, epinephrine deficiency proves most vulnerable because it relies on the most vitamins for its manufacture.

Many depressive illnesses arise from deficient epinephrine neurotransmitter levels. One clue to the immense scope of the problem concerns the clinical observation that many dieters taking ephedra (epinephrine-like) note a marked improvement in their depressive symptoms. Many other benefits derive from epinephrine-like medication, such as; diminished insulin secretion, allergy relief, and mental alertness.

One needs to keep these benefits in mind and contrast them against the many patented and expensive drugs that would no longer be in demand if the public ever found out about these benefits. Re-including these facts into the ongoing mainstream media campaign against ephedra begins to provide the other side of the story for why the complex feels so strongly against ephedra. After all, there are several over the counter drugs that have proven to be much more dangerous. Where is the consumer protection from these patented drugs?

Histamine (consciousness and arousal): Histidine is the amino acid building block. Pyridoxal phosphate (Vitamin B6) is needed for its biosynthesis (see earlier discussion about this important neurotransmitter).

GABA (calm states): Glutamic acid is the building block amino acid precursor needed. Pyridoxal phosphate (Vitamin B6) is the vitamin needed for biosynthesis of GABA to occur.

An important aside about GABA is that its production within the central nervous system depends on adequate progesterone levels. For this reason, people that have diminished progesterone levels for too long tend to be anxious and irritable. This situation commonly occurs in peri-menopausal females up to two weeks before their periods (PMS).

The other irritability factor that always needs to be considered involves the amount of sodium relative to potassium intake. Potassium has a calming effect within the central nervous system (CNS). It probably has to do with an adequate force field (cell voltage). Also, recall the ability of the nerve to concentrate potassium within depends on sufficient membrane pumps (Na-K ATPase). In turn, the number of these pumps throughout the body depends on the sufficient presence of thyroid hormone. Consequently, high normal thyroid replacement powerfully diminishes depressive symptoms by this mechanism (high voltage neurons are happy).

The advice of a nutritionally competent physician will facilitate the correct replacement dosages and regimens. In addition, some attention needs to be directed at the integrity of the digestive tract. Improperly functioning digestive tracts will frustrate attempts to heal nutrition deficiency caused depression. In some of these cases, intravenous vitamin therapy may be warranted until the digestive problem resolves.

A caveat now occurs regarding supplementation to correct certain neurotransmitter deficiencies. The salt of glutamic acid is known as glutamate. It is popularly known as monosodium glutamate (MSG) and it often hides within ingredients such as vegetable flavorings, hydrolyzed protein and spices. Glutamate is the most powerful neurotransmitter for nerve excitation. Consequently, too much glutamate can excite a nerve cell to death.

Nerve cell death results from over stimulation. Over stimulation of a nerve cell leads to a draining down of the nerve cell force field (cell voltage). When the nerve cell force field depletes, the massive in rushing of unwanted charged particles like calcium follows. Too much calcium within a cell binds to its enzymes and delicate structures and this causes cell injury.

Because of this fact, just eliminating this salt from one's diet can often enhance memory. This improvement occurs because nerve cells need to generate an adequate force field (cell voltage) to be able to work efficiently. Molecules like glutamate continually discharge the force field's energy. The memory nerve's force field depletes because the over stimulation of their membrane leads to the discharge of the concentration difference between important minerals. As the concentration difference between these important minerals about the nerve cell membrane decreases, the protection energy depletes (the force field has run down).

Acetylcholine (abstract thinking ability): The first building block precursor for this important neurotransmitter's manufacture comes from consuming adequate choline in the diet, mostly from fish and eggs. The second building block precursor is acetate, which can be derived from all fuel sources (protein, fat and carbohydrates) but only when adequate vitamin levels are present (chapter 1). However, within the brain, it derives only from carbohydrate.

Low fat diet adherents strain their methyl donor system. Recall, with appropriate types and amounts of fat intake, the methyl donor system donates a carbon at approximately one billion times a second. However, unless low fat diet adherents have even more methyl donors available than normal, their acetylcholine levels will tend to fall off. The acetylcholine levels will fall off because deficient fat intake leads to an increased need for the methyl donor system to synthesize choline from scratch. Consequently, the more severe the fat deficiency becomes, the greater the burden on one's methyl donor system. For this reason, the amount of methyl donor that one needs will sky rocket towards much higher levels per second.

An additional potential problem exists that regards the procurement of acetate within the brain for the manufacture of acetylcholine and other fat-building blocks within the brain. This problem arises from the fact that the brain only uses carbohydrate for its acetate creation (explained earlier). This limitation means that all five nutritional cofactors need to be present in order for the brain to convert glucose to acetate. Specifically, the rate-limiting step in question involves the conversion of pyruvate to acetate. Scientists call the enzyme complex that performs this task, pyruvate dehydrogenase.

This enzyme needs all five additional nutritional co-factors or acetate formation becomes impossible. The five cofactors necessary are: Vitamins B1, B2, B3, pantothenic acid, and lipoic acid. Unfortunately, processed food often proves depleted in pantothenic and lipoic acids. The fact that it has been re-fortified with a little of the B vitamins also proves unhelpful in many suffering owners. This consequence results from the fact that like other sequential chemical reactions in the body the depleted nutrient acts like a broken link in a chain. Here, deficiency of any of the five cofactors causes this important reaction to falter at this point and only lactic acid forms. Equally alarming, involves the fact that vitamin supplements often prove deficient in pantothenic and lipoic acids unless owners specifically take them individually.

Closely related to depression are the Autism spectrum disorders that include Attention Deficit Hyperactivity Disorder (ADHD). They are closely related but again the overused vernacular of biochemical imbalance takes the curious off the trail of nutrition and other culprits (see below). Consequently, millions of little people continue to suffer more than necessary at the hands of the complex.

Attention Deficit Hyperactivity Disorder and Other Childhood Disordered Brain Function Pathologies

More than 9 million children take stimulant medications for inattention and hyperactivity. An additional 500 thousand suffer from autism. In between attention deficit hyperactivity disorder and autism are other brain dysfunction syndromes like: obsessive-compulsive disorder (OCD) and dyslexia. Jeff Bradstreet, M.D. calls these the autism spectrum disorders. He points out that although they share overlapping common symptoms, which provide valuable clues for effectively treating them with holistic strategies, they also have their own unique features. The eventual outcome for a child with one of these disorders depends on whom the parents trust for their medical advice.

The human brain contains more fat weight than nerve weight. Brain fats are unique in their composition compared with other body structural fats. Because they are unique, their manufacture requires numerous minerals, cofactors and vitamins. An often-overlooked consequence of the brain's high fat composition arises from its rapid metabolic rate.

A high metabolic rate means that these tissues encounter free radicals more often. Free radicals cause oxidation to the structural fats that make up the brain. Ideally, throughout life, replacement processes remedy this ongoing problem. However, the replacement of damaged brain fats can only occur smoothly when adequate molecular replacement parts exist. One acquires adequate replacement parts through proper absorption of the dietary fats that the brain needs or through nutritional supplementation.

Numerous government studies have documented that the majority of American children are nutritionally deficient at multiple levels. Some common examples are: vitamin A, magnesium, essential fatty acids, zinc, vitamin C, B vitamins, and vitamin E. All these nutrients that American children so profoundly lack also comprise some of the nutrients critically needed to manufacture new structural brain fats. Children experience additional vulnerability because these brains not only need to replace damaged fats but they also need to grow.

Somehow a schism perpetuates between the children victims suffering with dysfunctional brains and the treatment offered by mainstream medicine. This fact is exemplified by the evisceration of basic brain nutritional science that points towards some healing possibilities for these children. Furthermore, the digestion impairments, toxic loads, metabolic and immune defects commonly found in these patients, are effectively downplayed or marginalized.

Fortunately, one pediatrician, Jeff Bradstreet, M.D. has devoted his practice to helping more than 1500 of these patients yearly to improve their brain function through focusing attention towards improved brain nutrition, immune function, liver detoxification and digestive tract healing. He reports success rates that leave prescription drugs, with all their side effects, in the undesirable and primitive category. In addition, pediatrician, Allen Lewis is medical director at the Pfeiffer clinic. He provides another beacon of light for the importance of applying nutritional biochemistry for those suffering from these disorders.

One of the consequences of living in a profit driven health care system concerns the vigorous attacks that arise towards people like Drs. Bradstreet and Lewis because they affect drug sales. Recall, healing has only one side effect.

Mechanisms for Brain Malfunction in Children:

Allergens, environmental toxins like mercury, persistent viral infections, maldigestion, intestinal inflammation, sulfation defects, inflammatory fats (the hydrogenated fats) that incorporate into the brain, altered mineral intake, and nutritional deficiencies.

Solutions to Consider (a brief overview)

Specific molecular parts that replace and stabilize the malfunctioning brain components

Special brain fats like; phosphatidal serine, phosphatidal choline (lecithin) and essential fatty acids. Avoid hydrogenated fats intake.

Specific molecular building components needed to make these specialized brain fats from, like, the methyl donor system (serine, methionine, folate, Vitamin B6 and Vitamin B12).

Specific minerals that the brain needs to power up its neurons and drive protective chemical reactions like; zinc, magnesium, selenium and potassium.

Digestive Enzymes that Deactivate Toxins, Help Assimilate Nutrients and Obliterate Allergens

Many of these brain dysfunction children continue to suffer because no one helps them improve their leaky gut and faulty digestive process. Orally supplementing with digestive enzymes helps with these three mechanisms of injury. In addition, some of these children need supplemental stomach acid so that they can digest protein more completely and hence starve the overgrowth of putrefaction producing organisms so rampant in this disorder.

Improve the Detoxification Abilities of the Liver

Environmental toxin exposures, which are "safe" for adults, are poorly handled in infancy during a critical period of brain development.

Liver detoxification ability impairs with: nutritional deficiencies, increased GI tract toxin load, increased environmental toxin load, and genetic predisposition for a defect to metabolize certain toxins (sulfation defects).

These are more completely explained in the liver chapter but the high prevalence of sulfation defects deserves brief mention. Decreased ability to sulfate biological molecules predisposes to leaky gut. Leaky guts allow toxins to seep towards the liver that are normally confined to the GI tract. Decreased sulfation ability also impairs the liver's ability to neutralize toxin loads. Extra toxins in the blood stream penetrate into the brain and cause injury there. One study showed that 100% of autism spectrum disorder children suffered from abnormal liver detoxification pathways.

Supplementing with various forms of sulfur in these children therefore proves cornerstone. Examples of these supplements are: MSM, N-acetyl cysteine, garlic, onions and methionine.

Mainstream medical doctors are taught to treat ADHD with counseling and stimulant prescriptions. Unfortunately, this approach ignores the basic nutritional science of what a healthy brain needs to maintain itself. It also ignores the common immune, metabolic and GI tract difficulties experienced by these children. In the end, the child's brain function will undoubtedly deteriorate until these holistic factors are addressed. Alarmingly, the mainstream literature admits that drugs have not proved of value in the long term. They further agree about the side effects from their use including high blood pressure and growth stunting. Drs. Bradstreet and Lewis, on the other hand, have proven the benefits of the above modalities but very few are listening. The health care revolution endeavors to change that.

The health care revolution also endeavors to raise awareness about the Seventh Principle: The energies that heal contrasted to the energies that maim. Recall, this principle proves to be the most difficult for the Western mind to grasp. Yet, the pursuit of happiness eventually evades all who fail to adhere to its tenets. Happiness is big so while reading the next few pages take a deeper look into this at first seemingly evasive principle as a preview to the physical needs of the heart.

CHAPTER TWENTY-FIVE

HEART

The Seventh Principle: The Energies that Heal Contrasted to the Energies that Maim the Heart

Science has not been pure in the pursuit of knowledge or understanding. Politics, social acceptance, vested interest; prejudice, money, etc have effected the conclusions and holdings of scientific inquiry. Consequently, some scientific theories have been based on incorrect analysis of the data. The data has been manipulated to serve many unscientific purposes. In the second half of this decade the data was manipulated by the tobacco industry for monetary purposes.

Five hundred years ago the data was manipulated to appear consistent with the canons of a powerful religious system—read power. Scientific theories that were prevalent during the renaissance are laughable today because the data is reinterpreted in view of new knowledge. Einstein's cosmological constant has been interpreted and reinterpreted several times during the century of its first postulation because of new data, observation, or the persuasive power of the most recent and prevailing theory.

The most consistent element of scientific inquiry has been the intellectual tenacity of some members of the scientific community. These people did not accept a popular scientific theory that was inconsistent with the data. Their curiosity and intellectual integrity was stronger than their sense of professional survival; and in cases such as Galileo, their personal survival.

Ptolemy lived in the first century AD. He noted certain inconsistencies in the scientific dogma that the sun revolved around the earth. He methodically explained his conclusions. When he proposed the novel idea that the earth revolved around the sun he and his theory were rejected and ridiculed by his scientific peers. For the next fourteen hundred years the world's top scientist clung to the belief that the sun revolved around the earth.

More than 1400 years after Ptolemy, Copernicus (1473-1543), noted similar inconsistencies. He methodically studied the data and observations. Copernicus reached the same conclusion as Ptolemy. The Church initially persecuted him. Copernicus' tenacity eventually won acceptance for his at first seemingly preposterous theory.

Galileo (1564-1642) made observations of unequally weighted falling bodies that were inconsistent with Aristotle's theories of gravity. Galileo's findings resulted in his dismissal from the faculty at the

University of Pisa. Aristotle's theory was still alive and powerful amongst the University of Pisa faculty. Today, basic physics include Galileo's observation that bodies of the different weights fall at the same velocity.

Dr. Ignatius Semmelweis, a Hungarian physician, who practiced in Vienna in the 1800's, demanded that his hospital colleagues and support staff wash their hands, especially when moving from autopsies and sick patient wards to the child birthing wards. Following this, the incidence of post-delivery fever and ensuing death from this illness plummeted to well below that of the wealthy women's childbirth hospital. The western germ theory was not even a speculation until Semmelweis perceived them; even before Lois Pasteur. Dr. Semmelweis had noted the inconsistencies of the scientific understandings of his day. He successfully developed this understanding into a primitive, but accurate germ theory.

Semmelweis was fired and ostracized from the medical community of his time. His ability to practice and his source of income was gone. Some say he cut off his finger and jammed the wounded stump into a corpse at autopsy. He then died from the infection attempting to prove his new theory. Others say he committed suicide from the despair and isolation.

Dr. Robert Becker, in the 'Body Electric' says,"science is a bit like the ancient Egyptian religion, which never threw old gods away but only tacked them on to new deities until a bizarre hodgepodge developed. For some strange reason science is equally reluctant to discard worn out theories". Later on Dr. Becker adds,"the healers' job has always been to release something not understood, to remove obstructions (demons, germs, despair) between the sick patient and the force of life driving obscurely towards wholeness".

The material provided in this section offers a theory of health that is based on an energy theory. The energy theory proposed in this section is similar, in some respects, to the previously described historical antidotes. This theory is supported by scientific data and mathematical theory that remains unrecognized by mainstream medicine. The conclusions described in this section have a devastating monetary impact on the medical industry. These conclusions also diminish the power and prestige of the medical industry. For these reasons, the energy theory of life will not receive immediate acceptance by the medical industry.

Independent of western thought, the Chinese medical scientists observed a pattern of energy flow within the human body ages ago. After thousands of years of observation these scientist decided that this energy pattern is invariable in the healthy human body. The early Chinese scientists determined disharmony or disruption in these energy flow qualities were associated with disease.

After further meticulous observation the specific imbalances were correlated with certain chronic degenerative diseases. Heart diseases were one of these disease patterns discovered. Several thousand years later, the followers of this system developed methods that are intended to restore the energetic balance found in the healthy state.

Today, this Chinese medical system is popularly known as acupuncture. The western scientific community was ignorant of this medical system until the 1970's until an American journalist, in China, became afflicted with an acute appendicitis. The journalist was a high profile case because he was there to document President Nixon's historic tour. The journalist, following the removal of his appendix, was impressed by the pain control achieved by acupuncture techniques. He was allowed to witness Chinese citizens undergoing surgical operations with acupuncture needles as their only anesthesia! When the journalist published his experience and observations of acupuncture techniques, the Western scientific community was caught off guard. Western scientific medical theory could not offer an explanation for the medical phenomenon described in the article.

According to the western medical theory, needles placed in the skin would not have an anesthetizing effect during surgical procedures. Western medical theory contradicted many documented cases where Chinese patients undergo various surgeries without any injected or inhaled anesthesia. Instead, they receive strategically placed needles. These surgical patients remain conscious and conversant while the operation occurs. When the operation is over they walk to the recovery room. These observations are well documented. The western scientific medical theory, however, does not have an explanation for this phenomenon.

The National Institute of Health was mobilized to remedy this embarrassing deficiency of Western scientific understanding. One of the scientists engaged by the NIH was Robert Becker, MD of Syracuse, New York. Dr. Becker's credentials are impressive. He was instrumental in discovering the electrical device used to heal fractures that had failed to respond to mechanical or surgical techniques. His work also led to the understanding that fracture sites need to generate an adequate electric field in order for the bone to heal.

When Dr. Becker began to work with acupuncture, he discovered the existence of electrical grids on or in the body. Dr. Becker proved the existence of the meridians themselves. He did this by measuring the electrical resistance difference between the meridians and the surrounding skin. He also developed a method to document the existence of these unvarying electrical grids. These grids were present within all the numerous subjects tested. He noted the presence of periodic "jump stations" along these electrical pathways. He documented that these "jump stations" corresponded to the acupuncture points of the ancient Chinese system.

One of Dr. Becker's theories was that the acupuncture meridians carried injury messages electrically to the brain. The brain responded by sending direct current to stimulate the healing process in the injured area. He postulated that the conscious mind perceives these messages as pain.

He knew that any electrical current grows weaker as the distance from the source of the electrical current increases. This is due to resistance along the transmission medium. He also knew that the smaller the amperage and voltage of the electrical charge then the faster the current would diminish as it moved away from its source. Electrical engineers solve this problem by building booster amplifiers along a power line to restore the strength of the electrical current. For currents measured in nano-amperes and microvolts, however, these boosters would have to be no more than several inches apart from one another.

He had more elaborate experiments planned but suddenly the NIH withdrew funding for further research into the matter.

A metal needle placed in an amplifier will short it out and stop the pain message. The Chinese believe that balanced circulation of energy through this constellation of points is a prerequisite to health. Proper placement of various patterns of needle placement brings these currents into harmony.

Realize Western medicine has no corresponding anatomical structures to Becker's grid (acupuncture meridian points). Western science is based upon molecular structure and the forces contained within these structures. This reductionism approach is too narrow to include an explanation of Becker's grid. The western scientific theory needs an anatomical structure to explain the energy moving within the meridians. The effectiveness of acupuncture without a convincing western scientific explanation is an ongoing credibility problem for western medicine.

Recall, the western medical approach can be likened to the slab of meat approach. The slab of meat describes all that is left when Western medical theory ignores the existence and effect of life energy. However, alternative medicine addresses ways to re-invigorate the flow of the life energies within a human body. This often forms the common denominator between chiropractic manipulation, acupuncture therapy, message modalities, homeopathy, yoga and prayer. Each of these disciplines, in their own way, causes a healing response by imparting a more harmonious energy flow.

Many a good scientist's life work continues to collect dust because their work reintroduced the concept of an organizing energy contained within living systems. In contrast the western scientific approach preoccupies itself with DNA and the information that it contains. However, the information contained in the DNA is not useful within the body unless the life energy directs its activation and silence in a coherent way.

Coherence of informational direction, describes how life violates the laws of physics. Life processes violate the laws of physics because living things convert simple molecules into complex molecules in a coherent manner. However, the western scientific community panders no believable explanation for this basic fact of life.

Modern science asked it's devotees to believe the similar analogy that there is this wonderful computer hard drive that can intake raw data without the direction of good software or a programmer! In other words garbage in is equal to garbage out. If DNA is the computer hard drive then where is the programmer?

In contrast, the Chinese system of acupuncture theory directly addresses the importance of honoring the need for a healthy 'organizing force'. The organizing force contained within living things is supplied by the proper flowing of *intelligent energy*. The possession by living things of an *intelligent energy*, which organizes and directs life's complex processes, is one theory, which explains the ability for life to violate the physical laws of nonliving systems. *Intelligent energy* is responsible for satisfying the ever present need to organize the flow of how the body spends its energy.

The theory of *intelligent energy* as a determinate of one's health involves a continuum between rhythm and chaos. This occurs within the energetic template. The energies that heal contrasted to the energies, which maim owner's cells, describe this process. Healing energies are thought to contain rhythm while harmful energies impart chaotic forces. Examples of healing energies are the positive emotions such as joy, forgiveness, love, kindness, and courage. Conversely, examples of the negative emotions are hatred, fear, jealousy, and self-entitlement. The heart as a rhythmical organ can facilitate a better understanding of the effect of these energies on one's health.

The Heart and the Seventh Principle

Scientific evidence for 'life rhythms' casts doubt towards completeness of mainstream thought that regard the life process. Mainstream viewpoints regarding life appear less complete because this explanation of the universe does not include the evidence for life's rhythmical energies. Strong evidence exists that the life process contains rhythmical energies (see intelligence behind the intelligence). This evidence points to the fact that rhythmical energies make life possible.

The erroneous mainstream scientific assumption started years ago. The western paradigm for the life processes was thought to be explainable by the molecules that make up the body structure. Hence the energies that heal contrasted to the energies that maim were relegated to the religious belief systems. Even when the rhythmical energies are discussed, they are only discussed in a peripheral way (the EKG or the EEG). However, many good scientists have demonstrated the folly of this approach (see intelligence behind the intelligence).

To understand the matters of the heart is to maintain one's personal power (rhythm). In order to understand healing paths of the heart, a discussion of rhythmical energy versus' chaotic energy needs to be undertaken.

Think of the heart as a rhythmical engine. Realize the performance of the body cells diminishes when rhythm deteriorates. Consequently, processes that facilitate rhythm energize the body while processes that diminish rhythm harm the integrity of the body's cells. Body cells including heart cells suffer from chaotic energies.

Chaotic energies inflict harm by their effect on body rhythm. These chaotic waves impart unique ways of injuring cells. Cells become diseased when the disorganizing energies exceed the body's ability to neutralize them. Rhythmic energies, on the other hand, originate within the heart and serve as a major source of rhythm for all other body cells.

This chapter contains an unusual approach to common ways that the heart becomes injured and diseased. The seventh principle of health/longevity describes the relationship of heart rhythm with the physical structure of the heart. Healing energies promote rhythmical forces while maiming energies hamper these forces.

The heart involves much more than a pump for swishing blood back and forth. For example, when rhythm occurs within the heart it provides the background energy, which all the body cells need. Rhythm causes the oscillations necessary for the efficient transfer of molecules from one cell to another. In addition, the cells outside of the blood stream use the pressure wave generated by the heart. Consequently, the quality of the pressure wave generated beyond the blood vessels determines much about the cellular health. Unfortunately, all too often, mainstream medicine ignores the obvious consequences when this energy wave proves sub-optimal at the level of the cell.

For example, the cartilage cell dilemma discussed in section five illustrated the necessity of the pressure wave's ebb and flow. Another important aspect of this dilemma concerns the consequences to body health when rhythm fails. Recall (section five) that the cartilage cell does not have a direct blood supply. Instead, these cells rely on the ebb and flow of fluids within the joint. The pressure wave from the beating heart causes the ebb and flow of fluids to the cartilage cell (the body periphery). Here it is the ebb and flow that causes the exchange of nutrients and waste in contrast to the cells that are closer to the blood vessels. Even so, all cells depend on the pressure wave created by the beating heart.

Realize, the pressure wave created by the heart creates 'squishing forces'. Squishing forces are the mechanical squeeze within body's cells. These squishing forces are similar to the forces of gravity, which augment nutrient delivery and waste removal. In addition, gravitational effects on joint tissue due to body motion lead to the ebb and flow of molecules. Similarly, the ebb and flow occurs in the body cells from the mechanical effects of the heart's rhythm. For this reason, optimal heart rhythm creates just the right force that improves energy transfer beyond the obvious movement of blood.

Sometimes truth is so simple that it remains overlooked. In medicine when truth continues to be overlooked healing possibilities fail to be realized. The red blood cell's deformability process, (chapter two) when it arrives at the level of the capillary, provides as one such example. Capillaries are a tight squeeze for red blood cells. Consequently, in order for a red blood cell to successfully squeeze through the capillary it needs to be sufficiently deformable. All red blood cells must do this or they will plug up the capillary. When this happens it is called micro-vascular disease (chapter two).

One of the consequences of decreased deformability of the red blood cells is high blood pressure. As a consequence, only when the heart elevates its pressure will the stiffened red blood cells squeeze

through the tight capillary spaces. Here, healing requires attention to the reasons that red blood cells become stiff (chapter two). Healing does not involve lowering the blood pressure with drugs without also endeavoring to understand the reason for the elevated blood pressure.

The presence or absence of the heart rhythm and the consequent pressure wave form an important determinant of a healthy cell. Healthy cells receive adequate nutrients. Healthy cells also coordinate an efficient reloading of waste onto the red blood cells. For this reason, processes that encourage the effectiveness of the heart rhythm will enliven the body cells. In other words, optimal heart rhythm generates efficient pressure waves and this allows the recipient cells to become more alive because they receive nutrition and eliminate waste more effectively.

Ignoring the importance of the energy wave reduces the discussion of the heart to its pump function. The seventh principle of health concerns itself with the quality of this rhythm inside the body. Specifically, the seventh principle involves the presence or absence of balance between the energies that heal contrasted to the energies that maim cells.

Cognizance here explains how restoring rhythmical energies forms a common denominator between several alternative-healing modalities. Effective alternative modalities for improving the rhythmical energies include: chiropractic, acupuncture, homeopathy, meditative prayer and body message. Each of these modalities uses its specific techniques towards improving the life rhythms. Paradoxically theses energies are almost always ignored by the mainstream view of the universe.

Rhythm

Several common themes exist among the great violinist, athletes, poets, and songwriters. A truth exists, which they all employ to achieve greatness. Without mastery of this single prerequisite, advancement beyond mediocrity proves impossible. All great performers or every great performance includes rhythm. Rhythm is an important element contained in every great performance.

Rhythm is not a linear skill that can be learned. It must be felt, used and exercised. Consistently the great performers possess a mastery of rhythm. Great violinists must feel the rhythm of the music before a remarkable performance exudes from their instrument. Likewise, great athletes tap into a higher rhythm that shows their grace. Rhythm causes the efficient use of available energy. The less wasted energy then the greater the achievement possible. When cells feel rhythm, less precious life energy is wasted. Ample life energy allows for a peak performance in the pursuit of happiness.

Healthy cells contain rhythm. Healthy owners enjoy rhythm in their lives. The heart is the metronome that creates a harmonic resonance throughout the body. Doc Childre and Howard Martin of Heart Math Institute, point out that the heart is the body's main energetic oscillator, and in health an efficient, heart generated, pressure wave penetrates each organ.

The energies that heal are the energies that promote rhythm. It helps to conceptualize the power in rhythm by considering different emotional energies and their effect on body rhythm qualities. For example, the emotion of forgiveness imparts energetic rhythm. In contrast, the negative emotions contain chaotic energies which are destructive to body rhythm. For these reasons, many owners waste precious life energy carrying around the energetic baggage of past grudges, guilt feelings, failures, and fears.

Emotions can be understood as thought forms. Thought forms contain energy. The presence of rhythm or chaotic waves depends on the thought form. With the passage of time the chaotic energies tend to localize in their preferred body tissues (see below). The energies that maim do so by imposing chaotic forces on the body's underlying rhythm. As the chaotic energies accumulate within the body they present clinically as stiff and sore body tissues. Realize, many alternative medical therapies effectuate their healing effect by facilitating the removal of accumulated chaotic energies within the body.

The negative chaotic energies begin in the mind. The importance of this fact explains why coaches often spend considerable effort in attempting to clear the athlete's minds before a performance. When the athlete's mind clears the rhythm of their performance improves. Rhythmical energies help them to enhance their athletic performance.

As life happens most owners tend to accumulate significant negative, chaotic energies within their body tissues. All owners experience periods of emotional pain. The seventh principle of health promotes life rhythm energies in the face of adversity. The rhythmical energies are promoted in two ways. First, minimize the accumulation of the chaotic energies such as: hate, anger, jealousy, impatience, and sadness. Second, maximize rhythmical energies such as: forgiveness, love, thankfulness, kindness and patience. In addition, increased rhythmical emotional energies can be thought of as spiritual growth. Conversely, increased chaotic energies can be thought of as spiritual wilting.

Spiritual growth is painful but it will not harm the body. Spiritual growth can be described as the process of energetically releasing old toxic patterns of chaotic energies. The transition from accumulated chaotic energies towards the ability to release them from the body is a heartfelt process. However, spiritual stagnation creates physical pain. Pain arises from the congestion of chaotic energies within body tissues.

Staying stuck in one's illusions requires increasing life energy to maintain until one day the owner falls off into another painful reality check. Reality checks describe growth of the spirit. A growing spirit manifests as the increased ability to forgive, love, give, surrender, accept, help and be kind.

Doctors witness this common thread between pain release and the process of spiritual growth among their patients and themselves. Some have concluded that owners are here to learn. Some owners learn their lessons faster than others. Some waste less life energy. Reducing chaotic energy also reduces the waste of life energy.

Minimizing chaotic energies turns out to be a very selfish understanding when pursuing health and longevity. Owners, who stay fresh in the rhythm of the moment, benefit from the health advantage of the seventh principle of longevity. In addition, owners who accomplish this are also able to release the energies that maim. This conservation allows even more energy for the present. More energy for the present day results from the increased body rhythm that the positive emotions confer. When an owner enjoys internal rhythm, they are intensely alive. They are alive down to the level of their vibrating cells.

Master owners down through the ages have consistently maintained their own rhythm despite adverse life experiences occurring. Awareness of their own rhythm during painful times allowed them to stay centered. Centeredness describes a state of maintaining one's personal rhythm despite the temptation for the chaotic energies to arise. Staying centered describes how the masters of life refrain from reacting emotionally in ways that have negative energetic consequences to their body tissues.

Healing into longevity, despite adverse life events, involves the understanding of how one deflects the chaotic emotions. In contrast, the common unhealthy experience is typified by reacting to each and every crisis. Unfortunately, frequent indulgence in negative emotional reactivity leads to the accumulation of the chaotic energetic debris. In turn, the chaotic energetic debris weighs down the cells. Eventually it accumulates to the point of affecting inner rhythm. The masters understood that no matter what happens one has a choice to react or not to react. It comes down to keeping personal power (rhythm).

The Energetics of Enlightenment

In general, as human beings progress towards enlightenment there seems to be an increased conservation of energy within their body cells. The energy conservation within these cells arises from their optimizing rhythmical vibrations. Optimal rhythmical vibrations occur when the energies that heal form the predominant emotions. The 'masters' knew the secrets of maintaining their personal power in the face of negative events.

The masters were aware of the temptation to experience negative emotions. The masters viewed these temptations as learning opportunities. In adverse circumstance, the master knew how to choose personal power. Personal power involves the rhythm of living energy that allows health to continue.

Healing involves allowing the processes that facilitate increased rhythm to penetrate to the level of the body cells. So much disease results from the disharmonious chaotic energies. The chaotic energies can be thought of as stagnant and swirling in nature. Chaotic energies absorb into the body tissues when the owner indulges in negative emotions. Eventually, negative emotions, absorb beyond one's tolerance threshold and disease processes begin their destructive effect.

Many owners become involved in a vicious cycle of emotional highs and lows. Owners caught in this drama of emotional reactivity have good days. However, the willingness to indulge in negative emotions guarantees there will certainly be bad days. Eventually, it becomes an increasing challenge to have a good day as more emotional negative baggage accumulates within the tissues. 'Gray' emotional tone typically sets in around middle age. Survival mode occurs at this time. These owners feel trapped in a gray and cold world.

Fortunately, some forms of knowledge exist that are accessed by being in touch with common sense. Accessing the 'collective mind' was what the life work of pioneers like Carl Jung was about. However, the dominant frenzy to hoard and amass more in industrial based societies often forgets men/women that contemplated higher knowing paths.

In contrast, listening to a heart felt path is of great value in some cultures. These societies place great importance on its members discovering their uniqueness. They believe this is a teaching planet and that humans are created to learn. They believe that only one human worry exists. It involves that a given owner honors his/her reason for asking to be born. They believe in asking to be born into the human domain. They believe that each person receives unique talents and abilities. In these cultures it is up to the individual to re-discover why they are here.

Their only worry concerns whether they honor their gifts. All other worries in these societies prove as an illusion. As a consequence, the orientation within these cultures channels conscious energy into discovering why an owner chose to be born and what it is he/she can contribute.

However, the Western mindset often forgets its member's personal missions as a primary factor of the human experience. Some argue that this trait results in a decrease in common sense and personal empowerment. The life of being a doctor in clinical practice reveals that most adults are stressed out. Most of the time owners are in a series of days typified by the need to hurry. Often the hurry involves pursuit of what they believe will make them happy.

Exceptions exist to this common observation. These exceptional people encourage physicians continuing to work. These exceptional people make a difference in all who are sensitive enough to perceive their beauty. They are beautiful because these owners have not lost their rhythm (personal power) and consequently remain awake to what life has to offer. Often they are described as exuding a particular freshness.

Some mystics opine that as a culture, the relationship between happiness and rhythm seems to be forgotten. However, without rhythm operating in one's life, there can be no happiness. Perhaps other cultures have something to teach Western people about more fulfilling lives. These cultures possess knowledge of the importance of rhythm and its relationship to health and happiness. These cultures possess knowledge of processes that facilitate rhythm. These cultures look within and understand the kind of emotional baggage that destroys health and happiness.

The energies that maim congregate within certain body tissues. These chaotic energies tend to accumulate with the passage of time. If one understands this, a healing path becomes possible. Thankfully, this path does not require a suffering patient to wait until they become enlightened.

Rather, alternative medicine modalities facilitate a flushing out of the tissues of the energies that maim (the painful and chaotic energies). These methods include chiropractic cranial sacral therapy, acupuncture, different types of massage therapies (body work), homeopathy, and prayerful meditation. Each of these modalities shares the common denominator that they cleanse the life field. Consequently, each in their own way, they cleanse the body of the emotional baggage, the energies that maim.

These techniques can be applied as an owner works to consciously learn how to forgive. These modalities also buy time while one learns how to avoid the reactive indulgence in the negative emotions. Also, these treatment modalities offer a way of keeping things in an energetic balance. It becomes a personal choice as to how one feels most comfortable flushing their chaotic energetic debris.

Ideally, there will come a time in each owner's life when the ability to forgive enhances. This ability allows the experience of freshness and openness to life. Many theologians believe this is where one begins to awaken to life and its true meaning.

Without forgiveness, joy in life is not possible. The Chinese have known for several millennia that joy is the preferred emotion of the heart. Ample joy operating in one's life allows rhythm to continue.

The peculiar thing about life that physicians witness first hand is that the owners who choose joy each day very often have some of the most difficult lives and circumstance. This fact describes one of the truly awe-inspiring advantages of a life devoted to helping owners to heal. Physicians often witness a joyful owner who confronts the painful moments in life with a faith that things will get better. Accompanying this faith is the belief that what seems like misfortune often turns into an opportunity.

An old parable illustrates this point and goes something like this: There was an old poor man living high in a mountain valley with his only son. One day he and his son came upon a group of horses corralled in a narrow canyon. The young son was so excited and exclaimed 'father what wonderful luck to have come on these horses trapped in this canyon'. The father was older and wiser and he took this opportunity to say 'good luck or bad luck who knows'. The son was quite puzzled by his father's words. The next day the son attempted to work with the horses when suddenly he was kicked and suffered a terrible fracture to one of his legs. To this he cried out to his father 'oh what terrible luck'. His father patiently responded while splinting up the son's leg, 'good luck or bad luck, who knows'. The son just looked at his father in disbelief at this statement. Then in the next little while a terrible war broke out in the kingdom and while the young man was lying in his bed recovering an emissary came to recruit all young men to fight in the king's war. When he left because he saw that this young man would be crippled for quite some time the son said to the father 'good luck or bad luck who knows'.

What does an openness and freshness to life look like in every day terms, so that an owner can apply this principle towards a more healing life rhythm? Cultivating a consciousness of the energy that they, and those around them, exude provides a meaningful clue. Conceptually it is a question. Is there 'lantern' energy or 'vacuum' energy in operation? Most people are a blend of both. Very few exist on either extreme of the energy spectrum.

The lantern energies result from those who have accessed the gift of their hearts, allowing joy to touch those that they contact. Almost all owners have encountered people that have an abundance of love, courage, passion and faith. It is truly a joy to be in their presence. They become the trusted friends that people seek out and rely on during the challenges of their life experience. These people have accessed the gifts of the heart and are able to touch others lives in a powerful way. Less obvious is the energetic rhythm that permeates those that possess this wisdom.

The energetic lanterns of the world have accessed the gifts of their heart. Doctors see these owners. Many have had challenging lives. Many are materially poor. Many experience ongoing problems that they face with courage. The difference between them and the energetic vacuums seems to be that they choose to forgive and therefore greet each day with freshness. They realize that hanging on to the negative emotional energies did them harm. Freed by this understanding, they possess the ability to touch the lives of those all around them.

In contrast, there are those who seem to suck energy from all they contact. These types typify the other extreme on the energetic spectrum. A powerful component of the healing process is gained when an owner becomes sensitive to the energetic dynamics in operation and consciously begins to promote ways to facilitate their own rhythm.

It takes all types of energetic shades, between the vacuum and lantern types, to make up a world. It also takes an openness to see this dynamic played out in so many ways between so many different owners each and every day. Less obvious is the rhythm-versus-chaos that transfers with each interaction, down into the owner's cells. Healing can begin to occur when a given owner begins to make conscious decisions that facilitate the healing energies.

The energies that heal contrasted to the energies that maim are a difficult concept for the Western mind to grasp. Jesus' Sermon on the Mount summarizes, in many ways, the path to the healing energies that confer a rhythm to the cells. The love chapter in 11 Corinthians also helps one to grasp how to access the gifts of the heart.

It comes down to living the truth of the gifts from the heart. What does it look like when one lives in heart wisdom? Mother Theresa provides an inspiring example. She was able to live out her life in the wisdom of the gifts from the heart and give to those in need. Mahatma Gandhi lived a life of non-violence and tolerance through which he was able to accomplish

585

much good for his fellow countrymen. Patch Adams, MD, whose message of laughter and non-violence, has led to a hospital providing for free patient care. Patch has continued to live on minimal dollars a month and the rest he donates to the gift of his free clinic. He decided many years ago that he was never going to have a bad day again. Here is a man living in the gifts from the heart.

The Physical health of the heart muscle

The seventh principle of longevity has unique application within one's heart. However, like other body organs the physical structure hungers for specific factors before healing occurs. For this reason, the additional principles, which need extra clarification as they pertain specifically to the heart, are briefly expanded below.

Principles 1 and 2

What is good for the blood vessels is also good for the heart (section one). However, the heart blood vessels prove unique in two ways. First, the heart receives its blood nourishment in diastole. Diastole denotes the resting phase pressure while the heart chambers fill with blood that will be ejected with the heart's next beat, systole.

Consequently, when the blood pressure lowers too far the heart blood supply may become vulnerable. In contrast, other body tissues depend on systolic pressure for their nourishment. Systole describes the forceful pressure of ejection of blood from the heart out into the body. Systolic pressure is measured by the upper blood pressure value. Diastolic pressure is measured by the lower blood pressure value. Sometimes   heart vulnerability occurs when blockages exist within the blood vessels that supply the heart. Blockages tend to increase risk because they promote a pressure drop past the area of constriction. Consequently, beyond the blockage, a lower initial pressure causes a lower downstream perfusion pressure. As a rule, this warrants a more modest decrease of diastolic pressure when one already has heart disease. Ensuring this step will tend to keep the perfusion pressure adequate past the diseased segment of the coronary artery. This fact results because whatever the pressure value before the blockage, it always diminishes past the blockage.

The second unique feature about the blood vessels (coronary arteries) that supply the heart muscle regards the amount of immune scavenger cells that line the inside of these vessels. These scavenger cells are called macrophages. Recall, these cells possess a propensity to collect LDL cholesterol. On the upside, this propensity provides the heart with an adequate fat fuel supply when the owner exercises. However, well-fed and sedentary types of owners very rarely cause these cells to discharge their fat contents. Rather, in these sedentary types the fat slowly collects after each feeding event. In addition, the higher the insulin levels, the higher the message content within the liver to make and dump LDL cholesterol into the blood stream (butter fat). Obviously, the more LDL cholesterol released into the blood stream, the more stuffed these macrophage cells become.

> As an aside, the work of Broda Barnes, MD, PhD, clearly suggests that less than higher normal thyroid function promotes the failure of sugar waste removal (mucopolysaccharides or GAG) overlying the endothelium (the innermost blood vessel cell). This process predates the actual accumulation of lipid. It also causes stiffening of the arteries (arteriolosclerosis). Dr. Barnes lectured that it was the excessive waste, which eventually slowed the ability of LDL to exit the arteries and as a consequence it abnormally accumulates within the macrophages secondary to its delayed exit time. Thankfully, at any time the gradual reintroduction of high normal thyroid states, once again allows the body to remove this waste and hence the cholesterol begins to leave the endothelial layer again.

Typically, around middle age these cells can become so laden with LDL cholesterol that they grow into foam cells. Foam cells do not go anywhere. The larger they grow the more the coronary arteries block off. Congregations of foam cells constitute the earliest recognized lesions in the development of heart disease, the fatty streak.

The ways to discourage foam cell growth in one's coronary arteries were reviewed in the blood vessel chapter, the digestion of fat subsection (section three) and in the liver chapter (section four). Attention to the ways one lowers blood vessel risk factors discussed in the first section will help to solve the foam cell growth problem. Progress can be followed by sequential cholesterol profiles, especially if one's profile was abnormal to begin with. This also applies to owners who have a more normal profile only because they ingest a cholesterol-lowering drug. Cholesterol lowering drugs lower LDL cholesterol production. However, these drugs cause the owner's body to experience the side effects mentioned in the first, third and fourth sections. More information about the statin drugs downside follows in the next subsection.

Principle 3: the Hormones Giveth and Taketh Away One's Heart

Several hormones prove important in the regulation of the blood supply within one's heart. The ability to increase the heart's supply of nutrient rich blood, on demand, is largely the role of the biogenic amine type hormones. **Histamine** is one such hormone, which is important to both blood supply and pump function of the heart muscle. Histamine seems to be the secret hormone within the heart.

One of the secrets about histamine regards its ability to increase the strength of the heart's beating. In fact, one of the main benefits to the failing hearts that ACE inhibitor type drugs provide involves their ability to increase the activation of the histamine receptors in the heart. Activated histamine receptors increase the force of contraction. The increased power of contraction increases the delivery of nutrients to the body.

Epinephrine is the second example of an important blood flow regulator to heart muscle from the biogenic amine hormone class. Increased epinephrine levels will cause the dilatation of coronary arteries to five times their resting diameter. During times of increased demand, dilatation greatly enhances cardiac work output. For this reason, processes that ensure adequate epinephrine availability protect the heart from inadequate vessel dilatation. Realize, epinephrine deficiency decreases the ability of the heart to increase its work output. Epinephrine deficiency results from nutritional deficiency. Nutritional deficiency commonly manifests when one chronically subsists on a processed food diet. As a consequence, when epinephrine deficiency occurs, the heart becomes unable to dilate its coronary arteries to increase its blood flow.

Realize some of these dietary deficiencies result in the increased production of norepinephrine, which proves much weaker because it is less able to dilate the coronary arteries. The additional consequence of increased nor-epinephrine production, secondary to the epinephrine deficiency that causes it, is that the systemic blood pressure rises considerably. In turn, the consequent blood pressure increase places a tremendous extra strain on the heart.

Recall, epinephrine deficiency usually involves a depleted methyl donor system (section one and three). Methyl is needed to turn norepinephrine into epinephrine. Methyl donation creates homocysteine unless the methyl donor system of nutrients remains intact. Consequently, an elevated blood homocysteine level provides a useful laboratory marker that the methyl donor system has depleted. Increased homocysteine levels prove easier to interpret than a twenty-four hour urine test for epinephrine breakdown products. In addition, since epinephrine has such a short half-life in the blood stream the testing for meaningful blood level averages becomes cumbersome.

Sufficient amounts of **thyroid hormone** are fundamental to normal heart function. Optimal thyroid message content directs the heart cells to do four important things. First, thyroid directs the heart cell DNA programs to make more epinephrine receptors. More epinephrine receptors allow the heart to increase its work performance, because its message directs increased blood supply within the coronary arteries by five fold.

Second, the thyroid message allows the heart to burn more fuel in the presence of oxygen because its message also directs heart DNA to invest in upgrades of the mitochondria (the power plants). Recall, the mitochondria often number over two thousand per heart cell. This high number causes massive amounts of energy to be generated for useful work. For this reason, sufficient thyroid hormone causes the energy generation abilities of the mitochondria to increase (see thyroid discussion in section two).

Thirdly, the thyroid message powerfully increases the membrane voltage of heart cells. The heart cell membrane voltage increases because thyroid message content directs other DNA programs to direct membrane pump synthesis (sodium-potassium ATPase). Important point: The more membrane pumps the higher the cardiac cell voltage possible. In turn, the higher the membrane voltage the less irritable (the more rhythmical) and the more work a heart cell produces.

Many physicians fear thyroid for its supposed heart palpitation potential. However, adequate magnesium and potassium supplementation lowers the occurrence of this problem. It helps to think of the acute situation of restoring sufficient thyroid message content as straining the already mineral depleted body. Initially, increased thyroid stresses the system because it directs more minerals like magnesium and potassium to enter the cells. Recall, the 2% percent tank of potassium is contained within the blood stream and the remainder (98%) resides inside body cells. One consequence of this fact is increased message content from thyroid drives the tiny blood stream amount of potassium into the cells. Therefore, insufficient dietary potassium and/or magnesium increase irregular heart rate possibilities. For these reasons, withholding appropriate dietary counseling causes heart palpitations to become likely.

A final point about mineral pumps deserves emphasis. The medical physiology textbooks allude to the fact that aldosterone message content also contributes to the cell voltage abilities of the nerve and cardiac cell types. Whether this effect proves to be a direct effect of aldosterone working with thyroid hormones to activate specific DNA programs remains to be seen. It may be that because aldosterone controls the rate of all body steroids manufacture rates; this drives the voltage in some other indirect way.

The fourth point that concerns thyroid hormone sufficiency determining cardiac health arises because it determines the amount of pituitary manufactured Growth Hormone. Growth Hormone levels provide the ability to defend protein (positive nitrogen balance control regulator). Muscle performance, like found in cardiac tissue, critically depends on adequate nitrogen balance. In addition, muscle tissue, like in cardiac cells, prefers IGF-1 for its fuel delivery requirements. Recall, Growth Hormone centrally determines IGF-1 release rates. Finally, as was mentioned earlier in this section, cartilage tissue, like found in heart valves, critically depends on sufficient Growth Hormone.

Cortisol helps thyroid direct the heart cell DNA (genes) to manufacture the epinephrine receptors. Extreme cortisol depletion results in Addison's disease and these patients present with a small and weakened heart. Both thyroid and cortisol message content are needed to instruct the heart cell DNA to manufacture the completed epinephrine receptor. Cortisol and thyroid are level one-type hormones and are therefore able to direct DNA activity. For this reason, insufficient levels of either hormone will produce a decreased ability to respond to epinephrine. A decreased epinephrine response results in a diminished ability to increase the nutrient supply within the heart muscle. In turn, decreased nutrient supply results in a diminished ability to increase the work output of the heart.

Testosterone primarily directs heart muscle cell build up (anabolism). Realize heart cell DNA, throughout life, critically depends on adequate build up message from testosterone. Functional buildup of any tissue, including heart, requires positive nitrogen balance. Positive nitrogen balance is another way of saying it requires sufficient gene activation because only active genes determine the protein synthesis rate. In turn, protein synthesis sufficiency is really what positive nitrogen balance is all about. When was the last time anyone heard about a conventionally trained physician considering these facts for their patients in heart failure?

A corollary to this fact concerns one of the most successful medications used to reinvigorate the failing heart, as a pump, the digitalis medications (Lanoxin). Digitalis medications' molecular structures consist of testosterone like steroids attached to a few sugars. These patented derivatives of the fox glove plant are second to no other heart medication in their ability to reinvigorate a failing heart.

Unfortunately, physicians are usually schooled about peripheral effects of this medication like its slowing conduction time. In addition this medication is presented with the abstraction of the Frank-Starling curve. This curve describes the improvement of pump function when digitalis-like medications are prescribed. However, the more powerful salient point that elucidates their mechanism of action is found in their molecular structure.

The molecular structure of the digitalis derivatives (cardiac glycosides) contains testosterone-like steroids. These molecular arrangements are similar to ginseng. However, the relation to digitalis and ginseng obscures by duplicitous scientific nomenclature. The nomenclature changes when it describes ginseng's active components as saponins. However, both of these substances are technically glycosides.

The digitalis-like medications have the side effect of breast enlargement. Also similarly, one of the big obstacles to successful testosterone replacement in middle-aged males concerns breast enlargement. Three common reasons explain why this occurs in middle-aged males.

First, involves the increased presence of body fat content. Increased body fat proves as a common feature in those owners that have a weakened heart. **One of the problems with increased body fat is that it has a propensity to convert testosterone to estrogen. Estrogen is made from testosterone with the enzyme called aromatase. Aromatase is found in fat cells.** Consequently, the breasts of obese males are stimulated to grow secondary to the increased estrogen that forms.

Recently there has been increased interest in aromatase inhibitors. So far this interest has been devoted towards inhibiting estrogen formation in women with breast cancer reoccurrence potential. Unfortunately, less commonly appreciated concerns the fact that the majority of men with enlarged or malignant prostates suffer from excessive prostatic estrogen exposure and this shows up in their 24-hour urine test results. Making this common observation even more alarming concerns the fact that estrogen causes cystic metaplasia (precancerous changes) and hypertrophy (enlargement) of prostate tissue. How effective the different aromatase inhibitors diminish the estrogen levels within the prostate, which often drives this disease problem remains to be seen.

The second reason that estrogen levels increase in middle-aged males involves zinc deficiency. Zinc inhibits aromatase activity. Zinc status in the body is best measured by hair or red blood cell analysis. Zinc also proves fundamental in immune cell function, skin health, retinal function, steroid hormones and thyroid hormones ability to bind DNA (zinc fingers), pH balance of blood, stomach acid manufacture ability and testosterone production rates.

The third reason that the middle-aged heart disease afflicted male will tend towards enlarged breast concerns the fact that they often prove methyl donor deficient. Methyl donor deficiency increases the conversion rate of testosterone to estrogen. This side effect occurs because this conversion creates methyl for other body processes. Recall that in the best of circumstances the body needs a methyl at the rate of one billion times a second!

Testosterone treatment exists in the mainstream for treating a failing heart in other parts of the world. Several years ago there was a study done in England that convincingly showed the benefit of testosterone replacement therapy for heart disease patients. The caveat here is to avoid testosterone's conversion into estrogen. One possible solution is to administer the more powerful dihydro-testosterone. Dihydro-testosterone ((DHT) that cannot be converted to estrogen. Chemists denote this property as non-aromatizable.

Important caveats occur for administering DHT or testosterone to male owners. The first concern involves the mercury additive sometimes found in the injectable forms of testosterone. The code name for this additive is thimerosal (see mercury discussion in the brain chapter). Mercury is toxic to body tissues and has no business being added to these preparations. Therefore any owner with heart disease considering testosterone therapy needs to obtain mercury free hormone. In addition, there is also the need to follow serial PSA values any time steroids are prescribed past middle age, in men, because of the possibility of stimulating abnormal prostate growth.

It is important to note that estrogen mimics (see hormone mimics, section two) within the prostate stimulate abnormal amounts of DHT receptor formation. DHT receives blame but often the true culprit proves as the increased estrogen message content. The European medical community spends more time unraveling the prostate problem's etiology. Over there, they realize that prostate tissue deteriorates when testosterone levels fall. Over here a knee jerk reaction occurs about how bad DHT is for the prostate. If this were true then being young would predictably be a risk for prostate cancer because young men have the highest levels of DHT. For these reasons, it seems prudent to begin to better assess each male owners unique prostate status. The 24-hour urine for steroids with estrogen status included provides a place to start. The definitive book on this subject is written by Jonathan V. Wright, M.D. and is called; ***Protect your Potency and Vitality for Men over age 45***.

William B. Ferril, M. D.

Inflammation and Heart disease: a Holistic Perspective

The amount of insulin within the body determines the amount of fat-maker message. Hormones, like insulin, carry information to the body cells. Hormone information always concerns how cells direct energy expenditure. Insulin carries information that instructs cells to store energy. Most body energy storage occurs as fat. Cholesterol is one type of body fat. The enzyme in the liver that makes sugar into cholesterol turns up its activity when insulin levels rise. Insulin levels rise following carbohydrate meals or excess mental stress (among several other promoters). Rather than educate doctors and the public about this simple cause and effect relationship, the story for the wonders of the statin drugs bombards media outlets.

Statin drugs work, in part, because they poison this liver enzyme's ability to listen to the insulin message. The trouble with poisons concerns their inevitable side effects and toxicities. One nasty side effect from these medications concerns the depletion of Co enzyme Q10 in the body. The heart needs the lion's share of this important nutrient. Deficiency here causes one type of heart failure.

Another emerging understanding for how statin drugs lower heart disease risk involves their ability to subdue inflammation. Rather than come clean and educate physicians about the most likely mechanism for how this occurs, the statin selling companies perpetrate the story that it remains largely a mystery. The argument for it being a mystery diminishes once a few critical clues add back into the discussion. Additionally, their rosy innocence fades as well, because their likely downside emerges.

The **first** clue involves the long-known association between heart disease and the Type A personality types. Type A personality types are classically described as hard driving, over achieving, and always worried about their next deal. Physiologically, these emotions when chronically expressed lead to a constant stress hormone response. The stress response was designed to survive physical stressors. In order to survive a physical stress, the massive dumping of fuel into the blood stream makes sense because exercising muscles consume the fuel. Additionally, physical stressors often lead to trauma. This explains why the acute phase reactants predictably elevate with the onset of the stressor. The acute phase reactants prove appropriate with trauma, but deleterious with mental stress. C-reactive protein are only one acute phase reactant. Others include complement, interferon, fibrinogen, ferritin, ceruloplasmin and amyloid. Fibrinogen directly increases the clotting tendencies of blood. Ferritin elevations increase iron absorption into the body tissues.

The trauma associated with physical stressors underscores the desirability for new blood cells' manufacture where-with-all. However, with mental stress, once iron absorbs into the body, it proves very difficult to remove. This detail may help explain the emerging realization that many heart disease patients have elevated ferritin levels. It further explains a potential reason that chelation therapy maintains its devotees, despite the ongoing criticism. Specifically, EDTA binds and removes iron from the body. This fact may prove as the number one benefit for this approach.

Lastly, concerning the acute phase reactants elevation in the setting of mental stressors, involves its inappropriate effect toward an increase in angiogenesis propensity. The angiogenesis propensity increases when the acute phase reactants elevate. This again makes sense with physical stressors because these traumas associate with the need for new blood vessel formation.

Chronic mental stress promotes two powerful processes that promote the angiogenesis critical to tumor growth: increased insulin needs and the heightened angiogenesis propensity described above. **These facts, taken together, provide a likely mechanism for why overweight and stressed individuals suffer increased morbidity and mortality from cancer.**

The **second** clue involves the emerging research results that document that the statin drugs lower C-reactive protein levels (CRP). However, once one recalls the connection between HMG Co A reductase activity and steroid synthesis rates, a more holistic picture emerges. Anything that subdues the ability of the adrenal glands to make steroids, will also diminish the magnitude of cortisol released for a given stressor. In turn, less cortisol release subdues the acute phase reactants' release. C-reactive protein (CRP) is only one of the acute phase reactants. The normalization of acute phase reactants, in the chronic mentally stressed state, leads to less inflammation for the reasons described above.

These facts initially sound too good to be true. This old adage once again proves useful because the downside to this scenario provides insight into the advantages of counseling Type A personality-type owners about the bigger picture of cause and effect relationships.

In order to better appreciate the downside of the statins, one needs to recall the typical body habitus of the Type A personality owner. The majority of them are large in the waistline, or at the very least, they have increased visceral fat. Currently, a waist measurement above 40 inches is felt to predict these metabolic syndrome types at risk for accelerated aging and blood vessel disease. Over forty years ago, obese individuals were found to have increased stress steroid metabolites in their urine.

Uniting these two facts together it becomes more likely to understand one of the metabolic syndromes individual's driving pathological forces: Exaggerated stress steroid release rate for a given stressor. Another way to look at this is, in the setting of chronic mental stress, those prehistorically equipped survival machines selected for down through the ages have become the metabolic syndrome victims from chronic sedentary-type stressors. What was once a survival benefit derived from mounting a strong fuel release and acute phase reactant release (both secondary to a strong cortisol release) in the setting of physical stress, now has become a curse, promoting excessive body fat accumulation and blood vessel inflammation.

Excessive cortisol release violently activates protein dismantling into more sugar (gluconeogenesis). Protein content within denotes the metabolically active constituent of body tissue. Defense of body protein content proves fundamental to healthful longevity. Healthy people have sufficient Growth Hormone release that protects their protein from excessive catabolism during these times. However, middle-aged individuals that chronically experience stress but have sedentary lifestyles begin to suffer various amounts of glandular decline.

One mechanism for glandular decline involves the inappropriate elevation of blood sugar caused by mental stress in the sedentary state. Elevated blood sugar suppresses Growth Hormone release. In turn, less Growth Hormone release leads to less defense of body protein ability. This fact ties in the observation about Syndrome X (metabolic syndrome) patients evidencing sarcopenia. It also elucidates the likely association between this Syndrome, and it underlying a variant presentation of Cushing's disease pathology (see testing below).

With mental stress, the increased blood fuel has nowhere to go. Hence, for these reasons, increased insulin amounts eventually release to normalize the blood sugar. Again, this same metabolic derangement operates within the classical Cushing's disease patient. Unfortunately, very few physicians appreciate the sequential release of first cortisol (catabolic) followed by increased need for insulin to correct the inappropriate rise in blood sugar. It is the increased insulin that makes the typical Cushing's disease patient fat. It is the increased cortisol that causes excessive catabolism of their body protein that leads to chronic surges in their blood sugar levels. These surges need excessive insulin to return the blood sugar towards normal.

Unfortunately, insulin releases into the portal vein and heads straight for the liver. HMG Co A reductase turns on with increasing insulin and off with increasing glucagon. Because the liver (also fat cells) cells have 200,000 pure insulin-type receptors per cell, insulin excess profoundly influences the cholesterol profile by this mechanism.

Consequently, a heightened stress response causes what was once protein, a few minutes before to now float within the blood stream as sugar. However, with mental stress a few minutes later, the pancreas senses the elevated blood sugar. Now the protein turned into sugar is changed yet again into cholesterol and fat.

A cognizance for this anatomical reality helps one to see that the liver functions as an insulin trap and only excessive amounts of insulin secretion can spill past the liver and out into the general circulation. Healthy people need less insulin because their livers secrete sufficient IGF-1 that largely negates the need for insulin between meals, while fasting or when exercising. Circulating IGF-1 levels directly depend on sufficient Growth Hormone release. Realize, only sufficient Growth Hormone release defends body protein between meals, while exercising or when fasting. All other counter regulatory hormones (cortisol, epinephrine and glucagon) make protein dismantling for fuel creation fair game.

The old name for IGF-1 clarifies its crucial role in sugar metabolism, the nonsuppressible insulin like activity of the blood stream. Many physicians remain unaware of this fact and it seems rather odd to this author that it fails to receive even cursory mention while reviewing Metabolic Syndrome (Syndrome X) pathology. The healthiest people possess the highest IGF-1 levels. A falling IGF-1 leads to increased insulin need (insulin resistance).

The very survival of the statin drug-selling rosy picture depends on eviscerating certain scientific consequences that result from a diminished glandular ability. When healthy, the adrenal glands make both catabolic and anabolic message content. A higher anabolic message content leads to a faster repair rate. The lower the antioxidants, the more repairs need to occur. Here lies the likely additional risk of chronically consuming statin drugs in place of healing lifestyles: They contribute to the lack of repair from ongoing wear and tear that the blood vessels encounter. Disrepair causes inflammatory damage despite their benefit from inducing decreased cholesterol and acute phase reactants levels.

Beyond the liver, HMG Co A reductase also occurs within the adrenals and gonads as well. Any drug or toxin that inhibits the steroid manufacture ability within the adrenals or gonads, will also decrease the repair rate that logically follows from diminished anabolic message content. Here lies another downside that remains ignored until one begins to examine the interrelatedness of steroid synthesis rates and HMG Co A reductase activity.

In one way or another, blood vessel disease results from the repair rate not keeping up with the injury rate. Statin drugs may in fact lower the injury rate by diminishing the acute phase reactants' caused inflammation and cortisol-related blood sugar spikes. In turn, the lessened blood sugar spikes lead to decreased insulin need despite a sedentary and stress-filled lifestyle. A subdued stress response means that less acute phase reactants release, as well. However, what is not being said concerns their probable negative influence on the repair rate of blood vessels and muscle tissue. The repair rate of muscles and blood vessels depend on androgen levels, like all other DNA-containing body cells. Since science has already documented subdued acute phase reactants with statin usage, it remains quite likely that other steroids' synthesis rates decrease, as well

The likely consequence of diminished testosterone, which results from statin drug usage, may help further elucidate the ongoing suspicion about their contribution to heart failure. Many in the holistic community attribute this tendency to the diminished Co enzyme Q10 levels that logically follow. However, maybe a fall off in testosterone in some chronic statin users, contributes to their pump failure as well.

Following serial 24-hour urine measurements for steroids would provide a logical next step for testing the severity of diminished anabolic message content. It also will further elucidate the before and after profiles of the stress steroid metabolites of Syndrome X patients. Recall, that over fifty years ago, obese patients were documented to have elevations in their 24-hour urine test for stress steroid metabolites. If each doctor in the holistic community began collecting baseline 24-hour urine specimens for steroids, and followed them serially, a new level of understanding would emerge about the association of a heightened stress response, increased insulin need, and elevated acute phase reactants in the development of blood vessel disease. At the very least, real hormone replacement therapy could be instituted to address these steroid defects before they weaken the statin drug user. Ideally, this test could be used to help better motivate the type A personality derived Metabolic Syndrome (Syndrome X) individual take a more active role in which hormones secrete.

Most cited references on statins effect on testosterone levels. Physicians confront the superficial veneer that suggests an intellectual dead end.

1) Z Kardiol. 2004 Jan;93(1):43-8.

Does statin therapy influence steroid hormone synthesis?

Bohm M, Herrmann W, Wassmann S, Laufs U, Nickenig G.

2) J Clin Pharm Ther. 2004 Feb;29(1):71-3.

Hormonal changes with cholesterol reduction: a double-blind pilot study.

Ormiston T, Wolkowitz OM, Reus VI, Johnson R, Manfredi F.

3) J Atheroscler Thromb. 2003;10(3):160-4.

Atorvastatin treatment does not affect gonadal and adrenal hormones in type 2
diabetes patients with mild to moderate hypercholesterolemia.

Santini SA, Carrozza C, Lulli P, Zuppi C, CarloTonolo G, Musumeci S.

4) Psychoneuroendocrinology. 2003 Feb;28(2):181-94.

Does simvastatin affect mood and steroid hormone levels in
Hypercholesterolemic men? A randomized double-blind trial.

Hyyppa MT, Kronholm E, Virtanen A, Leino A, Jula A.

5) Am J Med. 2002 Dec 15;113(9):723-7.

Cholesterol-lowering medication, cholesterol level, and reproductive
hormones in women: the Women's Ischemia Syndrome Evaluation (WISE).

Bairey Merz CN, Olson MB, Johnson BD, Bittner V, Hodgson TK, Berga SL, Braunstein GD, Pepine CJ, Reis SE, Sopko G, Kelsey SF; Women's Ischemia Syndrome Evaluation.

6) Metabolism. 2000 Sep;49(9):1234-8.

Effects of high-dose simvastatin on adrenal and gonadal steroidogenesis in men with hypercholesterolemia.

Dobs AS, Schrott H, Davidson MH, Bays H, Stein EA, Kush D, Wu M, Mitchel Y, Illingworth RD.

7) Metabolism. 2000 Jan;49(1):115-21.

Effects of simvastatin and pravastatin on gonadal function in male hypercholesterolemic patients.

Dobs AS, Miller S, Neri G, Weiss S, Tate AC, Shapiro DR, Musliner TA.

8) J Endocrinol Invest. 1998 May;21(5):310-7.

Effects of long-term pravastatin treatment on spermatogenesis and on adrenal and testicular steroidogenesis in male hypercholesterolemic patients.

Bernini GP, Brogi G, Argenio GF, Moretti A, Salvetti A.

9) Horm Metab Res. 1996 Apr;28(4):193-8.

Testicular function in hypercholesterolemic male patients during prolonged simvastatin treatment.

Azzarito C, Boiardi L, Vergoni W, Zini M, Portioli I.

10) Metabolism. 1993 Sep;42(9):1146-52.

Long-term endocrine function in hypercholesterolemic patients treated with pravastatin, a new 3-hydroxy-3-methylglutaryl coenzyme A reductase inhibitor.

Dobs AS, Sarma PS, Schteingart D.

In general, at first glance, these articles effectively cause the inquiring physician to lose enthusiasm about a negative consequence between statin usage and steroid levels. However, four main points (beyond the numerous methodological flaws that occurred with most of these individual studies) allow the resuscitation of integrative physicians collaborating further and providing less dubious conclusions. 1) All the above studies fail to differentiate between high cholesterol and the presence or absence of heart disease in their cohort groups. 2) 8 out of 10 of the above studies are of 24 weeks or less duration time. 3) The 2 studies that most convincingly demonstrate the diminution of steroids with statin drug use were the only studies longer than 24 weeks duration. 4) None of the above popularly cited studies utilized the gold standard of scientifically assessing steroid status-the GC mass spec derived values from 24-urine results. Only GC mass spec measures the important steroid metabolites that add predictive value.

Possibly, for these reasons the time is ripe for holistic physicians to begin spending less time initially persuading their patients against statin therapy but, for a short while, begin documenting the effects of such therapy by monitoring their 24-urine steroid profiles before and after treatment in their patients that prefer the pill approach. Preliminary findings of those patients on statin drugs with heart disease tend to support a negative correlation. This will prove helpful if there is truth in the long held suspicion that those individuals with lower testosterone to start with are the very ones that are at increased risk of atherosclerosis. Therefore, lowering cholesterol without maintaining testosterone will prove to be folly.

Principle 4: You are What You Absorb

Diet related deficiencies impair the work performance of the heart. **Carnitine deficiency** has long been known to produce a type of heart failure. Unfortunately, physicians often fail to even perform a rudimentary inquiry into their heart failure patient's carnitine status. Carnitine proves as a necessary carrier of most fatty acids into heart cell mitochondria. Only when a fatty acid successfully transports inside the furnace can it be further processed for combustion in the presence of oxygen. Heart cells are particularly vulnerable to carnitine deficiency because they prefer fatty acids for their fuel source. This probably explains why the macrophage cells line the coronary arteries. These cells probably store fat for the next time an owner physically performs.

Carnitine deficiency leads to a diminished ability of the heart mitochondria to burn their preferred fuel, fatty acids. In turn, the diminished ability to combust fatty acids diminishes the work performance of the heart cells. When work performance diminishes severely, heart failure occurs. In these cases, healing occurs when the carnitine again becomes available. How convenient, low fat diet adherents are the ones most vulnerable to this type of deficiency.

Co enzyme Q10 (ubiquinone) is needed in all the cells. However, the heart requires increased amounts of this nutrient (chapter one) because it combusts so much energy within its mitochondria. Only when owners eat a real food diet can they absorb this in sufficient quantities. Sushi provides an excellent source.

The backup system is the liver's ability to manufacturer Co enzyme Q10. Unfortunately, statin like drugs compromise this backup system because these drugs work by poisoning the liver enzyme, HMG Co A reductase. This enzyme makes both cholesterol and Co enzyme Q10. This fact means that unless an owner absorbs sufficient dietary derived Co enzyme Q10 an increased risk for deficiency of this important nutrient occurs while on the statin drugs. Again, how convenient to not educate physicians about this scientific fact. Problems drive demand for what the complex has for sale.

A smoldering suspicion exists that owners on the statin drugs, who become deficient in Co enzyme Q10, are at increased risk for both heart failure and cancer development. The facilitation of cancer's development is thought to be because the major advantage of the body's immune system against cancer cell formation involves its superior energy generation. Immune cells can generate energy much more effectively when adequate Coenzyme Q10 remains present. This occurs because early on cancer cells often lack a blood supply and hence live off anaerobic methods.

The heart failure is thought to occur because heart cells require the highest amount of this nutrient of anywhere in the body. Therefore a deficiency will show up here first. If Co enzyme Q10 becomes deficient while on the statin drugs, the powering up of both the immune system and heart function compromises.

Often statin drugs become unnecessary whenever the diet and lifestyle stimulate the secretion of appropriate hormones. In the case of HMG Co A reductase, cholesterol biosynthesis increases when insulin levels rise. As discussed before, the requirement for insulin increases with excess carbohydrates consumption, potassium deficiency, or chronic stress with a sedentary lifestyle to name a few. Alternatively, this enzyme's activity towards cholesterol manufacture retards when glucagon levels increase. Low carbohydrate diets encourage increased glucagon levels. Increased insulin levels inhibit glucagon release. Potassium deficiency increases the need for insulin (see below). Finally stress decreases the ratio between glucagon and insulin. It is the lowered ratio at the level of the liver that makes cholesterol synthesis more likely. These three common culprits often cause abnormal cholesterol profiles. Each one has been discussed in the previous sections of this book. However, potassium deficiency is important to review because it provides specific examples of diminished heart performance preventing longevity.

Note: Principle 5 was discussed in section 4

The Sixth Principle and the Heart: Avoid *low cell voltage syndrome*

Potassium deficiency will damage one's heart in eight different ways

Potassium deficiency can show clinically as a diminished EKG voltage. Potassium deficiency commonly occurs by the onset of middle age. Many owners remain unaware of this fact because their laboratory slip from their annual blood work clearly states that their serum potassium is normal. Recall, the serum potassium only measures the 2% tank that regards body potassium. The other 98% of body potassium occurs within the body cells. The 98% tank cannot be measured by this common test. In addition, the 2% tank (the blood stream) will not fall at all until total body potassium becomes severely diminished.

A decrease in total body potassium content will harm one's heart in eight different ways. Remember, the reason potassium deficiency is so common involves the fact that most owners in America consume processed food. Processed food in general has a greatly diminished potassium and magnesium content (mineral table). Also processed food tends to have huge amounts of sodium added. The sodium is added by the food industry to preserve shelf life. Shelf life prolongs because bacteria have just as hard of time with reversed minerals as human cells. The body was designed to intake about three times as much potassium as sodium per day. Here lies the problem in America today: The popular American diet consists of a processed food diet. However, unless food remains unprocessed, the ratio of these important minerals will alter (see section one for relative food mineral concentrations).

Because of this fact, an altered mineral intake ratio eventually subdues the heart's cellular charge. Both the heart and nerve cells, which innervate the heart, are extremely vulnerable to altered mineral balance. This fact occurs because the heart and nerve cells operate on a principle of exaggerated rapid exchange between these minerals in their work cycle. This means, the heart cells and nerve cells within the heart conduct more electrical activity about their cell membrane compared to other body cells.

When mineral flow increases these cells perform more work. The body, with the help of aldosterone and thyroid hormones, will direct the concentration of potassium and magnesium to be maximal within these cells. Simultaneously, these hormones facilitate the concentration of sodium and calcium outside these cells. Realize the functional ability of the heart cell relies on the preferred concentration of these four minerals about the heart cell membrane (section five).

Physicians are educated in a manner that compounds the problem of a low potassium diet. The physician's education does not directly emphasize the importance and methods to achieve adequate potassium intake. A vague emphasis occurs about trying a low sodium diet when a middle-aged patient begins to experience elevated blood pressure. Fresh fruits, unprocessed nuts, fresh meats, dried beans and vegetables are high in potassium. However, when an owner continues to eat processed food the increased sodium diminishes the beneficial ratio.

When stress occurs, even more potassium passes out of the body and into the urinal. Making matters worse, involves the fact that stress favors sodium retention! The consequent diminished ratio between potassium and sodium sets the stage for increasing blood pressure.

Remember, where minerals predominate determines the force of water being drawn towards. Because sodium predominates within the blood stream, its excess accompanied by simultaneous potassium deficiency within the cells causes the blood pressure to rise simply from this aberration alone (insufficient potassium to adequately draw water out of the blood stream and into the cells). Unless both physicians and owners become aware of this fact, a diminished likelihood of avoiding symptom control medicine occurs.

Before the brief discussion on how potassium deficiency injures the heart in eight different ways, one additional point deserves emphasis. The body's cells charge themselves by creating an optimal concentration ratio between four main electrolytes (minerals). The electrolyte ratio occurs between sodium, potassium, magnesium and calcium. In general, if one eats about 1000mg a day of sodium, 4000mg of potassium, 500mg of calcium and 300mg of magnesium the optimal ratio remains. This only stays valid when an owner has normal adrenals and kidney function. Sodium requirements will also increase with increased sweating or gastrointestinal losses. It should also be emphasized that individual variation exists for the need of these different minerals. Therefore the counsel of a competent physician is sometimes necessary if questions arise. Two useful methods used to monitor this ratio involve following the blood pressure and also how one feels. These two facts taken together will go along way for developing an effective plan for improving the quality of one's mineral ratio.

The eight ways that potassium deficiency will damage the heart are:
1. Diminished heart cell voltage generating abilities (section five).
2. Potassium deficiency accelerates syndrome X because it raises insulin requirements (chapter three).
3. Chronic potassium deficiency damages the kidneys and this begins blood pressure elevation. Blood pressure elevation wears out the heart muscle (chapter three).
4. Potassium deficiency causes insulin resistance. Insulin resistance means that for a given sugar load more insulin will need to be secreted before blood sugar will come down. The delay in returning blood sugar to normal will tend to 'rust' heart blood vessel.
5. A body potassium deficiency will lead to an increased activity of the liver enzyme, HMG Co A reductase. This enzyme's activity increases with rising insulin levels. Low potassium with a given sugar load will tend to promote greater insulin release. The increased insulin level will tend to activate HMG Co A reductase and begin the synthesis of cholesterol particles known as LDL cholesterol. The cholesterol manufacture process becomes greatly exaggerated because of the increased insulin level when one is insulin resistant (increased insulin need). Additionally, potassium proves necessary to create glycogen but not for fat and cholesterol manufacture (LDL cholesterol). Elevated LDL cholesterol is a known risk factor for the development of coronary artery blockages. Remember, the foam cells that eventually form here.
6. Low potassium states diminish one's tolerance for aldosterone secretion. Diminished potassium will affect aldosterone in three possible ways. First aldosterone levels will fall off because aldosterone increases potassium loss. However, when a given owner eats the correct mineral ratios then potassium loss involves a good thing. In these situations potassium loss allows the kidneys to flush out waste. However, when potassium becomes deficient then the increased sodium causes fluid retention whenever aldosterone increases.

The second problem related to aldosterone and potassium deficiency is blood pressure. Chronic potassium deficiency will require the aldosterone level to come down in order to normalize the blood pressure. The blood pressure comes down either through medication or the body's wisdom. Aldosterone will need to come down or blood pressure will rise whenever increased sodium and decreased potassium occurs within the body. The trouble with diminished aldosterone states caused by potassium deficiency or medication involves the fact that aldosterone levels determine biosynthesis rates for all other body steroids. Owners with higher aldosterone secretion will make more steroids than owners with low outputs of aldosterone.

The third consequence of diminished aldosterone with potassium deficiency is that aldosterone increases the heart cell's ability to fully charge its membrane (along with the help of thyroid hormone). Only when the body minerals remain balanced can the increased aldosterone, needed by the heart's cell charging mechanisms, be tolerated without high blood pressure problems. The one exception occurs in those owners who possess high levels of the override hormone, ANP (discussed in hormone chapter).

7. Adequate potassium is needed within all body cells to stabilize protein content. When the heart cell content of potassium proves insufficient, protein loss occurs from these cells. Both heart cells and other muscle cells contain high amounts of protein. This fact explains why a potassium deficiency leads to loss of muscle mass.

8. For this reason, potassium deficiency will make the nerves innervating the heart irritable. Irritable nerves excite more readily and therefore cause an irregular heart rate. Irregular heart rate provides one cause for sudden death. Sudden death becomes less likely when an optimal mineral concentration about the heart nerve membrane occurs. Owners that constantly push their luck by eating foods that will alter this ratio increase their risk of sudden death for this reason.

The seventh principle and the heart

The body hormones carry out message delivery initially within the blood stream. However, the *intelligent energy* within living bodies determines when and which body hormones secrete. As a consequence, processes that facilitate the harmony of this life energy (intelligent energy) promote the best hormones. Conversely, processes that interrupt the life energies flow will also disrupt the hormone types and amounts. Bottom line: Health consequences occur when this organizing life energy becomes static, disorganized, excessive or deficient.

The stasis, disorganization, or excessiveness of the life energy is the energies that maim heart cells. However, processes that confer rhythmic flow and optimal amounts of the life energy comprise the energies that heal heart cells. These considerations are also important within the context of the next chapter. Muscles and ligaments provide some of the major tissues that sequester and therefore become congested with static energies, the ones that maim.

CHAPTER TWENTY-SIX

MUSCLES AND LIGAMENTS

The Seventh Principle and the Muscles and Ligaments

Some physicians and alternative practitioners have noted the relationship between different life issues and different levels of back and neck pain. For example, emotional distress tends to disrupt level T9. More painful life issues tend to disrupt T6. Career issues tend to be felt in C3. Relationship issues tend to be felt in L5. Of course, back and neck pain also result from trauma, strain and degenerative processes. In contrast, the above correlations tend to result from trivial movements in bed, bending over, or twisting while grasping an object. These patients then present with varying degrees of incapacitating neck or back pain.

East Indian energy theory regarding the charkas seems to correlate with these cases of incapacitating back and neck pain. Former NASA researcher, Barbara Brennan wrote an excellent introduction to these theories in her book, "*Hands of Light*".

In addition, these ideas form the foundation of chiropractic theory. Chiropractic adjustment techniques facilitate the unbinding of the static energy (the energies that maim). The theory of static emotional energy collecting within the joint spaces explains a possible mechanism for these types of clinical presentation.

No western scientific explanation exists for why chiropractic medical modalities effectively relieve these symptoms. Western medicine fails to recognize that energy stasis describes how these energies maim tissues. The relief of pain by spinal adjustments provides just one example for the powerful healing effect contained in chiropractic techniques (see below).

Importantly, the alternative treatment modalities such as chiropractic, Charka energy theory, acupuncture, and homeopathy understand the need to optimize the mysterious life energy's flow before healing begins. The life energy flow is important within the muscles, ligaments and joints. Stasis within these tissues produces pain and stiffness.

Many alternative treatment modalities address the relief of the stasis within one's body tissues. Stasis occurs when the flow of one's life energy disrupts. Another description of static energy collection within body tissues is tension. For this reason, stressed owners tend to be particularly vulnerable to accumulations of static energy. When these aberrant energies collect they lead, initially, to painful body areas and only later diminish joint, ligament, and muscle function. Alternative modalities effectively release these static energies.

Chiropractic adjustment theory applied appropriately in the clinical setting effectively addresses these aberrant energy collections. Aberrant energy collections tend to occur within body tissues as negative emotions collect. The supplementation of these treatments with a competent message therapist is often synergistic.

As stated previously, the quality of the hormones reflects the health of an owner. However, the quality of life energy flow patterns form a determinate for which hormones become possible. For example, before stressed owners secrete cortisol an aberration in the life energy occurs, which causes the command for the cortisol secretion. Therefore alternative treatment modalities, which facilitate the normalization of energy flow patterns, will improve the hormone milieu in stressful situations.

On the opposite extreme, when considering muscle, ligament and joint health, are the healing powers contained within the positive emotions. Owners who have rewarding emotional experiences will tend to secrete optimal hormone mixtures. Alternative treatment modalities, like chiropractic, can be extremely helpful to those owners who experience chronic negative emotions in their lives. These owners have an increased likelihood of secreting sub-optimal hormone mixtures that reflect the distressed energetic state. The more quickly aberrant energy releases, the less damage caused by hormonal imbalance.

Different emotions have unique impacts within the body tissues. Emotions directly affect the types and amounts of hormones secreted into the blood stream. Athletic competitors enjoy an elevated testosterone level just before a competitive event. However, the only players who continue to have elevated testosterone levels just after the competition are the winning team.

Another example occurs in those owners who feel overwhelmed and trapped within a negative life situation. These owners will tend to have a much higher blood cortisol level. Recall, the chronic elevation of the cortisol level will direct body energy into survival pathways and out of the rejuvenation activities necessary for continued vitality.

While owners learn to improve their emotional energy quality in their daily life, these alternative treatment modalities can often release some of the accumulating static energies. They accomplish this, each in their own way (i.e. chiropractic, acupuncture, homeopathy, neural therapy, message therapy, yoga exercises, etc.), but the common denominator that they each seem to engage regards their optimizing the movement of the life energies into a direction of harmony.

Most owners agree that having a human experience is hard work at times. Many people find that there will always be new challenges and disappointments along the path of their life's work. Cultivating an awareness of the options of how to cope allows re-channeling of fresh new life energy. The use of new life energies, to reinvigorate one in times of hardship, allows healing paths to open up. Unfortunately, the Western medical model of health delivery is like the slab of meat approach. When the intelligent energy considerations are eviscerated from the treatment strategies human beings often become slabs of meat. The slab of meat describes all that remains when the life force has been removed.

Many owners eventually leave mainstream medicine. Many of these owners sense something missing from their conventional treatment. Some holistic physicians would argue that the common denominator between many alternative treatment modalities involves their manipulation of the intelligent life energies towards optimum (see above discussion and see below for further examples). The qualities of the life energies are an under-utilized approach in mainstream medicine today. Healing modalities, which consider the life energies, make more sense in the management of the numerous chronic degenerative diseases.

One adjustment technique, which has shown marked promise in the treatment of chronic degenerative disease, is called cranial sacral therapy. Cranial sacral therapy is a spinal adjustment technique that has great power to heal. It can be viewed as a mechanism for releasing static energy situations within the spine.

An M.D. in Missoula, Montana had an interesting encounter with the healing potentials within this discipline several years ago. While training in a cranial sacral therapy class he related the following story. Upon arriving, another M.D. addressed the class and informed them that he was only there because his wife insisted that he attend to help her. Apparently he reluctantly agreed. The Missoula physician was paired up to learn this alternative technique with this gentleman as his partner. While working on this man's spine in the mid-chest area (according to Chakra theory this is the area of the heart/lung energy center) the good doctor noticed an unusual energy release. At first he didn't say anything because he suspected it was only his imagination. Suddenly this skeptical doctor asked if he had felt the energy release that he was experiencing. The Missoula doctor informed him that he did notice an odd sensation. The next morning the previously skeptical doctor came in and exclaimed that he had terrible asthma that required regular intervals of medicine or he would need a rapid intervention in the emergency room to stabilize his breathing. He then said that during the previous evening he had forgotten to take his breathing treatment and medicines. He woke up in the middle of the night remembering his medication. He was pleasantly surprised to notice that he had no breathing difficulty what so ever!

Cranial-sacral theory would explain that this man suffered from a static energy imbalance within his spine, which was affecting his lungs. The lungs were energetically imbalanced to the point that he was not able to breath without a constant symptom control medical regime. The power contained in moving life energy around forms a very important point that this case illustrates.

However, the Western medical view has no explanation for this mans healing response. Scientific inconsistencies point the way to better methods of treating a disease. Cranial sacral medical theory maintains that human beings contain intelligent energy (life energy). Health can only occur when the life energy flows rhythmically and optimally.

When the life energy becomes static or imbalanced then the body becomes diseased.

Just as important as the energies that heal contrasted to the energies that maim are the physical requirements of muscles, ligaments, and joints. The rest of this chapter explores the other six principles as they pertain to these tissues.

BIG MUSCLES OR LOTS OF FAT

Muscle size and strength provide tangible evidence for the power contained in hormone quality and proper nutrition. Directly observing these two important determiners of muscle and ligament function reveals that something very important often turns up missing from the physical exam in America today.

The science exists to explain the importance of optimal hormone (types and amounts) and nutritional building blocks for muscle tissue. All other performance enhancers marginally affect muscle size without these primary determinants. Unfortunately, failure to include this in one's annual evaluation, in the clinical setting, often contributes to an unnecessary acceleration into old age.

The first determiner, the quality of hormones, involves the fact that muscle cells only perform secondary to the directions they receive. The most powerful directors concern the level one-type hormones. Mantra: they instruct a muscle cell's DNA program (genes) activity level. **Realize the types and amounts of these most powerful hormones determine which genes turn off and which genes turn on.** The steroids, vitamin A, and thyroid hormones comprise the only hormones that contain this direct ability. Recall the genes provide nothing until the right hormone arrives. Logically it follows that the quality and amounts of the different steroids determine whether the message to the muscle cell DNA provides coherence.

Coherence or incoherence to energy's direction is analogous to a cellular 'melody' or cellular 'noise'. The incoherent message of noise leads to old age. One way to avoid old age depends on which DNA programs activate or suppress. Consequently, the quality of the message content determines where in the continuum the owner lies between chaotic genetic programs all the way up to the message melody of health. For this reason, the DNA activity powerfully determines how big and strong a muscle cell becomes.

Muscle cells provide excellent examples of the importance for balance between anabolic and catabolic message content. Only when proper balance occurs between these two opposing messages can the DNA program direct buildup activities appropriately within the muscle cell. Extremely high anabolic message content occurs in the body builder. Large muscles only become possible with high androgen message content. High androgen message content directs the muscle cell DNA to increase cellular infrastructure investment activities. Muscle development provides an example of the central role of anabolic steroids. Anabolic steroids direct the

DNA program to increase cell building up activities (positive nitrogen balance).

Realize the muscle cell response to steroids is no different than the other cells throughout the body. Other cells in the body respond to appropriate amounts and timing of their preferred anabolic steroid. The difference between muscle cells and other body cells concerns the fact that each body cell type desires its preferred anabolic steroid. For example DHEA is the preferred steroid within the brain. Whatever the blood level of DHEA, the brain concentrates it by a factor of five to six. How many senile owners result solely from the failure to find that their DHEA has severely diminished? Specialized fat producing cells within the brain, the Schwann cells, need sufficient progesterone message content or they deteriorate. How many Multiple sclerosis owners needlessly suffer because their doctor fails to discover a diminished progesterone level?

DHT (dihydrotestosterone) is the preferred steroid for nice skin, organs, joints and bones. However, the muscles prefer testosterone (including heart) for their maximal development message.

Muscle cell message content needs to be counterbalanced by the catabolic steroid, cortisol. Appropriate but not excessive cortisol message content maximizes energy while an owner exercises. The cortisol message also prevents excessive soreness following exercise (an additional message content of cortisol called an anti-inflammatory effect).

Health fails when defense of body protein mechanisms fail. Remember that the adequate release of Growth Hormone moderates the catabolic protein combusting message of cortisol. Consequently, if Growth Hormone levels prove inadequate when an owner exercises or fasts excessive protein structure will dismantle. For this reason, healthy bodies contain appropriate amounts of both cortisol and Growth Hormone while their muscles exercise. Balance between opposing hormones fundamentally prolongs youthfulness. *The hormones giveth and the hormones taketh away.* In other words, in the youthful state they giveth and in the unhealthful state, the imbalanced message (noise) taketh away.

Muscles need adequate stimulus (exercise) before the gonads and adrenals respond and produce increased message content from the anabolic steroids. A relationship between muscle use and steroid message content exists. Maximal muscle development depends on both processes. Failure on either end of this equation leads to little muscles (sarcopenia).

Exercise results in soreness and annoying injuries (strains) when adrenal and gonad function impair. Any owner who suddenly begins to become excessively sore following modest workouts needs a comprehensive steroid hormone evaluation. Replacement with real steroids may be indicated when a severe hormone deficiency reveals itself. However, many out of shape owners who get in shape respond nicely to improved diets and nutrients alone (see below).

Once a complete inquiry into the muscle hormone status of the level one-hormone types occurs, the 'lesser' hormones can be considered (see the hierarchy of hormones). An example of a **level two-hormone type** is insulin-like-growth-factor (IGF-1). Mantra: IGF-1 occurs at amounts over 100 times more plentiful in the blood stream of healthy owners than those of insulin.

IGF-1 helps muscle cells obtain their nutrition within the blood steam. IGF-1 facilitates the anabolic steroids desire to build bigger and stronger muscles. Less IGF-1 within the blood stream means the anabolic steroid message contains diminished ability to build cells like muscle cells. Muscle cells cannot build themselves up without the proper nutritional molecular building blocks (see digestion section for specifics). IGF-1 and insulin (the fuel nozzles) facilitate the absorption of nutrition by muscle cells. Insulin needs increase when IGF-1 falls because insulin becomes the backup hormone (fuel nozzle) for muscle cell fuel intake.

The Half-truth about VO2 Max elucidates another piece of the fiction that doctors receive in their training. Consider that only monitoring the function of one's car air filter would prove as folly. Most everyone knows that either carburetor or fuel injection function plays an equally important role for performance. Similarly, human cells depend on fuel delivery in addition to O2 delivery. Textbook fact: exercise quickly leads to insulin levels falling towards zero in healthy owners. Yet, mainstream physicians actually believe that normally insulin delivers fuel to exercising muscle.

More recently, the GLUT story has been created to perpetuate even more confusion. Add to this the PPAR story and one begins to smell another groom job. It will take more work to ferret out what these two popular stories really say because there is no doubt these cover up a connection between IGF-1 and its binding proteins that the healthy body actually depends on to deliver fuel into muscle cells. Further bolstering this suspicion involves the fact that recently there are now seven binding proteins for IGF-1 and GLUT has seven as well. The reader is also cautioned that IGF-1 associates with additional proteins in the serum, like acid labile subunit (ALS). This fact makes it harder to dissect out the connection between these several ways to say the same thing that are so commonly used for perpetuating doctors practicing in the dark.

The relative roles of IGF-1 and insulin in muscle cell nutritional needs have been largely ignored within the mainstream medical approach. Even though, in the healthy owner, IGF-1 occurs at 100 times the normal insulin levels, the increase of insulin receives the advertising dollar. The trouble with this approach involves the fact that insulin produces many side effects, which IGF-1 does not share. Examples of the differences between the insulin message content compared to IGF-1 within the body are: insulin causes increased cholesterol and triglyceride synthesis within the liver, insulin more rapidly degrades without adequate IGF-1, increased insulin increases appetite, insulin rises after eating while IGF-1 rises during fasting.

Insulin and IGF-1 facilitate the uptake of muscle fuel. However, in healthy owners, insulin facilitates a relatively small amount of fuel uptake within muscle cells because it occurs in much smaller amounts (less than one percent of IGF-1 levels). Additionally, insulin only elevates maximally following a carbohydrate meal.

Conversely, IGF-1 levels in healthy owners tend to stay up between meals. IGF-1 has a half-life of 15 hours to four days while insulin's half-life is less than ten minutes. In addition, IGF-1 levels rise slightly between meals (fasting). The simultaneous rise in IGF-1 and the release of sugar and fat into the blood stream, which Growth Hormone commands, provides fuel to healthy muscles between meals.

Healthy muscles depend on adequate IGF-1 levels for their nutritional needs between meals. They also depend on adequate insulin following meals, which directs sufficient liver storage of sugar and fat in preparation for the next between meal states. Between meals Growth Hormone releases when the brain senses a fall in blood sugar. The Growth Hormone released causes the stored sugar, fat and IGF-1 to release. Sufficient IGF-1 between meals allows the muscles to receive nutrition without the need for insulin. For this reason, healthy people have no need for insulin in the fasting state.

Syndrome X (Metabolic Syndrome) individuals, because their IGF-1 has fallen, need insulin in exaggerated amounts between meals. Hungry body cells beyond the liver need a fuel nozzle, either IGF-1 or insulin. However, insulin increasing while the blood sugar falls is abnormal. Recall, because of simple anatomy the liver always receives the highest concentration of pancreatic hormonal secretions. In addition, liver and fat cells also have the highest amount of pure insulin type receptors occurring at 200,000 per cell.

Visualize the liver as an insulin trap. Consequently, even though the blood sugar is falling off, the majority of insulin trapped within the liver worsens the falling blood sugar before any of it escapes to serve as a fuel nozzle. Realize, insulin within the liver always delivers the message to store energy. Most energy storage occurs as cholesterol and fat. These details explain how the increased insulin output stimulates the liver's fat and cholesterol making machinery.

Visualize the conflict within the livers' of these desperate owners. Syndrome X owners suffer from conflicting message content within their livers during the fasting state. The first conflicting aberration concerns their diminished Growth Hormone out put while between meals. As a consequence, excessive epinephrine, glucagon and cortisol then need to release in order to maintain the blood sugar level (fuel level) between meals. **However, the fall in Growth Hormone has two health consequences.** One is that body protein stores become fair game for dismantling when Growth Hormone levels fall off (increased catabolism or also known as negative nitrogen balance). Second involves the fall off of

IGF-1 release. This last fact sets up the overall second conflicting message at the level of the liver.

Simplistically the conflict involves the competing message between the increased insulin needed to shore up a fallen IGF-1 level, which always arrives in the liver first. Visualize that fuel nozzles are scarce beyond the liver and this causes hungry cells. Unfortunately, very little insulin ever makes it past the billions of its pure insulin type receptors occurring within the liver. But remember by binding to insulin receptors within the liver the message directs them to store fuel. Visualize the liver as an insulin trap simply because of the basic anatomy of its secretion pathway. This worsens the falling blood fuel!

Keep in mind that this exacerbates the need for the simultaneous and competing process involving the release of excessive counter hormones, cortisol, glucagon and epinephrine, instructing the liver to release fuel. Also remember that these hormones are much more catabolic than the preferred Growth Hormone because they encourage gluconeogenesis, a catabolic process that if chronic leads to diminished protein content.

Diminished protein content provides one of the biomarkers for the aging process. Until someone helps these owners to realign their hormones that instruct their liver, these owners will continue on the accelerated path to an old body. Visualize the next level of violence within these owners' livers.

Popular strategies abound that purport to raise Growth Hormone secretion rates. All of them ignore the fact for why the pituitary secretes Growth Hormone in the first place: Growth Hormone secretes to protect body protein content yet keep the blood fuel level adequate between meals or when exercising. Cognizance of this fact allows one to see that the popular approaches have their effect by peripheral pathways.

For example, certain amino acids are fastidiously protected within the body from fuel combustion. Popular strategies raise Growth Hormone levels in some owners because these same amino acids when taken as supplements set off the pituitary alarm that important amino acid blood levels are elevated. Examples of important amino acids that the body fastidiously protects are: arginine, ornithine, glutamine and lysine. But what about those owners who have a pituitary defect acquired around middle age that no longer allows sufficient Growth Hormone release?

Many Syndrome X owners have such a defect. They are doomed to die prematurely unless they receive counsel on how to raise their Growth Hormone levels. Here again popular Growth Hormone replacement protocols fail to inquire about liver health and androgen levels before prescribing Growth Hormone replacement injections. Hence, all the media attention to the supposed risk for Growth Hormone induced diabetes. Healthy livers that receive adequate androgen message content will curtail a diabetes tendency with Growth Hormone treatments (see liver chapter).

Textbook fact: Growth Hormone synthesis rates within the pituitary gland depend on sufficient thyroid message content arriving

here. A cognizance here allows one to understand yet another reason that thyroid deficient patients age so quickly. This fact also explains another cause for the Syndrome X (metabolic syndrome) pathology. Sadly, most physicians fail to receive educations that contain this basic fact. Add in the dirty world environment that causes thyroid injury by numerous mechanisms and one begins to glean another epidemic cause of accelerated aging rates. Finally, normal thyroid function means that the test result checked out above the bottom 2.5% mark of a thyroid poisoned population (within two standard deviations of the mean). Hopefully, this far into this manual the reader can see that this 'normal' is not optimal.

Recall, IGF-1 levels depend on two basic factors. First, concerns the hormonal factor. The liver needs adequate direction from thyroid, DHEA or testosterone and cortisol. When all three of these hormone types occur at normal levels, these level one type hormones instruct the liver DNA to manufacture IGF-1 hormone and its binding proteins properly.

However, number two, the life style factor, allows the release of IGF-1 from the liver. The lifestyle factor controls Growth Hormone (GH) release rates. Growth Hormone releases when the blood fuel level decreases. Common situations for which the blood fuel falls are: exercise, fasting and between meal states. Conversely, increased estrogen levels inhibit the release of IGF-1 by GH (see liver chapter). Therefore, owners who have healthy levels of IGF-1 also have healthy levels of thyroid hormones, DHEA, testosterone, cortisol, estrogen and GH.

Nerd Corner:

High blood sugar stimulates insulin increases but low blood sugar stimulates IGF-1 release along with sugar and fat. The opposite is also true. High blood sugar eventually decreases IGF-1 levels but low blood sugar decreases insulin release. When IGF-1 releases there has been a preceding release of GH. The GH release response results from a falling blood sugar, which causes **stored** sugar to be dumped by the liver into the blood stream. The simultaneously released IGF-1 then causes the liver released sugar to be sucked up by cells beyond the liver. IGF-1 levels maintain body cell fuel levels between meals. Insulin maintains liver storage levels of sugar and fat following meals. In this way healthy muscles have access to fuel at all times.

Remember, only sufficient Growth Hormone release, while fasting or exercising defends body protein content. Youth depends on adequate protein. Therefore, processes that disrupt defense of body protein accelerate the aging rate. The other counter hormones to insulin provoke such a process (cortisol, glucagon, and epinephrine). Excessive amounts of these that occur in the unhealthy body increase catabolism. Consequently, these owners cannot defend their protein. Even though

---

> they attempt to fast and exercise they slowly unravel their body form. Remember, protein is the metabolically active component of body structure. The more of it one has the more power contained in their cells for participating in what life has to offer.

The *hormone report card* evaluates these when health diminishes. Paradoxically, mainstream medicine does not routinely inquire about these important hormone considerations. The suspicion is that mainstream doctors are not taught to think about these hormone relationships. I wasn't encouraged. The science is all there, although it presents in a convoluted and disjointed fashion. As long as there continues to be divergent and multiplicitas ways to say these important facts physicians will remain in the dark. Be kind to your physician and help him to learn anew.

For the above reasons, maintaining balance between IGF-1 and insulin form an important biochemical determinant of youthfulness within the muscles. It is also important to avoid the popular practice of receiving Growth Hormone injections without a proper evaluation of the IGF-1 levels. Without a proper evaluation of one's livers ability to increase IGF-1 levels, GH will tend to promote high blood sugars and therefore increase insulin output. Increased insulin output associates with all the negative effects on body physique discussed in the obesity chapter.

This last fact explains the negative publicity associating Growth Hormone injections with breast and abdominal fat growth. Normal livers respond to Growth Hormone by releasing stored IGF-1 along with sugar and fat. The released IGF-1 delivers the sugar and fat released to the organs and muscles thus negating the need for insulin in the fasting state. Unhealthy livers can still release sugar and fat but release diminished amounts of IGF-1 and insulin release rates consequently need to increase to pick up the slack in the elevated blood sugar. Higher insulin levels always arrive in the liver first and thus abnormally stimulate the fat and cholesterol making liver machinery. The extra fat and cholesterol deposits within the breast and abdomen. All these side effects could be avoided if someone first helped the liver to heal (see liver chapter).

The **level three hormones** (see hierarchy of hormones) affect muscle performance by opening up or closing down the blood supply within the exercising muscle. For this reason, deficiency of the level three hormones leads to diminished muscle performance. Adequate supplies of the level three hormones depend on adequate protein meals and many vitamins. Examples of level three hormones are: epinephrine, nor-epinephrine, histamine, serotonin, and dopamine. All of these hormones have short active life spans of several minutes. Therefore, the amount of the level three hormones constantly determines the tone of the blood vessels every few minutes.

The useful analogy here regards the water system network that underlies many large cities. Fluctuations in demand because of time of day and location necessitate that water engineers open up or tighten down available water supplies with numerous different and strategically located check valves throughout the city water supply system. Similar processes operate within the body. Understanding ways to direct maximal blood supply into the performing metabolically hungry areas of the body confers a performance advantage on its owner. Under optimal conditions, the body reroutes a tremendous increase in blood flow to the active area. Shunting blood away from the less active areas enhances the effect.

The adrenal gland contains two layers. The outer layer makes up the cortex. The adrenal medulla describes the inner layer and manufactures some of the level three hormones. In order to understand muscle performance the inner core (the adrenal medulla) of the adrenal gland's hormonal products needs to be understood.

Here powerful hormones release and prevent unconsciousness from occurring when one stands up. The arterial muscle layer needs to contract when one stands. Arterial muscles contract when enough level three hormones instruct them to do so. The ability for the arteries to contract or relax is determined in part by the adrenal medulla. The other part of contraction versus relaxation, in the blood vessels, concerns the autonomic nervous system. Here the discussion focuses on the hormone component of blood vessel caliber because nutrition powerfully affects this ability (see below).

The adrenal medulla is largely responsible for performing the task of the body's 'water engineers'. The city planners design the water system underneath the city but the water engineers constantly decide which valves to turn up and which to turn down in flow. Incompetent water engineers on the staff create inefficient water delivery to certain areas of the city. This analogy simplifies what the adrenal medulla does in regards to directing blood flow within the vessels.

The level three hormones task of directing blood flow requires the availability of certain molecular parts. Epinephrine proves the most desirable of the level three hormones in exercising muscle. Exercising muscle needs sufficient epinephrine levels to direct the blood vessels to open. When the blood vessels supplying muscle open an increased supply of fuel and oxygen delivery occurs. Some of the other level three hormones, if present, compete with this process (see below).

The second determinant of powerful muscles, alluded to above, concerns the nutritional status of the body. Epinephrine manufacture requires specific nutrients. The adrenal gland needs an adequate supply of either phenylalanine or tyrosine and also numerous cofactors (vitamins). If one or more cofactors become deficient then the adrenals cannot manufacture the most beneficial types of exercise performance enhancing hormone within this class, epinephrine. The necessary cofactors needed for the synthesis of epinephrine are: tetrahydrobiopterin (made from folate), vitamin C, vitamin B6, and SAMe. Since SAMe deactivates within the body at the rate of one billion times a second, it needs to be recharged with the following additional nutrients: vitamin B12, folate, serine and methionine.

Epinephrine is a member of the bioactive amines, listed above. Scientists call the bioactive amines either hormones or neural transmitters. Their site of action determines which class they are in. When bioactive amines are between two nerve endings, the synapse, scientists call them neural transmitters. If they discharge into the blood stream (the adrenal medulla is a major site for this but there are other sites through out the body) scientists call them hormones.

When bioactive amines course in the blood stream they act as the water engineers, as discussed above. All water engineers are not created equal. Peak performance athletes predictably receive only the best 'water engineers' directing their blood flow. Most owners fail to understand ways to enhance the level three-hormone mixture to obtain more competent water engineers. More competent water engineers lead to better blood flow to the exercising muscles. Nutritional deficiencies prevent the manufacture of adequate epinephrine, which leads to a prematurely diminished athletic performance.

For maximum performance abilities within the muscles epinephrine can be thought of as the master water engineer. It has the informational content to open up the blood vessel diameter leading to the exercising muscles, liver and the heart. Increasing blood flow within the areas of increased metabolic demand obviously allows for better delivery of oxygen, nutrients and the increased ability for waste removal (carbon dioxide, lactic acid, spent cofactors, etc.). The liver needs an increased blood supply during exercise because it removes and reprocesses the huge amounts of lactic acid generated within exercising muscles. Also remember the liver performs as the main fuel releasing organ in the body (see liver chapter).

Epinephrine requires all the above cofactors availability because its biosynthesis lies at the end of the assembly line for the bioactive amines manufacturing process. Consequently, when nutritional deficiencies cause the synthesis of epinephrine to decrease there becomes less instruction for the blood vessels to open up during exercise. Normally during exercise the blood supply to the heart, skeletal muscles and liver increases because of epinephrine's presence. However, when epinephrine becomes deficient nor-epinephrine levels will rise. The trouble with increased levels of nor-epinephrine concerns the fact that its message tightens down the blood supply to the heart, skeletal muscle and liver. The health consequence here results from less fuel and oxygen delivery to these metabolically active tissues during exercise. Also, the nasty side affect of abnormal blood pressure elevation occurs (explained in section one).

When optimum conditions prevail (youthfulness) the adrenal medulla will make 90% epinephrine. Under healthy conditions (to be reviewed shortly) the adrenal only makes 10% nor-epinephrine and dopamine. This has important implications for those owners who desire to feel as good as good as possible when they exercise.

Recall, one of the most common nutritional deficiencies within the adrenal medulla occurs in what is known as the methyl donor group of substances. When a methyl donor deficiency occurs within the adrenal medulla, there arises the inability to convert nor-epinephrine into epinephrine. Consequently, when these molecular part deficient adrenals secrete, during exercise, their ability to dump epinephrine into the blood stream diminishes.

Epinephrine release proves inadequate because of the methyl donor deficiency (see methyl donor system chapter three). Recall, only epinephrine contains the message to direct blood flow increases to exercising muscles, the heart, and the liver. For this reason, exercise performance critically depends on the epinephrine message content to increase blood supply to these areas. Unless epinephrine releases the exercising owner will suffer decreased blood supply to his heart, liver and muscles. In addition, his blood pressure will rise abnormally because only epinephrine will moderate blood pressure during exercise.

Many owners take the expensive SAMe in a pill to recharge their methyl donor status. This is not always necessary or best. Methyl deficient owners degrade SAMe to homocysteine. For this reason, elevated homocysteine levels provide an excellent marker for those owners who suffer with this deficiency. Supplementing with adequate serine, vitamin B12, vitaminB6 and folate often will recharge the deficient methyl donor state. Remember that these bioactive amines within the adrenal derive from tyrosine or phenylalanine. A functional digestive tract needs to be involved (see digestion section). In addition, there are other cofactors needed to manufacture epinephrine from tyrosine; tetrahydrobiopterin (made from folate), vitamin C and adequate cellular magnesium.

The exercising muscles discussion concludes the organ systems and longevity principles contained within this manual. The last section provides a perspective of what needs to be checked before healing paths can be created. Most owners wait until at least mid-life before they have the revelation about their demise being somewhere in the future. This realization leads some to begin to want renewed health. Others could care less and that's OK. The last section is for the owners who want to know some of the basic tests that can better evaluate how bad off they are. The body report card so generated provides a baseline from which healing can begin.

SECTION SEVEN

100,000 Mile Exam

SECTION SEVEN *617*

100,000 Mile Exam   **617**

CHAPTER TWENTY-SEVEN

100,000 MILE EXAM

Middle age to the body is analogous to a car with one hundred thousand miles on its odometer. How the car has been maintained, accident history, quality of replacement parts, quality of fuel, and how it has been used begins to show at the one hundred thousand mile point. It is the same with an owner's body at the middle age.

Many owners have experienced life-changing realizations at this point in their life cycle. Some receive their wake up when they take a long hard look at themselves naked in front of the mirror. They ask themselves the hard question that day that had been buried beneath layers of denial for years. How long will this body last? This question is usually followed by a second question regarding whether or not they will suffer as they near the end.

The doctor sees evidence that some things about the earthling experience are fairly typical. The hard question that occurs around middle age is one such example. Not all owners ask this question while they are naked in front of a mirror, but sooner or later they ask it. Sooner or later they also ask it honestly.

At this point of connection, with their need for a functional body, they usually seek guidance on how to repair some of the damage, which one hundred thousand miles of living inflicts. Who they trust and obtain advice from, forms a big determinant for success or failure in achieving healthful longevity.

This book has been about the other side of the story of what science reveals. It concerns the maintenance of health. This section applies all seven principles. Application occurs only when an owner reaches the point in their life where they are ready to ask the hard question. The one hundred thousand mile exam involves an assessment of where an owner stands in regard to the seven principles of longevity. If they can obtain a report card on all seven determinants, they are in a better position to take an active role in their own healing.

PRINCIPLE ONE: An assessment of rust promoting mechanisms

History:
1. Deficiency of anti-inflammatory fatty acids
2. Diabetes
3. Obesity
4. Excessive consumption of oxidized fats
5. Nutritional deficiencies that promote rust
6. Excessive exposure to oxidizing agents
7. Abnormal hormone message content exposure history
8. Tobacco abuse
9. Male gender

Physical signs of rust:

1. Premature gray hair
2. Reading glasses before age forty-five when compared to normal vision when younger
3. Premature wrinkles, sagging skin and skin discoloration
4. Shortness of breath
5. Protein in the urine
6. Retinal vessel changes
7. Certain nail changes
8. Leg hair distribution decrease

PRINCIPLE TWO: An assessment of the loss of flexibility mechanisms

High blood pressure is a sign of this problem, but there are many fixable causes.

History for high blood pressure causality:
1. Magnesium deficiency
2. Increased insulin level
3. Increased sodium intake and/or decreased potassium intake
4. Stiffened red blood cells
5. Methyl donor deficiency
6. Nitric oxide deficiency
7. Syndrome X (duet to increased insulin need)
8. Abnormal hormonal fats

EXTENSION OF PRINCIPLE ONE is the opportunistic mechanisms that accelerate rust formation, but require its initial presence from some other rust promoter.

1. The additional abnormal hormones that direct the liver to manufacture the sticky fats (LDL and VLDL cholesterol)
    c. Additional nutritional deficiencies that inhibit the burning of fat for energy
    d. Nutritional deficiencies that inhibit carbohydrate fuel combustion in the presence of oxygen.

Basic lab that concern principles one and two:

1. Fasting insulin and C-peptide levels
2. Fasting IGF-1 levels
3. Prolactin levels
4. Cholesterol, HDL, LDL, and triglycerides level
5. Blood sugar level
6. Homocysteine level
7. Dark field microscopy of blood cells
8. Hemoglobin A1C
9. Ferritin levels
10. CRP
11. Magnesium, potassium and sodium levels
12. UA with microscopy

PRINCIPLE THREE: The hormones giveth and the hormones taketh away

An assessment for the presence of obesity or emaciation and the amount of involvement of the seven different hormones

1. High insulin states
2. High cortisol states
3. Diminished androgen states
4. Increased estrogen states
5. Diminished thyroid states
6. Diminished epinephrine states with increased nor-epinephrine
7. Diminished IGF-1 levels

The health of the adrenal system

1. An assessment of the stress level
2. An assessment of the six links of their adrenal chain of health
3. A twenty-four hour urine test for adrenal steroids quality and amounts
4. A valuable clue about adrenal dysfunction concerns the appearance of either an increased eosinophil count or a right shift in the white blood cells. A right shift is evidenced by an increased lymphocyte and decreased leukocyte count. Also anemia without iron deficiency (the anemia of chronic disease) also provides a potential clue that adrenal defects underlie certain disease processes. Unfortunately, these changes are consistently present with autoimmune disease but conventional medicine fails to unite these clues of association.

Ovary health in women

1. Assessment inquires into the level of balance between estrogens and progesterone
2. Assessment also includes the sufficiency of androgen that is needed for rejuvenation by muscles, joints, organs, skin and skeleton.
3. This consideration also involves an assessment of the six links of the ovary chain of health

Informational substances: assess how wisely an owner spends available body energy. The informational substances (hormones) determine the direction of body energy expenditure.

Steroid tone and its six determinants:

1. Adrenal and gonad health
2. Nutritional adequacy
3. Genetics
4. Environmental toxins
5. Emotional qualities operating within
6. Secretogogues

The four misunderstood steroids inclusion in the evaluation by using a twenty-four hour urine test

1. Aldosterone
2. Thyroid
3. Vitamin A
4. Vitamin D

Thyroid health

1. The seven links in the thyroid chain of health need to be considered in all patients
2. Vitamin A adequacy - it is necessary for thyroid message content to manifest
3. Adrenal adequacy is a permissive determinant for normal thyroid function
4. Physical signs of an accelerated aging rate necessitate a thorough thyroid evaluation because its amounts in the pituitary determine how much Growth Hormone is made

Testicle health in men

1. Twenty-four hour urine test for testicle produced steroids
2. Assessment of estrogen mimics and estrogen status
3. IGF-1 levels interplay with the steroids
4. The joints, skeleton, skin, muscle mass, and personality provide valuable clues about testicle health

Hierarchy of hormones assessment

Level 1 - the generals of the hormones
Level 2 - the polypeptides
Level 3 – the biogenic amines
Level 4 – the 'vocal' hormones
\

THE FOURTH PRINCIPLE: you are what you absorb [two components to this]

1. Digestive tract integrity and adequacy for the different juices required in the different digestion chambers
2. Nutritional adequacy of the molecular replacement parts
   a. amino acid quality for all twenty different amino acids
   b. essential fatty acid intake

      c.   fiber
      d.   bacteria helpers
      e.   adequate fats in the diet
      f.   intact vitamins and amount
      g.   relative mineral intake ratios and amounts
      h.   appropriate carbohydrates consumption for activity and fitness level

3. Quality of body protein
4. Quality of body carbohydrate content (GAGs, glycogen)
5. Adequacy of the four different types of fat roles
6. Cell structure and H20 retention
7. Fuel
8. Pancreas hormones and the opposing counter regulatory hormone types
9. Assessment of the torture chamber effect in the diet

PRINCIPLE FIVE: Taking out the cellular trash adequacy

Sufficient thyroid message content allows all six-trash removal organ systems to function properly.

1. Kidney
2. Lungs
3. Skin
4. Liver
5. Colon (section three)
6. Immune system (section five)

Steroid Pressure - signs of deficiency show up on the periphery first.

1. Skin health
2. Joint health
3. Bone health

PRINCIPLE SIX: the adequacy of cellular charge assessment

1. Cellular charge depends on the optimal ratios of potassium, sodium, magnesium, and calcium. After middle age this can only occur with a consistent real food diet instead of a processed food diet.

2. Cellular charge in the brain and heart will decrease around middle age if the above minerals are not consumed in the proper ratios.

3. Chronic stress depletes cellular charge because the mineral ratios become altered.

4. Aldosterone levels need to be sufficient for the maintenance of cellular charge especially of the nerve and heart conduction systems. A separate benefit of adequate aldosterone is the stimulation of continued steroids biosynthesis.

5. Thyroid needs to be adequate for nerve and heart conduction health to occur.

6. Certain trace minerals like vanadium and chromium injure the red blood cells electrical charge by inhibiting the sodium and potassium ATPase pump. This increases serum potassium and is the reason that insulin sensitivity improves (insulin's fuel uptake role depends on available potassium).

7. The immune system is the prototypical organ system that illustrates the principle of cellular charge.

8. Fluoride and iodide inhibit energy packet formation in the red blood cell.

9. The digestive tract integrity affects cellular charge because it secretes over seven quarts of various concoctions of minerals daily. In all, it absorbs almost nine of these quarts of mineral and nutrients daily.

10. Pancreatic Beta cells release GABA, which hyperpolarizes (increases cellular charge) the alpha cells.

11. Calcium pummels sperm heads when cervical mucus contains progesterone.

12. Nerve cells relax and are fed when they encounter progesterone because GABA is released and these cells hyperpolarize with chloride (nerve cell voltage increases).

13. Niacin intake leads to increased red blood cell cellular charge because of the increased formation of NADH (this can lead to decreased potassium availability secondary to potassium sequestration that can lead to insulin resistance).

14. Red blood cell deformability and cellular charge.

15. Vitamin deficiency and its effects on cellular charge.

16. Hypoxia in the EMF environment.

17. Toxemia of pregnancy is secondary to a progesterone deficiency that leads to decreased GABA and a diminished chloride channel activity.

   a. Pancreas

   b. CNS

c. Red blood cells

18. There is an electrical sucking grid that pulls in adequate water to inflate cells that otherwise would become squished flat by gravitational forces. When this system fails the owner begins to have the look of old age. It manifest in:
    a. Joints
    b. Skin
    c. Lining of the inside surface of the blood vessels
    d. Lining of the respiratory tract
    e. Lining of the digestive tube
    f. The space between neighboring cells called the intersitial space

THE SEVENTH PRINCIPLE: the energies that heal contrasted to the energies that maim owners' cells

The rhythm of the heart beat

1. The intelligence behind the intelligence
2. Life is vibrational
3. Homeopathy and how it expands understanding of life's underpinnings
4. Acupuncture another clue about defects in the Western model of the universe
5. Certain emotional energies confer rhythm on cells.
6. Certain emotional energies confer chaos on cells.
7. The summation of the integrity of the energy template (intelligent energy field) determines which hormones secrete and therefore determines functional ability at the highest level.
8. Counseling needs to occur on which of the alternative disciplines (chiropractic, acupuncture, homeopathy, yoga, prayer, message, or breath work) is right for releasing the chaotic energies that maim the body cells. Each owner has unique needs and the discipline that works for one may be uncomfortable to another. Thankfully, numerous offerings for these modalities exist and flourish despite the complex's best effort to squelch this freedom of choice.

Finding a holistically trained medical doctor is rare. Fortunately, many mainstream doctors are leaving the brotherhood of the complex. As of this writing, there are several thousand alternatively minded medical doctors scattered throughout the country.   Many belong to either the American Holistic Medical Association, the American College for the Advancement of Medicine, A4M or Institute of Functional Medicine. The health care revolution endeavors to support those physicians currently feeling the heart felt urge to make things right and again become the healers they originally set out to be. Others will fight us all the way and that is O.K.   May the lantern energy burn brightly in all of you.

Good luck and God bless.

BIBLIOGRAPHY

Abou-Seif, MA., Youssef, AA. Oxidative Stress and Male IGF-I, Gonadotropin and Related Hormones in Diabetic Patients. *Clin Chem Lab Med*, July, Vol. 39, No. 7, 2001.

Anderson RA THE SCIENTIFIC BASIS FOR HOLISTIC MEDICINE: Annotated abstracts 2001 Edition *American Health Press, Wenatchee, Wa*

Abrams, William B., M.D., et al. *The Merck Manual of Geriatrics*. New Jersey: Merck Sharp & Dohme Research Laboratories, 1990.

Adams, Patch, M.D., et al. *Gesundheit!* Vermont: Healing Arts Press, 1993.

Adams MR. Oral L-arginine improves endothelium-dependent dilatation and reduces monocyte adhesion to endothelial cells in young men with coronary artery disease. Dept. of Cardiology, Royal Prince Alfred Hospital, Sydney, Australia.

Allolio, Bruno and Wiebke Arlt (2002) DHEA treatment: myth or reality? *Trends Endocrin* Vol 13 No 7

Arlan L. Rosenbloom, Jaime Guevara-Aguirre et. Al. Growth Hormone Receptor Deficiency in Ecuador *J Clin Endo Metab* (1999) Vol. 84 (12) 4436-4443

Arlt, Wiebke (1999) Biotransformation of Oral Dehydroepiandrosterone (DHEA) in Elderly Men: Significant Increase in Circulating Estrogens *J Clin Endocrin Metab* Vol 84 No 6

Adkins, Robert C., MD. *Dr Adkins' New Diet Revolution*. 2nd ed. New York: M. Evans and Company, Inc, 1999.

_____. *Dr Adkins' Vita-Nutrient Solution*. New York: Simon and Shuster, 1998.

Aiswa T Thyroid Hormone Metabolism in Patients with Liver Cirrhosis, as judged by urinary excretion of Triiodothyronine *J Am Geriatr Soc* 1980; 28(11): 485-91

Ames Company. *Modern Urine Chemistry*. Elkhart, IN: Miles Laboratories, Inc, 1982.

Arndt, Kenneth A., MD. *Manual of Dermatologic Therapeutics*. Boston: Little, Brown and Company, 1983.

Aoki, Kazutaka, et al. Dehydroepiandrosterone (DHEA) Suppresses the Elevated Hepatic Glucose-6-Phosphatase and Fructose-1, 6-Biophosphatase Activities in C57BL/Ksj-db/db Mice. *Diabetes*, Vol. 48, August 1999.

Arlt W Dehydroepiandrosterone (DHEA) Replacement in Women with Adrenal Insufficiency *New England J Med* September 30 1999; Vol. 341. No. 14: 1013-1020

Arlt W Dehydroepiandrosterone (DHEA) Supplementation in Healthy Men with an Age-Related decline of Dehydroepiandrosterone Secretion *J Clin Endocrinol & Metab* 2001; 86 (10): 4686-4692

Arvat E, Di Vito L, Lanfranco F, et al. Stimulatory effect of adrenocorticotropin (ACTH) on cortisol, aldosterone, and dehydroepiandrosterone (DHEA) secretion in normal humans: dose-response study. *Journal of Clinical Endocrinology and Metabolism.* 2000;85(9):3141-3146.

Ballentine, Rudolph, MD. *Radical Healing.* New York: Harmony Books,1999.

Baulieu E-E, Thomas G, Legrain S, et al. Dehydorepiandrosterone (DHEA), DHEA sulfate, and aging: Contribution of the DHEAge Study to a sociobiomedical issue. *Proc. Natl. Acad. of Sci. USA.* 2000;97(8)4278-4284.

Balch, James F. M.D., et al. *Prescription of Natural Healing.* New York: Garden City Park, 1990.

Barazzoni, R., et. Al. (2000) Increased Fibrinogen Production in Type 2 Diabetic Patients without Detectable Vascular Complications: Correlation with Plasma Glucagon Concentrations. *Journal of Clinical Endocrinology and Metabolism.* Vol. 85. No. 9 pages 3121-3125

Bareford, D., (1986) Effects of Hyperglycemia and sorbitol accumulation on erythrocyte deformability in diabetes mellitus. *Journal of Clinical Pathology.* Vol. 39 Issue 7

Bargen, J.A., MD, et al. *Every Woman's Standard Medical Guide.* Indianapolis: American Publishers' Alliance Corp., 1949.

Barret-Connor E. et al. A Prospective study of Dehydroepiandrosterone (DHEA) Sulfate, Mortality and Cardiovascular Disease. *N Engl J Med* 1986 Dec 11;315 (24):1519-24.

Barret-Conner E. Lower endogenous androgen levels and dyslipidemia in men with non-insulin dependent diabetes mellitus. *Ann Intern Med* 1992 Nov 15; 117(10):807-11

Bate-Smith, E.C., ed. *Chemical Plant Taxonomy.* London: Spotttiswoode, Ballantyne and Company Limited, 1963.

Baiser, W. V., Thyroid Insufficiency, Is TSH Measurement the Only Diagnostic Tool? *Journal of Nutritional & Environmental Medicine* (June 2000); 10, 2 pg. 105

Barnes B Basal Temperature versus basal metabolism *JAMA*

_____ Hypothyroidism: The Unsuspected Illness. London, Harper and Row, 1976

_____ Solved: The Riddle of Heart Attacks. Robinson Press Inc., 1976

Bauer, Cathryn. *Acupressure for Everybody.* New York: Henry Holt and Company, 1991.

Becker, Robert O., M.D., et al. The Direct Current Control System, A Link Between Environment and Organism. *New York State Journal of Medicine,* April 15, 1962.

Becker, Robert O., MD, et al. *The Body Electric.* New York: William Morrow and Company, Inc, 1985.

Beers, Mark H., MD, ed. *The Merck Manual of Diagnosis and Therapy.* Whitehouse Station, NJ: Merck Research Laboratories, 1999.

Bellack, Leopold, MD, ed. *Psychology of Physical Illness.* New York:Grune & Stratton, 1952.

Bellamy, MF et Al. (1998) Hyperhomocystinemia After an Oral Methionine Load Acutely Impairs Endothelial Function in Healthy Adults. *Circulation* 98:1848-1852.

Behrendt, H., M.D. *Chemistry of Erythrocytes.* Illinois: Charles C Thomas Publisher, 1957.

Bennett RM, Clark SR, Campbell SM, Burckhardt CS. Low levels of somatomedin C (IGF-1) in patients with fibromyalgia syndrome. *Arthritis&Rheumatism.*1992;35(10)1113-1116.

Bennett RM, Cook DM, Clark SR, et al. Hypothalamic-Pituitary-Insulin-like Growth Factor-1 Axis Dysfunction in Patients with Fibromyalgia. *Journal of Rheumatology.* 1997;24(7)1384-1389.

Bereket, Abdullah (1996) Regulation of the Insulin-like Growth Factor System by Acute Acidosis* *Endocrinology* Vol 137 No. 6:2238-2245

Berezina TL et. Al. (2002) Influence of storage on red blood cell rheological properties. *Surg. Res.* Jan 2002 Volume 102(1) 6-12

Bergman, Richard N., et al. Free Fatty Acids and Pathogenesis of Type 2 Diabetes Mellitus. *Trends In Endocrinology and Metabolisim,* 11, 2000.

Berkow, Robert, MD, ed. *The Merck Manual of Medical Information.* Whitehouse Station, NJ: Merck Research Laboratories, 1997.

Bensky, Dan, et al. *Chinese Herbal Medicine, Mateia Medica.* Seattle: Eastland Press, Inc, 1986.

_____. *Chinese Herbal Medicine, Formulas and Strategies.* Seattle: Eastland Press, Inc, 1990.

Berkow, Robert, MD, ed. *The Merck Manual.* 15th ed. Rahway, NJ: Merck, Sharp, & Dohme Research Laboratories, 1987.

Bernstein, Richard K., MD, F.A.C.E. *Diabetes Solution.* New York: Little, Brown and Company, 1997.

Binz K, Joller P, Froesch P, et al. Repopulation of the atrophied thymus in diabetic rats by insulin-like growth factor. *Proc Natl Acad Sci* USA 1990;87:3690-3694

Biondi B Effects of Subclinical Thyroid Dysfunction on the Heart *Ann Intern Med* 2002; 137: 904-914

Bland, Jeffery S., PhD, ed. *Clinical Nutrition: A Functional Approach.* Gig Harbor, WA: Institute for Functional Medicine, 1999.

Bland, Jeffrey, Ph.D., *Nutritional Endocrinology.* Washington: Metagenics Educational Programs, 2002.

Brand, Paul, MD, et al. *Fearfully and Wonderfully Made.* Grand Rapids, MI: Zondervan Publishing House, 1980.

Boothby, Lisa A. (2004) Bioidentical hormone therapy: a review *Menopause* Vol 11 No 3 pp 356-367

Bown, Deni. *Growing Herbs*. New York: Dorling Kindersley Publishing, Inc., 1995.

_____. *Encyclopedia of Herbs and Their Uses*. New York: Dorling Kindersley Publishing, Inc, 1995.

Bratman, Steven, M.D., et al. *Natural Health Bible*. 2nd ed. California: Prima Health, 2000.

Bremner, William J., MD (Feb 2004) Editorial: Serum Testosterone Assays---Accuracy Matters *Journal Clin Endo Metab* Vol 89 Number 2

Brennan, Barbara Ann. *Light Emerging*. New York: Bantam Books, 1993.

_____. *Hands of Light*. New York: Bantam Books, 1987.

Bricklin, Mark, ed. *The Practical Encyclopedia of Natural Healing*. Emmaus, PA: Rodale Press, 1976.

_____,et al. *The Practical Encyclopedia of Natural Healing New, Revised Edition*. Emmaus, PA: Rodale Press, 1983.

Brink, Marijke, et al. Angiotensin II Induces Skeletal Muscle Wasting Through Enhanced Protein Degradation and Down-Regulates Autocrine Insulin-Like Growth Factor I. *Endocrinology*, Vol. 142, No. 4, 2001.

Bruce, Debra F., et al. *The Unofficial Guide to Alternative Medicine*. New York: Macmillian, Inc, 1989.

Brueggemeir, Robert W. Effects of Phytoestrogens and Synthetic Combinatorial Libraries on Aromatase, Estrogen Biosynthesis, and Metabolism *Annals of New York Academy of Science*

Buchwald D, Umali J, Stene M. Insulin-like growth factor-1 (Somatomedin C) levels in chronic fatigue syndrome and fibromyalgia. *Journal of Rheumatology*. 1996;23(4)739-742.

Buffington CK et al. Case report: amelioration of insulin resistance in diabetes with dehydroepiandrosterone. *Am J Med Sci* 1993 Nov; 306 (5):320-24.

Bunevicius R Effects of Thyroxine as compared with thyroxine plus triiodothyronine in patients with hypothyroidism *N Eng J Med* 1999: 340: 424-9

Bunker VW, Lawson MS, Delves HT, et al. Metabolic balance studies for zinc and nitrogen in healthy elderly subjects. *Human Nutrition:Clinical Nutrition*.1982;36C:213-221.

Burke CW Thyroid Hormones *Br Med Bull* 1974; Vol. 30 No. 1

Burke CW Urinary triiodothyronine and thyroxine and their relationship to the serum free levels *Clin Sci* 1973; 44(2): 5P-6P

Burke CW Measurement of thyroxine and triiodothyronine in human urine *Lancet* 1972; 2: 1177-1179

Burke CW Triiodothyronine and Thyroxine in Urine. II. Renal Handling, and Effect of Urinary Protein *J Clin Endocrinol Metab* 1976; 42(3): 504-513

Burr, Harold S. *Blueprint for Immortality*. Essex, England: The C.W. Daniel Company

Limited, 1972.

Caine, Winston K., et al. *The Male Body: An Owner's Manual.* Emmaus, PA: Rodale Press, Inc, 1996.

Capra, Fritjof. *The Tao of Physics.* New York: Bantam Books, Inc, 1984.

Carey, Ruth, Ph.D., et al. *Common Sense Nutrition.* California: Pacific Press Publishing Association, 1971.

Carrol P, Christ E, Umpleby, M, *et al.* IGF-1 Treatment in Adults With Type 1 Diabetes-Effects on Glucose and Protein metabolism in the Fasting State and During a Hyperinsulinemic- Euglycemic Amino Acid Clamp. *Diabetes.* 2000;49:789-796

Castagnetta Giuseppe Carruba L.A.M Re: Urinary 2-Hydroxyestrone/16 alpha-Hydroxyestrone Ratio and Risk of Breast Cancer in Postmenopausal Women *Journal of the National Cancer Institute* November 3, 1999; Vol. 91, No. 21

Cattaneo, L., et al. Characterization of the Hypothalamo-Pituitary-IGF-I Axis in Rats Made Obese by Overfeeding. *Journal of Endocrinology*, February, Vol. 148, No. 2, 1996.

Chambers, John (1999) Demonstration of Rapid Onset Vascular Endothelial Dysfunction after Hyperhomocystinemia. *Circulation* 99:1156-1160.

Chan V Urinary thyroxine excretion as index of thyroid function *Lancet* 1972; 4-6

Childe, Doc L., *The HeartMath Solution.* New York: HarperCollins Publishers, 1999.

Ching-Chung C Autoantibodies to thyroid peroxidase in patients with type 1 diabetes in Taiwan *Euro J of Endocrin* 1998; 139 44-48

Choi, Cheol S., et al. Independent Regulation of in Vivo Insulin Action on Glucose Versus K+ Uptake by Dietary Fat and K+ Content. *Diabetes*, Vol. 51, April, 2002.

Chopra, Deepak M.D. *Ageless Body, Timeless Mind.* New York: Harmony Books, 1993.

Christ, Emanual R. et al. (1998) Dyslipidemia in adult Growth Hormone Deficiency and the Effect of GH Replacement Therapy. *Trends in Endocrinology and Metabolism* 9: 200-206

Christ ER, et al. Effect of IGF-1 therapy on VLDL apoliopprotein B100 metabolism in type 1 diabetes mellitus. *Am J Physiol Endocrinol Metab* 2002;282(5):E1154-1162.

Clasey, JL., et al. Abdominal Visceral Fat and Fasting Insulin are Important Predictors of 24-Hour GH Release Independent of Age, Gender, and Other Physiological Factors. *J Clin Endocrinol Metab*, August, Vol. 86, No. 8, 2001.

Clarke BL Predictors of Bone Mineral Density in Aging Healthy Men Varies by Skeletal Site *Calcified Tissue International* 2002; 70: 137-145

Clemente, Carmine, Ph.D. *Anatomy A Regional Atlas of the Human Body.* Maryland: Urban & Schwarzenberg, 1981.

Clemmons DR. IGF binding proteins: regulation of cellular actions. *Growth Regul. 1992;*2:80-87.

Clemmons, David R. (2000) The Combination of Insulin-Like Growth Factor I and Insulin-Like Growth Factor Binding Protein-3 Reduces Insulin Requirements in Insulin-Dependent Type 1 Diabetes: Evidence for *in vivo* Biological Activity* *J Clin Endocrin Metab* Vol 85 No 4:1518-1524

Clemmons, David R., (2004) The relative roles of Growth Hormone and IGF-1 in controlling insulin sensitivity *J Clin Invest* 113: 24-27

Coleman DL et al. Therapeutic effects of dehydroepiandrosterone (DHEA) in diabetic mice. *Diabetes* 1982 Sep; 31(9):830-33.

_____ et al. Therapeutic effects of dehydroepiandrosterone (DHEA) in Diabetic Mice. *Diabetes* 1984 Jan;33 (1):26-32.

Conti, Elena et al. Insulin-Like Growth Factor-1 as a Vascular Protective Factor, *Circulation* (2004) 110; 2260-2265

Cousins, Norman. *Anatomy of An Illness as Perceived By the Patient.* New York: Bantam Books, 1979.

Cusi, Kenneth, et al. Recombinant Human Insulin-Like Growth Factor I Treatment for 1 Week Improves Metabolic Control in Type 2 Diabetes by Ameliorating Hepatic and Muscle Insulin Resistance. *The Journal of Clinical Endocrinology and Metabolism,* Vol. 85. No. 9, 2000.

Crawford, Bronwyn A. (1996) Androgens Regulate Circulating Levels of Insulin-Like Growth Factor (IGF)-1 and IGF Binding Protein-3 During Puberty in Male Baboons *J Clin Endocrinol Metab* 81: 65-72

Cush, Keneth and Ralph DeFronzo (2000) Recombinant Human Insulin-Like Growth Factor 1 Treatment for 1 week Improves Metabolic Control in Type 2 Diabetes by Ameliorating Hepatic and Muscle Insulin Resistance. *The Journal of Clinical Endocrinology and Metabolism.* Vol. 85 No. 9 pages 3077-3084

Danese, Mark D., (2000) Effect of Thyroxine Therapy on Serum Lipoproteins in Patients with Mild Thyroid Failure: a Quantitative Review of the Literature. Vol. 85 No. 9. Pages 2993-3001

Danesh J et al. Association of Fibrinogen, C-reactive protein, Albumin, or leukocyte count with Coronary Artery Disease. *JAMA* 1998 May 13;279(18):1477-82.

Davenport, Horace W., DSc. *A Digest of Digestion.* 2nd ed. Chicago: Year Book Medical Publishers Inc, 1978.

Davidson P Growth Hormone replacement in adults and bone mineral density: a systematic review and meta-analysis *Clinical Endocrinology* 2004; 60. 92-98

Davis SR, Tran J. Testosterone influences libido and well being in women. *Trends in Endocrinology and Metabolism.* 200112(1):33-37.

DeBoer, H., et al. Changes in Subcutaneous and Visceral Fat mass During Growth Hormone Replacement Therapy in Adult Men. *Int. Journal of Related Metabolic Disorders*, June, Vol. 20, No. 6, 1996.

De Leo, Vicenzo. Effect of Metformin on Insulin-Like Growth Factor (IGF) I and IGF-Binding

Protein I in Polycystic Ovary Syndrome. *The Journal of Clinical Endocrinology & Metabolism*, December, Vol. 85, No. 4, 2000.

Dessein PH, Shipton EA, Joffe BI, et al. Hyposecretion of adrenal androgens and the relation of serum adrenal steroids, serotonin, and insulin-like growth factor-1 to clinical features in women with fibromyalgia. *Pain*. 1999;83:313-319.

De Wasch K Consequences of boar edible tissue consumption on urinary profiles of nandrolone metabolites. II. Identification and quantification of 10-norsteroids responsible for 19-norandrostrerone and 19-noretiocholanolone excretion in human urine *Rapid Communications Mass spectrometry* 2000; 15: 1442-1447

Dhatariya, Ketan (2005) Effect of Dehydroepiandrosterone Replacement on Insulin Sensitivity and Lipids in Hypoadrenal Women *Diabetes* 54: 765-769

Diamandis EP Selective determinations of urinary free cortisol by Liquid chromatography after solid-state extraction *Journal of* Chromatogrphy 1988; 426: 25-32

Diamond, John W., M.D. *An Alternative Medicine Definitive Guide to Cancer.* California: Future Medicine Publishing, Inc., 1997.

Dobelis, Inge N. *Reader's Digest Magic and Medicine of Plants.* Pleasantville, NY: The Reader's Digest Association, Inc, 1986.

Downing, Damien, Hypothyroidism: Treating the Patient not the Laboratory *Journal of Nutritional & Environmental Medicine* (2000) 10, 101-103

Dowsett, M. (1999) Drug and hormone interactions of aromatase inhibitors. *Endocrine Related Cancer* 6 181-185

Dunkelman SS, Fairhurst B., et al. Cortisol metabolism in obesity. *J Clin Endocrin Metab* 24: 832-841,1964. and quoted from Jefferies, William McK., MD, *Safe Uses of Cortisol* (1996) Thomas Publishing Pgs. 30-33.

Eden, Donna, et al. *Energy Medicine.* New York: Penguin Putnam Inc, 1998.

Ejima J et Al. (2000) Relationship of HDL cholesterol and red blood cell filterability: cross-sectional study of healthy subjects. *Clinical Hemorheological Microcirculation* 22(1): 1-7

Endocrtinology, 4th Edition, 2001 Edited by Leslie J. De Grout

Epstein, Donald, et al. *The 12 Stages of Healing.* California: Amber-Allen Publishing, 1994.

Er F, Michels G, Gassanov N, et al. Testosterone induces cytoprotection by activating ATP-sensitive K+ channels in the cardiac mitochondrial inner membrane. *Circulation.*2004:Nov,9:3100-3107.

Erickson MD, Robert A (2001) Testosterone-Its Real Impact. *Journal of Longevity* Vol 7 No. 9

Eskildsen PC Renal handling of iodothyronines in acromegaly *Scand J Clin Lab Invest* 1987; 47: 17-21

Etienne-Emile Baulieu. Dehydroepiandrosterone (DHEA): A Fountain of Youth?, *Journal of Clinical Endocrinology and Metabolism.* 1996;81(9):3147 – 3151.

Faber J urinary excretion of Free and Conjugated 3', 5'- Diiodothyronine and 3, 3'-diiodothyronine* *J Clin Endocrinol Metab* 1981; 53(3): 587-93

Fawcett, JP, (1994) Does cholesterol depletion have adverse effects on blood rheology? *Angiology* Volume 45 Issue 3

Felt V, Starka L. Metabolic effects dehydroepiandrosterone (DHEA) and atromid in patients with hyperlipidemia. *Cor et Vasa* 1966; 8 (1):40-48.

Feskens EJ, Kronhout D. Hyperinsulinemia, risk factors, and coronary artery disease. The Zutphen Elderly Study. *Arterioscler Thromb* 1994 Oct;14 (10):1641-47.

Firoozeh S The Influence of Hormones and Pharmaceutical Agents on DHEA and DHEA-S Concentrations: A Review of Clinical Studies *J Clin Pharmacol* 2002; 42: 247-266

Fitzpatrick, Thomas B., et al. *Color Atlas and Synopsis of ClinicalDermatology*. 3d ed. New York: Mcgraw-Hill Companies, 1997.

Fonesca V Can urinary thyroid hormone loss cause hypothyroidism? *Lancet* 1991; 338: 475-476

Fottner, C., et el. Regulation of Steroidogenesis by Insulin-Like Growth Factors (IGFs) in Adult Human Adrenocortical Cells: IGF-I and, more Potently, IGF-II Preferentially Enhance Androgen Biosynthesis Through Interaction With the IGF-I Receptor and IGF-Binding Proteins. *Journal of Endocrinol*, September, Vol. 158, No. 3, 1998.

Frankel, Edward. *DNA: The Ladder of Life*. 2nd ed. New York: McGraw-Hill Book Company, 1979.

Fredrick C. W. Wu and Arnold von Eckardstein, (2003) *End Rev* Androgens and Coronary Artery Disease 24 (2):183-217

Frost, Robert A., Lang, Charles H. Differential Effects of Insulin-Like Growth Factor I (IGF-I) and IGF-Binding Protein-1 on Protein Metabolism in Human Skeletal Muscle Cells. *Endocrinology*, Vol. 140, No. 9, 1999.

Gaby, Alan R., MD, et al. *Nutritional Therapy in Medical Practice*. Kent, WA: Wright/Gaby Seminars, 1996.

Gaitan JE Measurement of triiodothyronine in enextracted urine *J Lab Clin Med* Sept 1975 pgs. 538-546

Gangong, William F., MD. *Review of Medical Physiology*. 10th ed.   Los Altos: Lange Medical Publications, 1981..

_____. *Review of Medical Physiology*. Los Altos: Lange Medical Publications, 1971

_____. *Review of Medical Physiology*. 19th ed. Stamford, CT: Appleton&Lange, 1999.

_____. *Review of Medical Physiology*. 20thed. McGraw-Hill Companies, Inc., 2001.

Gardner, Joy. *Healing Yourself*. Freedom, CA: The Crossing Press, 1989

Gharib H Radioimmunoassay for Triiodothyronine (T3): I. Affinity and Specificity of the Antibody for T3* *J Clin Endocrinol Metab* 1971; 33: 509-516

Garnero P Biochemical Markers of Bone Turnover, Endogenous Hormones and the Risks of Fractures in Postmenopausal Women: The OFELY Study *Journal of Bone and Mineral Research* 2000; Vol. 15, No. 8

Gdansky, E., et al. Increased Number of IGF-I Receptors on Erythrocytes of Women with Polycystic Ovarian Syndrome. *Clinical Endocrinal*, August, Vol. 47, No. 2, 1997.

Genazzani AD, Stomati M, *et* al. Oral dehydroepiandrosterone (DHEA) supplementation modulates spontaneous and Growth Hormone-releasing hormone- induced Growth Hormone and insulin-like growth factor-1 secretion in early and late postmenopausal women. *Fertil Steril,* 2001;76:241-248.

Gerber, Richard MD. *Vibrational Medicine*. Sante Fe: Bear and Company, 1996.

Gerras, Charles, ed. *The Complete Book of Vitamins*. Emmaus, PA: Rodale Press Inc, 1977.

_____, et al. *The Encyclopedia of Common Diseases*. Emmaus, PA: Rodale Press, Inc., 1976.

Giller, Robert M., MD, et al. *Natural Prescriptions*. New York: Ballentine Books, 1994.

Glowacki, Rosen CJ, et al. Sex steroids, The Inuslin-Like Growth Factor Regulatory System, and Aging Implications for the Management of Older Postmenopausal Women. *J Nutr Health Aging*, Vol.2, No. 1, 1998.

Gokce MD, Noyan, (1999) Long Term Ascorbic Acid administration reverses Endothelial Vasomotor Dysfunction in Patients with Coronary artery Disease. *Circulation*;99 pages 3234-3240

Goldberg Group, Burton, ed. *Alternative Medicine The Definitive Guide*. Washington: Future Medicine Publishing, Inc., 1994.

Golden GA et al (1999) Rapid and opposite effects of cortisol and estradiol on human erythrocyte Na+, K+-ATPase activity: relationship to steroid intercalation into the cell membrane. *Life Science* 65(12):1247-55

Golden GA et Al. (1998) Steroid hormones partition to distinct sites in a model membrane bilayer: direct demonstration by small-angle X-ray diffraction.

Goodman, David, 'Soy toxins', press release

Goodman, Paul, *Compulsory Mis-education and the Community of Scholars*. New York: Vintage Books, 1962.

Gori F *et al*. Effects of androgens on the Insulin-like growth factor system in an androgen-responsive osteoblastic cell line. *Endocrinology*. 1999;140:5579-5586.

Graham, Ian M (June 11 1997) Plasma Homocysteine as a Risk Factor for Vascular Disease. *JAMA* Vol 27, No. 22

Grant Ph D, William (November 1998) The role of milk and sugar in heart disease. *The American Journal of Natural Medicine.*

Greendale GA Endogenous Sex Steroids and Bone Mineral Density in Older Women and Men: The Rancho Bernardo Study *Journal of Bone and Mineral Research* Nov 11 1997; Vol. 12

Greenspan, Francis S.,MD, et al., eds. *Basic and Clinical Endocrinology.* Stamford, CT: Appleton&Lange, 1997.

Griffin, Tom, M.D., et al. *The Physicians Blueprint Feeling Good For Life.* Arizona: New Medical Dynamics Inc., 1983.

Grinspoon S, Corcorran C, Stanley T, et al. Effects of Androgen Administration on the Growth Hormone-insulin-like growth factor-1 axis in men with acquired immunodeficiency syndrome wasting. *Journal of Clinical Endocrinology and Metabolism.* 1998;88(12):4251-4256.

Guler HP, Zapf J, Froesch ER. Short-term metabolic effects of recombinant human insulin-like growth factor-1 in healthy adults. *N Engl J Med.* 1987;317:137-140.

Guler H-P, Zapf J, Schmid C, et al. Insulin-like growth factors I and II in healthy man. Estimations of half-lives and production rates. *Acta Endocrinologica.* 1989;121:753-758.

Guler HP, Schmid C, Zapf J, et al. Effects of Insulin-like growth factor I in man. *Acta Paediatr Scand..* 1990;367:52-54.

Gurnell, Eleanor M., (2001) Dehydroepiandrosterone (DHEA) replacement therapy. *European Journal of Endocrinology.* 145 pages 103-106

Guyton, Arthur C., M.D. *Textbook of Medical Physiology.* 7th ed. Pennsylvania: W.B. Saunders Company, 1986.

Haden ST Effects of Age on Serum Dehydroepiandrosterone (DHEA) Sulfate, IGF-1, and IL-6 Levels in Women *Calcified Tissue International* 2000; 66: 414-418

Haffner SM et al. Relationship of sex hormones to lipids and lipoproteins in nondiabetic men. *J Clin Endocrinol Metab* 1993 Dec; 77(6): 1610-15.

Halmos, Gabor, et. al. (2000) Human Ovarian Cancer Express Somatostatin Receptor. *The Journal of Clinical Endocrinology and Metabolism.* Vol. 85 No. 10 pages3509-3512

Hamel, Frederick G., et al. Regulation of Multicatalytic Enzyme Activity by Insulin and the Insulin-Degrading Enzyme. *Endocrinology*, Vol. 139, No. 10, 1998.

Hamano K Increased Risk for Atherosclerosis Estimated by Pulse Wave Velocity in Hypothyroidism and its Reversal with Appropriate Thyroxine Treatment *Endocrin J* 2005; 52;95-101

Hammer, Fabrian *Journal of Clin End and Metab* (March 8, 2005) No Evidence for Hepatic Conversion of dehydroepiandrosterone sulfate (DHEAS) to DHEA-*in vivo* and *in* vitro studies as doi:10.1210/jc,2004-2386.

Handelsman DJ and Peter Y. Liu (March 2005) *Trends in Endocrinol Metab* Andropause: invention, prevention, rejuvenation Vol. 16 No. 2

Handelsman, DJ, Crawford, BA. Androgens Regulate Circulating Levels of Insulin-Like Growth Factor (IGF)-I and IGF Binding Protien-3 During Puberty in Male Baboons. *Journal of Clinical Metabolism*, January, Vol. 81, No. 1, 1996.

Hanley, Anthony J.G., et al. Increased Proinsulin Levels and Decreased Acute Insulin Response Independently Predict the Incidence of Type 2 Diabetes in the Insulin Resistance Atherosclerosis Study. *Diabetes*, Vol. 51, April, 2002.

Hansten, Philip. *Drug Interactions.* 4th ed. London: Henry Kimpton Publishers, 1979.

Harper, Harold A., PhD. *Review of Physiological Chemistry.* 7th ed. Los Altos: Lange Medical Publications, 1959.

Harris, J.R., ed. *Blood Cell Biochemistry, Erythroid Cells.* New York: Plenum Press, 1990.

Harrington, James and Christin Carter-Su (2001) Signaling Pathways activated by the Growth Hormone receptor. *Trends in Endocrinology*. Vol. 12 No. 6 August 2001

Harrison, George R. *How Things Work.* New York: William Morrow and Co., 1941.

Hayes, Francis J., (2000) Aromatase Inhibition in the Human Male Reveals a Hypothalamic Site of Estrogen Feedback. *Journal of Clinical Endocrinology and Metabolism*. Vol. 85 No. 9 pages 3027-3035

Heitzer, Thomas (2000) Tetrahydrobiopterin Improves Endothelium-Dependent Vasodialtion in Chronic Smokers. *Circulation Research*;86:e36

Heller, Richard F., MS, PhD, et al. *The Carbohydrate Addict's Healthy Heart Program.* New York: Ballentine Publishing Group, 1999.

Hendrickson, James E., MD. *The Molecules of Nature.* New York: W.A. Benjamin, 1965.

Herrington DM et al. Plasma dehydroepiandrosterone (DHEA) and dehydroepiandrosterone sulfate in patients undergoing diagnostic coronary angiography. *J Am Coll Cardiol* 1990 Nov; 16(4):862-70.

Herrington J Carter-Su C. Signaling pathways activated by the Growth Hormone receptor. *Trends in Endocrinology and Metabolism.* 2001;12(6):252-257.

Hilding A, Hall K, *et al.* Serum Levels of Insulin-Like Growth Factor 1 in 152 Patients with Growth Hormone Deficiency, Aged 19 – 82 Years, in Relation to Those in Healthy Subjects. *Journal of Clinical Endocrinology and Metabolism.* 1999;84(6):2013-2019.

Hiramatsu R, and Nisula BC (1987 June) Erythrocyte-associated cortisol: measurement, kinetics of dissociation and potential physiological significance. *Journal of Clinical Endocrinology and Metabolism.* Vol. 64 No. 6 pages 1224-32

Hiramatsu, Ryoh and Bruce C. Nisula (1990) Uptake of erythrocyte-associated component of blood testosterone and corticosterone to rat brain. *Journal of steroid biochemistry.* Pages 383-87

Hiramatsu, R (1991) Uptake of erythrocytes-associated component of blood testosterone and corticosterone to rat brain. *J of Steroid Biochemistry Mol Biol* Mar 38: 383-7

William B. Ferril, M. D.

Hoffman, David. *The Complete Illustrated Holistic Herbal*. New York: Barnes&Noble, Inc, 1996.

Hogate ST et al. Leukotriene antagonists and synthesis inhibitors: new directions in asthma therapy. *J allergy Clin Immunol* 1996 Jan; 97 (1): 1-8.

Holly JMP. The Physiologic role of IGFBP-1. *Acta Endocrinol* (Copenh), 1991;71:1632-1636.

Horton, Richard et. al. (1982) 3alpha, 17beta-Androstanediol Glucuronide in Plasma: A Marker of Androgen Action in Idiopathic Hirsutism *J Clin Invest* Vol 69 1203-1206

Howland RH. Thyroid dysfunction in refractory depression: implication for pathophysiology and treatment *Journal of Clinical Psychiatry* 1993; 54: 47-54

Hufner M Radioimmunoassay for Triiodothyronine in Human Serum *ACTA Endocrinologica 1973;* 72: 464-474

Hufner M Tri-iodothyronine Determination in Urine *Lancet* 1975; 1: 101-102

Hunt PJ, Gurnell EM, Huppert FA, et al. Improvement in mood and fatigue after Dehydroepiandrosterone replacement in Addison's disease in a randomized double blind trial. *Journal of Clinical Endocrinology and Metabolism.* 2000;85(12):4650-4656.

Hunt, Valerie V. *Infinite Mind: The Science of Human Vibrations of Consciousness.* Malibu, CA: Malibu Publishing Co, 1996.

Hwu CM, Kwok CF, *et al.* Growth Hormone (GH) Replacement Reduces Total Body Fat and Normalizes Insulin Sensitivity in GH-Deficient Adults: A Report of One –Year Clinical Experience. *Journal of Clinical Endocrinology and Metabolism.* 1997;82(10) 3285-3292.

Isaacson, Robert L., et al. Toxin-Induced Blood Vessel Inclusions Caused by the Chronic Administration of Aluminum and Sodium Fluoride and Their Implications for Dementia. *Annals New York Academy of Sciences,*

Iversen E Unconjugated thyroxine and triiodothyronine in urine: influence of age, sex, drugs and thyroid function *Scand J clin Lab Invest* 1979; 39: 7-13

Jacob, Stanley, M.D., et al. *The Miracle of MSM The Natural Solution for Pain.* New York: G.P. Putnam's Sons, 1999.

Jacobson GM (1975) 17 Beta-estradiol transport and metabolism in human red blood cells. J Clin Endocrinology and Metab. Feb 40 Issue 2

Jaffe MD. Effect of testosterone cipionate on the postexercise ST segment depression. *Br Heart* J 1977 Nov;39(11): 1217-22.

Jawetz, Ernest, MD, PhD, et al. *Review of Medical Microbiology.* 15th ed. Los Altos: Lange Medical Publications, 1982.

Jin, Weijun et Al. (2002) Lipases and HDL metabolism. *Trends in Endocrinology* Vol 13 No. 4 May 2002

Joffe RT. Thyroid Hormone treatment of depression *Thyroid* 1995; 3: 235-9

Jones, DS editor in chief Textbook of Functional Medicine 2005 *Institute of Functional Medicine, Gig Harbor, Wa.*

Jones J, Clemmons, D. Insulin-Like Growth Factors and Their Binding Proteins: Biological Actions. *Endocrine Reviews*. 1995;16(1):3-34.

Jones, T.W.H. *Dictionary of the Bach Flower Remedies*. Essex, England: C.W. Daniel Company Limited, 1995.

Jorge E Measurement of triiodothyronine in unextracted urine *J Lab Clin Med* 1975: 86 (3) 538-536

Jose Agusto Soares Barreto-Filho, Marta Regina S. Alcantara et. Al. Familial Isolated Growth Hormone Deficiency is Associated with Increased Systolic Blood Pressure, Central Obesity and Dyslipidemia. *J Clin Endo Metab* (2002) Vol. 87 (5) 2018-2023

Junqueira, Luis C., MD, et al. *Basic Histology.* 3rd ed. Los Altos: Lange Medical Publications, 1980.

Kamat, Amrita, et. Al. (2002) Mechanisms in tissue-specific regulation of estrogen biosynthesis in humans. *Trends in Endocrinology and Metabolism*. Vol. 13 April 2002 pgs. 122-128

Kang JX, Li Y, Leaf, A. Manose-6-phosphate/insulin-like growth factor-II receptor is a receptor for retinoic acid. *Proc. Natl. Acad. Sci. USA*. 1998;95:13671-13676.

Kann PH Clinical effects of growth hormone on bone: a review *The Aging Male* 2004; 7: 290-296

Kellner, Michael, et al. Atrial Natriuretic Factor Inhibits the CRH-Stimulated Secretion of ACTH and Cortisol in Man. *Life Sciences*, Vol. 60, 1992.

Kemper, Donald ed. *Healthwise Handbook.* Idaho: Healthwise, Inc. 1976.

Keymolen V., J Endocrinol. 1976 Nov; 71 (2):219-229 Output of oestrogens, testosterone, and their precursors by isolated human adrenal cells as compared with that of glucocorticoids.

Keough, Carol, ed. *Future Youth*. Emmaus, PA: Rodale Press, Inc, 1987.

Khalsa, Dharma Singh, MD, et al. *Brain Longevity*. New York: Time Warner Company, 1997.

Kim, Min sun (2004) Suppression of DHEA sulfotransferase (Sult2A1) during the acute-phase response *Am J Physiol Endocrinol Metab* 287:E731-E738

Kirpichnikov, Dmitri, and James Sowers (2001) Diabetes mellitus and diabetes-associated vascular disease. *Trends in Endocrinology and Metabolism*. Vol. 12 No. 5 July 2001.

Kishi, Yutaka, et al. Alph-Lipoic Acid: Effects on Glucose Uptake, Sorbitol Pathway, and Energy Metabolism in Experimental Diabetic Neuropathy. *Diabetes*, Vol. 48, October, 1999.

Kitamura S Anti-thyroid hormone activity of tetrabromobisphenol A, a flame retardant, and related compounds: Affinity to the mammalian thyroid receptor, and effect on tadpole metamorphosis *Life Sciences* 76 (2005) 1589-1601

Klaassen, Curtis D., Ph.D. *Casarett & Doull's Toxicology.* 6th ed. McGraw-Hill Medical Publishing Division, 2001.

Klatz, Ronald, et al. *Grow Young with HGH.* New York: Harper Perennial, 1997.

Klien I Thyroid hormone and the Cardiovascular System *N Engl J Med* Feb 15, 2001 Vol 344, No 7

Khosravi MJ, Diamandi A, *et al.* Acid-Labile Subunit of Human Insulin-Like Growth Factor-Binding Protein Complex: Measurement, Molecular, and Clinical Evaluation. *Journal of Clinical Endocrinology and Metabolism.* 1997;82(12)3944-3951.

Kotelchuck, David, ed. *Prognosis Negative.* New York: Vintage Books, 1976.

Kraemer W.J., et el. Effects of Heavy-Resistance Training On Hormonal Response Patterns In Younger VS. Older Men. *Journal of Applied Physiology,* September, Vol. 87, No.3, 1999.

Krupka RM and R Deves (1980) Asymmetric binding of steroids to internal and external sites in the glucose carrier of erythrocytes. *Biochim biophys Acta* Vol 598 Issue 1

Labrie, Fernand (2003) Endocrine and Intracrine Sources of Androgens in Women: Inhibition of Breast Cancer and Other Roles of Androgens and their Precursor Dehydroepiandrosterone *Endo Reviews* 24(2): 152-182

Labrie, Fernand (1997) Marked Decline in Serum Concentrations of Adrenal C19 Steroid Precursors and Conjugated Androgen Metabolites During Aging *J Clin Endocrin Metab* Vol 82: No8

Lacayo, Richard (April 24, 2000) Testosterone. TIME Magazine: Page 58

Lasley, Bill L., et al. The Relationship of Circultating Dehydroepiandrosterone (DHEA), Testosterone, and Estradiol to Stages of the Menopausal Transition and Ethnicity. *The Journal of Clinical Endocrinology and Metabolism,* Vol. 87, No. 8, 2002.

Laughlin, Gail and Elizabeth Barret-Conner (2000) Sexual dimorphism in the Influence of Advanced Aging on the Adrenal Hormone levels: The Rancho Bernardo Study. *The Journal of Clinical Endocrinology and Metabolism* pgs 3561-3568

Lavallée B, Provost PR, *et al.* Effect of insulin on serum levels of dehydroepiandrosterone metabolites in men. *Clinical Endocrinology* (Oxf). 1997 46:93 – 100.

Leavelle, Dennis E., MD, ed. *Mayo Medical Laboratories Interpretive Handbook.* Rochester, MN: Mayo Medical Laboratories, 1997.

Lee, John R., MD, et al. *What Your Doctor May Not Tell You About Premenopause.* New York: Warner Books, Inc, 1999.

_____. *Natural Progesterone: the Multiple Roles of a Remarkable Hormone.* Sebastopol, CA: BLL Publishing, 1993.

Lehninger, Albert L. *Biochemistry.* New York: Worth Publishers, Inc, 1975.

_____ *Biochemicstry*. New York: Worth Publishers, Inc., 2000.

Leong SR, Baxter RC, Camerato T, et al. Structure and functional expression of acid labile subunit of the insulin-like growth factor binding protein complex. *Mol Endocrinol*. 1992;6:870-876.

Le Roith D, Scavo L, Butler A. What is the role of circulating IGF-1? *Trends in Endocrinology and Metabolism.* 2001;12(2)48-52.

LeShan, Lawrence, Ph.D. Psychological States as Factors in the Development of Malignant Disease: A Critical Review. *New York Journal of Medicine*, August 24, 1958.

Levitt, B.B. *Electromagnetic Fields*. New York: Harcourt Brace and Company, 1995.

Lewis, John G., et al. Caution on the use of saliva measurements to monitor absorption of progesterone from transdermal creams in postmenopausal women. *Maturitas*, 4, 2002.

Ley, Beth. *DHEA: Unlocking the Secrets to the Fountain of Youth.* California: BL Publications, 1996.

Liu, Peter Y., (2003) *Endocrine Rev* Androgens and Cardiovascular Disease 24(3):313-340.

Lovern, J.A., *The Chemistry of Lipids of Biochemistry Significance.* London: Methuen & Co. LTD, 1955.

Lowe, John C., et al. *The Metabolic Treatment of Fibromyalgia*. Boulder, CO: Mc Dowell Publishing Company, 2000.

Lowenthal, Albert A., MD. *Endocrine Glands and Sexual Problems*. Chicago:_____, 1928.

Lorand, Arnold, MD. *Old Age Deferred*. Philadelphia: F.A. Davis Publishers, 1911.

Maciocia, Giovanni. *Tongue Diagnosis in Chinese Medicine*. Seattle: Eastland Press, Inc, 1987.

Mantzoros CS et al. Relative androgenicity, blood pressure levels, and cardiovascular risk factors in young healthy women. *Am J Hypertension* 1995 Jun; 8(6):606-14.

Martel C Predominant androgenic component in the stimulatory effect of dehydroepiandrosterone on bone mineral density in the rat *J Endocrinol* 1998; 157: 433-442

Martin, Janet L., et al. Insulin-Like Growth Factor Binding Protein-3 Is Regulated by Dihydrotestosterone and Stimulates Deoxyribonucleic Acid Synthesis and Cell Proliferation in LNCaP Prostate Carcinoma Cells. *Endocrinology*, Vol. 141, No. 7, 2000.

Maskarinec G Urinary Sex Steroid Excretion Levels During a Soy Intervention Among Young Girls: A Pilot Study *Nutrition and Cancer* 2005; 52(1): 22-28

Mauras N, Martinez V, *et al.* Recombinant Human Insulin-Like Growth Factor 1 Has Significant Anabolic Effects in Adults with Growth Hormone Receptor Deficiency: Studies on Protein, Glucose, and Lipid Metabolism. *Journal of Clinical Endocrinology and Metabolism*, 2000; 85(9):3036-3042.

Mauras, Nelly, et. al. (2000) Estrogen Suppression in Males: Metabolic Effects. *The Journal of Clinical Endocrinology and Metabolism.* Vol85 No. 7 pages2370-2377.

Mawatari S and Murakami K. (1999) Effects of ascorbic acid on peroxidation of human erythrocyte membranes by lipoxygenase. *Nutrition Science vitaminology* (Tokyo) Dec 45(6)687-99

McCarty, MF. Modulation of Adipocyte Lipoprotein Lipase Expression as a Strategy for Preventing or Treating Visceral Obesity. *Med Hypotheses,* August, Vol. 57, No. 2, 2001.

Merck Company &. *The Hypercholesterolemia Handbook.* Pennsylvania: Merck Sharp & Dohme, 1989.

McCann, Una D. (August 27, 1997)Brain Serotonin Neurotoxicity and Primary Pulmonry Hypertension From Fenfluramine and Dexfenfluramine. *JAMA* Vol.278, No 8

McEvoy, Gerald K., Pharm.D, ed. *AHFS Drug Information, 2001.* Bethesda, MD: American Society of Health-System Pharmacists, Inc, 2001.

_____. *AHFS Drug Information, 1986.* Bethesda , MD: American Society of Health-System Pharmacists, Inc, 1986.

McIntosh, M., et al. Opposing Actions of Dehydroepiandrosterone (DHEA) and Corticosterone in Rats. Proc Soc Exp Biol Med, July, Vol. 221, No. 3, 1999.

Mchedlishvili, G, New evidence for involvement of blood rheological disorders in rise of peripheral resistance in essential hypertension. *Clinical Hemorheology Microcirculation* Vol 17 Issue 1

McLaughlin, T, et Al. (2000) Carbohydrate Induced Hypertriglyceridemia: An Insight into the Link between Plasma Insulin and Triglyceride Concentrations. *The Journal of Clinical Endocrinology and Metabolism.* Vol85. No. 9 pages 3085-3088

Mease, Philip J., Ellen M. Ginsler (2005) Effects of Prasterone (DHEA) on Bone Mineral Density in Women with Systemic Lupus Erythematosus Receiving Chronic Glucocorticoid Therapy *Journal of Rheum* 32:4

E. Melian, B. Gonzalez et. Al *J Endo* Tissue-specific response of IGF-1 mRNA expression to obesity associated GH decline in the male Zucker rat (1999) 160, 49-56

Mellon, Cynthia H. and Lisa D. Griffin (2002) Neurosteroids: biochemistry and clinical significance. *Trends in Endocrinology and Metabolism* 13 pages 35-43

Mendelsohn, Robert S., M.D. *Confessions of a Medical Heretic.* New York: Warner Books Inc., 1979.

Michalak, Patricia S. *Rodale's Successful Organic Gardening, Herbs.* Emmaus, PA: Rodale Press, 1993.

Miralles-Garcia JM Urinary Kinetics of Triiodothyronine and their modification with Aging *Hormone metabol Res* 1985: 17: 366-369

Morley J.E., et al. Potentially Predictive and Manipulable Blood Serum Correlatives of Aging in the Healthy Human Male: Progressive Decreases in Bioavailable Testosterone, Dehydroepiamdrosterone (DHEA) Sulfate, and the Ratio of Insulin-Like Growth Factor 1 to Growth Hormone. *Pro Natl Acad Sci* USA, July, Vol. 94, No.14, 1997.

Mindell, Earl L., R.Ph.D, Ph.D., et al. *Dr. Earl Mindell's Secrets of Natural Health.* Illinois: Keats Publishing, 2000.

Mokken FC, et. Al. (1992) the clinical importance of erythrocyte deformability, a hemorheologically parameter. Annals of Hematology Volume 64 Issue 3

Mooradian, J. E. (1987) Biological Actions of Androgens, *Endocrine Reviews* Vol. 8 No. 1

Morin, Laurie C., (2000) Endocrine and Metabolic Effects of Metformin vs. Ethinyl-Cyproterone acetate in Obese Women with Polycystic Ovary Syndrome: A Randomized Study. *The Journal of Clinical Endocrinology and Metabolism.* Vol. 85 No. 9 pages 3161-3168

Moss, Ralph W. *The Cancer Industry.* New York: Paragon House, 1989.

Monte, Tom, et al. *World Medicine.* New York: F.P. Putnam's Sons, 1993.

Morales A J, Nolan J J, Nelson J C, Yen, SSC. Effects of Replacement Dose of Dehydroepiandrosterone (DHEA) in Men and Women of Advancing Age. *J. Clin. Endocrinol. Metab.* 1994;78:1360–1367.

Morales, AJ. et al. The Effects of Six Months Treatment with a 100 mg Daily Dose of Dehyroepiamdrosterone (DHEA) on Circulating Sex Steroids, Body Composition and Muscle Strength in Age-Advanced Men and Women. *Clinical Endocrinology* (Oxf), October, Vol. 49, No. 4, 1998.

Mullenix, Phyllis J., Neurotoxicity of Sodium Fluoride in Rats. *Neurotoxicology and Teratology*, Vol. 17, No. 2, 1995.

Munoz-Gurerra J GC/MS/MS Anaalysis for Anabolic Steroids in Urine for Athletic Testing *GC/MS Varion Application Update* Number 60

Muramoto, Naboru. *Healing Ourselves.* New York: Avon Books, 1973.

Murialdo G, *et al.* Relationship between cortisol, dehydroepiandrosterone (DHEA) sulphate and insulin-like growth factor-1 system in dementia, *Journal of Endocrinology Investigation.* 2001;24:139-146.

Murray, Michael, N.D., et al. *Encyclopedia of Natural Medicine.* California: Prima Health, 1998.

Munzer, T., et al. Effects of GF and/or Sex Steroid Administration on Abdominal Subcutaneous and Visceral Fat in Healthy Aged Women and Men. *J Clin Endocirinol Metab*, August, Vol. 86, No. 8, 2001.

Myss, Caroline, PhD, et al. *Creation of Health.* New York: Three Rivers Press, 1993.

Nafziger, AN, et al. Dehydroepiandrosterone (DHEA) and dehydroepiandrosterone sulfate: their relation to cardiovascular disease. *Epidemiol Rev* 1991; 13:267-93. Review.

Nam, S.Y., et al. Low-Dose Growth Hormone Treatment Combined with Diet Restriction

Decreases Insulin Resistance by Reducing Visceral Fat and Increasing Muscle Mass in Obese Type 2 Diabetic Patients. *Int J Obes Relat Metab Disord*, August, Vol. 25, No. 8, 2001.

Nelson, David L., et al. *Lehninger Principles of Biochemistry*. 3rd ed. New York: Worth Publishers, 2000.

Nestler JE et al. Dehydroepiandrosterone (DHEA): the "missing link" between hyperinsulinism and atherosclerosis. *FASEB J* 1992 Sep; 6(12):3073-75

Netzer, Corinne T. *Encyclopedia of Food Values*. New York: DellPublishing, 1992.

Nicklas, B.J., et al. Testosterone, Growth Hormone and IGF-I Response to Acute and Chronic Resistive Exercise in Men Aged 55-70 Years. *Int. Journal of Sports Medicine*, October, Vol. 16, No. 7, 1995.

Nitenberg A. Acetylcholine induced coronary vasoconstriction in young, heavy smokers with normal coronary arteriographic findings. *Service d'Explorations Fonctionnelles*, Unite 251, France.

Ody, Penelope. *The Complete Medicinal Herbal*. New York: Dorling Kindersley Inc, 1993.

Older SA, Battafarano DF, Danning CL, et al. The effects of Delta Wave Sleep Interruption on Pain Thresholds and Fibromyalgia-like Symptoms in Healthy Subjects; Correlations with Insulin-like Growth Factor-1. *Journal of Rheumatology*. 1998;25(6):1180-1186.

Okada, Hidetaka, et. al. (2000) Progesterone Enhances Interleukin-15 Production in Human Endometrial Stromal Cells in Vitro. *Journal of Clinical Endocrinology and Metabolism*. Volume 85. No. 12 pages 4765-4770

Om P. Ganda, MD (Diabetologist at Joslin Diabetes Center, Boston, MA) Chapter 5 Prevalence and Incidence of Secondary And Other Types of Diabetes

Orden I Thyroxine in unextracted urine *Acta Endocrinologica (Copenh)* 1987; 114: 503-508

Ornstein, Robert, et al. *The Amazing Brain*. Boston: Houghton Mifflin Company, 1984.

O'Rourke, P.J. *Parliament of Whores*. New York: The Atlantic Monthly Press, 1991.

Osius N Exposure to polychlorinated biphenyls and levels of thyroid hormones in children *Environmental Health Perspective* 1999; 107: 843-9

Owino V, Yang SY, Goldspink G. Age-related loss of skeletal muscle function and the inability to express the autocrine form of insulin-like growth factor-1 (MGF) in response to mechanical overload. *FEBS Letters*. 2001;505:259-263.

Page, Kate, ND (Feb/March 2005) Natural Management Options for Menopause *Integrative Medicine* Vol 4 No 1

Paolisso, Giuseppe (1997) Serum Levels of Insulin-Like Growth Factor-I (IGF-1) and IGF-Binding Protein-3 in Healthy Centenarians: Relationship with Plasma Leptin and Lipid Concentrations, Insulin acition, and Cognitive Function *J Clin Endocrin Metab* Vol 82 No 7: 2204-2209

Paolisso G., et al. Insulin Resistance and Advancing Age: What Role For

Dehydroepiandrosterone Sulfate (DHEA-S)? *Metabolism*, November, Vol.46, No.11, 1997.

Pascal, Alana. *DHEA the Fountain of Youth Discovered?* California: Ben-Wal Printing, 1996.

Peeke, Pamela, MD, MPH. *Fight Fat After Forty*. New York: Penguin Group, 2000.

Persson SU (1996) Correlations between fatty acid composition of the erythrocyte membrane and blood rheology data. *Scandinavian Journal of Clinical Laboratory Investigation*. April 96 vol. 56 Issue 2

Pfeifer, Margia (1999) Growth Hormone (GH) Treatment Reverses Early Atherosclerotic Changes in GH-Deficient Adults* *J Clin Endocrin Metab* Vol 84 No 2: 453-457

Pert, Candace B., PhD. *The Molecules of Emotion*. New York: Simon and Schuster, Inc, 1997

Petersdorf, Robert G., M.D., et al. *Harrison's Principles of Internal Medicine tenth edition.* McGraw-Hill Book Company, 1983.

Philippe F. Backeljauw, Louis E. Underwood Therapy for 6.5-7.5 Years with Recombinant Insulin-Like Growth Factor I in Children with Growth Hormone Insensitivity Syndrome: A Clinical Research Study *J Clin Endo Metab* (2001) Vol. 86 (4) 1504-1510

Phillips GB et al. The association of hypotestosteronemia with coronary artery disease in men. *Arterioscler Thromb* 1994 May; 14(5):701-06.

Pillar TM Thyroid hormone and gene expression in the regulation of mitochondrial respiratory function *European J Endocrin* 136 231-239

Pinchera, Aldo, MD, ed. *Endocrinology and Metabolism*. London: McGraw-Hill International(UK) Ltd., 2001.

Pino, Ana M. et. al. (2000) Dietary Isoflavones Affect Sex Hormone Globulin levels in Postmenopausal Women. *The Journal of Clinical Endocrinology and Metabolism*. Vol 85. No.8 pages 2797-2800

Prezio JA, Ccarrion G, et al. Influence of body composition on adrenal function in obesity. *J Clin Enddocrinol Metab* 24: 481-485, 1964

Pries, Axel R., et al. Structural Autoregulation of Terminal Vascular Beds. *Hypertension*, 1999.

Quillin, Patrick, PhD, RD, CNS, et al. *Beating Cancer with Nutrition*. Rev ed. Tulsa, OK: Nutrition Times Press, Inc, 2001.

Quin JD, Fisher BM, Paterson KR, Inoue A, et al. Acute response to recombinant insulin-like growth factor-1 in patients with Mendenhall's syndrome. *N Engl J Med*. 1990;323:1425-1426.

Rajaram S, Baylink D, Mohan S. Insulin-Like Growth Factor-Binding Proteins in Serum and Other Biological Fluids: Regulation and Functions. *Endocrine Reviews*. 1997;18(6):801-831.

Rastogi GK Srum Urinary Levels of Thyroid Hormones in Normal Pregnancy *Obstet Gynecol* 1974; 44(2): 176-180

Rath, Matthias, MD. *Eradicating Heart Disease*. San Francisco: Health Now, 1993.

Ravaglia, G., et al. Regular Moderate Intensity Physical Activity and Blood Concentrations of Endogenous Anabolic Hormones and Thyroid Hormones in Aging Men. *Mech Aging Dev*, February, Vol. 122, No. 2, 2001.

Ravel, Richard, MD. *Clinical Laboratory Medicine.* 6th ed. St Louis: Mosby-Year Book, Inc, 1995.

Raynaud-Simon, A., et al. Plasma Insulin-Like Growth Factor I (IGF-1) Levels in the Elderly: Relation to Plasma Dehydroepiandrosterone (DHEA) Sulfate Levels, Nutritional Status, Health and Mortality. *J Gerontology*, July-August, Vol.47, No. 4, 2001.

Reaven, Gerald, M.D., et al. *Syndrome X.* New York: Simon & Schuster, 2000.

Reid, Daniel. *The Complete Book of Chinese Health & Healing.* Massachusetts: Shambhala Publications, Inc. 1994.

Reiss, Uzzi, M.D., et al. *Natural Hormone Balance for Woman.* New York: Pocket Books, 2001.

Remington, Dennis, M.D., et al. *Back to Health.* Utah: Publishers Press, 1986.

Ridker PM et al. C-reactive protein and other markers of inflammation in the prediction of cardiovascular disease in women. *N Engl J Med* 2000 Mar 23; 342 (12):836-43.

Rifkind, Richard, et al. *Fundamentals of Hematology.* 2nd ed. Illinois: Year Book Medical Publishers, Inc. 1980.

Rizzo M Resting Metabolic Rate and Respiratory Quotient in Human Longevity *J Clin Endocrin & Metab* 2005; 90(1): 409-413

Robbins, John. *Reclaiming Our Health: Exploding the Myth and Embracing the Source of True Healing.* Tiburon, CA: HJ Kramer Inc, 1998.

Robbins, Stanley L., MD, et al. *Pathologic Basis of Disease.* 2nd ed. Philadelphia: W.B. Saunders Company, 1979.

Rodale, J.I., et al. *The Health Seeker.* Emmaus,PA: Rodale Books, Inc. 1972.

Roggenkamp HG (1986) Erythrocyte rigidity in healthy patients and patients with cardiovascualr disease risk factors. KWH Oct 1986 64: 1091-6

Rojo ND, Ruth (2001) Why is it harder to lose weight as we age? *Journal of Longevity* Vol 7 No 9

Rolleman EJ Changes in renal tri-iodothyronine and thyroxine handling during fasting *European J Endocrinol* 2000; 142: 125-130

Rosedale MD, Ron Presentation at the Health Institute's Boulder-Fest, August 1999 seminar

Rosenfalck AM, Maghsoudi S, Fisker S, et al. The effect of 30 months of low-dose replacement therapy with recombinant human Growth Hormone(rhGH) on insulin and C-peptide kinetics, insulin secretion, insulin sensitivity, glucose effectiveness, and body composition in GH-deficient adults. *Journal of Clinical Endocrinology and Metabolism.* 2000;85(11):4173-4181.

Rosenfeld, Isadore, M.D. *The Complete Medical Exam.* New York: Simon & Schuster, 1978.

Rosmond, R, Bjortorp, P. The Interactions Between Hypothalamic-Pituitary-Adrenal Axis Activity, Testosterone, Insulin-Like Growth Factor I and Abdominal Obesity with Metabolism and Blood Pressure in Men. *Int Journal Obes Relat Metab Disord*, December, Vol. 22, No. 12, 1998.

Rosmond, Roland (1998) Stress-Related Cortisol Secretion in Men: Relationships with Abdominal Obesity and Endocrine, Metabolic and Hemodynamic Abnormalities* *J Clin Endo Metab* Vol 83, No 6 pages 1853-59

Ross, A.C. Gordon, M.B., Chb, MFHom. *Homeopathy An Introductory Guide.* Northamptonshire: Thorsons Publishers Limited: 1976.

Rowgowski P Radioimmunoassay of thyroxine and triiodothyronine in urine using extraction and separation on Sephadex columns *Scand J clin Lab Invest* 1977; 37: 729-734

Rubin, Philip, ed. *Clinical Oncology sixth edition.* American Cancer Society, 1983.

Ruiz, Gomez F. (1998) Treatments with progesterone analogues decreases macrophage Fcgamma receptors expression. *Clinical Immunopathology* Dec; 89(3): 231-9

Russell, A.L. Glycoaminoglycan (GAG) Deficiency in Protective Barrier as an Underlying, Primary Cause of Ulcerative Colitis, Crohn's Disease, Interstitial Cystitis and Possibly Reiter's Syndrome. *Medical Hypotheses*, Vol. 52, No. 4, 1999.

Ryan, Graeme B., MB, BS, PhD, et al. *Inflamation.* Kalamazoo, MI: The Upjohn Company, 1977.

Safer JD Defective Release of Corepressor by Hinge Mutants of the Thyroid Hormone receptor Found in Patients with Resistance to Thyroid Hormone *J Biolog Chem* 1998; Vol. 273 No 46: 30175-30182

Sategna-Guidetti C Autoimmune thyroid disease and coeliac disease *European Journal Gastro & Hepatology* 1998; 10:927-931

Samsioe, G., (2004) Transdermal hormone therapy: gels and patches *Climacteric* 7:347-356

Sapolsky, Robert M. *Stress, the Aging Brain, and the Mechanisms of Neuron Death.* Cambridge, MA: The MIT Press, 1992.

_____. *The Trouble with Testosterone.* New York: Simon and Shuster, Inc, 1997.

Sarno, John E., MD. *The Mindbody Prescription.* New York: Warner Books, Inc, 1998.

Schoenle EJ, Zenobi PD, Torresani T, et al. Recombinant human insulin-like growth factor-1 (rhIGF1) reduces hyperglycemia in patients with extreme insulin resistance. *Diabetologia.* 1991;34:675-679.

Schofield, Janice F. *Discovering Wild Plants.* Bothell, WA: Alaska Northwest Books, 1989.

Simpson, E. R. (April 7 2005) Estrogens-The Good, The Bad, and the Unexpected *Endo*

Reviews doi:10.1210/ep.2004-0020

Simpson, Leslie O. (1987) Red cell and hemorheological changes in multiple sclerosis. *Pathology*, 19 pp51-55

Secomb, T. W. (1998) A model for red cell motion in glycocalyx-lined capillaries. *American Journal of Physiology* 274 H1016-H1022

Sahelian MD, Ray (October 1996) DHEA Youth in a Bottle? *Lets Live*

Schechter M. D. , Michael, et. Al. (2000) Oral Magnesium Therapy Improves Endothelial Function in Patients with Coronary Artery Disease. *Circulation* Nov. 7 2000. Pages 2353-2358

Scholl, B.F., PhG, MD, ed. *Library of Health*. Philadelphia: Historical Publishing, Inc, 1932.

Schoneshofer M Increased Urinary Excretion of Free 20alpha and 20beta- dihydrocortisol in a Hypercortisolemic but Hypocortisoluric Patient Causing Disease *Clin Chem* 1983; 29/2 385-389

Schwarzbein, Diana, MD, et al. *The Schwarzbein Principle*. Deerfield Beach, FL: Health Communications, Inc, 1999.

Sears, Barry, PhD, et al. *Enter the Zone*. New York: HarperCollins Publishers, Inc, 1995.

Shackleton C.H.L. Use of Sep-pak cartridges for urinary steroid extraction evaluation of the method for use prior to gas chromatographic analysis *Clinica Chimica Aeta* 1980: 107: 231-243

Shackleton C.H.L Profiling Steroid Hormones and Urinary Steroids *Journal of Chromatography* 1986; 379: 91-156

Shakespear RA Triiodothyronine and thyroxine in Urine. I. Measurement and Application *J Clin Endocrinol Metab* 1976; 42(3) 494-503

Sheally, C.N., MD, PhD, ed. *The Complete Family Guide to Alternative Medicine*. New York: Barnes&Noble, Inc, 1996.

Shippen, Eugene, MD, et al. *The Testosterone Syndrome*. New York: M.Evans and Company, Inc, 1998.

Signorello, LB., et al. Hormones and Hair Patterning In Men: A Role for Insulin-Like Growth Factor 1? *Journal of the American Academy of Dermatology*, February, Vol. 40, No. 2, 1999.

Sinha MK, Buchanan C, Leggett N, et al. Mechanism of IGF-1 stimulated glucose transport in human adipocytes. Demonstration of specific IGF-1 receptors not involved in stimulation of glucose transport. *Diabetes*. 1989;38:1217-1225

Sites, Cynthia K. et. al. (2005) The Effects of Hormone Replacement Therapy on Body Composition, Body Fat Distribution, and Insulin Sensitivity in Menopausal Women: A Randomized, Double-Blind, Placebo-Controlled Trial *J Clin Endocrinol Metab* 90: 2701-2707

Skinner GRB Thyroxine should be tried in clinically hypothyroid but biochemically euthyroid patients *BMJ* 1997; 314: 1764

Slowinska-Srzednicka J et al. Decreased plasma dehydroepiandrosterone (DHEA) sulfate and dehydroepiandrosterone concentrations in young men after myocardial infarction. *Atherosclerosis* 1989 Sep; 79(1):197-203.

Snyder DK, Clemmons DR. Insulin-dependent regulation of insulin-like growth factor binding protein-1. *Journal of Clinical Endocrinology and Metabolism*. 1992;71:1632-1636.

Sobel, David S., MD, et al. *The People's Book of Medical Tests*. New York: Simon and Schuster, 1985.

Solerte, Sebastiano Bruno, et al. Dehydroepiandrosterone (DHEA) Sulfate Enhances Natural Killer Cell Cytotoxicity in Humans Via Locally Generated Immunoreactive Insulin-Like Growth Factor I. *The Journal of Clinical Endocrinology & Metabolism*, Vol. 84, No. 9, 1999.

Song, Linda Z.Y.X., M.D. et al. Heart-Focused Attention and Heart-Brain Synchronization: Energetic and Physiological Mechanisms. *Alternative Therapies*, September, Vol. 4, No. 5, 1998.

Spallarossa, Paolo, MD (Jan 15, 1996) Insulin-Like Growth Factor −1 and Angiographically Documented Coronary Artery Disease *Amer J Cardio* Vol 77

Spector, Walter G. *An Introduction to General Pathology*. 2nd ed. Edinburgh, Scotland: Churchill Livingstone, 1980.

Sterling K Thyroid Hormone Action at the Cell Level *New Engl J Med* 1979; Vol. 300, No. 3

Stelfox, Henry Thomas, M.D., et al. Conflict of Interest in the Debate Over Calcium-Channel Antagonists. *The New England Journal of Medicine*, January 8, 1998.

Stewart, Paul M. and Tomlison, Jeremy W. (April 2002) Cortisol, 11B-hydroxysteroid dehydrogenase type 1 and central obesity. *Trends in Endocrinology and Metabolism* pgs.94-96

Steinberg D et al. Beyond cholesterol modification of low-density lipoprotein that increase its atherogenicity. *N Engl J Med* 1989 April 6;320(14):915-24.

Stites,Daniel P., MD, et al., eds. *Medical Immunology*. 9th ed. Stamford, CT: Appleton&Lange, 1997.

Stuart, J. (1985) Erythrocyte rheology. J Clinical Pathology Vol. 38 Issue 9

Studd, J. and Panay, N. (2004) Hormones and depression in women *Climacteric* 7:338-346

Studd, John, (2004) Personal View Second thoughts on the Women's Health Initiative study: the effect of age on the safety of HRT *Climacteric* 7; 412-414

Study Links high Carb to Cancer, Associated Press (April 2002)

Sun Yipang Treatment of osteoporosis in men using dehydroepiandrosterone (DHEA) sulfate *Chinese Medical Journal* 2002; 115 (3): 402-404

Sutton-Tyrrell K et al. High homocysteine leveles are independently related to isolated systolic hypertension in older adults. *Circulation* 1997 Sep 16;96(6):1745-9.

Szathmari J Dehydroepiandrosterone (DHEA) Sulfate and Bone Mineral Density *Osteoporosis International* 1994; 4: 84-88

Tagami T Mechanisms That Mediate Negative Regulation of the Thyroid-stimulating Hormone alpha Gene by the Thyroid Hormone Receptor *J Bilog Chem* 1999; Vol 274, No. 32 22345-22353

Taieb, Joelle (2003) *Clinical Chemistry* Testosterone Measured by 10 Immunoassays and by Isotope-Dilution Gas Chromatogrphy-Mass Spectrometry in Sera from 116 Men, Women and Children 49:8 1381-1395

Takaya, Kazuhiko, et. al. (2000) Ghrelin Strongly Stimulates Growth Hormone (GH) Release in Humans. *The Journal of Clinical Endocrinology and Metabolism.* Vol. 85. No. 12 pages 4908-4911

Tchernof, A., Labrie, F. (1996) Obesity and metabolic complications: contribution of dehydroepiandrosterone (DHEA) and other steroid hormones *J Endocrin* 150 S155-S164

Theodosakis, Jason, MD, MS, MPH, et al. *The Arthritis Cure.*
New York: Affinity Communications Corporation, 1998.

Thomas, Lewis, *The Lives of a Cell.* New York: Bantam Books, 1974.

Thrailkill, K.M. Insulin-Like Growth Factor-I in Diabetes Mellitus: its Physiologic, Metabolic Effects, and Potential Clinical Utility. *Diabetes Technol Ther, Spring*, Vol. 2, No. 1, 2000.

Tilford, Gregory L. *Edible and Medicinal Plants of the West.* Missoula: Mountain Press Publishing Company, 1997.

_____. *From Earth to Herbalist.* Missoula: Mountain Press Publishing Company, 1998.

Tiller, William A. (1996) Cardiac Coherence: A New, Noninvasive Measure of Autonomic Nervous System Order. Alternative Therapies Jan 96, Vol. 2, No 1

Tissandier, O., et al. Testosterone, Dehydroepiandrosterone (DHEA), Insulin-Like Growth Factor 1 (IGF-1), and Insulin in Sedentary and Physically Trained Aged Men. *Eur J Appl Physiol,* July, Vol.85, No. 1-2, 2001.

Toscano V Importance of Gluten in the Induction of Endocrine Autoantibodies and Organ Dysfunction in Adolescent Celiac Patients *Amer J Gastoenterology* 2000: Vol. 95, No. 7

Tsuda K et al (2001) Electron paramagnetic resonance investigation on modulatory effect of 17 Beta-estradiol on membrane fluidity of erythrocytes in postmenopausal women. *Arteriosclerosis Thromb Vasc Biol* Aug:21(8):1306-12

Tsuji, K. Specific Binding and Effects of Dehroepiandrosterone Sulfate (DHEA-S) on Skeletal Muscle Cells: Possible Implication for DHEA-S Replacement Therapy in Patients with Myotonic Dystrophy. *Life Science*, Vol. 65, No.1, 1999.

Tuomainen TP et al. Cohort study between donating blood and risk of myocardial infarction in 2,682 men in eastern Finland. *BMJ* 1997 Mar 15; 314 (7083):793-94.

Tyler, Varro E., PhD, ScD. *Herbs of Choice.* New York: Pharmaceutical Products Press, 1994.

Tuzcu A Subclinical Hypothyroidism may be Associated with Elevated High-sensitive C-Reactive Protein (Low Grade Inflammation) and Fasting Hyperinsulinemia *Endocrine Journal* 2005; 52(1), 89-94

Van Boxtel MPJ Thyroid Function, depressed mood, and cognitive perfromance in older individuals: the Maastricht Aging Study *Psychoneuroendocrinology* 2004; 29, 891-898

Van Den Beld AW, De Jong FH, Grobbee DE, et al. Measures of Bioavailable serum testosterone and estradiol and their relationships with muscle strength, bone density, and body composition in elderly men. *Journal of Clinical Endocrinology and Metabolism.* 2000;85(9):3276-3282.

VanHaaften, M., et al. Identification of 16-alpha Hydroxyestrone as a Metabolite of Estriol. Gynecol, Endocrinol 2, 1988.

Veldhuis, Johannes D., et al. Estrogen and Testosterone, But Not a Nonaromatizable Androgen, Direct Network Integration of the Hypothalamo-Somatotrope (Growth Hormone)-Insulin-Like Growth Factor I Axis in the Human: Evidence from Pubertal Pathophysioogy and Sex-Steroid Hormone Replacement. *Journal of Clinical Endocrinology and Metabolism*, Vol. 82, No.10, 1997.

Veldhuis, Johannes D. *J Clin Endo and Metabolism* (April 5,2005) Joint Mechanisms of Impaired GH Pulse Renewal in Aging Men as doi:10.1210/jc.2005-0336

Vendola, K., et al. Androgens Promote Insulin-Like Growth Factor-I and Insulin-Like Growth Factor-I Receptor Gene Expression in the Primate Ovary. *Hum Reprod,* September, Vol. 1, No. 9, 1999.

Ventura A Gluten-dependent diabetes-related and thyroid-related autoantibodies in patients with celiac disease *J Pediatrics* 2000; Vol. 137, Issue 2

Verheist JA Use of ketoconazole in the treatment of a virilizing adrenal cortical carcinoma *Acta Encrinologica (Copenh)* 1989; 121: 229-234

Villareal D Effects of DHEA replacement on bone mineral density and body composition in elderly women and men *Clin Endocrinol* 2000; 53, 561-568

Villareal D Effects of Dehydroepiandrosterone on Bone Mineral Density *Trends Endocrin* 2002: 1 (6): 349-357

Villareal DT, Holloszy JO (2004) Effect of DHEA on abdominal fat and insulin action in elderly women and men: a randomized controlled trial, *JAMA* 292:2243-2248

Viveiros MM, Liptrap RM. ACTH treatment disrupts ovarian IGF-1 and steroid hormone production. *Journal of Endocrinology.* 2000;164:255-264.

Volek J.S., et al. Body Composition and Hormonal Responses to a Carbohydrate Restricted Diet. *Metabolism,* July, Vol. 51, No. 7, 2002.

Vondra, K., et al. Role of the Steroids, SHBG, IGF-I, IGF BP-3 and Growth Hormone in Glucose Metabolism Disorders During Long-Term Treatment with Low Doses of Glucocorticoids. *Cas Lek Cesk,* February, Vol. 141, No. 3, 2002.

Von Petrykowski W urinary Free T4 and T3 in Healthy Infants and during Noise Exposure *Hoemonw Res* 1982; 16: 56-60

Wallach, Jacques, MD. *Interpretation of Diagnostic Tests.* 6th ed.

New York: Little, Brown and Company, 1996.

Wang, Christina (2004) *Journ Clin Endo Metab* Measurement of Total Serum Testosterone in Adult Men: Comparison of Current Laboratory Methods versus Liquid Chromatography-Tandem Mass Spectrometry Vol 89 Numb 2: 534-543

Wardle CA Pitfalls in the use of thyrotropin concentration as a first-line thyroid-function test March 31 2001 *Lancet* Vol. 357

Watkins, Alan D., et al. The Impact of a New Emotional Self-Management Program on Stress, Emotions, Heart Rate Variability, DHEA and Cortisol. *Integrative Physiological and Behavioral Science*, April-June, Vol. 33 No. 2, 1998.

Warrier, Gopi. *The Complete Illustrated Guide to Ayurveda*. New York: Barnes&Noble, 1997.

Weast, Robert C., PhD. *Handbook of Chemistry and Physics*. 56th ed. Cleveland, OH: CRC Press, Inc, 1975.

Weil, Andrew, MD. *Natural Health, Natural Medicine*. Boston: Houghton Mifflin Company, 1990.

_____. *Health and Healing*. New York: Houghton Mifflin Company, 1995.

_____. *Spontaneous Healing*. New York: Alfred A. Knopf, Inc, 1995.

_____. *Eating Well for Optimum Health*. New York: Alfred A Knopf, 2000.

Welsh TH Jr, (1982 Dec: 27 (5): 1138-46) Biol Reprod Mechanism of glucocorticoid-induced suppression of testicular androgen biosynthesis in vitro.

Wheelwright, Edith G. *Medicinal Plants and their History*. New York: Dover Publications, Inc, 1974.

Wen-Chao Song *Annals New York Academy of Science* (2006) Certain hydroxylated polychlorinated biphenyls are potent inhibitors of human estrogen sulfotransferase enzyme raises the possibility that environmental chemicals can cause endocrine disruption by enhancing endogenous estrogen activity through inhibition of steroid transformation enzymes such as estrogen sulfotransferase

Whitaker, Julian MD. *Dr Whitaker's Guide to Natural Healing*. Rocklin, CA: Prima Publishing, 1995.

Whitaker MD, Julian (September 1998) DHEA helps regulate the immune system. Health and Healing Vol 8 No 9

Wild, Russell, ed. *The Complete Book of Natural and Medicinal Cures*. Emmaus, PA: Rodale Press, 1994.

Wilson, Helen E and Ann White (1998) Prohormone: their Clinical Relevance. *Trends in Endocrinology and Metabolism* 9:396-402

Wood WI, Cachianes G, Henzel WJ, et al. Cloning and expression of the GH dependent insulin-like growth factor binding protein. *Mol Endocrinol*. 1988;2:1176-1185.

Wood, D.& J. *The Incredible Healing Needles*. New York: Samuel Weiser Inc., 1974.

Wood, Ian (2002) Pro-inflammatory mechanisms of a nonsteroidal anti-inflammatory drug. *Trends in Endocrinology* Vol 13 No. 2 March 2002

Wright, Jonathan V., MD, et al. *Natural Hormone Replacement for Women Over 45*. Petaluma, CA: Smart Publications, 1997.

_____, et al. *Natural Hormone Replacement*. California: Smart Publications, 1997.

_____, et al. *The patient's Book of Natural Healing*. California: Prima Health, 1999.

------------------------ and Alan Gaby MD (October 16-19) Nutrional Therapy in Medical Practice, Doubletree Seattle Airport Hotel

Wrutniak-Cabello C Thyroid Hormone action in mitochondria *J Mol Endocrin* 2001; 26: 67-77

Wu S-Y Triiodothyronine (T3)-Binding immunoglobulins in a Euthyroid Woman: Effects on Measurement of T3 (RIA) and T3 Turnover *J Clin Endocrinol Metab* 1976; 42(4): 642-52

Wudy SA, Hartmann MF. Gas Chromatography-Mass Spectrometry Profiling of Steroids in Times of Molecular Biology. *Hormone Metabolism and Research*. 2004:36:415-422

Xu X, Duncan AM, Merz-Demlow BE, et al. Menstrual cycle effects on urinary estrogen metabolites. *Journal of Clinical Endocrinology and Metabolism*. 1999;84(11):3914-3918.

Xu X Soy consumption Alters Endogenous Estrogen Metabolism in Postmenopausal Women *Cancer Epidemiology, Biomarkers & Prevention* August 2000; Vol. 9: 781-786

Yamaguchi Y, Tanaka S, *et al,* Reduced serum dehydroepiandrosterone levels in diabetic patients with hyperglycemia. *Clinical Endocrinology* (Oxf). 1998;49:377-383.

Yen SSC Replacement of DHEA in Aging Men and Women *Department of reproductive Medicine, UC San Diego, La Jolla, Ca. 92093 Annals New York Academy of Sciences*

Yen, SS. Replacement of DHEA in aging men and women. Potential remedial effects. <u>*Fam Pract News*</u> 1995 Aug 15; 25(16):6.

Yen, SS, Laughlin GA. Aging and the Adrenal Cortex. *Exp. Gerontol*, Nov-Dec, Vol. 33, No. 7-8, 1998.

Yen, Samuel S.C. Dehydroepiandrosterone sulfate and longevity: New clues for an old friend. *Proc. Natl. Acad. of Sci. USA*. 2001;98(15)8167-8169.

Youl, Kang H., et al. Effects of Ginseng Ingestion on Growth Hormone, Testosterone, Cortisol, and Insulin-Like Growth Factor I Responses to Acute Resistance Exercise. *J Strength Cond Res*, May, Vol. 16, No. 2, 2002.

Young J Panhypopituitarism as a Model to Study the Metabolism of Dehydroepiandrosterone (DHEA) in Humans* *J Clin Endocrinol Metab* 1997; Vol. 82. No. 8

Yoshida K Measurement of triiodothyronine in urine *J Exp Med* 1980; 132(4): 389-95

Zachrisson, I., et al. Determinants of Growth in Diabetic Pubertal Subjects. *Diabetes Care,* August, Vol. 20, No. 8, 1997.

Zager PG et Al. (1986) Distribution of 18-hydroxycorticosterone between red blood cells and plasma. *J Clin Endocrinology Metab* Jan 62: 84-9

Zenobi PD, Jaeggi-groisman SE, Riesen WF, et al. Insulin-like growth factor-1 improves glucose and lipid metabolism in type 2 diabetes mellitus. *J Clin Intest.* 1992;90:2234-2241.

Zoncu S Cardiac function in boderline hypothyroidism: a study by pulsed wave tissue Doppler imaging *European J Endocrin* 2005; 152; 527-533

Zulewski H Estimation of Hypothyroidism by a new clinical score: evaluation of patients with various grades of hypothyroidism and controls *J Clin Endocrionol Metab* 1997; 82: 771-6

Zitzmann M, Nieschlag E. Testosterone levels in healthy men and the relation to behavioural and physical characteristics: facts and constructs. *European Journal of Endocrinology.* 2001;144:183-197.

ABOUT THE AUTHOR

William B. Ferril, M.D. earned a Bachelor of Science degree in Biochemistry and doctorate in medicine at UC Davis, California. He completed his postgraduate education at Sacred Heart Medical Center in Spokane Washington in 1986. Most of the past 22 years, he has practiced on the Flathead Indian Reservation. It was there; during this posting that he gained experience for the topics in his books. He works with chiropractors, acupuncturist, homeopaths and naturopaths attempting to bridge forgotten science with the mainstream. He has also written two other books since the first edition of *The Body Heals; Glandular Failure Caused Obesity* and *Healing Has One Side Effect*

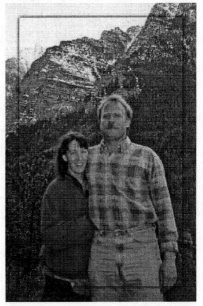

Dr. Ferril Co-founded the Bio-identical Hormone Society with Jonathan Wright, M.D. in January 2005. In this capacity, he lectured hundreds of doctors on the biochemistry of the steroids and the best testing methods. Since childhood he has remained fascinated with answering the mystery for why some people age gracefully while others do not. The biochemistry of the steroids provides part of the answer.

His wife Brenda received her doctorate at Western States Chiropractic College in Portland, Oregon. They live with their sons in Western Montana.

Would you like more copies of *The Body Heals?*

The Bridge Medical Publishers
P. O. Box 324.
Whitefish, MT 59937

www.thebodyheals.com

406 863-9906

Please send me _____ copies of *The Body Heals.*
$40.00 per book _____ enclosed
$ 7.00 per book _____ shipping and handling
     Total   _____

Name   : _____

Address: _____

City   : _____

State   : _____   Zip: _____

To avoid damaging your book, we suggest you photocopy
this page and send us the completed copy with your check*